Register Now for O
to Your Bo

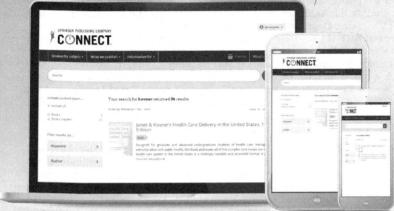

William Rosa, MS, RN, AGPCNP-BC, ACHPN, FCCM, Caritas Coach is currently an RWJF Future of Nursing Scholar, University of Pennsylvania, School of Nursing, PhD Program, Philadelphia, PA, and Nurse Practitioner, Supportive Care Service, Memorial Sloan Kettering Cancer Center (MSKCC), New York, NY. Mr. Rosa received his BSN magna cum laude from NYU Rory Meyers College of Nursing (2009) and was valedictorian of his MSN class, Hunter College (2014). He recently completed the MSKCC Palliative Care Fellowship (2016–2017); other specialties or board certifications include holistic nursing, critical care, nurse coaching, and global health. Mr. Rosa spent one year with the Human Resources for Health Program in Rwanda, East Africa (2015–2016), contributing to the curriculum content for the first Masters-prepared nursing cohort in the country. He is the editor of two previous books related to leadership and global health and has more than 100 publications in a host of diverse forums. Mr. Rosa has been recognized with numerous awards, including the American Association of Nurse Practitioner's New York State Award for Excellence (2018); NYU's Young Distinguished Alumnus Award (2018); and Sigma's Daniel J. Pesut International Spirit of Renewal Award (2017). He was also named one of America's Most Amazing Nurses by *The Doctors* television show and *Prevention* magazine. Mr. Rosa serves on the national Nominating Committee for the American Holistic Nurses Association and the editorial board for the *Journal of Hospice & Palliative Nursing*. He is a proud member of the American Association of Critical-Care Nurses' Circle of Excellence Society. Mr. Rosa is a Fellow of the American College of Critical Care Medicine and the New York Academy of Medicine. He will be inducted as a Fellow into the American Academy of Nursing in November 2018.

Sara Horton-Deutsch, PhD, RN, PMHCNS, FAAN, ANEF, Caritas Coach, is a professor at the University of San Francisco, School of Nursing and Health Professions. She also holds an adjunct appointment at the University of Colorado College of Nursing where she mentors doctoral students in the PhD program's Caring Science focus area. Prior to joining the University of San Francisco, she served as the Watson Caring Science Chair at the University of Colorado College of Nursing. Upon earning her doctorate, she completed a postdoctorate in psychoneuroimmunology and spent the next 7 years on faculty as a practitioner/teacher and assistant professor at Rush University, Chicago, Illinois. Her career included a joint appointment to the School of Nursing (SON) and School of Medicine at Indiana University (1999) where she taught nursing students, medical students, and psychiatric residents and served as co-chief of a psychiatric consultation/liaison program at University Hospital. In 2004, she assumed a full-time position in the SON, where she coordinated the graduate psychiatric nursing track and served as interim department chair. Her honors include nomination as Nurse Educator of the Year (2012), induction as an Academy of Nursing Education Fellow (ANEF) in 2014, and Fellow in the American Academy of Nursing (FAAN). From 2014 to 2015, she served as president of the International Society of Psychiatric Mental Health Nurses (ISPN) and worked with the national association of Quality and Safety Education for Nurses (QSEN). She has been recognized with international, national, and regional awards recognizing her excellence in creative work in reflective practice and leadership. Her other co-edited publications include *Reflective Practice: Transforming Education and Improving Outcomes; Reflective Organizations: On the Front Lines of QSEN and Reflective Practice Implementation;* and *Caritas Coaching: A Journey Toward Transpersonal Caring and Informed Moral Action in Healthcare.*

Jean Watson, PhD, RN, AHN-BC, FAAN, is distinguished professor emerita and dean emerita of the College of Nursing at the University of Colorado, Denver. She is the founder of the Center for Human Caring in Colorado, a fellow of the American Academy of Nursing, and the past president of the National League for Nursing. Her current activities include founder and director of Watson Caring Science Institute, a nonprofit international organization foundation, committed to furthering caring science in the world. Dr. Watson has earned undergraduate and graduate degrees in nursing and psychiatric–mental health nursing with a PhD in educational psychology and counseling. She is a widely published author and recipient of numerous awards and honors, including an international Kellogg Fellowship in Australia, a Fulbright Research Award in Sweden, and 14 honorary doctoral degrees, including 11 honorary international Doctor of Science awards from Sweden, Spain, the United Kingdom, Japan, Canada (British Columbia and Quebec), Turkey, and Colombia. Clinical nurses and academic programs throughout the world use her published works on the philosophy and theory of human caring and the art and science of caring in nursing. Dr. Watson's Caring Science/Philosophy Theory is used to guide new models of caring and healing practices in diverse settings worldwide. At the University of Colorado, Dr. Watson held the title of distinguished professor of nursing, the highest honor accorded its faculty for scholarly work. In the period of 1998 to 1999, she assumed the nation's first endowed Chair in Caring Science, based at the University of Colorado. In 2013, Dr. Watson was inducted as a Living Legend by the American Academy of Nursing, its highest honor. Her work continues through the Watson Caring Science Institute (www.watsoncaringscience.org).

A Handbook for Caring Science
Expanding the Paradigm

Editors

William Rosa, MS, RN, AGPCNP-BC, ACHPN, FCCM, Caritas Coach

Sara Horton-Deutsch, PhD, RN, PMHCNS, FAAN, ANEF, Caritas Coach, HeartMath Trainer

Jean Watson, PhD, RN, AHN-BC, FAAN

Associate Editors

Marilyn A. Ray, PhD, RN, CTN-A, FAAN

Marlaine C. Smith, PhD, RN, AHN-BC, FAAN

Marian C. Turkel, PhD, RN, NEA-BC, FAAN

Assistant Editors

Diane L. Gullett, PhD, MSN, MPH, RN

Grissel Hernandez-Kertland, MPH, BSN, RN, HNB-BC

SPRINGER PUBLISHING COMPANY

Springer Publishing Company, LLC
11 West 42nd Street
New York, NY 10036
www.springerpub.com

Acquisitions Editor: Margaret Zuccarini
Associate Managing Editor: Kris Parrish
Compositor: Graphic World

ISBN: 978-0-8261-3388-5
ebook ISBN: 978-0-8261-3389-2

18 19 20 21 22 / 5 4 3 2 1

The author and the publisher of this Work have made every effort to use sources believed to be reliable to provide information that is accurate and compatible with the standards generally accepted at the time of publication. The author and publisher shall not be liable for any special, consequential, or exemplary damages resulting, in whole or in part, from the readers' use of, or reliance on, the information contained in this book. The publisher has no responsibility for the persistence or accuracy of URLs for external or third-party Internet websites referred to in this publication and does not guarantee that any content on such websites is, or will remain, accurate or appropriate.

Library of Congress Cataloging-in-Publication Data
Names: Rosa, William, 1982- editor. | Horton-Deutsch, Sara, editor. |
    Watson, Jean, 1940- editor.
Title: A handbook for caring science : expanding the paradigm / editors,
    William E. Rosa, Sara Horton-Deutsch, Jean Watson ; associate editors,
    Marilyn A. Ray, Marlaine C. Smith, Marian C. Turkel ; assistant editors,
    Diane L. Gullett, Grissel Hernandez-Kertland.
Description: New York, NY : Springer Publishing Company, [2019] | Includes
    bibliographical references and index.
Identifiers: LCCN 2018015086 (print) | LCCN 2018015896 (ebook) |
    ISBN 9780826133892 | ISBN 9780826133885 (sof) | ISBN 9780826133892 (ebook)
Subjects: | MESH: Philosophy, Nursing | Empathy | Nurse-Patient Relations |
    Nursing Care—ethics
Classification: LCC RT84.5 (ebook) | LCC RT84.5 (print) | NLM WY 86 | DDC
    610.7301—dc23
LC record available at https://lccn.loc.gov/2018015086

Contact us to receive discount rates on bulk purchases.
We can also customize our books to meet your needs.
For more information please contact: sales@springerpub.com

Printed in the United States of America.

*For the whole of the global nursing village,
carrying the light of humanity
and human caring into the future.*

Contents

Contributors   *xiii*
Foreword   *xix*
Preface   *xxv*
Acknowledgments   *xxvii*

1. **Introduction: Ontology, Epistemology, and the Lived Experience of Caring Science**   *1*
   Marilyn A. Ray, Marlaine C. Smith, Marian C. Turkel, and Grissel Hernandez-Kertland

I. THE DISCIPLINARY DISCOURSE: THEORIES AND FRAMEWORKS EVOLVING TO UNITARY CARING SCIENCE   *19*

2. **Unitary Caring Science: Disciplinary Evolution of Nursing**   *21*
   Jean Watson, Marlaine C. Smith, and W. Richard Cowling, III

3. **The Evolution of Nursing's Ethics of Caring**   *37*
   Peggy L. Chinn

4. **Caring as Emancipatory Nursing Praxis: The Theory of Relational Caring Complexity**   *53*
   Marilyn A. Ray and Marian C. Turkel

5. **Caring in African Ontology—Ubuntu**   *73*
   Anna Nolte and Charlene Downing

6. **Caring Science–Native Science: Paving Pathways of Courageous Authenticity, Advocacy, and Agency**   *85*
   Shawna M. McDermott

7. Developing the Knowledge of Human Caring   *103*
    Jacqueline Fawcett

II. CONVERGING PARADIGMS: CONSTRUCTING NEW WORLDVIEWS   *117*

8. Caring Science and Heart Science: A Guide to Heart-Centered Praxis   *119*
    Jean Watson and Robert Browning

9. Expanding Global Reach Through a Massive Open Online Course in Mindfulness
    and Caring   *133*
    Kathleen Sitzman

10. Conscious Dying: Human Caring Amid Pain and Suffering   *145*
    William Rosa, Tarron Estes, Stephanie Hope, and Jean Watson

11. Reflective Practice and Caring Science   *163*
    Sara Horton-Deutsch and William Rosa

12. Linking the Unitary Paradigm to Policy Through a Synthesis of Caring Science
    and Integrative Nursing   *173*
    Mary Koithan, Mary Jo Kreitzer, and Jean Watson

III. CARING SCIENCE LITERACY: FROM CARITAS TO GLOBAL COMMUNITAS   *187*

13. Ways of Being/Knowing/Becoming   *189*
    Jean Watson and Sara Horton-Deutsch

14. Curriculum Development Processes and Pedagogical Practices for Advancing
    Caring Science Literacy   *197*
    Marcia Hills and Chantal Cara

15. Loving-Kindness and Equanimity: Illuminating the Nursing Literature Through
    a Caring Lens   *211*
    Zane Robinson Wolf and Marian C. Turkel

IV. CARITAS LITERACY AS A FOUNDATION FOR NURSING EDUCATION   *223*

16. Teaching From the Heart   *225*
    Nancy Vitali

17. Developing Values and Philosophies of Being   *243*
    Lisa Lally Flack and Donnean Thrall

18. Fostering Metamorphosis Through Caring Literacy in an RN-to-BSN
    Program   *257*
    Mark D. Beck

19. **Nurturing Doctorally Prepared Caring Scientists**   *277*
Sara Horton-Deutsch, Kathy Oman, and Karen Sousa

20. **Advancing Caring Science Through the Missions of Teaching, Research/
Scholarship, Practice, and Service**   *285*
Marlaine C. Smith

V. AUTHENTICATING CARING SCIENCE THROUGH SCHOLARLY INQUIRY   *303*

21. **Leading From the Heart: Caring, Love, Peace and Values Guiding
Leadership**   *305*
Marian C. Turkel

22. **Evaluation of Authentic Human Caring Professional Practices**   *317*
Barbara B. Brewer and Jean Watson

23. **The Evolution of Knowledge Development Related to Caring in Online Classrooms
and Beyond**   *327*
Kathy Sitzman

VI. TOUCHING THE SPACE OF PRAXIS   *341*

24. **Caring Inquiry Methodology: The Aesthetic Process in the Way of
Compassion**   *343*
Marilyn A. Ray

25. **Holding Sacred Space for Loving-Kindness and Equanimity for Self/Others**   *355*
Joseph Giovannoni

26. **Mutual Vulnerability: Creating Healing Environments That Nurture Wholeness
and Well-Being**   *373*
Beth M. King and Charlotte D. Barry

27. **Integrating Caring Science and Caritas Into Professional Practice**   *385*
Linda Ryan

VII. REDEFINING HEALTHCARE THROUGH HEART-CENTERED WISDOM   *399*

28. **A Blueprint for Caritas Health "Care"**   *401*
Jacqueline G. Somerville and Susan M. Lee

29. **Kaiser Permanente Patient Care Services Northern California: The Adaptation
of Caring Science**   *413*
Anne M. Foss-Durant and Shawna M. McDermott

30. Nursing as Love: A Hermeneutical Phenomenological Study of the Creative Thought Within Nursing   433
Marlienne Goldin

VIII. GLOBAL CARING SCIENCE   447

31. The Essential Nature of Caring Partnerships: Contextual Relevance and Cross-Cultural Ethical Considerations   449
Michele J. Upvall, Diane L. Gullett, and William Rosa

32. Scandinavian Caring Sciences   461
Charlotte Delmar

33. Caring Practices in an Era of Conflict: Middle East Nurses   475
Julie Benbenishty and Jordan R. Hannink

34. Caritas, Peace, and Change in Japan   485
Mayumi Tsutsui, Rina Emoto, and Jean Watson

35. Caritas Nursing and Professional Practice in Peru   493
Patrick A. Palmieri

36. Toward Planetary Caring: Sustainable Health and Well-Being for All   511
William Rosa

IX. EMERGING INQUIRY: THE EVOLUTION OF A SCIENCE   527

37. Unitary Caring Science Inquiry   529
Marian C. Turkel, Joseph Giovannoni, and Jean Watson

38. Unitary Caring Science and Multicultural Perspectives   539
Joyce B. Perkins

39. Unitary Caring Science: Evolving Society Toward Health, Healing, and Humanity   555
Jean Watson, Sara Horton-Deutsch, and William Rosa

X. JOURNEYS INTO THE TRANSPERSONAL: AESTHETIC WAYS OF KNOWING   563

40. Caritas Coaching: The Future of Health and Well-Being   565
Jan Anderson

41. Creative Healing Arts   577
Mary Rockwood Lane

42. **Narrative Healing** *587*
    A. Lynne Wagner

43. **The Power of Ritual in Nurses' Everyday Lives: Personal and Professional Exemplars** *599*
    Zane Robinson Wolf

44. **Photovoice: Qualitative Research Strategy for Theory-Guided Nursing Practice** *609*
    Gayle L. Casterline

45. **Music and Poetry for Healing** *619*
    Patrick Dean

46. **The Interplay of Integrative Nursing, Caring Science, and Healing Environments** *627*
    Mary Jo Kreitzer and Terri Zborowsky

47. **Remembering Purpose: An Autoethnography** *633*
    Anna Biley

48. **Caring Science and Yoga: The Human Caring Science-Kosha Model** *643*
    Andy Davies

49. **The Embodiment of a Caring Nature** *653*
    William Rosa

50. **Conclusion: Going Forward in Interconnectedness and Compassion** *657*
    Jeanne Anselmo

Bridge to the Future: Frontier or Fantasy? Nursing Caring in the Artificial Intelligence Ecosystem *663*
Appendix A: Tools for Caring Science Measurement and Research *669*
Appendix B: Caritas Coach Abstracts *695*
Appendix C: Caring Science Literature: The Annals of Caring *709*
Index *741*

Contributors

Jan Anderson, EdD, RN, AHN-BC, Caritas Coach Director, Caritas Coach Education Program, Watson Caring Science Faculty Associate, Watson Caring Science Institute, Boulder, Colorado

Jeanne Anselmo, BSN, RN, HNB-BC, BCIA-SFC Holistic Nurse Educator/Consultant, Sea Cliff, New York; Co-Founder, Contemplative Urban Law Program, School of Law, City University of New York, Long Island City, New York; Faculty, Merton Contemplative Initiative, Iona Spirituality Institute, Iona College, New Rochelle, New York; Dharma Teacher, Order of Interbeing, Plum Village Tradition of Vietnamese Zen Master Venerable Thich Nhat Hanh, Green Island Sangha: Community of Mindful Living—Long Island, Syosset, New York

Emily Barr, MSN, RN, CPNP, CNM, Caritas Coach Senior Instructor With Distinction, University of Colorado Children's Hospital Colorado, Department of Pediatric Infectious Disease, Aurora, Colorado

Charlotte Barry, PhD, RN, NCSN, FAAN Professor and Master Teacher, Florida Atlantic University, College of Nursing, Boca Raton, Florida

Mark D. Beck, DNP, MSN, BS, RN-BC, CENP, HeartMath™, Caritas Coach Assistant Professor, RN to BSN Program, Samuel Merritt University, Santa Rosa, California

Julie Benbenishty, PhDc, MSN, RN Nurse, Hadassah Hebrew University Medical Center, Jerusalem, Israel

Anna M. Biley, DCSc, MSc, DipN Dorchester, United Kingdom

Barbara B. Brewer, PhD, MBA, RN, MALS, FAAN Associate Professor, College of Nursing, The University of Arizona, Tucson, Arizona

Lyn Brown, MA, RN-BC   Atlanta Veteran Affairs Medical Center, Decatur, Georgia

Robert Browning, PhD (hc)   Co-Director & Master Trainer, HeartMath Healthcare; Faculty & Board Member, Watson Caring Science Institute, Boulder, Colorado; Adjunct Faculty, University of Colorado, College of Nursing, Anschutz Medical Campus, Denver, Colorado; Co-VP, Pathways to Peace, UN Consultative Status (ECOSOC), UN Peace Messenger

Michelle Camicia, MSN, RN, CRRN, CCM, NEA-BC, FAHA, Caritas Coach   Director of Operations, Kaiser Foundation Rehabilitation Center, Kaiser Permanente Vallejo Medical Center, Vallejo, California

Chantal Cara, PhD, RN   Full Professor, Faculty of Nursing, Université de Montréal, Montréal, Québec, Canada; Distinguished Caring Science Scholar, Watson Caring Science Institute, Boulder, Colorado

Gayle L. Casterline, PhD, RN, AHN-BC   Associate Professor of Nursing, Hunt School of Nursing, Gardner-Webb University, Boiling Springs, North Carolina; Faculty Associate, Watson Caring Science Institute, Boulder, Colorado

Peggy L. Chinn, PhD, RN, FAAN   Professor Emerita, University of Connecticut, Storrs, Connecticut; *Advances in Nursing Science*, Editor

W. Richard Cowling, III, PhD, RN, AHN-BC, ANEF, FAAN   Dean of College of Nursing, Argosy University, Orange, California

Andy Davies, PhD, MEd   Deputy Director of Nursing – Nursing Education, Prince Sultan Cardiac Centre, Riyadh, Saudi Arabia

Patrick J. Dean, EdD, MSN, RN, OSTJ   Clinical Associate Professor ad Honorem, School of Nursing, University of Minnesota, Rochester, Minnesota; President, International Association for Human Caring

Charlotte Delmar, PhD, MSc, RN, MPG, FEANS, FAAN   Professor and Chair, Head of Department of Nursing Science, Department of Nursing Science, Institute of Public Health, Health Faculty, Aarhus University, Aarhus, Denmark; Adjunct Professor, Faculty of Medicine, Aalborg University, Aalborg, Denmark; Professor II, Norway Arctic University, Tromsø, Norway; Professor II, Diakonova University College, Oslo, Norway

Charlene Downing, PhD, RN, RM, RPN, RNA, RNE, RCN   Senior Lecturer, Department of Nursing, Faculty of Health Sciences, University of Johannesburg, Johannesburg, South Africa

Rina Emoto, PhD, RN   Professor, Japanese Red Cross College of Nursing, Tokyo, Japan

Tarron Estes, BA, RN   Founder, Conscious Dying Institute, Boulder, Colorado; Transformational Learning Consultant for Health Care Systems; Palliative Innovation Specialist and End of Life Education Design and Curriculum Development

Jacqueline Fawcett, PhD, ScD (Hon), RN, FAAN, ANEF   Professor, Department of Nursing, University of Massachusetts, Boston, Massachusetts

Lisa Lally Flack, DNS, MS, RN, Watson Caring Postdoctoral Scholar   Director/Founder and Associate Professor, Baldwin Nursing Department, Sienna College, Loudonville, New York

Anne M. Foss-Durant, MSN, MBA, NP, RN, NEA-BC   Regional Director of Adult Services and Caring Science Integration, Kaiser Permanente Northern California, Oakland, California

Joseph Giovannoni, DNP, APRN, PMHCNS-BC, Caritas Coach   Watson Caring Science Scholar—Postdoctorate, Watson Caring Science Institute, Boulder, Colorado; Owner, Joseph Giovannoni, Inc., Honolulu, Hawaii

Marlienne Goldin, DSc, RN, MPA, BSN, CNML, Caritas Coach   Director, Trauma and Neurosurgical Intensive Care Unit, Moses Cone Memorial Hospital, Cone Health System, Greensboro, North Carolina

Diane L. Gullett, PhD, MSN, MPH, RN   Instructor, Christine E. Lynn College of Nursing, Florida Atlantic University, Boca Raton, Florida

Jordan R. Hannink, BA   Hebrew University of Jerusalem, Jerusalem, Israel

Grissel Hernandez, MPH, BSN, RN, HNB-BC, Caritas Coach   Nursing Professional Development Specialist, Center for Education and Professional Development, Stanford Health Care, Stanford, California

Marcia D. Hills, PhD, RN, FAAN   Professor, School of Nursing, University of Victoria, Victoria, British Columbia, Canada; Watson Caring Science Distinguished Scholar, Watson Caring Science Institute, Boulder, Colorado

Stephanie Hope, BSN, RN, NC-BC   DNP Student, Integrative Health and Healing, University of Minnesota, Minneapolis, Minnesota; Nurse Coach, NBN Group, Kingston, New York

Sara Horton-Deutsch, PhD, RN, PMHCNS, FAAN, ANEF, Caritas Coach, HeartMath Trainer   Full Professor, University of San Francisco, School of Nursing and Health Professions, San Francisco, California; Adjunct Professor, University of Colorado-Denver, College of Nursing, Denver, Colorado

Hirokazu Ito, PhD, RN   Assistant Professor of Nursing, Institute of Health BioSciences, Department of Nursing Science, University of Tokushima, Tokushima Prefecture, Japan

Beth M. King, PhD, ARNP, PMHNP-BC   Florida Atlantic University, Christine E. Lynn College of Nursing, Boca Raton, Florida

Mary Koithan, PhD, CNS-BC, FAAN   Anne Furrow Professor, College of Nursing, University of Arizona, Tucson, Arizona

Mary Jo Kreitzer, PhD, RN, FAAN   Director, Earl E. Bakken Center for Spirituality and Healing, Professor, School of Nursing, University of Minnesota, Minneapolis, Minnesota

Mary Rockwood Lane, PhD, RN, FAAN   Associate Clinical Professor, College of Nursing, University of Florida, Gainesville, Florida

Susan M. Lee, PhD, RN, CNP   Senior Nurse Scientist and Caring Science Scholar, Brigham and Women's Hospital, Boston, Massachusetts

Rozanno C. Locsin, PhD, RN, FAAN   Professor Emeritus, Christine E. Lynn College of Nursing, Florida Atlantic University, Boca Raton, Florida; Professor of Nursing, Institute of Health BioSciences, Department of Nursing Science, University of Tokushima, Tokushima Prefecture, Japan

Shawna McDermott, MBA   Watson Caring Science Institute Doctoral Candidate, Boulder, Colorado

Kelly Morrow, MSN, RN-BC, CNE   Instructor, Nevada State College, Henderson, Nevada

Debra Morton, RN, MLDR, Caritas Coach and HeartMath Trainer   Chief Nurse Executive, Patient Care Services, Kaiser Permanente Vallejo Medical Center, California

Anna Nolte, PhD   Professor, Department of Nursing, Faculty of Health Sciences, University of Johannesburg, Johannesburg, South Africa

Kathleen S. Oman, PhD, RN, FAEN, FAAN, Caritas Coach   Professor, College of Nursing, University of Colorado-Denver, Denver, Colorado; Chair of Pediatric Nursing, Children's Hospital Colorado, Denver, Colorado

Patrick A. Palmieri, DHSc, EdS, MBA, MSN, RN, FACHE, FISQua, FAAN   Core Faculty, Doctoral Program, School of Nursing, Walden University, Minneapolis, Minnesota; Professor and Primary Investigator, Universidad Privada del Norte, Lima, Peru

Joyce B. Perkins, PhD, MA, MS, RN, AHN-BC, CHTP, RMP-T   Associate Professor, Department of Nursing, St. Catherine University, St. Paul, Minnesota

Marguerite Purnell, PhD, RN, AHN-BC   Editor Emeritus, *Journal of Art and Aesthetics in Nursing and Health Sciences,* Boca Raton, Florida

Marilyn A Ray, PhD, RN, CTN-A, FAAN, FESFCH (Hon), FSFAA   Professor Emeritus, Christine E. Lynn College of Nursing, Florida Atlantic University, Boca Raton, Florida

Robert Reynoso, MSN/Ed, BSN, AAS, RN, CEN, Caritas Coach   Lecturer, School of Nursing, Nevada State College, Henderson, Nevada

William Rosa, MS, RN, AGPCNP-BC, ACHPN, FCCM, Caritas Coach   Robert Wood Johnson Foundation Future of Nursing Scholar, School of Nursing, University of Pennsylvania, Philadelphia, Pennsylvania; Nurse Practitioner, Supportive Care Service, Memorial Sloan Kettering Cancer Center, New York, New York

Linda Ryan, PhD, RN, AHN-BC   Assistant Professor, College of Nursing & Health Professions, Lewis University, Romeoville, Illinois

Kathleen Sitzman, PhD, RN, CNE, ANEF, FAAN   Professor, College of Nursing, East Carolina University, Greenville, North Carolina

Marlaine C. Smith, PhD, RN, AHN-BC, FAAN   Dean and Helen K. Persson Eminent Scholar, Christine E. Lynn College of Nursing, Florida Atlantic University, Boca Raton, Florida

Jacqueline A. Somerville, PhD, RN, FAAN   Faculty Associate, Watson Caring Science Institute, Boulder, Colorado

Karen Sousa, PhD, RN, FAAN   Professor, College of Nursing, University of Colorado-Denver, Denver, Colorado

Donnean Thrall, ND, RN, Watson Caring Postdoctoral Scholar   Assistant Professor of Nursing; Siena College, Loudonville, New York

Mayumi Tsutsui, PhD, RN   Professor Emeritus, Director of International Collaboration Center, Japanese Red Cross College of Nursing, Tokyo, Japan

Marian C. Turkel, PhD, RN, NEA-BC, FAAN, Watson Post-Doctoral Scholar   Associate Professor, Christine E. Lynn College of Nursing, Florida Atlantic University, Boca Raton, Florida

Michele J. Upvall, PhD, RN, CNE   Professor of Nursing, Program Director, MSN Nurse Educator Programs, College of Nursing, University of Central Florida, Orlando, Florida

Nancy Vitali, PhD, RN, Caritas Coach   Associate Professor, Tulsa Community College, Tulsa, Oklahoma

A. Lynne Wagner, EdD, MSN, RN, FACCE, CHMT   Professor Emeritus of Nursing, Fitchburg State University, Fitchburg, Massachusetts; Faculty Associate, Watson Caring Science Institute, Boulder, Colorado

Jean Watson, PhD, RN, AHN-BC, FAAN   Distinguished Professor and Dean Emerita, College of Nursing Anschutz Medical Center, University of Colorado-Denver, Denver, Colorado

Danielle Wofford, PhD and DNP-FP Student, RN   Arizona State University, Phoenix, Arizona

Zane Robinson Wolf, PhD, RN, FAAN   Dean Emerita and Professor, School of Nursing and Health Sciences, La Salle University, Philadelphia, Pennsylvania; Editor-in-Chief, *International Journal for Human Caring*

Terri Zborowsky, PhD, EDAC   Design Researcher, HGA Architects & Engineers, Minneapolis, Minnesota; Teaching Specialist, Center for Spirituality & Healing, University of Minnesota, Minneapolis, Minnesota

Foreword

Of all the professions, it is perhaps nursing that is most decisively leading the way toward a reorientation of values and behaviors that promote wellness and the continuity of humanity on Earth. This is a fitting development because "nurse" is derived from the Latin *nutrire*, meaning "nourish," and it is nurses whose empathy, compassion, caring, and wisdom have nourished countless humans in their journeys from birth to death. Now nurses and their leaders are nourishing the human species in a worldwide effort.

Dr. Jean Watson, one of the most distinguished and widely honored nurses in the world, has been awarded 15 honorary doctorates, 12 of which are international. She is distinguished professor and Dean Emerita, University of Colorado-Denver, College of Nursing, where she held the nation's first endowed chair in Caring Science for 16 years. She is the founder of the original Center for Human Caring in Colorado and the founder and director of Watson Caring Science Institute, a nonprofit foundation. The Caring Science philosophy and clinical practice model that Watson has pioneered include but transcend the needs of individuals. They also promote health in the largest sense—the health of the Earth itself. Caring Science philosophy and practice have been embraced by nursing organizations worldwide.

Through the courage and wisdom of Dr. Watson and her colleagues represented in this volume, we see the dawning of a concept that is powerful enough to catalyze a solution not only to health-related issues but also to the challenges that affect humanity's very survival. The origin of the problems we face can be expressed succinctly: *We have tried as a species to secede from nature, and we have failed. In so doing, we have misconstrued our relationship to one another and to all sentient life.* "The twenty-first century will be spiritual or it will not be," said André Malraux (1901–1976), France's former Minister of Cultural Affairs (Dennis, 2017, p. 41). Malraux's observation dates to the second half of the 20th century, and it appears more accurate now than ever before. As the planetary dilemma Malraux predicted plays out, it is no longer possible to be a passive bystander. As global citizens, if we are passive toward the problems we now face, we contribute to them. In our era, neutrality is not an honorable option. As Mahatma Gandhi put it, "To believe something and not live it is dishonest" (Dewal, 2015, p. 29).

We confront threats to our existence our forebears never imagined. The evidence for our global predicament is based in abundant science, not on some sidewalk lunatic wearing a sandwich board yelling, "The end is near!" Our challenges include climate change and global warming; polluted air and water; exploding populations; habitat and species loss; water scarcity; deforestation; desertification; murderous ideologies; resource depletion; grinding poverty; endless wars of choice; ethnic and religious hatreds; lack of decency, love, and kindness toward others; on and on, all abetted by the materialistic "I've got mine/every man for himself" philosophy with which our society is currently septic. This is a hell from which, experts say, beyond a certain point there may be no escape. As author John Graves wrote in his elegy *Goodbye to a River*, "That long and bedrock certainty of thoughtful men that regardless of the race's disasters the natural world would go on and on is no longer a certainty" (Graves, 1974).

What do these dismal facts have to do with Watson's Human Caring Science? The answer is, *everything*.

There is an ancient belief that during times of crisis, the Earth produces or raises up a solution. It may be in the form of a great heroine or hero, or it may be a new belief or concept that is powerful enough to steer things back on course. What is our current crisis? As the mythologist Joseph Campbell wrote toward the end of the past millennium, "The old gods are dead or dying and people everywhere are searching, asking: What is the new mythology to be, the mythology of this unified earth as one harmonious being?" (Campbell, 2002, p. xix). Nowadays we hunger for a culture that transcends the suffocating narrowness and intellectual strangulation resulting from the prejudice, bigotry, greed, and crass materialism that threaten our future. We are vision starved and myth hungry. As cultural historian Morris Berman writes, we long for a future culture that "will have a greater tolerance for the strange, the nonhuman, for diversity of all sorts, both within the personality and without" (Berman, 1981, p. 275). Also, Kingsley L. Dennis, the British sociologist, observes, "We will reconnect with the sacred or we will stagnate" (2017, p. 49). Many believe we have turned the corner in the right direction. As Dennis writes, "The magical, mysterious sacred revival is already underway, it just isn't paraded by the mainstream yet. But the spores are seeding all over the holy ground of this blessed planet. It will come to pass—it has already been born" (2017, p. 49). We contend that the Human Caring Science that Jean Watson has midwifed is part of this process of rebirth. It is part of "the knowing, accepting, and the seeking out the sacred aspects of life that bring the revitalizing energies surging and coursing through our spirit veins" (Dennis, 2017, p. 51).

Our online dictionary suggests that "care" is related to the assurance of health; welfare; maintenance; and protection of a person or thing (Online Dictionary, 2011). We in the healing professions usually translate this into our professional roles, responsibilities, and skills toward sick and suffering individuals, but the "health, welfare, maintenance, and protection" of the "something" apply also to Earth itself. For if our environment is degraded beyond reclaim, it will not matter much what our blood pressure or cholesterol levels are. Human health is impossible if the Earth cannot sustain us. Only by sensing at the deepest emotional, psychological, and spiritual levels our connections with one another and the Earth itself can we summon the courage necessary to make the tough choices that are required to survive. This is Human Caring Science writ large.

But the connections implicit in Human Caring Science are not human- or Earth-limited; they are infinite. As French philosopher René Guénon put it, "The human order and the cosmic order are not in reality separated, as they are nowadays all too readily imagined to be; they are on the contrary closely bound together, in such a way that each continuously reacts on the other so that there is always correspondence between their respective states" (Guénon, 1953, p. 140). This view is ancient. As the Greek philosopher Parmenides famously asserted in the 5th century BCE, "No mind, no world" (Singh, 2014).

The fact of our oneness and connectedness suggests that we revise the Golden Rule from the customary "Do unto others as you would have them do unto you," to "Be kind to others because in some sense they *are* you" (Dossey, 2013a, p. xxviii). As novelist Alice Walker said, "Anything we love can be saved" (Walker, 1998)—including the Earth and its creatures, our children, and generations yet unborn. Also, as poet W. H. Auden bluntly said in the 1930s, as if peering into the present, "We must love one another or die" (Auden & Mendelsson, 1977, p. 246). Love is a natural accompaniment of our inherent unity, connectedness, and oneness. Love helps us resacralize our world. Love helps us survive.

Extending Human Caring Science to all our interactions in the world is a way of recalibrating our collective response to all the problems we face, a move that permits a cascade of solutions to fall into place. As Watson has consistently emphasized, this approach requires a shift in our consciousness. It entails reorienting our ethical and moral compass toward the Earth and one another. It is about changing channels, redialing our basic concepts of who we are and how we are related to one another and to the terrestrial crucible that sustains us.

When caring includes all of life, it becomes a vision powerful enough to make a difference in how we approach *all* the challenges we face—not as a mere intellectual concept, but as something we feel in the deepest way possible. As Herman Hesse said in the prologue to *Demian*, "I have been and still am a seeker, but I no longer seek in stars and books; I have begun to listen to the teachings my blood whispers to me" (Hesse, 1919, p. ii).

Jean Watson sees that *caring* and *science* must be wedded, thereby producing a force greater than either factor can achieve in isolation. Her vision is affirmed by developments in the physical sciences that portend a revolution in how we conceive our relationships with one another.

It is now clear that, owing to advances in modern physics and the biological sciences, we live in a *nonlocal* world in which apparently separate elements are intrinsically connected or entangled (Dossey, 2013b, p. 30; Radin, 2006). These intimate connections defy separation in space and time. They operate at both an invisible subatomic level and, we have recently learned, in the everyday, macroscopic biological domain as well (Vedral, 2011). Our existence is based not in separation, competition, and rugged individuality, but in unity, connectedness, and cooperation. The sheer fact of *caring* arises naturally from these intrinsic relationships.

It is beginning to dawn on our society that the implications of nonlocality are enormous. As renowned historian of religions Huston Smith expressed the relevance of this development, "[If] nonlocality holds for the material world, what about the world of the human mind? If both mind and matter are nonlocal, we are on our way to regaining what was lost in Newton's time—a complete, whole world in which we can live complete, whole lives, in the awareness that we are far more interrelated than we had thought" (Jauregui, 2007, p. xiv).

But we do not require modern physics to inform us of our unity. This wisdom is ancient. We merely detoured from this knowledge in the modern era in our attempted withdrawal from nature and one another. The thread of oneness runs through human history, from ancient times through the present. The pedigree of this concept is extensive. As Plato wrote, "[H]uman nature was originally One and we were a whole" (Wilber, 1983, p. 234). Hippocrates stated, "There is one common flow, one common breathing, all things are in sympathy" (Watson, 1992, p. 27). Pico della Mirandola, the Renaissance philosopher, believed that the world is governed by a "unity whereby one creature is united with the others and all parts of the world constitute one world" (Watson, 1992, p. 27). In the 19th century, the German philosopher G. W. F. Hegel called distant mental exchanges between humans "the magic tie." He believed that "the intuitive spirit oversteps the confines of time and space; it beholds things remote; things long past, and things to come" (Inglis, 1992, p. 158). Arthur Schopenhauer, the 19th century German philosopher, suggested that a single event could figure in two or more different chains of circumstance, linking the fates of different individuals in profound ways. He believed in a form of communication that took place between humans during dreams (Watson, 1992, p. 27). Walt Whitman, America's 19th century bard, proclaimed, "All these separations and gaps shall be taken up and hook'd and link'd together.... Nature and Man shall be disjoin'd and diffused no more" (Whitman, 1917). His contemporary, philosopher-essayist Ralph Waldo Emerson, wrote, "There is one mind common to all individual men ... [a] universal mind...." Emerson called this universal mind the "Over-soul" which, he said, is "that unity ... within which every man's particular being is contained and made one with all other.... [W]ithin man is the soul of the whole ... the eternal ONE" (Emerson, 1987). Among the poets in Emerson's camp was William Butler Yeats: "[T]he borders of our minds are ever shifting, and ... many minds can flow into one another ... and create or reveal a single mind, a single energy.... [T]he borders of our memories are ... shifting, and ... our memories are part of one great memory" (Pierce, 2000, p. 62). Swiss psychiatrist Carl G. Jung's concept of the collective unconscious and the collective conscious paralleled the views of Emerson and Yeats (Jung, 1968). These various observers are saying that everything is connected, including minds.

Caring awareness is spreading. We have allies. For example, Vaclav Havel, the playwright, poet, and first president of the Czech Republic, said: "I have been given to understand how small this world is and how it torments itself with countless things it need not torment itself with if people could find within themselves a little more courage, a little more hope, a little more responsibility, a little more mutual understanding and love" (Havel, 1995). In other words, a little more caring.

Caring is not something we have to invent. It is our nature to care. Caring must merely be rekindled. That is what Jean Watson has done. She reminds us of who we are and of what we are capable. In her perspective, reality is interconnected, multidimensional, mindful, relational, and loving (Radin, 2013, p. 310).

It is appropriate that Watson launched her Human Caring Science nursing, for all the human professions it is nursing that provides the soil and the soul that can best nurture the wisdom on which our future likely depends. In so doing, Watson stands in the tradition of Florence Nightingale (1820–1910), a towering genius of both intellect and spirit who streaked like a fiery comet across the sky of 19th-century England, transforming nursing in world culture with her philosophical "art and science" nursing legacy (Dossey, 2010). In

Nightingale's tradition, Dr. Jean Watson has herself streaked across the 20th- and 21st-century skies with an equally precious gift—her Human Caring Science that is now an emerging paradigm. Her vision calls us to ethically informed caring and love—praxis in action. It is difficult to imagine a greater contribution.

Barbara Montgomery Dossey, PhD, RN, AHN-BC, FAAN, HWNC-BC
Co-Director, International Nurse Coach Association
International Co-Director, Nightingale Initiative for Global Health

Larry Dossey, MD
Executive Editor, Explore: The Journal of Science and Healing

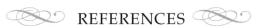 REFERENCES

Auden, W. H., & Mendelson, E. (Ed.). (1977). *The English Auden: Poems, essays and dramatic writings, 1927-1939.* London, UK: Faber.

Berman, M. (1981). *The reenchantment of the world.* New York, NY: Cornell University Press.

Campbell, J. (2002). *The inner reaches of outer space* (3rd ed.). New York, NY: New World Library.

Dennis, K. L. (2017). *The sacred revival: Magic, mind & meaning in a technological age.* New York, NY: Select Books.

Dewal, O. S. (2015). *MK Gandhi: The educationist par excellence.* New Delhi, India: Prabhat Prakashan.

Dossey, B. M. (2010). *Florence Nightingale: Mystic, visionary, healer.* Philadelphia, PA: F. A. Davis.

Dossey, L. (2013). *One mind: How our mind is part of a greater consciousness and why it matters.* Carlsbad, CA: Hay House.

Emerson, R. W. (1987). *The essays of Ralph Waldo Emerson* (Rev. ed.). Cambridge, MA: Harvard University Press.

Graves, J. (1974). *Goodbye to a river.* New York, NY: Alfred A. Knopf.

Guénon, R. (1953). *The reign of quantity and the signs of the times.* New Delhi, India: Munshiram Manoharlal.

Havel, V. (1995, May 12). Radical renewal of human responsibility. Commencement address at Harvard University. Retrieved from http://www.humanity.org/voices/commencements/vaclav -havel-harvard-university-speech-1995

Hesse, H. (1919). *Demian.* Berlin, Germany: S. Fischer Verlag.

Inglis, B. (1992). *Natural and supernatural.* Bridport, Dorset, UK: Prism Press.

Jauregui, A. (2007). *Epiphanies: Where science and miracles meet.* New York, NY: Atria.

Jung, C. G. (1968). *The archetypes and the collective unconscious* (2nd ed., R. F. C. Hull, Trans.). Princeton, NJ: Princeton University Press.

Online Dictionary. (2011). Macintosh Word version 14.7.7.

Pierce, D. (Ed.). (2000). *Irish writing in the twentieth century.* Cork, Ireland: Cork University Press.

Radin, D. (2006). *Entangled minds.* New York, NY: Paraview/Simon & Schuster.

Radin, D. (2013). *Supernormal.* New York, NY: Deepak Chopra Books/Crown.

Singh, V. (2014). *All is mind: The Skolimowskian philosophy of the participatory mind.* New York, NY: Penguin/Partridge Publishing India.

Vedral, V. (2011). Living in a quantum world. *Scientific American, 304*(6), 38–43. doi:10.1038/ scientificamerican0611-38

Walker, A. (1998). *Anything we love can be saved.* New York, NY: Penguin/RandomHouse.

Watson, L. (1992). *Dreams of dragons.* Rochester, VT: Destiny Books.

Whitman, W. (1917). Passage to India. In D. H. S. Nicholson & A. H. E. Lee (Eds.). *The Oxford book of English mystical verse.* Oxford, UK: The Clarendon Press. Retrieved from https://www.bartleby.com/236/120.html

Wilber, K. (1983). *Eye to eye: The quest for the new paradigm.* Garden City, NY: Anchor/Doubleday.

Preface

As the title suggests, *A Handbook for Caring Science: Expanding the Paradigm* is an inclusive and broadly encompassing text—the encyclopedia, if you will—of Caring Science. This book is the realization of over 30 years of Caring Science scholarship and a guidepost for the next stages of emerging paradigm.

Over 20 books by Dr. Jean Watson, along with hundreds of scholarly articles and additional publications by Caring Science scholars and authors, have validated Caring Science as a starting point for nursing as a field of study. As Caring Science nears its 40th anniversary of development, innovation, and continued emergence, nursing is preparing to celebrate its 150th anniversary as a profession. Never has a detailed and expansive guide for ethical philosophical nursing practices, across specialties and cross-cultural settings, been more needed.

In building upon and furthering Caring Science as the philosophical foundation and core of professional nursing, there is the opportunity to recalibrate the discipline to the healing art and science it was always meant to be. It does so despite the bureaucratic constraints and dictates that have dehumanized the healthcare scenario.

Caring Science as disciplinary foundation resounds the call for nurses to fulfill their covenant with society as peacemakers, the vanguards of human dignity, and the advocates for human betterment. Outdated institutional norms in healthcare are rapidly unraveling, and nurses must be equipped with a clear moral compass for effective leadership. Caring Science gives voice to that compass, offering a guide as a deeper practice consciousness for authentic human caring and healing throughout health systems for the future.

This book will be the first of its kind, guided by the disciplinary maturity of nursing, from theorists, from Caring Science educators and researchers, from practice insights, and from expert clinicians and accomplished administrators. These foundational Caring Science principles, strategies, and values serve to extend and transform health policy change.

These changes will continue to emerge from the hearts of Caring Science activists, cross-cultural colleagues, and global moral actions and applications from international/national caring scientists, and inspired voices from frontrunners in Caritas and integral health coaching, the creative healing arts, spirituality, self-care, and the next generation of Caring Science scholars and Caring Science praxis.

This book merges the full spectrum of Caring Science evolution and identifies a clear path for future growth and development. By illustrating the detailed connections between theory and practice, this book provides an opportunity to experience that delicate space of praxis, as the examples of a living philosophy are made accessible to the reader through the expert writing of contributing authors.

The ability to cross-reference Caring Science leaders across specialties and identify links between research and practice, practice and education, education and theory development, and global action in the world, makes this book a unique and essential partner in Caring Science scholarship for nurses and all other health and human service professionals. Through personal narrative, exemplars, and discourses on Caring Science, the reader will come to understand the history, accomplishments, and vision of human caring as a serious ethical, ontological, epistemological, practical endeavor; it is an art and science, celebrating the landscape of our shared humanity. In short, the reader will understand how to transform systems with a caring consciousness and a commitment to ethically informed action.

A Handbook for Caring Science is for all students who are forming or evolving their own philosophy of nursing; experts who are looking to renew or redefine their practice; educators, researchers, and scientists hoping to reconnect with the mature disciplinary foundation of nursing while adopting a greater purpose. Likewise, it is a gift for any health professional searching to regain his or her authentic identity as a caring-healing advocate and informed leader working toward an evolved moral community of caring and peace.

May this handbook be a source of wisdom, reflection, self-growth, and self-discovery along the path. May it bring you encouragement in your efforts to promote healing and wholeness. May it also offer solace in the knowledge that there is a place—a global village of the heart—that offers nourishment to the caring spirits of our nurse leaders, educators, scholars, and clinicians. May this book offer your work the reliable shelter and sustenance that emerges from a foundation of human caring and compassion.

William Rosa
Sara Horton-Deutsch
Jean Watson

Acknowledgments

This work started with a vision to create a handbook that would provide readers with a rich and comprehensive literary source rooted in Human Caring Science wisdom. I believe we have successfully compiled a substantial, heart-centered guide to inform the future unfolding of Caring Science scholarship. I am deeply honored and humbled to have had a small hand in its journey toward the light.

My sincerest gratitude to Springer Publishing Company and Margaret Zuccarini for your shared belief and trustworthy partnership in accomplishing this vision.

My sincerest gratitude to the chapter authors; your words enlighten with your unabashed commitment to caring-healing. The entire editorial team bows to each of you for your inspiration and relentless advocacy of Caring Science dissemination.

Dr. Sara Horton-Deutsch, your friendship helped to guide me through this project with love, compassion, and understanding. I am so grateful to and continue to learn from you in so many ways.

Dr. Jean Watson, you continue to amaze and humble me with your generous heart and mentorship. I am forever awed by your willingness to elevate the next generations of Caring Science leaders and to help usher all of us to our next levels of self-growth and self-discovery.

Drs. Marilyn Ray, Marlaine Smith, and Marian Turkel, and Grissel Hernandez, your fierce dedication to Caring Science is palpable throughout this volume of vision. Endless thanks for trusting me to spearhead this book and for your myriad contributions to its realization.

Dr. Diane Gullett—our "hub" of Caring Science communication—please believe me when I say that none of this would be possible without you. How honored we are to know and have you!

Mom and Dad, you always have a hand in every word. I love you.

Michael—whole, perfect, and complete—and so deeply, deeply loved.

To nurses everywhere who may read and come to embody this work, please know you are always cared for and supported.

Wishing you all endless waves of compassion and caring for the road ahead.

—William

I humbly and gratefully acknowledge the cocreators of this handbook—editors, authors, mentors, students, friends, Caritas colleagues. I have grown from your knowledge and wisdom to understand and appreciate there is always more to Caring Science than we can ever imagine. Collaborating with you has enriched my life by teaching me the value of opening myself—to surrender as an act of power and courage; this conscious choice leading to new energy, to new creation, to present forward.

I am honored to share this collection of works with our nurse and healthcare colleagues around the world as a source of scholarship for healing, hope, and wholeness—enlightening the world to "seeing" how healthcare as a healing art nurtures and sustains humanity.

Thank you, I love you.

—Sara

First, my dedication with deep gratitude to my beloved historic Caring Science scholars/ colleagues who were the original faculty associates of Watson Caring Science Institute (WCSI), who birthed and journeyed WCSI with me, cocreating, and implementing the Caritas Coach Educational Program (CCEP). They include Dr. Jim D'Alfonso, Dr. Jan Anderson, Dr. Gayle Casterline, Dr. Marliene Goldin, Dr. Lois Kelly, Dr. Mary Rockwood Lane, Dr. Linda Ryan, Dr. Marian Turkel, Dr. Lynne Wagner, Dr. Sharon Cumbie, and Marilyn Fogerty, Mary Jane McGraw, Terri Woodward. Without this group of dedicated Caring Science scholars, educators, and caring-healing practitioners, along with the original board of directors believing in me and this work, WCSI and the nature and extent of local, national, and global Caring Science programs would not have come into existence.

Second, my sincere bow to Mr. Rosa and Dr. Sara Horton-Deutsch for their leadership and vision for this manuscript as an important contribution to the growing global scholarship in Caring Science; their prescience is already legendary by generating such a comprehensive tome of collective works by experts in Human Caring Science. Enduring heart thanks for your devotion to this field of study, as you continue on your path of living Caring Science scholarship. Your gifts of self and sacrifice for this work stand out in our world—a world in need of new voices for a new generation, for a new era for humankind. You are showing the way.

Finally, but ironically first in my heart, I dedicate my deep love and awe to nurse partners, colleagues, and human caring practitioners all over the world, wherever you may be in the world, and wherever you may be in the work of compassionate Caring Science, human service. You are the ones who inspire me, inform me, teach me, guide me, touch me, and affirm my writings, my theory, my teachings, my vision and voice for Human Caring Science. I am in gratitude to the human caring you each offer, often behind the scenes, as nursing's gift to humanity to sustain Human Caring Science. You, wherever you are in the world, are the ones contributing to nursing coming of age as a distinct caring-healing health profession for our world and a new era for humanity. I offer you, all, my love and light!

—Jean

1

Introduction: Ontology, Epistemology, and the Lived Experience of Caring Science

Marilyn A. Ray, Marlaine C. Smith, Marian C. Turkel, and Grissel Hernandez-Kertland

The editors' intent of *A Handbook for Caring Science: Expanding the Paradigm* is to create a compendium of cutting-edge literature related to Caring Science from scholars in nursing and other disciplines for the purpose of reflecting on its foundations, inspiring continuing knowledge development, and sparking the creative use of Caring Science to inform and transform nursing practice. Throughout the book, all ways of knowing are used to grasp the many contours of being and becoming within this tradition. We introduce this work with a reflection on the associate editors' personal journeys into Caring Science to ground this work and establish a scholarly premise upon which to expand the paradigm. Their stories reflect the power of Caring Science to influence scholarship, research, education, administration, practice, and personal challenges that confront the human experience on our individual and collective journeys.

PERSONAL JOURNEYS INTO CARING SCIENCE

Marilyn A. Ray

Two nurse-anthropologists, the late Dr. Madeleine Leininger and Dr. JoAnn Glittenberg-Hinrichs, declared at the American Nurses Association Conference in 1976 that "caring: [is] the essence and central focus of nursing" (Leininger, 1977, p. 1). From Leininger's perspective, it was the first time that nurses talked directly about caring attitudes and activities related to nursing care at a conference (Foreword of the first Three National Caring Conferences, Leininger, 1981). This introduction to *A Handbook for Caring Science: Expanding the Paradigm* is the story of the thoughtful evolution of nursing as a Caring Science by scholars who share their philosophies, research, and practice experiences about a movement that *formally* began in Leininger's doctoral program in 1977, in which caring was a primary concentration and of which I, Dr. Marilyn Ray, was a part. Historically, the study of caring started many years earlier, developing foundational work by defining concepts; providing conceptual frameworks; creating models; identifying paradigms; and advancing theories (Alligood, 2018; Smith & Parker, 2015).

I was a master of science student of Leininger in 1969 and was enthralled with the fact that she declared nursing as a human science. She was committed to caring because she had studied the lifeways and care/caring behaviors of the Gadsup people of the Eastern Highlands of New Guinea for her PhD in cognitive anthropology, thus becoming the first nurse-anthropologist. She identified that, in the maintenance of health, caring behaviors were practically all within the purview and leadership of women, whereas men were concerned with curing behaviors (Leininger, 1979). She stated that from an anthropological perspective, caring is one of the oldest and most universal expectations for human development and survival throughout human history (Leininger, 1970, 1978, 1991). Archaeologists validated the claim that caring is as paramount in human development as is the evolution of the brain (Ray, 1981a, 1981b). After my introduction to nursing as a human and anthropological science, I completed a master's degree in cultural anthropology focusing on the contemporary culture of nurse decision making in the hospital. Dr. Leininger admitted me into the first transcultural nursing PhD program, with a focus on caring at the University of Utah (U of U) College of Nursing (CON). Under her mentorship, my passion continued in the study of nursing in the contemporary hospital culture, with emphasis on the ways of knowing of caring in nursing practice.

In 1978, a small group of faculty and doctoral students had the privilege of being invited to the first conference on human caring, "The Phenomena and Nature of Caring." A highlight of my life was meeting Dr. Jean Watson from the University of Colorado (UCO), my alma mater, who was working on her first book on caring and Carative Factors (later enhanced to the Caritas Processes®). Watson was seeking the core of nursing that forms a structure for studying, understanding, and implementing the science of caring. Her first book, *Nursing: The Philosophy and Science of Caring* (1979), is in its third edition. I presented on the philosophical analysis that engaged the metaphysics of first principles or what is related to meaningfulness and understanding, determining that, in nursing, *caring* and *love* are synonymous (Ray, 1981a, p. 32). At that time in nursing science, methods to study nursing were more positivistic, but at the U of U, qualitative research methods were emerging as a systematic way of inquiry. My work focused on the *meaning* and *action* of caring using three qualitative research methods: ethnography (study of the organizational culture), phenomenology (study of the meaning of life-world caring experience), and grounded theory (discovering substantive theory and generating formal theory; Glaser & Strauss, 1967; Morse et al., 2009; Ray, Morris, & McFarland, 2013; van Manen, 2014). It was the first caring research study in the hospital culture (Ray, 1981b, 1989, 2010a; Ray & Turkel, 2015).

The strength of these integrated methods in nursing practice was the generation of the widest variety of descriptive and reflective understanding of data gleaned from multiple participants laying the foundation for the discovery of the grounded theories. As Smith (2014) pointed out, "A theory provides a particular way of seeing phenomena of concern to the discipline" (p. 8). Two theoretical codes emerged to formulate theory. First, the **substantive** theory code was discovered from the experiential *and conceptual patterns of meaning* of caring and their categories and properties within all units of the hospital culture—the Theory of Differential Caring (Ray, 1981b, 1984, 1989, 2010a). Second, the **formal** theory code, the *conceptual model* emerged from analysis of the caring relationship that was discovered from the substantive codes and discerned through the Hegelian dialectic of thesis, antithesis, synthesis—thus, the synthesis of the *paradox* of caring and the hospital as a bureaucratic system (The Theory of Bureaucratic Caring; Coffman, 2014, 2018; Glaser, 1992; Glaser & Strauss, 1967; Hegel in Stace, 1955; Ray, 1981b, 1984, 1989, 2010a; Ray & Turkel, 2015; Turkel, 2007). This work showed how important the concept of spiritual-ethical caring, or creativity, love, and moral choice were related to the context, the physical, technological, economic, political, legal, and social-cultural (Ray, 2010a, 2010b, 2016). The theories identified a universal meaning, or, in part, "theoretical transparency" (van Manen, 1997, p. 17) in the context of the hospital. Research in this sense was "a caring act" (van Manen, 1997, p. 5); it showed what is most essential or substantive to persons as well as went to the heart of institutional caring. Finally, the use of the theory in practice is ongoing, with new theoretical approaches emerging from additional research, such as the Theory of Relational Complexity (Turkel & Ray, 2000, 2001) and the Theory of Relational Caring Complexity (Ray & Turkel, 2014). The Theory of Bureaucratic Caring is now being used as a structural model for the United States Air Force Patient-Centered Caring Model. The economics of caring was critical to understanding sustaining caring in complex systems. Thus, in the early 1990s, Dr. Marian Turkel and I conducted the first studies on the economics of caring.

My academic career included joining Dr. Jean Watson, dean at UCO CON in the 1980s, as a faculty member to develop Caring Science, human science, and qualitative research methodologies. Watson's leadership in the scholarship of caring philosophy and science is an unparalleled developing Caring Science at the UCO. In 1989, I joined the faculty of Florida Atlantic University (FAU) under the leadership of Dean Anne Boykin as the Christine E. Lynn Eminent Scholar in Nursing to facilitate the development of Caring Science. I continued teaching human science/qualitative research in the doctoral program at UCO until the death of my caring husband and soul mate, James Droesbeke, in 2005. (Jim was the creator of the Droesbeke Caring Award for international students in the International Association of Human Caring [IAHC].)

Throughout the 1980s, Leininger and others continued the evolution of the caring movement, educational developments, and the national caring research conferences with many publications of proceedings by Leininger. She initiated the first advisory board and was appointed the founder and chair of the IAHC with charter membership in 1987. During the creation of the IAHC, there was a lively discussion about whether the organization would be called the International Association for Human *Caring* or *Care*. It was determined that "caring" was the most expressive and scholarly name for the advancement of Caring Science for the organization. I was a charter member of the IAHC and designed the first set of goals of the bylaws, finalized in 1990 at the IAHC annual conference. Dr. Doris Riemen designed the first logo of the IAHC, and Drs. Delores Gaut and Doris Riemen were business officers. Drs. Gaut and Gwen Sherwood launched the first quarterly newsletter of the organization until it emerged as a peer-reviewed journal, the *International Journal for Human Caring* in 1997, under the coeditorship of Dr. Kathleen Valentine, a caring scholar dedicated to understanding how caring and cost structures were integrated. Drs. Anne Boykin and Patricia Benner were also part of the caring movement that illuminated caring, clinical judgment from novice to expert, and ethics (Benner, Tanner, & Chesla, 1996). It is important to note that Caring Science was a global movement. While Caring Science was developing in North America, the Caring Science movement was evolving in Scandinavia in 1970 under the pioneering efforts of Drs. Kari Martinsen, Katie Eriksson, and Charlotte Delmar who highlighted the essential meaning of caring as collectively caritative caring, love, mercy, and the ethical demand (Delmar & Johns, 2008; Eriksson, 2006; Martinsen, 2006).

Marlaine C. Smith

From the very beginning of my education, I was introduced to nursing as a discipline focused on the health of unitary human beings. My Fundamentals of Nursing teacher at Duquesne University was Rosemarie Parse. In the early 1970s, she taught us the difference between the "nursing model" and the "medical model." One of those differences, she said, was that medicine's goal was "cure," whereas nursing's was "care." After I received my master's degree, I returned to my alma mater to teach. I attended a provocative presentation on caring in nursing from Anne Davis, the noted nursing ethicist, in which she argued that the essence of nursing was caring. I remember being impressed with the clear connections between the relational dimensions of caring and the practice of nursing. At several nursing theory conferences, I heard Madeleine Leininger speak about the centrality of caring to nursing and Jean Watson presented her work on the art and science of human caring. Tenets related to existential-phenomenology (E-P) reflected in Watson's theory resonated with me since I was exposed to this philosophy at Duquesne University and was studying Parse's theory of man-living-health (now human becoming).

During my doctoral work at New York University (NYU), I studied Rogers's Science of Unitary Human Beings and healing modalities such as relaxation, guided imagery, music, and therapeutic touch. After completing my PhD at NYU and teaching at Duquesne, Penn State, and LaRoche College in the late 1970s and 1980s, I moved to Colorado and accepted a faculty position at the UCO. Jean Watson was the dean of the school at the time. She was a visionary, transformational leader, establishing a Center for Human Caring and a caring-based Doctor of Nursing (ND) program that was a 4-year postbaccalaureate professional entry program modeled after other professional degrees like medicine and law. Scholars from a variety of disciplines came to the Center so that caring scholars in nursing could be informed by poets, artists, engineers, and scientists in quantum physics. The curricula of the degree programs were grounded in Caring with courses such as Caring in Art, Caring in Music, and Caring in Literature. PhD students engaged in research using a range of innovative methodologies to understand the nature of human caring. Faculty (Dee Ray, Janet Quinn, Fran Reeder, Sally Gadow, Peggy Chinn, and others) was working at the intersection between caring and ethics, healing, and social-political reform. This was a nurse-led, caring theory–guided Center for persons with HIV/AIDS. My time there was like living in Camelot for Caring Science.

I stayed in Colorado for 18 years, growing my thinking about Caring Science, its relationship to unitary science, and studying healing from a unitary and Caring Science perspective, specifically conducting research related to the outcomes of touch therapies for people with life-limiting diseases. Jean developed a certificate program in Caring and Healing that attracted nurses from around the world, thirsty for this content, and the opportunity to study with her and others. I immersed myself in my work with brilliant PhD students who were eager to conduct their research and scholarship on caring philosophy, science, and art. I progressed to become a tenured full professor and became the director of the master's program. During my sabbatical, I studied with Margaret Newman and Richard Cowling, following which I published "Caring and the Science of Unitary Human Beings" as a response to Rogerian scholars about the place of caring in the discipline and the nature of caring from a unitary theoretical perspective. This became my seminal work. In 2000, I revamped the ND into the new doctor of nursing practice program grounded in caring.

I loved Colorado; it was my home. I grew up there as a scholar and my family grew up there, but I also had a passion to advance Caring Science in a place that was dedicated completely to that mission. I was further inspired hearing Dr. Boykin, dean at FAU, speak at the IAHC conference in Denver of her vision and leadership. FAU was establishing an innovative caring-based program, and it was launching a PhD program. In 2005, Anne invited me to speak at the opening of FAU's new building, and in 2006 I accepted a position as associate dean for Academic Programs and the Helen K. Persson Eminent Scholar at the CON at FAU. I was in awe of the faculty; they were dedicated to "advancing caring as a science, practicing the art, studying its meaning and living caring day-to-day." This became our mission statement that continues to guide us to this day. I advanced my work, developing unitary caring into a middle-range theory. In coediting *Nursing Theories and Nursing Practice* with Marilyn Parker, we featured middle-range theories in Caring Science. Marian Turkel, Zane Wolf, and I coedited *Caring in Nursing Classics,* a text containing classic literature in Caring Science. As an associate dean, I led the caring-based curricular development in the College.

In 2011, I became the second dean of the CON. I could never replace Anne Boykin, but I followed in her footsteps, continuing to advance the College to be the preeminent leader in Caring Science in the world. During my deanship, I honored the traditions of excellence in our caring-based education, expanded our influence and visibility, and demonstrated caring in our community engagement. We reformed our PhD program to focus on the advancement of Caring Science and nurtured the development of our two nurse-led centers as demonstration models for Caring Science in action. In 2018, I will step down from the deanship to a new season of my life where I hope to continue my writing about caring and healing work with PhD students.

Marian C. Turkel

My journey into Caring Science began in 1989 when I read an advertisement in the local Fort Lauderdale newspaper about a new master of science in nursing (MSN) program at FAU, grounded in caring. I was working in a leadership role at a local hospital and thought of myself "as a caring nurse and caring leader," so I applied and was accepted into the Nursing Administration Concentration. I soon learned that there was an ontology and epistemology of caring, and that caring was informed by multiple ways of knowing, and that nursing was being and becoming through caring. It was a very exciting time, as Dean Boykin was committed to advancing caring into the nursing curriculum at the undergraduate and graduate levels. The graduate courses were explicitly grounded in caring and had innovated names such as "Creative Leadership" and "Values and Financing: Nursing Strategies." I took the first course, "Caring as Foundational to Advanced Nursing Practice" in 1989 under Dean Boykin. I remember that we had to find five articles on caring per week over the course of 12 weeks and analyze them in the multiple ways of knowing (not easy in an era prior to online journals, the Internet, and electronic search engines).

Dr. Savina Schoenhofer was associate dean for the graduate program and was very passionate about nursing theory. She organized nursing theory conferences at a Miami-based hospital in 1989, 1990, and 1991. Nursing theorists who presented at these conferences included Drs. Boykin, Dorothy Johnson, Margaret Newman, Betty Neuman, Dorothea Orem, Rosemarie Parse, Martha Rogers, Savina Schoenhofer, Sister Callista Roy, and Jean Watson. Drs. Schoenhofer and Parker inspired my love and passion for nursing theory. Reflecting on my personal journey through the lens of the Janus perspective, the past truly informed my future. I was inducted as a fellow in the American Academy of Nursing in 2012, joined the Nursing Theory Guided Practice Expert Panel, and served in a leadership role for 3 years. In this role, I was very fortunate to become a professional colleague and friend of Drs. Peggy Chinn, Jacqui Fawcett, Dorothy Jones, and Sister Callista Roy. They are true leaders of nursing theory and nursing knowledge advancing the disciplinary focus of nursing.

In 1996, I was invited to participate in meetings when the outside surveyors (deans and nurse leaders) from the National League for Nursing (NLN) came to the college to accredit the MSN Program. At the end of the visit when members of the survey team discussed their findings, they started with saying, "When we came on this site visit we did not think that a graduate program focused on caring/caring theory could be accredited but after talking with students and hearing their understanding of how caring is knowledge and can be integrated into practice, leadership, and research we changed our perspective and will be recommending full accreditation."

I remember Dr. Ray was hired in 1990 as the Eminent Scholar within the CON. As students, we knew that it was an important title, but we did not know whether we were allowed to talk with her. I was fortunate that she was my professor and we immediately bonded over our passion for studying caring and economics within complex healthcare systems. Upon graduation, I entered the PhD program at the University of Miami. In the first class I took, all students were invited to share our definitions of nursing and I proudly said, "being and becoming through caring." I was met with blank stares from my colleagues and my professor said, "What kind of definition is that?" I recall being in other classes and discussing our substantive areas of study and I said mine was "caring." The immediate response from my professors was "perhaps you mean 'comfort'?" I said no, "I mean 'caring'." I returned to Dr. Schoenhofer's office, upset about the responses I received to caring, and thought perhaps it was not the place for me to study. She said "No, you will go back, they don't understand caring and you will help them understand the meaning."

Dr. Ray and I wrote our first grant together, *Nurse-Patient Relationship Patterns: An Economic Resource,* over Thanksgiving 1994. We could not use the "C" word in the title but Ray's Theory of Bureaucratic Caring served as the nursing theoretical framework. Over the course of our research careers with Dr. Ray as principal investigator (PI) and myself as co-PI, we have received almost $1 million in federal funding to study caring and economics in complex systems (Ray & Turkel, 2012, 2014).

I met Dr. Watson for the first time in 1989 at a candle-lighting ceremony at FAU for students and faculty with her candle that traveled all over the world. I find it amazing that I now do that same ritual with colleagues, nurses in practice, and nursing students. In 2007, my husband and I moved to Philadelphia where I became director of Professional Practice/Magnet and Research at Einstein Hospital in Philadelphia and began the integration of Watson's Theory of Human Caring into the practice setting. I also joined the faculty of the

Watson Caring Science Institute (WCSI) teaching in the Caritas Coach Education Program (CCEP), mentoring nurses doing WCSI Caring Science doctorates, publishing, and assisting Dr. Watson with planning of international conferences. Einstein hospital was designated as a WCSI Affiliate hospital in 2010 for the intentional and authentic integration of Watson's Theory of Human Caring into practice.

In 2014, I returned to academia and am currently an associate professor with the CON at FAU. I teach Advanced Nursing Practice, grounded in caring, for graduate students and Creating Healing Environments for undergraduate students. I am also doing a postdoctorate with Dr. Watson with the focus on advancing the epistemology and ontology of nursing science and Caring Science. The second part of my postdoctoral work includes the submission of two book proposals. One book is related to Unitary Caring Science and the other is collaborating with my husband, Brooks Turkel (senior vice president of a healthcare system), on a book for healthcare executives framed within Caring Science. My husband has always been a part of my Caring Science journey. He loves to say that he knows more nursing theorists than any chief executive officer and many chief nursing officers.

Grissel Hernandez-Kertland

My journey into Caring Science began in 1996 during my Nursing Research course at the University of Pennsylvania (U of Penn). We were introduced to "nursing theorist" and watched the video series *The Nurse Theorists: Portraits in Excellence* by Jacqueline Fawcett. Although I barely understood anything Jean Watson shared about her Theory of Human Caring, it still made a profound impact on me. This theory resonated and aligned with my reasons for becoming a nurse and from that moment on, the theory became my philosophical and ethical-moral compass informed by my nursing student experience and eventually my professional life.

Caring Science reconnected me with the moral and ethical dimensions of caring in nursing, reminding me that as a nurse I have a social covenant with the public to advocate for my patients at all levels and above all preserve their humanity and dignity. Moreover, Watson's Theory of Human Caring, with its strong emphasis on caring for the caregiver, gave me permission to slow down, engage in self-care practices, and become a much better version of myself as I engaged with others. Its core principles have informed my many nursing roles from student, direct care provider, educator, and administrator, particularly Caritas Processes 1, 2, 3, 4, 8, and 10. And yet, my journey with Caring Science extends beyond my professional nursing career into personal experiences that transformed the way I viewed the nursing profession as a consumer and as a nurse. It began with my parents' experiences with cancer in the United States and in Puerto Rico, my own experience with cancer at age 38, and finally the untimely death of my beloved husband, John, at age 53.

In 1997, during my last semester of nursing school at U of Penn, my mother was diagnosed with thyroid cancer. A few months later, when she needed her first radioactive iodine treatment, she worried she was not going to be able to deal with it. When she was told she could not take communion that Sunday, she even considered leaving against medical advice. Luckily, her nurse had the presence to see her distress and requested a consultation with a Catholic chaplain who explained the situation to my mother. Rather than giving her communion, she received the sacrament of the sick prior to treatment. This simple act of acknowledgment and meeting her basic needs allowed my mother to remain calm and complete her treatment successfully. Years later, she was diagnosed with breast and uterine cancers. I witnessed both extraordinary displays of kindness as well as extreme indifference and disregard for her as a human being. She hated hospitals and every encounter became a source of stress and anxiety for her. To keep her mind preoccupied, I shared information related to caring and particularly Watson's Caring Science. She always commented how much she agreed with "la Señora Watson's" view of nursing as caring and how the work connected with her somehow. She encouraged me to view my practice of nursing as a sacred vocation and above all "to have charity for patients and listen to their stories."

In 2005, my father, who lived in Puerto Rico, was diagnosed with end-stage pancreatic cancer at age 60. He relied on his faith and prayer to sustain him, but unlike my mother, decided to keep his illness a secret. His hospitalizations were physically painful and, at times, neglectful, with incidences of overmedication with morphine. Whenever I tried to discuss any of these issues, he would beg me "not to stir the pot and get them angry because they will get mad and take it out on me in the hospital." Those statements and the realization that my father felt unsafe in the hospital were very distressing. He died within 6 months of receiving his diagnosis. By the end, he witnessed an outpouring of love, friendship, acts of kindness and charity from family, friends, and total strangers. His death too was peaceful, as he was surrounded by people who loved him.

In early 2008, I was diagnosed with renal cell carcinoma. This diagnosis came during a visit to the emergency department (ED) preceded by acute chest and right-sided flank pain. I remember asking, "Why me?," crying, and at the same time, surrendering and detaching from the outcome. I was horrified, afraid, embarrassed, angry, curious, grateful, hopeful, and thankful all at the same time. Unlike my father's decision, I chose love and told my family, friends, and colleagues and asked for help and prayers. I also embraced several caring-healing modalities to support me through my patient experience such as laughter, visualization, guided imagery, poetry writing, journaling using CarePages, and chronicled my journey as a way to keep everyone informed. I even named my tumor "Pearl."

I had the practice of Caring Science to help me frame and make sense of my feelings and was determined to use my parents' and my own experiences as examples of how to be with patients. I have integrated the theory into patient care and nursing educational activities, including nursing orientation, preceptor development, new nurse residency program, nursing leadership development program, and my own personal nursing leadership practice.

In 2005, I completed the Integrative Nursing Practice Certificate from the BirchTree Center for HealthCare Transformation, began the process of becoming a nationally certified holistic nurse and I attended the American Holistic Nursing Association conference in Philadelphia where Jean Watson was the keynote speaker. In 2008, AtlantiCare adopted Jean Watson as our nursing theorist. Once again, I was inspired to continue to infuse her work into my nursing leadership practice and in 2010, I began the CCEP—Cohort 5. My Caritas Coach project included the integration of Caring Science into our newly developed Nurse Manager Leadership Development program and the development of our organization's Professional Practice Model, integrating Caring Science as our foundational theoretical framework. In 2012, AtlantiCare hosted the 19th International Caritas Consortium and became a Watson Caring Science Affiliate (WCSA) Hospital.

For the past 4 years, I have been working at Stanford Healthcare in Palo Alto, California. Caring Science was already integrated into our Professional Practice Model and part of my role is to provide a road map for full practice integration into the fabric and DNA of the organization. We conducted a Caring Science needs assessment using the Caring Hospital criteria as outlined by Jean Watson and Barbara Brewer and created a 5-year Caring Science Integration Plan. In 2015, Stanford Healthcare became a WCSA Hospital, and this past October 2017, we hosted the 23rd International Caritas Consortium.

In 2014, I began my PhD in nursing at UCO CON in the Caring Science track. My research interest is the perceptions of nurse leaders regarding their influence on creating a caring, healing environment for their staffs. I am interested in conducting qualitative Caring Science research using Relational Caring Inquiry (RCI) and Photovoice on Caritas Process #8: Caring, healing environment.

This past June 2017, my beloved husband, John, died unexpectedly at home of a heart attack. His death left me heartbroken and in a deep depression and grieving. John suffered for many years with depression and panic and anxiety attacks. However, during the past year of his life he began integrating Watson Caring Science Caritas Processes, practicing lovingkindness, meditation, and spending countless hours in his garden tending to his Jersey tomatoes, bell peppers, and herb garden. His favorite Caritas Process was #5, allowing for positive and negative feelings! He called gardening his spiritual practice and attributed his practice of lovingkindness with his new-found sense of peace. Caring Science, along with my deep faith, has provided me with all the coping strategies I needed during these challenging times. It has given me the opportunity to pause, take a life inventory, prioritize, and refocus. It made me more resilient with a deeper capacity to handle anything that comes my way with a trusting spirit. It has provided me a road map for my professional and personal life mission to share my patient's experiences and teach healthcare providers about the need to reclaim the art and science of caring and the healing power of compassion, authentic presence, reflection, intentionality, and gratitude in every human encounter. It allowed me to feel love from others and more importantly allow others to love and care for me. Caring Science is lived in every encounter and these experiences have reaffirmed how, as a philosophical and ethical foundation, it has the potential to apply to any situation in which nursing occurs.

SECTION OVERVIEWS

The following part of the introduction provides section overviews for this Handbook, with detailed information about its structure, content, sections, and themes. The purpose of this overview is to give you a brief synopsis of the focus of the chapters in each section.

This book is structured with 10 sections, each focused on a particular theme. Each section contains several chapters written by expert scholars who offer some perspective on the theme. Sections I through IX include 38 chapters. Section X features personal journeys illuminating the power of aesthetic knowing in Caring Science, and is composed of 10 shorter pieces. These sections reflect substantive areas of disciplinary-specific knowledge in Caring Science.

- Section I: The Disciplinary Discourse: Theories and Frameworks Evolving to Unitary Caring Science

- Section II: Converging Paradigms: Constructing New Worldviews

- Section III: Caritas Science Literacy: From Caritas to Global Communitas

- Section IV: Caritas Literacy As a Foundation for Nursing Education

- Section V: Authenticating Caring Science Through Scholarly Inquiry

- Section VI: Touching the Space of Praxis

- Section VII: Redefining Healthcare Through Heart-Centered Wisdom

- Section VIII: Global Caring Science

- Section IX: Emerging Inquiry: The Evolution of a Science

- Section X: Journeys Into the Transpersonal: Aesthetic Ways of Knowing

SECTION I: THE DISCIPLINARY DISCOURSE: THEORIES AND FRAMEWORKS EVOLVING TO UNITARY CARING SCIENCE

The editors' assumption is that nursing knowledge is evolving toward a unitary-transformative worldview, and the ontology of Caring Science is embracing the tenets of this unitary worldview. There are six chapters in this section. Chapter 2, "Unitary Caring Science: Disciplinary Evolution of Nursing," by Jean Watson, Marlaine C. Smith, and W. Richard Cowling, III, is both a reprise of their previous work together and a deeper reflection on the foundations of an emerging Unitary Caring Science. Both Smith and Cowling are experts in Martha Rogers's Science of Unitary Human Beings and, of course, Watson's theoretical work reflects unitary tenets and has been informed by an ethic of belonging as well as metaphysical and Eastern philosophical thought. Chapter 3, by Peggy L. Chinn, the noted meta-theorist, critical-feminist scholar, and editor of *Advances in Nursing Science*, is titled, "The Evolution of Nursing's Ethic of Caring." In this chapter, Chinn provides a critical synopsis of the literature in the discipline on nursing ethics and its relationship to caring, and argues that caring is central to a nursing ethic. Chapter 4 is a reprint of Marilyn A. Ray and Marian C. Turkel's article on their Theory of Relational Complexity. Their theory draws on complexity theory as a metaphor to capture the dynamic process of caring within organizations, and the power of caring to influence both the valued outcomes of the organization and the persons served. Chapter 5, "Caring in African Ontology," is written by Anna Nolte and Charlene Downing, prominent South African nurse scholars. These authors introduce the readers to Ubuntu, the African worldview that originates from the primacy of belonging to a village, tribe, or community where actions come from the heart and manifest in love for each other. The authors recognized the close alignment of this cultural worldview with Watson's Caritas Processes, and they explicate these similarities. Shawna M. McDermott, a Native American nurse scholar, is the author of Chapter 6, "Caring Science—Native Science." McDermott apprehends the connection between the indigenous beliefs of interconnectedness, wholeness, discovery, and being in right relationship with Watson's Caritas Processes, and concludes with a call for action based in authenticity, agency, and advocacy. The final chapter in this section, Chapter 7, "Developing the Knowledge of Human Caring," is written by Jacqueline Fawcett, a renowned meta-theorist and prolific author on nursing theory.

Fawcett's focus is on the place of caring in nursology, the discipline-specific knowledge for nursing. She elaborates the structure of nursology, including the metaparadigm, philosophies, conceptual models, theories, and empirics and how this structure relates to the advancement of Caring Science.

SECTION II: CONVERGING PARADIGMS: CONSTRUCTING NEW WORLDVIEWS

The contributing authors developed explicit connections between established programs or initiatives and Caring Science. Chapter 8, by Robert Browning and Jean Watson, is titled "Caring Science and Heart Science: A Guide to Heart-Centered Caritas Praxis." Browning is a master teacher with the HeartMath Institute. Through the WCSI, he and Watson have re-formed HeartMath methods within a Caring Science framework as Caritas Heart Praxis. In Chapter 9, "Expanding Global Reach Through a Massive Open Online Course on Mindfuless and Caring," Kathleen Sitzman provides a report of the Massive Open Online Course (MOOC) called Caring Science, Mindful Practice (CSMP) that she created to bring Watson's theory and Caritas Processes and mindfulness praxis to people all over the world. Chapter 10, "Conscious Dying: The Sacred and Subtle of Living and Dying," by William Rosa, Tarron Estes, Stephanie Hope, and Jean Watson contains a vision of conscious dying within a Caring Science ontology, reflecting a deepening awareness of dying and death as part of the sacred cycle of life. Sara Horton-Deutsch and William Rosa authored Chapter 11, "Reflective Practice and Caring Science." Horton-Deutsch, a scholar of both reflective practice and Caring Science, is well-positioned to identify the synchrony between these two fields of study. Horton-Deutsch and Rosa provide a comprehensive review of the literature related to reflective practice and models for the structured reflection process. Chapter 12 is a reprinted article authored by Mary Jo Kreitzer, Mary Koithan, and Jean Watson. Kreitzer and Koithan are leading scholars in the field of integrative nursing. They present the tenets of integrative nursing and relate these tenets to Watson's Caritas Processes.

SECTION III: CARITAS SCIENCE LITERACY: FROM CARITAS TO GLOBAL COMMUNITAS

In Chapter 13, "Ways of Being/Knowing/Becoming," Jean Watson and Sara Horton-Deutsch invite each one of us to seek understanding of our ways of being, knowing, and becoming through knowledge of the meaning of Watson's 10 Caritas Processes. This understanding emerges through deep reflection on the processes to facilitate the beginning of illumination of our whole person presence with a perception of our evolving consciousness that opens us to the higher levels of an energetic, infinite spiritual field within us—universal Love. Chapter 14, "Curriculum Development Processes and Pedagogical Practices for Advancing Caring Science Literacy," by Marcia D. Hills and Chantal Cara, focuses not only on *what* we teach but also on *how* we teach that promote Caring Science literacy in nursing. From the ideas of Watson, Caring Science literacy deepens our ways of attending to and cultivating how we are to be deeply human, be caring, and have a healing presence. Chapter 15, "Loving Kindness and

Equanimity: Illuminating the Nursing Literature Through a Caring Lens," by Zane Robinson Wolf and Marian C. Turkel, addresses the roots and major influences of select Caritas Processes: first, "Cultivating the practice of loving kindness" and second, "Equanimity within the context of caring consciousness." By means of reviewing the literature, Wolf and Turkel highlight the fact that the cultivation of loving kindness and equanimity requires caregivers to act purposefully with kindness and calmness in the moment directed toward self and others by going on an inner journey of self-understanding to create healing environments.

Section IV: Caritas Literacy As a Foundation for Nursing Education

Chapter 16, "Teaching From the Heart," by Nancy Vitali, identifies ways to be present to students to help them engage in caring-healing relationships and to actually hear the stories of others in an educational setting. Vitali points out that the climate of nursing education in the United States is one of constant change and complexity, and resounds, "Teaching from the heart is a transpersonal experience." Chapter 17, "Developing Values and a Philosophy of Being," by Lisa Flack and Donnean Thrall, identifies ways to embody thought, being, and becoming, caring literacies in nursing education to promote the development of caring-healing nurses. In this chapter, Flack and Thrall develop a new Caring Science curriculum in a Franciscan College dedicated to opening the heart to love as well as opening the mind to truth. Chapter 18, "Fostering Metamorphosis Through Caring Literacy in an RN-to-BSN Program" is written by Mark D. Beck. As a Caritas Coach and educator, Beck describes a transformative unitary Caring Science curriculum and the many ways it has transformed relationships with self, others, the healthcare team, and the organization or system. Both students and educators experienced profound transformation in their personal and professional lives based on their relational encounters of caring and how they grounded themselves in the principles and framework of Watson's Caring Literacy. Chapter 19, "Nursing Doctorally Prepared Caring Scientists" by Sara Horton-Deutsch, Kathy Oman, and examines the role of the Caring Science researcher within a contemporary, socially progressive pedagogy of Caring Science and scholarship of an interprofessional PhD program. The significance of the PhD pedagogy and credential brings forth the qualities of a caring scholar and stewardship for the discipline of nursing through a Caring Science lens. Chapter 20, "Advancing Caring Science Through the Missions of Teaching, Research/Scholarship, Practice and Service," by Marlaine Smith, is a description of FAU Christine E. Lynn's CON programs from baccalaureate-, master's-, and doctoral-level programs of study where the core concept of caring over almost four decades ago emerged as the essence of nursing. Smith, as dean for nearly a decade, outlines the vision, mission, and philosophy of the CON and how caring has grounded the core values within the vision, mission, and philosophy. Sustaining and growing the culture of caring is a living tribute to the leadership over the years of many faculty scholars, especially former dean, Dr. Anne Boykin, and current dean, Dr. Marlaine Smith.

Section V: Authenticating Caring Science Through Scholarly Inquiry

The chapters written for this section focus on how scholarly inquiry advances the epistemology of Caring Science in the areas of leadership, research, and education. In Chapter 21, "Leading From the Heart; Caring, Love, Peace and Values Guiding Leadership," Dr. Marian C. Turkel offers a unique perspective on leadership from the unitary-transformative paradigm and a Caring Science perspective. Practice exemplars are presented to highlight how tenets from the unitary-transformative paradigm are guiding the practice of nursing leadership and how Caring Science can be used to reframe the traditional organizational language. In Chapter 22, "Evaluation of Authentic Human Caring Professional Practices," Drs. Barbara Brewer and Jean Watson expand the epistemology of Caring Science through development of the *Watson Caritas Patient Score©™*. The *Watson Caritas Patient Score (WCPS)* is a five-item measurement assessment to capture the patient's experience of caring based on Watson's 10 Caritas Processes. This measurement tool is in contrast to the traditional patient surveys that focus on the traditional biomedical view and customer service approaches. In Chapter 23, "The Evolution of Knowledge Development Related to Caring in Online Classroom and Beyond," Kathleen Sitzman provides an overview of core concepts of Watson's Theory of Human Caring. The unique and innovative perspective of this chapter is the creation of the 10 Caritas Processes for faculty to support caring comportment during online teaching (Sitzman & Watson, 2014).

Section VI: Touching the Space of Praxis

The chapters in this section are written by caring scholars whose scholarship has advanced the epistemology of research, aesthetic knowing (healing environments), and Caritas Praxis. In Chapter 24, "Caring Inquiry Methodology: The Esthetic Process in the Way of Compassion," Dr. Marilyn A. Ray illuminates a methodology for research grounded in caring. In this chapter, Dr. Ray makes explicit the connection among caring, love, compassion, esthetics, theology, and spirituality in nursing (caring) inquiry. In Chapter 25, "Holding Sacred Space for Loving-Kindness and Equanimity for Self/Others," Dr. Joseph Giovannoni writes about the metaphysical realm of Caring Science affirming that being still, silent, and connected with Source allows for a consciousness of humanity that is holographic, pandimensional, nonlocal, universal, and a true expression of love. In Chapter 26, "Mutual Vulnerability: Creating Healing Environments That Nurture Wholeness and Well-Being," Drs. Charlotte Barry and Beth King explore the concept of mutual vulnerability from the perspective of the nurse and the one nursed, and view the concept of mutual vulnerability as being an integral component of a healing environment. Their conceptualization of vulnerability is not a problem "to fix" but an opportunity to come to know each other as personal filled with potential. In Chapter 27, "Integrating Caring Science and Caritas Into Professional Practice," Dr. Linda Ryan focuses on the integration of Caring Science and Caritas Praxis within healthcare systems to create caring-healing environments and provides evidence of the outcomes related to increased patient satisfaction, nursing satisfaction, and improved patient outcomes when the role of the Caritas Practitioner becomes integrated within the healthcare system.

Section VII: Redefining Healthcare Through Heart-Centered Wisdom

Chapters in this section are written by Caritas nurse leaders who made the commitment to authentically and intentionally integrate Caring Science grounded in Watson's Theory of Human Caring and the 10 Caritas Processes into large complex healthcare systems. In Chapter 28, "A Blueprint for Caritas Health 'Care'," Drs. Jacqueline A. Somerville and Susan M. Lee share their experiences at Brigham and Women's Hospital in Boston. The transformation included the specific nursing practices of setting intentions at the start of each shift, posting Caritas Processes over the entrances to patients' rooms, practicing loving kindness to self and others during interdisciplinary team conferences, creating Caritas Rooms, and integrating Caritas Heart Math. In Chapter 29, "Kaiser Permanente Patient Care Services Northern California: The Adaptation of Caring Science," Anne M. Foss-Durant and Shawna M. McDermott share the process of integrating Caring Science across the Kaiser System in Northern California. The authors described the process of intentionally integrating Caring Science into the hiring process, orientation, and ongoing educational offerings for all registered nurses. In Chapter 30, "Nursing As Love: A Hermeneutical Phenomenological Study of the Creative Thought Within Nursing," Dr. Marlienne Goldin asserts that love of humanity, compassion, caring, and love are all qualities manifested by nurses when providing nursing care. Goldin's research question "How does love manifest itself in the day to day practice of nursing?" serves as the conceptual basis for a qualitative research study with registered nurses.

Section VIII: Global Caring Science

Chapters in this section reflect the process of Caring Science and cross-cultural (transcultural) ethical significance that is being developed in many parts of the world. Chapter 31, "The Essential Nature of Caring Partnerships: Contextual Relevance and Cross-Cultural Ethical Considerations," by Michele J. Upvall, Diane Gullett, and William Rosa, illuminates the concept of partnerships in terms of a global context and shared humanity. *Developing and sustaining loving trusting-caring partnership* (Watson, n.d.) provides the ethical foundation to the meaning, characteristics, and process for partnerships across cultures as practiced by the Caritas nurse. Chapter 32, "Scandinavian Caring Sciences" by Charlotte Delmar of Denmark, demonstrates the development of Caring Science in Scandinavia beginning in 1970 with the scholarship of Professor Katie Eriksson of Finland and Sweden, and Professor Kari Martinsen of Norway culminating in the scholarship of Charlotte Delmar. Chapter 33, "Caring Practices in an Era of Conflict: Middle East Nurses" by Julie Benbenishty and Jordan R. Hannink, illuminates the conflict situation in the Middle East between Israel and Palestine. The chapter highlights the nurse as a political and social being, the nurse as part of the political and social conflict and landscape, as well as the nurse as the organizer of the chaos of disease, mental states, nutrition, mobility, and so forth. The authors state, "the complexity of life in the Middle East has brought us together," and is represented by Nurses in the Middle East, a non-profit organization supported by Jean Watson. The organization helps nurses to come together and dialogue about conflict situations and how caring and Caritas Processes can mediate conflict to determine life chances and good health outcomes for the cross-cultural population. Chapter 34, "Caritas, Peace, and Change in Japan," by Mayumi Tsutsui, Rina Emoto, and

Jean Watson, illustrates the evolution of Caring Science within Japan over the past two to three decades. From the time that Watson was first in Japan as a Caring Science scholar in 1989 until the International Hiroshima Caring and Peace Conference in 2012, development of caring knowledge, values, theories, and practices of human caring have been embraced and advanced. Chapter 35, "Caritas Nursing and Professional Practice in Peru" by Patrick A. Palmieri, identifies the historical evolution of a sociomedical, paternalistic, "machismo" culture in healthcare and its influence on nursing to a new phase of development of Caritas-informed nursing and healthcare renaissance. The effort within Peruvian nursing in the past decade was initiated by Dr. Palmieri who has dedicated his professional life to changing the landscape of nursing within Peru. Chapter 36, "Towards Planetary Caring: Sustainable Health and Wellbeing for All," by William Rosa, addresses an ethical-spiritual starting point for human-centeredness, a planetary theory and way of being that encompasses and fosters a deep connection to the spiritual-metaphysical oneness of all, the human–environment integrality. Rosa outlines global problems in the 21st century that impact concerns about environmental and planetary health, and concludes that the 2030 Sustainable Development Goals of the United Nations need to be used as a guiding framework for multidisciplinary teams, especially nursing as a planetary partner, to implement planetary solutions to many global health and environmental problems—One Mind, One Health, One Planet. Caritas nursing is the answer—Love, and compassion, the ethic of Caritas, a new planetary caring and citizenship that honors the sacredness of planetary life for humans and all species on the planet.

Section IX: Emerging Inquiry: The Evolution of a Science

The chapters written for this section focus on advancing disciplinary-specific knowledge grounded in a relational unitary worldview within the context of Unitary Caring Science. In Chapter 37, "Unitary Caring Science Inquiry," Drs. Marian C. Turkel, Joseph Giovanni, and Jean Watson advance definitions of Unitary Caring Science, and expand the field of inquiry and the discussion related to what counts as knowledge within the Unitary Caring Science paradigm. Calling the Circle of Reflection, Videography and Photography, and Metaphysical and Non-Physical Inquiry are presented as forms of creative scholarly inquiry to advance, inform, and transform unitary Caring Science knowledge. In Chapter 38, "Unitary Caring Science and Multicultural Perspectives," Dr. Joyce B. Perkins addresses Unitary Caring Science through the lens of holistic healing and the multicultural perspectives of ancient traditions and indigenous culture. She presents an extensive description of Unitary Caring Science from the perspective of the Unitary/Transformative Paradigm and the scholarly writings of Rogers, Parse, Leininger, and Watson and integrates concepts from complexity science into the chapter. In Chapter 39, "Unitary Caring Science: Evolving Society Toward Health, Healing and Humanity," Dr. Jean Watson, Dr. Sara Horton-Deutsch, and William Rosa frame the discourse on Unitary Caring Science as an expanded worldview where all are connected to include the convergence of activism, caring economics, global human service, human rights, and social justice and reform. They invite us to return to our core values of caring, compassion, and LOVE, and to use Unitary Caring Science to guide moral actions toward health and healing to preserve humanity and planet Earth.

Section X: Journeys Into the Transpersonal: Aesthetic Ways of Knowing

The chapters written for this section focus on how Caring Science can become a journey of personal and professional transformation engaging in aesthetic ways of knowing. In Chapter 40, "Caritas Coaching: The Future of Health and Well-Being," Dr. Jan Anderson explores Caritas Coaching as a way to preserve dignity and to integrate Caring Literacy into transpersonal relationships honoring and finding purpose and meaning in persons' lives. In Chapter 41, "Creative Health Arts," Dr. Mary Rockwood Lane uses her personal traumatic experience to reflect on the healing aspects of art as caring-healing creative practices exploring the lived experiences. Her beautiful art and guided imagery provide a living portrait of how the Caritas Processes support the practice of art as a way of caring and healing. In Chapter 42, "Narrative Healing," Dr. A. Lynne Wagner explores the power of reflective practice through four lenses of storytelling/listening: (a) Knowing self through self-story, (b) knowing other through other's story, (c) honoring connected humanity through shared- connected story, and (d) discovering new possibilities through expanded story. In Chapter 43, "The Power of Ritual in Nurses' Everyday Lives: Personal and Professional Exemplars," Dr. Zane Robinson Wolf uses nursing literature and nursing experience to explore exemplars of both personal and professional rituals performed by professional nurses as reflective practice. In Chapter 44, "Photovoice: Qualitative Research Strategy for Theory-Guided Nursing Practice," Dr. Gayle L. Casterline describes the qualitative methodology of photovoice and its value to human Caring Science and theory-guided nursing practice. Using her professional experience integrating photovoice as a transformative educational strategy, Dr. Casterline provides us with an innovative way to create a caring learning environment providing students with a meaningful learning experience and enhancing the science of nursing practice. In Chapter 45, "Music and Poetry for Healing," Patrick Dean explores the intersection between music and poetry and Caring Science as essential artistic and scientific means of human healing. In Chapter 46, "The Interplay of Integrative Nursing, Caring Science, and Healing Environments," Mary Jo Kreitzer and Terri Zborowsky provide us with a road map to understand the six principles of integrative nursing through the lenses of Caring Science and the role of nurses in cocreating and promoting a caring, healing environment for self and others. In Chapter 47, "Remembering Purpose: An Autoethnography," Anna Biley reflects on how her professional experience studying Caring Science provided her the strategies she needed while caring for her terminally ill husband, Dr. Francis Christopher Biley, and ultimately how her personal experience provided a catalyst for her graduate research and informed her choice of autoethnography as an innovative Caring Science methodology to give meaning to her lived experienced and personal transformation. In Chapter 48, "Caring Science and Yoga: The Human Caring Science Kosha Model," Andy Davies shares his personal and professional journey integrating Watson's Human Caring Science with a Yoga Model to develop an educational experience for first year Bachelor of Nursing students in Australia providing a framework to evolve nursing consciousness within the context of human life complexity. In Chapter 49, "The Embodiment of a Caring Nature," William Rosa provides a personal reflection of what it means to fully embody a caring nature in our personal and professional lives. Through thought-provoking questions, he invites readers to reflect on what it means to be the embodiment of a caring nature and reminds us that this way of being requires fortitude and commitment.

ONWARD

Jeanne Anselmo's conclusion by way of meditation helps readers to breathe in and assimilate this Caring Science Handbook with integrity and reflection. Drs. Rozazano C. Locsin, Marguerite Purnell, and Hirokazu Ito's "Bridge to the Future" prepares us to embrace and live caring in the ecosystem of artificial intelligence. Appendix A provides several tools for Caring Science Measurement and Research from Caring Science pioneers Drs. Marilyn A. Ray, Marian C. Turkel, John Nelson, and Jean Watson. Appendix B offers a small sampling of abstracts by graduates of the CCEP to assist leaders and practitioners in developing Caring Science interventions to promote healing in their professional settings. Finally, Appendix C offers a reference list, to date, of the available Caring Science literature as a source and guide for ongoing Caring Science scholarship.

The editors of this Handbook wish you, the reader, peace and caring on your journey. We hope this collection of Caring Science thought and passion will impact your life and work with the caring-healing intentions it carries.

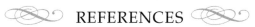 REFERENCES

Alligood, M. (2018). *Nursing theorists and their work* (9th ed.). St. Louis, MO: Elsevier.

Benner, P., Tanner, C., & Chesla, C. (1996). *Expertise in nursing practice: Caring, clinical judgment and ethics*. New York, NY: Springer Publishing.

Coffman, S. (2014). Marilyn Anne Ray's theory of bureaucratic caring. In M. R. Alligood (Ed.), *Nursing theorists and their work* (8th ed., pp. 98–119). St. Louis, MO: Mosby/Elsevier.

Coffman, S. (2018). Marilyn Anne Ray's theory of bureaucratic caring. In M. R. Alligood (Ed.), *Nursing theorists and their work* (9th ed., pp. 80–97). St. Louis, MO: Elsevier.

Delmar, C., & Johns, C. (Eds.). (2008). *The good, the wise and the right clinical nursing practice*. Aalborg, Denmark: Aalborg Hospital, Arhus University Hospital.

Eriksson, K. (2006). *The suffering human being* (C. Peterson & J. Zetterlund, Eds.; K. Olsson & C. Peterson, Trans.). Chicago, IL: Nordic Studies Press.

Glaser, B. G. (1992). *Basics of grounded theory analysis*. Mill Valley, CA: Sociology Press.

Glaser, B. G., & Strauss, A. L. (1967). *The discovery of grounded theory: Strategies for qualitative research*. Chicago, IL: Aldine.

Leininger, M. (1970). *Nursing and anthropology: Two worlds to blend*. New York, NY: John Wiley & Sons.

Leininger, M. (1977). The phenomenon of caring. Part v. caring: The essence and central focus of nursing. *Nursing Research Report, 12*(1), 2, 14.

Leininger, M. (1978). *Transcultural nursing: Concepts, theories and practices*. New York, NY: John Wiley & Sons.

Leininger, M. (1979). *Transcultural nursing*. New York, NY: Masson.

Leininger, M. (Ed.). (1981). *Caring: An essential human need*. Thorofare, NJ: Charles B. Slack.

Leininger, M. (Ed.). (1991). *Culture care diversity and universality: A theory of nursing*. New York, NY: National League for Nursing Press.

Martinsen, K. (2006). *Care and vulnerability*. Oslo, Norway: Akribe.

Morse, J. M., Stern, P. N., Corbin, J., Bowers, B., Charmaz, L., & Clarke, A. (2009). *Grounded theory: The second generation.* Walnut Creek, CA: Left Coast Press.

Ray, M. A. (1981a). A philosophical analysis of caring within nursing. In M. Leininger (Ed.), *Caring: An essential human need* (pp. 25–36). Thorofare, NJ: Charles B. Slack.

Ray, M. A. (1981b). *A study of caring within the institutional culture.* Doctor of Philosophy, University of Utah, Salt Lake City. *Dissertation Abstracts International, 42*(06) (University Microfilms No. 8127787).

Ray, M. A. (1984). The development of a nursing classification system of caring. In M. Leininger (Ed.), *Care: The essence of nursing and health* (pp. 93–112). Thorofare, NJ: Charles B. Slack.

Ray, M. A. (1989). The theory of bureaucratic caring for nursing practice in the organizational culture. *Nursing Administration Quarterly, 13*(2), 31–42. doi:10.1097/00006216-198901320-00007

Ray, M. A. (2010a). *A study of caring within an institutional culture: The discovery of the theory of bureaucratic caring.* Saarbrüken, Germany: Lambert Academic.

Ray, M. A. (2010b). *Transcultural caring dynamics in nursing and health care.* Philadelphia, PA: F. A. Davis.

Ray, M. A. (2016). *Transcultural caring dynamics in nursing and health care* (2nd ed.). Philadelphia, PA: F. A. Davis.

Ray, M. A., Morris, E . & McFarland, M. (2013). Leininger's Ethnonursing Method. In C. T. Beck (Ed.), *The Routledge international handbook of qualitative nursing research.* New York, NY: Routledge.

Ray, M. A., & Turkel, M. C. (2001). Federal nursing service award. Impact of TRICARE/managed care on total force readiness. *Military Medicine, 166*(4), 281–289. doi:10.1093/milmed/166.4.281

Ray, M. A., & Turkel, M. C. (2012). A transtheoretical evolution of caring science within complex systems. *International Journal for Human Caring, 16*(2), 28–49.

Ray, M. A., & Turkel, M. C. (2014). Caring as emancipatory nursing praxis: The theory of relational caring complexity. *Advances in Nursing Science, 37*(2), 137–146. doi:10.1097/ANS.0000000000000024

Ray, M. A., & Turkel, M. C. (2015). The theory of bureaucratic caring. In M. Smith & M. E. Parker (Eds.), *Nursing theories and nursing practice* (4th ed., pp. 461–482). Philadelphia, PA: F. A. Davis.

Sitzman, K., & Watson, J. (2014). *Caring science, mindful practice.* New York, NY: Springer Publishing.

Sitzman, K., & Watson, J. (2017). *Watson's caring in the digital world.* New York, NY: Springer Publishing.

Smith, M. (2014). Disciplinary perspectives linked to middle range theory. In M. J. Smith & P. Liehr (Eds.), *Middle range theory for nursing* (3rd ed., pp. 3–14). New York, NY: Springer Publishing.

Smith, M., & Parker, M. (Eds.). (2015). *Nursing theories and nursing practice* (4th ed.). Philadelphia, PA: F. A. Davis.

Turkel, M. A. (2007). An overview of the theory of bureaucratic caring. *International Journal for Human Caring, 11*(4), 57–67.

Turkel, M. C., & Ray, M. A. (2000). Relational complexity: A theory of the nurse-patient relationship within an economic context. *Nursing Science Quarterly, 13*(4), 307–313. doi:10.1177/08943180022107843

Turkel, M. C., & Ray, M. A. (2001). Relational complexity: From grounded theory to instrument development and theoretical testing. *Nursing Science Quarterly, 14*(4), 281–287.

Van Manen, M. (1997). *Researching the lived experience.* Walnut Creek, CA: Left Coast Press.

Van Manen, M. (2014). *Phenomenology of practice: Meaning-giving methods in phenomenological research and writing.* Walnut Creek, CA: Left Coast Press.

Watson, J. (1979). *Nursing: The philosophy and science of caring.* Boston, MA: Little, Brown.

Watson, J. (n.d.). 10 Caritas processes. Retrieved from http://www.watsoncaringscience.org/jean-bio/caring-science-theory/10-caritas-processes

I

The Disciplinary Discourse: Theories and Frameworks Evolving to Unitary Caring Science

2

Unitary Caring Science: Disciplinary Evolution of Nursing

Jean Watson, Marlaine C. Smith, and W. Richard Cowling, III

CARITAS LITERACIES

By the end of this chapter, the caring-healing nurse will be able to

1. Describe the elements of the foundational cosmology of a unitary-transformative worldview.

2. Analyze the ontological foundations of Unitary Caring Science within nursing.

3. Explain the meaning of metaphysics as a branch of philosophy relevant to study for Unitary Caring Science.

4. Appreciate the relevance of Unitary Caring Science as a reflection of the maturation of the discipline of nursing.

5. Envision the future of the discipline and profession informed by the philosophical foundations of Unitary Caring Science.

In this chapter, we elaborate the philosophical foundations of science, and the relevance of its metaphysical, cosmological, and ontological elements to the evolution of a Unitary Caring Science. Metaphysics is a branch of philosophy that addresses meaning regarding the fundamental nature of reality and Being going beyond the physical. Metaphysics is often understood only in terms of addressing the realm beyond the physical without appreciating metaphysics as the starting point for understanding and grasping what is real, what is the fundamental nature of Being, and of reality itself.

Cosmology and ontology are subsumed under the umbrella of metaphysics. Cosmology is the branch of metaphysics that addresses the nature of the universe, whereas ontology is the branch of metaphysics that studies the nature of being, becoming, existence, and reality. Ontology provides perspectives on the nature of being-in-relationship and often deals with questions concerning what entities exist or are proposed to exist. Ontology as a philosophical enterprise has both theoretical and practical applications. The ontological foundation of nursing provides an explication of the nature of the specific phenomena of concern to the discipline of nursing. So, although a particular cosmology informs the human-universe worldview of Unitary Caring Science, ontology informs the understanding of nursing phenomena such as human being-belonging in the world, health, and healing and caring.

Therefore, the starting point for understanding philosophy of science is to understand that theory and inquiry, the components of science, are shaped by varying philosophies (Lather, 2007), and the metaphysical starting point of an "ontology of Being and reality" is relevant for Unitary Caring Science and the discipline of nursing. The reflections and understandings offered in this chapter illuminate the philosophical–metaphysical foundations of a Unitary Caring Science, revealing how paradigms of science can be critiqued in relation to their metaphysical philosophical grounding. We believe that embracing and applying Unitary Caring Science for the betterment of humankind requires an appreciative immersion into its core philosophical underpinnings.

The meaning of science is not the same in all paradigms in terms of ethics, ontology, epistemology, methodology, and praxeology (Lather, 2007, p. 164). For example, the dominant worldview or ontology of medical science is grounded in an unstated definition of metaphysics: that the nature of reality is made up of parts and separate entities. This metaphysics of parts-thinking intersects with some of the early theoretical developments in nursing, prior to the emergence of a unitary worldview. With nursing's historical grounding of human-environment connectedness originating with Nightingale and followed by Rogers's (1970, 1992) introduction of the Science of Unitary Human Beings (SUHB), a revolutionary perspective redefined the nature of reality as unitary-versus-particulate or even integrative. This shift generated more and more discourse in nursing that challenged the predominance of the particulate-reductionistic view. Theoretical thinking in nursing has shifted to embrace the metaphysics of a unitary ontology, creating a greater understanding of the phenomena of whole human health and healing in which caring is recognized as more than just physical. With the advent of this conceptual thinking of wholeness, nursing's ontological shift moved toward a greater acknowledgment of human wholeness in nursing as incompatible with a reduction of persons to the sum of their parts.

Finally, in this chapter, we affirm a perspective on the disciplinary foundations of nursing that once and for all places Caring within the metaparadigm of nursing and invites the conceptualization of Unitary Caring Science as a reflection of a maturing discipline. We describe caring theories within the unitary-transformative paradigm and offer a conceptual synthesis of philosophies grounding Unitary Caring Science with implications for praxis and inquiry in the discipline of nursing.

With a metaphysical unitary ontological grounding for the discipline of nursing, we are committed to nurses practicing from the philosophical, theoretical, and scientific framework for the betterment of humankind. We fully embrace the ideals of freedom and the liberating power of education, knowledge, evolving consciousness, voice, and language.

Knowledge is power when nurses can articulate, inquire, and practice with disciplinary clarity stemming from their philosophical foundation in service to humankind.

Nursing's disciplinary embodiment of the full meaning of the philosophy of metaphysics as its foundation affirms the alchemy and majesty of human caring in evolving health and healing within well-becoming (Phillips, 2017), thereby embracing a unitary worldview or ontology. This means nursing education, research, and practice are aligned philosophically, ethically, theoretically, and scientifically with the phenomena of unitary wholeness and human caring.

BACKGROUND OF THE DISCOURSE

For several decades, scholarly works in nursing have described the convergence between two historically parallel, nonintersecting developments within the discipline: The SUHB (Rogers, 1970, 1992) and Caring Science (CS; Smith, 1999; Watson, 1979, 1985, 2008, 2012). This contemporary convergence emerged following critiques of the original, dominant disciplinary metaparadigm posed by Fawcett (1984) of Person–Environment–Health–Nursing. Nursing scholars (Conway, 1985; Cowling, Smith, & Watson, 2008; Newman, Sime, & Corcoran-Perry, 1991; Newman, Smith, Pharris, & Jones, 2008; Smith, 1994, 1999; Stephenson & Tripp-Reimer, 1990; Watson & Smith, 2002) have asserted that Caring is the fourth metaparadigm concept, replacing Nursing. We agree that Caring belongs in the nursing metaparadigm. Nursing is the study of human-environment health and healing through caring (Smith, 1994) or caring in the human health experience (Newman et al., 1991). These definitions reflect nursing's disciplinary focus on human wholeness, the significance of person-environment relationships to health, healing, well-becoming (Phillips, 2017), human betterment, and the centrality of caring to the health-healing process and experience. Nursing's ethical–moral covenant with humanity includes human caring and all the vicissitudes of wholeness, consciousness, and the human health and healing experience.

In 1991, Newman, Sime, and Corcoran-Perry identified three paradigms in the discipline of nursing, each with disparate ontologies about the nature of personhood, human-universe connectedness, health, and caring. These authors posited that through the lens of the unitary-transformative paradigm, human beings are viewed as whole and irreducible, continuously evolving with the environment through mutual patterning. Health is a dynamic process, rather than a state, perhaps, best articulated as "healing" or subjectively defined well-being, or what Phillips (2017) named, well-becoming. Newman et al. (1991) stated that caring is more difficult to characterize in the unitary-transformative paradigm, but might be understood as "synchrony and mutuality of nurse-client encounters that transcend time and space limitations of a present situation" (p. 6). The unitary-transformative paradigm has a distinctive ontology, epistemology, and ethic that inform an approach to science. Indeed, Whitehead (1953) indicated that all science starts with ontological assumptions. In the conventional science framework, the ontology is one of separation, in contrast to the nursing ontology of unity—of relation—which unites the SUHB as well as CS.

Levinas's (1969) philosophy of science asserted that "ethics comes before ontology" by acknowledging the "Ethic of Belonging" (to an infinite field of Cosmic Love) as the first principle and starting point for true science. These ethical philosophies of science place unitary science and CS within the same philosophical paradigm; this signifies a reality of both definitions of metaphysics: physical and nonphysical phenomena. This is a reality where wholeness is a given within a reality of universal infinity—all converging with an ethic and ontology of belonging. This evolution invites a metaphysical context as a deeper exploration of underlying caring theories, philosophy, ontology, and worldview. So we ask the reader to consider a starting point that is philosophical and goes beyond the physical, which may be unfamiliar to conventional scientific thinking. This is essential because the starting point will dictate where you will likely end up. If you seek to understand the human being as a whole, unitary being, fully connected and evolving with the infinite field of universal consciousness, and your starting point is static physicality of Western science, you cannot get there. In other words, if your orientation to humanity begins with only physical existence, you are limited in what can be understood or explained, and in danger of reducing humanity to the moral status of an object. R.D. Laing reminded us, "it is like trying to make ice by boiling water" (Laing, 1965, p. 24).

This chapter is not the first time that an analysis of the philosophical metaphysics of a group of nursing theories, considered more or less "unitary," has been conducted. In 1987, Barbara Sarter examined the philosophical/theoretical systems underpinning of Rogers's SUHB, Parse's theory of Human Becoming, Newman's Theory of Expanding Consciousness, and Watson's Transpersonal Caring Science. At the conclusion of her analysis, she identified five themes that constituted the development of a shared distinctive worldview: (a) an evolutionary process that portends constant change and transcendence, (b) health as evolution or transcendence, (c) open systems, (d) nonlinear space-time, and (e) pattern. Sarter (1988) concluded, "these themes together form a potentially powerful … metaphysical and epistemological foundation for the further development of a variety of nursing theories" (p. 58). She implied an emergent science with the potential for a coherent worldview from which other theories might merge—a Unitary Caring Science.

Another article (Cowling et al., 2008) was structured as a dialogue focused on the ontological convergence among several nursing theories. In that article, we reflected on the evolution of the discipline and how recent transtheoretical discourse revealed wholeness, consciousness, and caring as emergent concepts that were forming a Unitary Caring Science, at that time unnamed as such. The authors recognized this convergence in Transpersonal Caring science (Watson, 1985, 1999/2006, 2008, 2012; Watson & Smith, 2002), the SUHB (Rogers, 1988, 1992, 1994), and Health As Expanding Consciousness (Newman, 1997, 2002, 2003; Smith, 1999). The expanded discourse of this chapter returns us to this starting point—a reality that includes physical and nonphysical phenomena, a reality where wholeness is a given, and a reality of universal infinity—all converging with an ethic and ontology of belonging.

COSMOLOGY OF UNITARY CARING SCIENCE

As we return to this starting point, we begin with an elaboration of the cosmology of Unitary Caring Science. The term "cosmology" is used to reflect the nature of the entire universe, not just phenomena central to nursing. The cosmology of Unitary Caring Science is a portrait of the universe and human participation in it that emerges from the unitary-transformative worldview. There are five common elements to this cosmology: (a) interconnectedness and undivided wholeness, (b) eternal here and now, (c) evolutionary and participatory nature of change, (d) paradox, and (e) love.

INTERCONNECTEDNESS AND UNDIVIDED WHOLENESS

The cosmology of the unitary worldview is one of interconnectedness and undivided wholeness. "Unitary" refers to the view that humans and the environment are irreducible and integral. It is based on the assumption of a universe composed of contiguous, interpenetrating energy fields. Rogers (1992) states, "The energy field is the fundamental unit of the living and non-living" (p. 29). The universe consists of indivisible fields within fields, all vibrating. These energy fields have no boundaries; by their nature they are open, flowing, and continuously changing. Without boundaries and extending to infinity, fields are interconnected. This means that everything in the universe is interconnected; it is one whole. Each individual field as well is coextensive with the entire universe (Rogers, 1992). The universe is composed of "open energy systems constantly interacting and evolving with each other" (Newman, 1994).

This cosmology is supported by the ideas in both quantum physics and Eastern philosophies. McTaggart (2002) chronicles the scientific findings initiated by quantum physics in the 20th century and examines their implications in many areas of human life. She says,

> The world of the separate should have been laid waste once and for all by the discovery of quantum physics … in the early part of the twentieth century. Physicists peered into the heart of matter and were astounded by what they saw. The tiniest bits of matter weren't even matter. (p. 15)

McTaggart (2002) goes on to state,

> And even stranger, subatomic particles had no meaning in isolation, but only in relationship with everything else … Matter … was completely indivisible. You could only understand the universe as a dynamic web of interconnection. (p. 15)

Physicist-philosopher Bohm (1980) purported that the universe is an undivided whole composed of two orders: the implicate and explicate. The "implicate" is the primary order, the vast sea of pulsating and patterned energy that is not normally seen, felt, heard, or otherwise accessed through our more familiar five senses. This "metaphysical ground of being is a multidimensional pattern, unseen, yet generating, the visible world" (Sarter, 1988, p. 55). The implicate order precipitates the "explicate" order, which is accessible to us through the five senses. Bohm gives us a framework that corresponds to our experience of living in a three-dimensional, linear, often predictable world, even though we know that the underlying implicate order is vastly different.

Some scientists scoff, firmly believing it is not possible to apply quantum mechanics (the behavior of subatomic particles) outside that realm of subatomic particles, but others disagree. The role of human consciousness in mediating change has been studied extensively. The Copenhagen interpretation (named after Niels Bohr who lived there) is one of the most mysterious aspects of quantum theory, and according to this theory,

> an electron doesn't exist as an entity, but exists as a potential or the sum of all probabilities until someone measures or observes it, at which point the electron freezes into

a particular state. Once there is no observation occurring the electron goes back to its sea of possibilities. (Bohr, 1913; McTaggart, 2002, p. 102)

Human consciousness collapses wave functions or brings from this range of possibilities one possibility that emerges. The "observer phenomenon" suggests that reality emerges from a primordial soup or field with the involvement of living consciousness (McTaggart, p. 104). This happens through coherence of consciousness, the ability to come into resonant relationship with another field of consciousness, "This coherence may help to shape and create order … on the most profound level … reality is co-created by each of us only by our attention." (McTaggart, p. 122)

Eastern mysticism offers a similar cosmology. Watson (1985, 1999/2006, 2008) arrived at the assumptions of this cosmology from her grounding in these spiritual traditions. For example, in Hinduism, Maya is the illusion of mistaking shapes, structures, things, and events as reality (Capra, 1975, p. 88). Buddhist thought has as a central theme the unity and the interrelation of all things and events (Capra, 1975, p. 88). This unitary cosmology from Eastern mysticism and quantum physics has raised the awareness of mainstream thinking through popular books such as *The Dancing Wu I Master* (Zukav, 1979, 2013) and *The Tao of Physics* (Capra, 1975, 2013). In nursing, we see evidence of this mindset in the text and teachings of *Quantum Leadership* (Porter O'Grady & Malloch, 2011, 2015, 2018) and quantum-caring consciousness (Watson, 1999/2006). More broadly, we see the quantum cosmological perspective of oneness evident at the environmental-planetary level, with climate changes and threats to the survival of all species, including the human species (Gore, 2006, 2007; Watson, 2014).

The evolution of an awakening Consciousness of oneness is prominent in Unitary Caring Science. Consciousness is the information capacity of the field (Newman, 1986/1994) or the embedded intelligence/wisdom of the field. Fields are interconnected, so all knowledge of the universe or Absolute Consciousness is encoded or patterned into any field. The entire universe is conscious, and there are differences in the ability to respond to, be aware of, or access the encoded information; therefore, fields exhibit a range of consciousness. As consciousness expands, there is a growing awareness of the interconnectedness and oneness of All. There is an expanded ability to take in a broader range of information, to access more fully the true nature of the universe, open to appreciate the wholeness and interconnectedness of All There Is. It is like having a more sensitive receiver able to access a broader band of frequencies that are always available (McTaggart, 2002).

ETERNAL HERE AND NOW

Linear conceptions of time and space are not consistent with a cosmology underpinning Unitary Caring Science. In the SUHB (Rogers, 1988, 1992, 1994), the postulate of pandimensionality reflects this quality and is defined as "a non-linear domain without spatial or temporal attributes" (Rogers, 1992, p. 29). In a unitary cosmology, "absolute space-time is rejected and replaced by a multidimensional web in which patterns unfold" (Sarter, 1988, p. 57). Parse (1998) states, "The human-universe mutual process is lived relatively at many realms of the universe …. Space and time are unbounded and non-sequential. The structure of space-time is related to the flow of patterns of interconnections of all that is in the universe" (p. 52). According to Bohm (1980), the implicate order is omnipresent.

Watson and Smith (2002) described a cosmology not confined by objective space-time with the universal field of consciousness connected with Infinity (p. 459). In the unitary universe, there is no time or space as we know it. Everything is in the present, the here, and now. Similarly, Whitehead's (1953) philosophy discussed the eternal now, whereby the past, present, and future are present in a given moment, transcending time, space, and physicality, thus transpersonal, with unbounded connections to all in the moment (Watson, 1985, 1999/2006, 2008, 2012).

EVOLUTIONARY AND PARTICIPATORY NATURE OF CHANGE

In a unitary cosmology, the nature of change is participatory and evolutionary. Rogers described change as continuous, innovative, and unpredictable, qualities reflecting an open-system view of the universe (Rogers, 1992). Because of this continuous, mutual patterning, there is always uncertainty. In a universe of interconnectedness, predictability is not possible. Vibrating, contiguous fields are unpredictable in their interactions. Change in this conscious Universe is unfolding increasingly more complex and diverse patterning. The principles of helicy and resonancy offer descriptions of change as creative, with continuous change with lower to higher frequency wave patterns (Rogers, 1970, pp. 5–7). According to Rogers (1992), "This evolutionary change emerges from non-equilibrium and exhibits punctualism, not gradualism" (p. 32). The imbalances or disruptions in the field shift it to the next level or order. Newman (1994) states, "Evolution thrives on tension. … The disequilibrium is important in maintaining active exchangement with the environment, and active exchangement with the environment is essential for growth. New order appears when a giant fluctuation becomes stabilized by exchange of energy with the environment" (p. 21). Newman (1994) also states, "A critical event creates a giant fluctuation which propels disorganized unpredictable fluctuation to a higher level of organization" (p. 36).

Evolution is a process of expanding consciousness, and change is shaped by greater connection to Absolute Consciousness or the Source or Cosmic Universal Love (Levinas, 1969) with the integration of more complex information. Newman (1994) helps us reconcile the paradox of change in the timeless, eternal present, "Change is not linear; it is transformational and occurs all-at-once. … Consciousness shifts the field, and this morphic resonance manifests change without temporo-spatial connection" (Newman, 1994, p. 82). Evolution is about the movement from potential to actual, the unfolding of possibility. Parse (1998) describes this process of becoming as transcending multidimensionally with the possibles. Watson (1999/2006) discusses the evolution of the universe toward higher consciousness. She draws on Teilhard de Chardin's (1955) notions of evolving toward the omega point or union with the Divine, the Source, or Absolute Consciousness, Cosmic Universal Love.

PARADOX

A Unitary Caring Science cosmology is full of contradictions that are irreconcilable, so paradox is another of its dimensions. The universe manifests qualities that are apparent opposites but reflect the nature of the whole. Both sides and opposites are reflections of this more comprehensive whole. Eastern cosmologies such as Taoism have this embedded in their teachings of the yin and yang—opposite qualities contained in the whole. In a unitary cosmology, we are confronted with the paradox of subatomic particles being both wave and particle-matter simultaneously. We must reconcile a universe of the eternal now, yet we discuss change and evolution within it. How can this happen without time? Moreover, how do we understand atemporality when we experience time passing and witness its effects. Similarly, is it possible to account for nonlocal events like morphic resonance (Sheldrake, 1983) when we know we experience moving and acting in three-dimensional space? Causality cannot exist in a universe of open systems, and yet we rely on its assumptions each day as we live our lives. All this might be explained by Bohm's (1980) theory of one universe with both implicate and explicate orders. Newman (1994) states that all opposites are reconciled with Absolute Consciousness (p. 48). So in this cosmology, we dwell in the mysteries presented by paradox, trusting that within the larger infinite field of unity they are reconciled.

Love

The final common foundation in the cosmology of Unitary Caring Science is love, meaning unconditional love or agape. In all we know so far from the foundations of this cosmology, we can deduce that there are patterns reflected in the consciousness of the field, its information coding. The consciousness of love has a particular quality. This quality produces the most coherence or what is called "superradiance" (McTaggart, 2002, p. 93). "Coherence" is defined as the capacity to come into meaningful relationship. Absolute Consciousness is equated with Love (Newman, 1986/1994).

Watson (1985, 2008) places love or caring at the center of her cosmology. For her, love is primary. "Care and love are the most universal, the most tremendous and mysterious of cosmic forces" (Watson, 1985, p. 50). For Watson, Absolute Consciousness and love as the universal Force precede being-in-the-world. It is first order; the universe is loved into existence. Levinas's (1969) philosophy and ethic of belonging are tied to the unity of Cosmic Universal Love. Before existence there is love; after existence, there is love. Watson (2003) says, "love is originary. … being for the other precedes being with the other" (p. 201). Love, then, becomes a powerful force for existence, creativity, transformation. If love is the attribute of Absolute Consciousness, then abiding in it is transformative, and creates the coherence of consciousness to experience ultimate relationship, alignment, and awareness of All-There-Is, "humanity is ultimately floating in, trusting in … the energy (or Consciousness) of Cosmic love" (Watson, 2002, p. 202).

Summary Points: Unitary Views of Science Within the Cosmology and Metaphysics of Science

The most recent summary of the convergence of unitary views of science within the cosmological-metaphysical context is perhaps best summarized by Phillips (2017) in his description of emerging scientific knowledge which he labels "Selected Views of Science" (p. 223).

- Everything manifests wave frequencies, vibrations, resonances of patterns, and fields.

- The human body manifests wave frequencies and diversity.

- Spirit and soul are of the universe and are integral.

- Time and space do not exist in a unitary, integral universe.

- The universe manifests consciousness/awareness.

- The universe manifests thought information and knowledge.

- The universe has a process of communication, and communication can be nonlocal.

- Humans have a mind that is not confined to the brain.

- Humans are holoids of a holographic universe.

THEORIES AND FRAMEWORKS EVOLVING WITHIN UNITARY CARING SCIENCE

Moving from metaphysics, cosmology, and philosophy of science within a unitary perspective, we enter theories and the evolution of theories and frameworks within this articulated broader view of science. Theories and philosophies of science are what frame disciplinary knowledge; they transcend specific events and seek to provide universal explanations that can reflect the ethical–ontological–philosophical foundation and values for the entire field of study (Reed & Shearer, 2011).

Likewise, nursing theories contain underlying ontological–philosophical–ethical assumptions, knowledge, and values that explicate what it means: to be human; to engage in human caring, healing, and health experiences; and to be connected with the environment and the universe. For example, different ontologies of unitary versus particulate/separatist worldviews have existed in the evolution of nursing and CS. The unitary-transformative paradigm is required for the maturing of the discipline of nursing to address fully the phenomena of the wholeness of human-environment, health healing, and caring.

THEORY OF UNITARY CARING

The meaning of caring can be shaped by its framing within various theoretical perspectives. Smith (1999) sought to situate the meaning of caring within the SUHB. She analyzed the caring literature for meanings that were consistent with a unitary worldview and then analyzed the literature within the SUHB, identifying concepts that reflected the meaning of caring. Through this process, five constitutive meanings of caring were uncovered: manifesting intention, appreciating pattern, attuning to dynamic flow, experiencing the Infinite, and inviting creative emergence. The work evolved into a middle-range Theory of Unitary Caring (Smith, 2010, 2015). This theory development explicitly situated caring within the unitary worldview. A summary of the constitutive meaning of the concepts illuminates the meaning of caring from a unitary theoretical perspective:

- *Unitary Caring is manifesting intention*: What we hold in our heart matters (Cowling et al., 2008). Everything is energy. Our pattern of consciousness manifested through our feelings, thoughts, perceptions, attitudes, and values cocreates the evolving, dynamic patterning of the environment. This constitutive meaning suggests that intentions are powerful, so we need to be mindful of what we are bringing with us as we relate to others face to face or virtually. Intentions are nonlocal because of the interconnectedness of all. Caring is being aware of holding intentions for well-being, healing, peace; for enfolding loving kindness and compassion in our hearts; and in trusting that through the quality of this intentional engagement we are participating meaningfully in healing and well-becoming (Smith, 1999, 2010, 2015).

- *Unitary Caring is appreciating pattern*: This concept was appropriated directly from Cowling's (1999, 2000) work. He differentiated the process of "appreciating" from "assessing." Appreciating is apprehending the beauty and complexity of human wholeness with gratitude and awe. Cowling (1999, 2000) suggested, in contrast to a stance of identifying problems or making judgments, that caring is entering into a relationship with the curiosity to come to know the uniqueness of the other (person, family, or community), affirming the humanity/divinity revealed in relationship, and seeing the other as whole and complete in the moment (Smith, 1999, 2010, 2015).

- *Unitary Caring is attuning to dynamic flow*: Rhythmic relating occurs in the caring relationship. There is a sensing of where to place focus and emphasis, what to say, how to move in the between. This sensing of vibration is amplified by finely tuning the heart in connection with the other. It is a phenomenon of resonance or vibrating in synchrony. Caring is the ability to move in concert with the evolving patterning of healing and well-becoming (Phillips, 2017; Smith, 1999, 2010, 2015).

- *Unitary Caring is experiencing the Infinite*: In the intimate, caring relationship, there is a perception of the transcendence of the physical and material world and an expansion of time and space. There is an expanded sense of self, including transcendent awareness. Higher consciousness and evolving patterns of knowing are potentiated. Living caring is surrendering to the enfolding and unfolding mystery of spiritual connectedness and divine love (Smith, 1999, 2010, 2015).

- *Unitary Caring is inviting creative emergence*: Healing is a dynamic process of transformation involving change and growth. Unitary caring is nurturing that growth through exploring and supporting the person's chosen journey; helping the other to articulate what matters most in the moment; identifying strengths and obstacles to change; and mobilizing internal and external resources to support healing and well-becoming (Phillips, 2017). It is bearing witness to suffering and holding space for this transformation to evolve. In unitary caring, there is no prescribed outcome; instead, there is a process of guiding, sojourning with, and tending the birth of healing and well-becoming (Phillips, 2017; Smith, 1999, 2010, 2015).

As nursing continues to advance and mature with the clarity of its disciplinary foundation and these converging caring literacies, we affirm experiences such as "experiencing the Infinite," inviting a deeper philosophical ethic and evolving worldview. This CS as sacred science (Watson, 2005) affirms French philosopher Levinas's (1969) explication that the *"Ethic of Belonging"*—to Infinity of Universal Love—comes before *"Ontology of Separation"*

(Watson, 2005). Levinas's infinity of Love expands and converges with Smith's (1999) concept of Caring as "Experiencing the Infinite" and "Inviting Creative Emergence."

REFLECTING AND REFERENCING METAPHYSICAL AND NONLOCAL REALITIES IN NURSING

Can nursing create a science that makes room for the senses and the soul?
Cowling, 1999, p. 132.

Once we converge cosmology of Unitary Caring Science and themes of human-caring theories with the ethic of belonging and Infinity, we can embrace and invite nonphysical metaphysical phenomena, such as nonlocal consciousness, unknowing, and transcendence; we open to wonder, awe, mystery, miracles, mysticism, spirit, and sacred unknowns, the holy. These nonphysical phenomena, connecting humans with universals of Infinity, occur worldwide, across thousands of years, in human experiences of healing. This evolution of philosophy, science, and theory opens space for a metaphysical worldview embracing, more explicitly, a deeper understanding of spiritual healing.

NONPHYSICAL REALITIES

Until recently, many proponents of the unitary-transformative paradigm had difficulty with reconciling the role of soul/spirit as a phenomenal domain of concern within nursing science. Even recent attention to the significance of human spirituality has its limitations because of conceptualizations of spirit as a belief accompanied by attitudes and behaviors, rather than as an aspect of reality from a metaphysical sense. This denial of the reality of spirit often leads unintentionally to a disregard by nurses for the fullest and richest expression of the human experience when providing care. However, even without the deepest metaphysical and philosophical understandings, we see many nurses embracing and validating spirit with the people for whom they provide care, relying on the credibility of their senses.

WHOLENESS

Nursing's persistent concern has been focused on the wholeness of human experience contextualized in creating conditions for maximal well-being and healing. The context of healing as moving toward wholeness is abandoned in favor of healing as appreciating wholeness (Cowling, 2000). Appreciating wholeness as healing accepts that the nature of life is wholeness revealing itself in experiential patterning in a unity of physical/physiological, mental/emotional, social/cultural, spiritual/mystical phenomena. It is proposed that the well-worn message of "the whole is greater than the sum of the parts" is misleading because, in a world where wholeness is given, there are no parts. Rather, phenomena relegated to a part-conceptualization are expressions of wholeness and are clues to wholeness when looked through the lens of patterning. Newman (2003) proposed that we live in a world of no boundaries and for nursing the focal point is wholeness and suggests that healing is the realization of inherent wholeness in the form of patterning. Watson and Smith (2002) refer to the unitary nature of the universe, which implies wholeness placing caring in a unitary-transformative context.

INFINITY

Moss (1995) refers to a concept called "unitive consciousness" that describes a state of being where people become referent to infinite and experience a realization of their infinite potential and infinite time-space-movement-change—experienced as being "in a great sea of being infinite in all directions" (p. 65). Moss implies that in this state feeling, sensation, and thinking are experienced as not limited by the body where "every moment is a new birth and what is being born is not merely the product of the past, not merely the cause of some earlier effect, but rather part of a ceaseless cosmos of revelation" (p. 66). The metaphysics of a Unitary Caring Science is congruent with and supports this experience of "reality." The empowerment of people encountering the challenges and opportunities of life in health and illness can be accentuated when nurses allow themselves to embrace the ontological potential for healing aligned with the wishes and desires of the people with whom they engage in care. The potential for liberation through empowering infinite potentials in people is done from a perspective of wholeness that considers and contextualizes the social factors and forces of discrimination and inequality that confront us.

BELONGING

The metaphysical notion of a universe of belonging acknowledges the connectedness of all things in implicit and explicitly manifested wholeness. Ontologically speaking, reality is one of belongingness that evokes the participatory nature of all phenomena reflected in a patterning of wholeness. The ethical aspects of a universe of belongingness are obvious but are not evident in much of human relatedness, including medical-health-nursing endeavors and environments. Caring as an expression of belongingness to/with others and the world realized in attitudes, acts, and actualizations of loving kindness signify a living ethic. The ontology of belonging parallels the ontology of the cosmos as participatory, wholeness put forth by Laszlo (1996). He offers a provocative metaphorical image of the "whispering pond" where scientists see nature everywhere acting and evolving as a self-consistent, self-created whole fully integrated and not as a set of interdependent parts. This image evokes the explicit, overarching metaphysics of the unitary nature of the world that forms the foundation of the CS we propose.

Humans participate in the process of change. They do so through their choices manifest in intentions and actions. So the consciousness of the participant is central to what emerges in change. Rogers's (1988, 1992, 1994) principle of helicy purports that humans participate knowingly in the process of change. Newman (1986/1994) states that the movement of evolution is from potential freedom to real freedom. Insight and choice enhance movement from restriction to freedom in the process of expanding consciousness. Watson (1999/2006) refers to quantum theory explaining that there are infinite wave-like possibilities that exist in the field of consciousness waiting to become actualities. "Once we observe them, participate in seeing them with intention, the possible reality may become an actuality. Thus, we participate in co-creating reality, partially through our intentionality" (Watson, 1999, pp. 121, 123).

We honor and recognize the significance of metaphysics in the evolution of Unitary Caring Science as we enter this extended dialogue to explore and illuminate Unitary Caring Science phenomena. Within the metaphysics of Unitary Caring Science, we move beyond the physical domain of physical body care and cure at the material level alone. The body biophysical-machine view of human diagnosis and treatment has been referred to Era I thinking (Dossey, 2004)—highlighting the particulate-deterministic paradigm thinking (Newman et al., 1991). Indeed, Era II thinking, an integrative-interactive paradigm, also is incomplete with respect to perceiving wholeness. The metaphysics of Unitary Caring Science creates a new explanatory ethical, ontological, epistemological, and praxis model to recognize and appreciate the deep healing dimensions of Cosmic Love as the greatest source of all healing, returning us to our shared humanity for an evolved unitary consciousness.

Energy, spirit, evolving unitary, transcendent consciousness is by its nature metaphysical. Here in metaphysics we appreciatively embrace a universe of concepts and phenomena exemplifying Infinity, which has been reported and experienced across time by millions of people. However, until very recently, these universal human experiences have been discarded or dismissed by the dominant Western worldview and Western medicine.

Conventional physical-objective Era I, and even Era II science, have been unable to deal with these so-called "metaphysical phenomena" because they cannot be explained in the so-called medical-physical mindset; indeed, they have been ignored, laughed at, criticized, and even punished. Our conventional physical-objective Western-science ontology of separation has precluded curiosity, interest, and has resisted serious exploring or researching such nonphysical realities. The metaphysics of Unitary Caring Science is in sharp contrast to outdated principles of objective science alone—acknowledging our unitary connection to the higher universal consciousness of Cosmic Love.

We now see a new convergence of unitary views across time and worldviews. For example, in nursing, Rogers (1970, 1992), Newman (1994, 2003), Smith (1994, 1999), Cowling, Smith and Watson (2008) and Watson (2005) are intersecting with the philosophy of Levinas (1969), quantum realities from physics (Plotinsky, 2016), ancient indigenous and Eastern wisdom traditions and teachings, and enlightened views from other medical practitioners and noetic scientists (Dossey, 2004; Radin, 2015; van Lommel, 2011).

UNCONCLUDING POSTSCRIPT

New Openings for Philosophies of Science, Theory, and Knowledge Development

Metaphysics, as a branch of philosophy, acknowledges a Unitary Caring Science cosmology and relational ontological worldview. By further exploration of metaphysics of Unitary Caring-Healing, we open to new explanatory models for spiritual healing phenomena that transcend Western science.

This Unitary Science cosmology has implications for the way that the universe is viewed and has allowance for spirit, miracles, and cosmic Love to enter. When we move to the full definition and meaning of metaphysics as the core philosophy of Unitary Caring Science, we advance the consciousness of all of humanity. In this in-between space, nursing is transcending time, space, and physicality, creating a Unitary Caring universe for sustaining humanity and Mother Earth.

NEXT ERA POSSIBILITIES

Education

- How can we approach teaching and learning within a Unitary Caring Science ontology?
- What is knowing and understanding from a Unitary Caring Science ontology?
- How do we support evolved patterns of knowing in nursing education?

Research

- What research methodologies are consistent with a Unitary Caring Science ontology and epistemology?
- Identify a research question that might be studied from a Unitary Caring Science perspective.

Praxis

- How do Unitary Caring literacies shape nursing praxis?
- Share a story of practice that illustrates a Unitary Caring literacy.

Theory and Knowledge Development

- Describe the emerging metaparadigm or focus of the discipline of nursing.
- What concepts underpin the cosmology of a Unitary Caring Science?
- What existing nursing theories are encompassed within Unitary Caring Science?

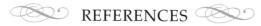 REFERENCES

Bohm, D. (1980). *Wholeness and the implicate order*. London, UK: Routledge & Kegan Paul.

Bohr, N. (1913). *On the quantum theory*. New York, NY: Springer Publishing.

Capra, F. (1975). *The tao of physics: An exploration of the parallels between modern physics and eastern mysticism*. Boston, MA: Shambhala.

Capra, F. (2013). *The tao of physics* (5th ed.). Boston, MA: Shambhala.

Conway, M. E. (1985). Toward greater specificity in defining nursing's metaparadigm. *Advances in Nursing Science*, 7(4), 73–81. doi:10.1097/00012272-198507000-00010

Cowling, W. R., III. (1999). A unitary-transformative nursing science: Potentials for transcending dichotomies. *Nursing Science Quarterly*, 12(2), 132–137. doi:10.1177/08943189922106774

Cowling, W. R., III. (2000). Healing as appreciating wholeness. *Advances in Nursing Science*, 22(3), 16–32. doi:10.1097/00012272-200003000-00003

Cowling, W. R., III, Smith, M. C., & Watson, J. (2008). The power of wholeness, consciousness, and caring: A dialogue on nursing science, art, and healing. *Advances in Nursing Science*, 31(1), E41–E51. doi:10.1097/01.ANS.0000311535.11683.d1 de Chardin, P. T. (1955). *The phenomenon of man.* London, UK: Harper & Row.

Dossey, L. (2004). *One mind.* Carlsbad, CA: Hay House.

Fawcett, J. (1984). The metaparadigm of nursing: Present status and future refinements. *Image the Journal of Nursing Scholarship, 16*(3), 84–89. doi:10.1111/j.1547-5069.1984.tb01393.x

Gore, A. (2006). *An inconvenient truth: The planetary emergency of global warming.* New York, NY: Viking Books.

Gore, A. (2007). *An inconvenient truth: The crisis of global warming.* New York, NY: Viking Books.

Laing, R. D. (1965). *The divided self: An existential study in sanity and madness.* London, UK: Penguin Books.

Laszlo, E. (1996). *The whispering pond: A personal guide to the emerging vision of science.* Rockport, MA: Element Books.

Lather, P. (2007). *Getting lost: Feminist efforts toward a double(d) science.* Albany, NY: SUNY Press.

Levinas, E. (1969). *Totality and infinity.* Pittsburgh, PA: Duquesne University.

Malloch, K., & Porter-O'Grady, T. (2010). *The quantum leader: Applications for the new world of work.* Boston, MA: Jones & Bartlett.

McTaggart, L. (2002). *The field: The quest for the secret force of the universe.* New York, NY: HarperCollins.

Moss, R. M. (1995). *The second miracle: Intimacy, spirituality, and consciousness relationships.* Berkeley, CA: Celestial Arts.

Newman, M. A. (1994). *Health as expanding consciousness* (2nd ed.). New York, NY: National League for Nursing. (Original work published 1986)

Newman, M. A. (1997). Experiencing the whole. *Advances in Nursing Science, 20*(1), 34–39. doi:10.1097/00012272-199709000-00006

Newman, M. A. (2002). The pattern that connects. *Advances in Nursing Science, 24*(3), 1–7. doi:10.1097/00012272-200203000-00003

Newman, M. A. (2003). A world of no boundaries. *Advances in Nursing Science, 26*(4), 240–245. doi:10.1097/00012272-200310000-00002

Newman, M. A., Sime, A. M., & Corcoran-Perry, S. A. (1991). The focus of the discipline of nursing. *Advances in Nursing Science, 14,* 1–6. doi:10.1097/00012272-199109000-00002

Newman, M. A., Smith, M. C., Pharris, M. D., & Jones, D. (2008). The focus of the discipline revisited. *Advances in Nursing Science, 31*(1), E16–E27. doi:10.1097/01.ANS.0000311533.65941.f1

Parse, R. R. (1998). *Human becoming school of thought: A perspective for nurses and other health professionals.* Thousand Oaks, CA: Sage.

Phillips, J. R. (2017). New Rogerian theoretical thinking about unitary science. *Nursing Science Quarterly, 30*(3), 223–226. doi:10.1177/0894318417708411

Porter-O'Grady, T., & Malloch, K. (2011). *Quantum leadership: Advancing innovation, transforming health care* (3rd ed.). Burlington, MA: Jones & Bartlett.

Porter-O'Grady, T., & Malloch, K. (2015). *Quantum leadership: Building better partnerships for sustainable health* (4th ed.). Burlington, MA: Jones & Bartlett.

Porter-O'Grady, T., & Malloch, K. (2018). *Quantum leadership: Creating sustainable value in health care* (5th ed.). Burlington, MA: Jones & Bartlett.

Radin, D. (2015). Meditation and the nonlocal mind. *Explore: The Journal of Science and Healing, 11*(2), 82–84. doi:10.1016/j.explore.2014.12.011

Reed, P. G., & Shearer, N. B. (2011). *Nursing knowledge and theory innovation: Advancing the science of practice.* New York, NY: Springer Publishing.

Rogers, M. E. (1970). *An introduction to the theoretical basis of nursing.* Philadelphia, PA: F. A. Davis.

Rogers, M. E. (1988). Nursing science and art: A prospective. *Nursing Science Quarterly, 1*(3), 99–102. doi:10.1177/089431848800100304

Rogers, M. E. (1992). Nursing science and the space age. *Nursing Science Quarterly, 6,* 27–34. doi:10.1177/089431849200500108

Rogers, M. E. (1994). The science of unitary human beings: Current perspectives. *Nursing Science Quarterly, 7*(1), 33–35. doi:10.1177/089431849400700111

Sarter, B. (1988). Philosophical sources of nursing theory. *Nursing Science Quarterly, 1*(2), 52–59. doi:10.1177/089431848800100205

Sheldrake, R. (1983). *A new science of life.* Los Angeles, CA: Tarcher.

Smith, M. C. (1994). Arriving at a philosophy of nursing: Discovering? Constructing? Evolving? In J. Kikuchi & H. Simmons (Eds.), *Developing a philosophy of nursing* (pp. 43–60). Thousand Oaks, CA: Sage.

Smith, M. C. (1999). Caring and the science of unitary human beings. *Advances in Nursing Science, 21*(4), 14–28. doi:10.1097/00012272-199906000-00006

Smith, M. C. (2010). Nursing theory and the discipline of nursing. In M. C. Smith & M. E. Parker (Eds.), *Nursing theory and nursing practice* (3rd ed., pp. 3–16). Philadelphia, PA: F. A. Davis.

Smith, M. C. (2015). Nursing theory and the discipline of nursing. In M. C. Smith & M. E. Parker (Eds.), *Nursing theory and nursing practice* (4th ed., pp. 1–18). Philadelphia, PA: F. A. Davis.

Stephenson, J. S., & Tripp-Reimer, T. (Eds.). (1990). Knowledge about care and caring. In *Proceedings of a Wingspread Conference* (1–3 February 1989). Kansas City, MO: American Academy of Nursing.

van Lommel, P. (2011). *Consciousness beyond life: The science of the near-death experience.* New York, NY: HarperCollins.

Watson, J. (1979). *Nursing the philosophy and science of caring.* Boston, MA: Little, Brown.

Watson, J. (1985). *Human science: Human care: A theory of Nursing.* Norwalk, CT: Appleton-Century Croft. Reprinted (1988). New York, NY: National League for Nursing. Reprinted (1999). Boulder: University Press of Colorado.

Watson, J. (2002). *Assessing and measuring caring in nursing and health science.* New York, NY: Springer Publishing.

Watson, J. (2003). Love and caring: Ethics of face and hand: An invitation to return to the heart and soul of nursing and our deep humanity. *Nursing Administration Quarterly, 27*(3), 197–202. doi:10.1097/00006216-200307000-00005

Watson, J. (2005). *Caring science as sacred science.* Philadelphia, PA: F. A. Davis.

Watson, J. (2006). *Postmodern nursing and beyond.* New York, NY: Elsevier. (Original work published 1999).

Watson, J. (2008). *Nursing philosophy and science of caring* (2nd ed.). Boulder: University Press of Colorado.

Watson, J. (2012). *Human caring science.* Boston, MA: Jones & Bartlett.

Watson, J., & Smith, M .C. (2002). Caring science and the science of unitary human beings: A transtheoretical discourse for nursing knowledge development. *Journal of Advanced Nursing, 37*(5), 452–461. doi:10.1046/j.1365-2648.2002.02112.x

Whitehead, A. N. (1953). *Science and the modern world.* Cambridge, UK: Cambridge University Press.

Zukav, G. (1979). *The Dancing Wu Li Masters.* New York, NY: HarperCollins.

Zukav, G. (2013). *The Dancing Wu Li Masters.* New York, NY: HarperCollins.

3

The Evolution of Nursing's Ethics of Caring

Peggy L. Chinn

CARITAS LITERACIES

By the end of this chapter, the caring-healing nurse will be able to

1. Describe how caring evolved as central to nursing's ethics.

2. Identify the necessity of caring ethics as central to creating healing encounters and environments.

3. Describe the elements of caring in the human health experience from which moral action in nursing arises.

Nursing, by definition, is a profession that calls for clear ethical and moral standards. Nurses are responsible for the very life of people and their families. Nurses have knowledge and skills needed to protect the well-being of the public and the environment we all inhabit and are in positions that can influence the political and cultural contexts from which social determinants of health arise. These are obligations of tremendous importance, and can be fulfilled only if nurses, individually and as a profession, earn the trust of the public by living up to the highest of ethical and moral standards.

The terms "ethics" and "morality" are often used interchangeably, but there is a subtle distinction. "Ethics" generally relates to knowing and the sources from which knowledge is derived; it is the epistemological grounding from which codes and principles are developed that reflect a particular group's views of right and wrong, duties, good and evil. "Morality" generally relates to behavior and comportment—the ontological, lived actions that are considered responsible and correct, or bad and unacceptable.

This chapter begins with an overview of the evolution of ethical thought that appears in the literature since the time of Florence Nightingale and the establishment of nursing as a profession. The discussion then explains how nursing came to embrace an ethic of caring as central to the discipline, ways in which this ethic defines nursing as a unique discipline while contributing to the broader knowledge of caring in the realm of human relationships. Finally, the chapter concludes with a discussion of the primary determinants of moral choice derived from a nursing ethic of caring.

NURSING ETHICS

EARLY INDICATORS OF ETHICS IN NURSING LITERATURE

Nurse scholars have addressed the matter of ethics, either implicitly or explicitly, from the earliest of times, in part because nursing has been viewed as deriving from a sense of duty to care with compassion for the sick and injured, even those who are strangers (Fowler, 2016). As religious and societal groups emerged, which took on this obligation from a sense of service to either God or people in general, nursing began to be seen as a social obligation, a moral duty for those who were willing to dedicate their lives to this kind of service. Nightingale's writings clearly affirm this social and religious foundation from which her ideas about nursing emerged. Her best-known work, "Notes on Nursing," was written to inform any person caring for the sick of basic principles from which best practices derived, and to guide the actions arising from these principles (Nightingale, 1860/1969). For example, Nightingale explained why, on the basis of what was known at the time, fresh air was beneficial to the sick, and on the basis of this knowledge, admonished those caring for the sick to open the windows to let in fresh air. Her writing also focused explicitly on the moral character that those who care for the sick must demonstrate to earn the trust and authority to manage the care of the sick and injured. Even though she did not explicitly present ethical codes that define good nursing practice, her writing established clear principles of beneficence and fidelity as core ideals of comportment (Clements & Averill, 2006; Hoyt, 2010). It is clear that Nightingale struggled with the underlying ethical issues involved in providing care for the sick and preventing illness and disease. In a footnote on page 106 of *Notes on Nursing*, she stated: "It is a much more difficult thing to speak the truth than people commonly imagine" (Nightingale, 1860/1969). In explaining this difficulty, it is clear that Nightingale associated "truth" with what is objectively observed and corroborated by reliable multiple observations.

Isabel Hampton Robb, who was instrumental in founding both the National League for Nursing and the American Nurses Association in the United States, published the first book on *Nursing Ethics* in 1900 (Robb, 1900; "The Isabel Hampton Robb Collection," 2002). In the Introduction, Robb (1900) explains the importance of this book for the profession:

> Any ideas of special moral responsibilities have been vague and indefinite to the many, while the few have evolved them for themselves as a result of observation and experience. Now, however, not only as individuals but as a profession, we are beginning to feel an increasing necessity for some such definite moral force or laws that shall bind us together in this work of nursing, and that will bring us into more uniform and harmonious relations. (p. 11)

The content of Robb's landmark book reflects the tradition set by Florence Nightingale in that it focuses on the character and characteristics that nurses must cultivate in themselves.

These include practical duties of nurses in their personal hygiene, dress, and proper comportment, specific duties of nurses serving in various hierarchical capacities, and finally the proper relationship of the graduate nurse with physicians, other nurses, and the public in caring for the patient. Robb, like Nightingale, spoke of a nurse's duty to "obey" physician orders, a principle rooted in the broader mores of the relationship between women and men of the time. More importantly (and often overlooked), Robb set forth principles of justice, equity, and respect for the humanity of each individual as foundations for the ethics of care. In the first paragraph of her final chapter on the care of the patient, she stated:

> Thus I would have the pupil nurse understand that from the first duty she is assigned in the hospital, from the first simple service which she is called upon to perform for some poor patient in the free ward, she begins the training which will fit her, after her graduation, to take care of the sufferers in the alley or the rich in their mansions. From the very outset let her determine that she will be no respecter of persons, but will treat all her patients with impartiality. While in the hospital, the nurse should always make it her rule to think of every patient—even the poorest and most unattractive—not as a mere case, interesting only from a scientific standpoint, but as an individual sick human being, whose wishes, fancies and peculiarities call for all consideration possible at her hands. (Robb, 1900, pp. 213–214)

Of course, nursing is not the only discipline that has an ethical and moral tradition of at least claiming to treat all people equally with respect for their humanity. However, because of the unique position that nurses hold in their relationships with other people, this fundamental ethic provides particular significance for nursing, as will become apparent as this discussion moves to the modern era.

THE MID-20TH CENTURY TURN

By the middle of the 20th century, social norms that governed the relationship between women and men began to shift in Western society, and the accompanying social changes arising from this shift began to change the landscape of sex-segregated occupations (Greenleaf, 1980). In part, because of this social shift, nurses began to pay attention to, and question, many of the early gender-related traditions and norms that governed the development of nursing and that had been advocated as proper behavior of nurses in deference to physicians. One of the first authors to acknowledge the influence of this shift was Wilma Scott Heide, nurse and social activist. At the time of her article in the *American Journal of Nursing*, titled "Nursing and Women's Liberation," Heide (1973) was the third president of the National Organization for Women. Her article explained how the traditional roles of women and men had limited the humanity of all people, and she urged a change for women and nurses to become more fully human. Although her article does not speak directly to ethics, she argued that nursing could be at the forefront of creating a fully human and humane healthcare system. Heide's (1973) conclusion to the article stated:

> Nurses and nursing can be leaders in bringing about a humanist society as well as in humanizing healthcare. In my view, one cannot be a humanist without the

feminist insights and convictions. They are essential for individual integrity, for the empowerment of women, for fully human and humane health practitioners and systems, and thus for a healthy society. (p. 827)

Jo Ann Ashley's groundbreaking dissertation research on the evolution of the apprenticeship model of nursing education was the first to examine specific ways in which the relationships of medicine and nursing, men and women, damaged the humanity of nurses and physicians, and the quality of healthcare in general (Ashley, 1976). Her later speeches and articles, although not addressing ethics directly, sparked a landmark shift in the culture of nursing that opened the way for nurses to more clearly address the kind of ethical perspective that uniquely derives from nursing, one that focuses primarily on the nature of the relationship between the nurse and those the nurse serves, rather than the nurse–physician relationship. Ashley spoke to the urgency of overcoming the many social and political barriers that prevented women and nurses from realizing their full human potential, the damage rendered by devaluing women's experiences of human relationships, and the promise inherent in seeking full humanity for all regardless of gender (Ashley, 1980; Kagan, 2006; Wolf, 1997).

As nurses and nursing began to experience the social, cultural, and political shifts accompanying the women's movement, not surprisingly, a wellspring of nursing knowledge, derived from nursing experience and intellect, began to emerge. Nursing philosophies and theories appeared in books and journal articles, some of them embedded in texts that retained a focus on nursing tasks and duties (Harmer & Henderson, 1960; Peplau, 1952; Rogers, 1970).

As Twomey (1989) noted, in the 1960s and 1970s, nurses began to recognize and conceptualize nursing as having distinct obligations to the patient and roles that contributed in significant ways to patient well-being, apart from the role of medicine. Thus unfolded a period of energetic debate and dialogue concerning the nature of nursing's ethical obligation and the foundation from which nursing's obligation arises—to identify the essential basis for moral behavior, which cannot be adequately communicated in ethical codes alone. The possibility began to emerge that nursing ethics is distinct from the bioethical basis for moral behavior that guides medical ethics—that there is a distinct basis guiding the moral behavior of nurses. As Twomey (1989) stated:

ultimately the question arises whether there are any subfields of normative bioethics at all or if nurses and physicians, as well as businesspersons, are simply subject to the same moral code that exists in society. The simple answer on a normative and descriptive level seems to be that the only factor that provides uniqueness to a professional's moral behavior is his or her role. Yet metaethical reasoning provides a firmer foundation for the claim for distinctive non-role-based bioethical perspectives for the healthcare professions. (p. 28)

In the literature that began to focus explicitly on nursing and ethics, the distinctive characteristic that began to emerge as central to nursing is the complex nature of the nurse–patient relationship. The relationship between medicine and nursing began to be viewed as a power dynamic institutionally situated and as part of the context in which nurses practice, rather than as a matter of the relationship between practicing nurses and physicians. It became increasingly clear that nursing relationships with patients are central to nursing's concern, and that these relationships are shaped by consistent and clear ethical and moral norms. By the same token, these same relationships began to be seen as providing the foundation for nursing's ethic of caring (Bishop & Scudder, 2003; Hess, 1996, 2003; Twomey, 1989, p. 28).

EARLY EXPLORATIONS OF ETHICS IN NURSING

The landmark article by Carper (1978) delineating nursing's fundamental patterns of knowing is among the most frequently cited works in nursing, in which she identified ethical knowing as one of four patterns of knowing that are essential for nursing practice. Just 1 year later, Carper also authored a less-known article focusing specifically on "The Ethics of Caring" in which she stated that the professional and personal value of caring provides the normative ethical standard that governs the actions and attitudes of all healthcare providers—values that have been eroded by specialization and technological advances. Carper proposed that technology and specialization have created a superstructure that is inherently depersonalizing. She drew on Mayeroff's examination of the concept of caring as urgent and essential in contexts shaped by specialization and technology. Carper (1978) explained:

> One experiences what is cared for as having a dignity and worth in its own right with potentialities and need for growth. Caring is the antithesis of possessing, manipulating or dominating, a process which requires devotion and trust. In any actual instance of caring there must be someone or something specific that is cared for. Caring cannot occur by sheer habit; nor can it occur in the abstract. (p. 14)

The relationship Carper alluded to in this quote is associated with key issues that Carper believed are closely aligned with the ethics of caring for all healthcare providers: (a) the nature of the relationship, (b) informed consent, (c) determination of the quality of life, and (d) participation in ethical decision making (Carper, 1979, pp. 15–16). Carper noted that existing models of the nature of relationships between physicians and patients do not provide sufficient assurance that the relationship will be a humane, caring relationship. She pointed to the study of the humanities as a potential means to encourage empathy and compassion in the face of another's pain and suffering. Nevertheless, Carper acknowledged that caring is not learned in a classroom. Rather, it emerges from the practitioner's belief in the dignity and worth of each person, and from critical self-examination of one's own personal values that influence the ability to care.

Unrelated to the publication of Carper's article, Leah Curtin, editor of *Supervisor Nurse*, published an editorial addressing the effect of technology on nursing practice in her April editorial titled "The Prostitution of CPR" (Curtin, 1979b). The response of readers was immense, prompting Curtin to follow up in the August issue of the journal with articles addressing this issue, and another editorial titled "CPR Policies in Perspective" in which she stated:

> Today's hospitals are seeking ways to humanize the care they offer; to moderate the conflicting demands of medical technology and human emotional need; and to reduce stress by adjusting policies. (Curtin, 1979a, p. 9)

Curtin (1979b) reaches this conclusion after reading the barrage of letters following the publication of the April editorial, "The Prostitution of CPR." The vast majority of respondents requested help—model policies, guidelines, techniques—so that they could adjust their policies to reflect a humane and rational approach to CPR (Curtin, 1979a, p. 9).

Four years after Carper's examination of the ethics of caring, and prompted in part by the 1979 *Supervisor Nurse* content, Roland Yarling and Beverly McElmurry published an article titled "Rethinking the Nurse's Role in 'Do Not Resuscitate' Orders: A Clinical" in *Advances in Nursing Science* (Yarling & McElmurry, 1983). Their article used the situation in which "do not resuscitate" (DNR) orders existed as a microcosm of the larger challenges in practice, implicitly exploring the claim made by Carper regarding the influence of technology in providing humane care. This article set in motion widespread dialogue concerning the unique role of nursing and the nature of nursing's obligation, which returned again and again to an emerging ethic of caring in nursing.

Yarling and McElmurry (1983) pointed out that the decision to use a DNR directive is clearly a decision that can be made only by the patient (or patient surrogate) by virtue of the fact that it is a moral decision guided by the moral principle of autonomy. The medical decision involved is a judgment of the irreversibility of a condition. It is not a legal decision, even though there may be legal ramifications. The proper role of the nurse, they believed, is to assist the patient and family in their struggle to understand the situation in the context of their reality, and to reach their own autonomous decision. Yarling and McElmurry (1983) proceeded with a review of historical and contemporary evidence related to the constraints placed on nursing by institutional policies, norms, and practices, including the uneasy relationship between nurses and physicians. They summarized the situation as follows:

> The fundamental moral predicament of hospital nurses is that they often are not free to be moral because they often are not free to exercise their commitment to the patient through excellence in patient care. Legal and institutional constraints hinder the practice of nursing sometimes in minor matters and sometimes in major matters of life and death. For the sake of patient care, the nurse must be set free to practice nursing, ie, set free to be moral. (Yarling & McElmurry, 1983, p. 8)

Yarling and McElmurry clearly situated nursing's ethical commitment to the relationship with the patient as nursing's core ethical responsibility. They concluded that institutional policies and practices must change to grant nurses the moral agency and autonomy required to engage in a meaningful relationship. Nurses have a responsibility to make themselves heard within the institution on these issues, but fundamentally, Yarling and McElmurry (1983) called for "the moral maturation of the hospital as a responsible social institution" (p. 11).

Three years later, Yarling and McElmurry elaborated on this conclusion in an article titled "The Moral Foundation of Nursing" (Yarling & McElmurry, 1986). Here they identified two remedies for the situation: the emergence of a strong sense of professional autonomy for nurses, and a shift in the locus of accountability for moral decisions from the provider to the patient. In examining what needs to happen to achieve these remedies, they concluded that

> If the fundamental moral problem of nursing is a consequence of the structure and policies of the social institution in which nursing is, for the most part, practiced, then any ethic that seeks to address this problem must seek reform of the policies and structures of that institution. An ethic that is concerned with structures and policies of social institutions is a social ethic. (Yarling & McElmurry, 1986, p. 71)

The Yarling and McElmurry articles spurred a significant response that lasted almost a decade, in which a number of nursing scholars critically examined their conclusions and proposed alternative views of nursing ethics and morality. The following account of this period in the development of nursing ethics shows a clear and growing commitment to an ethic of caring.

THE SEARCH FOR NURSING'S DISTINCT MORAL FOUNDATION

The first article to appear in response to those authored by Yarling and McElmurry (1983, 1986) was titled "Nursing Ethics in an Age of Controversy" by Bishop and Scudder (1987). They situated their analysis in the controversy between "curing," which demands ongoing advancement of technology and increasing specialization, and "caring," which demands cooperation between physicians and nurses to accommodate the growing demands of technology and specialization, but that maintains what they viewed as the essential nature of healthcare. They advocated for a caring model in which nurses have a privileged "in-between" position that nurses exercise in their day-to-day work, and wherein nurses fulfill their moral obligation to care. In their thoughtful analysis of the claims made by Yarling and McElmurry (1983, 1986), Bishop and Scudder (1987) made a significant contribution to the processes that Chinn and Kramer associated with the development of ethical knowledge in nursing—dialogue and justification (Chinn & Kramer, 2015) by expanding the possibilities for the development of ethical knowledge in nursing.

A key element of the Bishop and Scudder (1987) article is their proposal that nursing's "in-between" position is a privileged one that contributes to a cooperative process for reaching moral decisions. From a perspective that seeks autonomy, an in-between position seems offensive. Bishop and Scudder argued that instead, an in-between position focuses on the well-being of the person cared for, not the role of the provider or the exclusive rights of the patient. They explained this as follows:

> In short, the nurse, rather than being a facilitator of compromise, is an advocate of communal decisions that bring together expert medical advice and treatment, sound hospital policy and procedure, and the realizable hopes and aspirations of the patient into the concrete practice of health care that fosters the well-being of the patient. (Bishop & Scudder, 1987, p. 42)

They concluded that

> This approach affirms the traditional view of nursing as care and suggests that all health care is essentially what the name implies—the moral practice of caring for persons who need help restoring, maintaining, and promoting good health. (p. 43)

In the Bishop and Scudder discussion, there was a growing affirmation of caring as central to an ethic of nursing. They acknowledged the importance of the need for reform that Yarling and McElmurry (1983, 1986) advanced, but they believed that the reform that is needed is greater excellence in nursing and expansion of nursing's legitimate authority to care. Their view does not focus explicitly on the nature of caring, but it does, as their previous quote demonstrates, acknowledge the centrality of caring in relationship with those who are cared for.

The following year, in 1988, two articles (Cooper; Packard & Ferrara) appeared in *Advances in Nursing Science* offering further dialogue based on the 1986 Yarling and McElmurry article, and the 1987 Bishop and Scudder article. Cooper (1988) acknowledged the important contributions of both Yarling and McElmurry (1986) and Bishop and Scudder (1987) but pointed out the fact that neither of these publications addressed the nature of the nurse–patient relationship and the fundamental experience of moral agency of the nurse within the relationship. Cooper set out to move the dialogue in the direction of the essence of the nurse–patient relationship, which, as she affirms, had been a long-standing substantive basis for understanding the nature of nursing:

> It is argued here that covenantal relationships between the nurse and the patient provide a more substantial foundation for the nursing ethic. Arising from the moral principle of fidelity, this model furnishes guidance for the nurse, a link for the nursing ethic with traditional moral theory, and, most important, a grounding in the unique experience of the nurse-patient relationship. (Cooper, 1988, p. 48)

Cooper developed her justification for a covenantal relationship by examining the works of William May focusing the physician–patient covenantal relationship concept derived from a Judeo-Christian ethic, Robert Veatch's triple contract perspective for medical ethics, and nurse–philosopher Sally Gadow's caring relationship concept. Cooper identified three factors that are common in the works of May, Veatch, and Gadow—features that form a sound basis for a nursing ethic. First is the insistence on mutuality and reciprocity in the relationship. Second, all three authors view a covenantal relationship as distinct from one formed by way of a contract, which promotes self-interest, or a professional code, which easily becomes couched in philanthropic terms that are gratuitous rather than genuine. Third, the works of May and Veatch identify fidelity and promise-keeping as central ethical principles for covenantal relationships, and Gadow's work implicitly supports fidelity by her insistence that the nurse must "be there" for the patient using every dimension of the self. Drawing on the common elements of these three perspectives, Cooper described the importance of the unique nurse–patient relationship as a beginning point for developing an ethic of nursing—an ethic that is unique because it is grounded in the relationship.

Packard and Ferrara (1988) focused on the idea of nursing as the proper grounding for nursing ethics. They offered a detailed discussion of the main arguments presented by Yarling and McElmurry, pointing to ideas on which they agree, ideas that remain unclear and open for varying interpretation, and ideas that seem to be misplaced in relation to establishing a moral foundation for nursing. Packard and Ferrara contended that the idea of nursing is not derived from nursing jobs, tasks, collective identity, or legal or professional authority. Rather, the idea of nursing is derived from four components of nursing:

1. The right actions, the effects of which are productive of health and a life well lived

2. The talents needed to perform right acts

3. The knowledge of when to act and when not to act and what acts to perform

4. The will to act in such a manner as to serve the good (Packard & Ferrara, 1988, p. 63)

By "acts," Packard and Ferrara did not mean techniques or skills—they implied a deeper meaning of that which arises from a whole of knowing, insight, and wisdom, resulting in a way of being. They illuminated this point in their discussion of the inadequacy of defining the idea of nursing by what nurses do:

> The work of nursing is more than the nurse's (hospital) job. There is widespread recognition among practicing nurses that their jobs interfere with and misdirect their work, in the same sense that the job of postcard painter does not permit the artist to do art. All this illustrates a most difficult point, that nursing is other than what most nurses do. (Packard & Ferrara, 1988, p. 68)

Their discussion of the political nature of nursing was the first explicit recognition of the political dimension of nursing's ethic. They stated:

> If nursing comprises right desire, right knowledge, right talent, and right action, then, by its very nature, it is unavoidably political. Nursing struggles for, aims toward, knows about, and knows how to conduct right action, all of which is political and derives from the moral foundation of the very idea of nursing. (Packard & Ferrara, 1988, p. 65)

By 1989, and the publication of two more signature articles related to the development of nursing ethics, the concept of caring in the human relationship had taken a firm position (Fry, 1989; Twomey, 1989, p. 28). Both of these articles made a case for a distinct nursing ethic that is not derivative of, or a subset of, biomedical ethics.

John Twomey defended the argument that the basis for a distinct nursing ethic arises from persistent threads in nursing theories, including that health is more than the absence of illness, that humans interact with their environment, and insistence on the whole of human experience. Because of these threads, nurses are by definition dealing with human responses to unhealthy stressors, the contexts in which they live and work, and the meaning of the experience—all of which give rise to ethical problems that are apart from illness and the isolated process of disease and treatment of disease.

Fry (1989) analyzed various perspectives on the idea of caring in nursing and models of caring developed in other disciplines, and from her analysis concluded that theories of biomedical ethics are inadequate as a basis for nursing ethics. She justified caring as central in the development of nursing ethics because of the nature of nursing's relationship of caring. She explains this distinction as follows:

The context of nursing practice requires a moral view of persons rather than a theory of moral action or behavior or a system of moral justification. Present theories of medical ethics tend to support theoretical and methodologic views of ethical argumentation and moral justification that do not fit in with the practical realities of nurses' decision making in patient care and that, as a result, tend to deplete the moral agency of nursing practice rather than enhance it. Any theory of nursing ethics should consider the nature of the nurse-patient relationship within health care contexts and should adopt a moral point of view that focuses directly on this relationship, rather than on theoretical interpretations of physician decision making and their associated claims to moral justification for this decision making.

Second, the value of caring ought to be central to any theory of nursing ethics. There is a commitment to the role of caring in several conceptions of nursing ethics and nursing science. There also appears to be an important link between the value of caring and nurses' views on persons and human dignity... If a theory of nursing ethics is to have any purpose, it must espouse a view of morality that not only truly represents the social role of nursing as a profession in the provision of health care but also promises a moral role for nursing in the care and nurture of individuals who have health care needs. For theory to achieve this purpose, its view of morality ought to turn on a philosophical view of caring that posits caring as a foundational, rather than a derivative, value among persons. (Fry, 1989, pp. 20–21)

In 1991, a landmark article appeared that clearly positioned caring as central to nursing as a discipline. The article was titled "The Focus of the Discipline of Nursing," authored by Margaret Newman, A. Marilyn Sime, and Sheila Corcoran-Perry (Newman, Sime, & Corcoran-Perry, 1991). They drew on the body of nursing literature that explicitly or implicitly identified the proper scope of concern for nursing scholarship, including nursing's theoretical and philosophical literature, and the focus areas reflected in the content of scholarly nursing journals. They stated the following with respect to the focus they proposed:

We submit that nursing is the study of *caring in the human health experience.* This focus integrates into a single statement concepts commonly identified with nursing at the metaparadigm level. This focus implies a social mandate and service identity and specifies a domain for knowledge development. The social mandate and service identity are conveyed by a commitment to caring as a moral imperative. (Newman, Sime, & Corcoran-Perry, 1991, p. 3)

It is important to note that in this first declaration of their proposed focus for the discipline of nursing, Newman and colleagues referred specifically to caring as a moral imperative. In the years since the publication of this statement, there has been a widespread acknowledgment of the utility and the significance of this statement (Cook & Peden, 2017). Almost two decades later, Newman joined with Marlaine Smith, Margaret Dexheimer Pharris, and Dorothy Jones to revisit the focus of the discipline, and examined the progress made in defining the discipline (Newman, Smith, Pharris, & Jones, 2008). Notably, they included a footnote that stated that their use of the term "patient" refers not only to an individual but also to families and communities, which relates to the shift in the evolution of caring ethics that has dominated discussion of nursing's ethical and moral foundation over the past two decades. This same type of claim that "patient" refers not only to individuals and groups is found in other documents related to nursing ethics and scope of practice, but as Bekemeier and Butterfield (2005) pointed out in their analysis of such texts, the predominance of the person-to-person relationship far outweighs that given to system-level relationships and action. In the section to follow, I examine evidence of the shift toward social justice as a crucial element of the ethics of caring and propose a model that identifies the basis for moral choice in nursing that is derived from both the individual and the social human encounter.

NURSING ETHICS AND THE POLITICAL REALM

After the decades of scholarship that led to increasing clarification and development of a nursing ethic, and placing caring as a central element of nursing ethic, much of the literature related to nursing ethics was characterized by research reports and narrative analysis of experiences in education or practice (Bishop & Scudder, 2003; Hess, 1996, 2003; Minicucci, Schmitt, Dombeck, & Williams, 2003; O'Connor, 2017; Schneider & Ramos, 2012; Sorrell, 2006). These contributions offered insights and explored meanings that provided further development of the foundational ideas developed prior to 1990, but the most notable contribution of this literature was that which addressed the necessity for an ethic that focuses on the responsibility of nursing to the social, environmental and political dynamics that affect health (Austin, 2007; Bekemeier & Butterfield, 2005; Easley & Allen, 2007; Falk-Rafael & Betker, 2012; Ivanov & Oden, 2013; Kagan, Smith, & Chinn, 2014; Kangasniemi, 2010; Thompson, 2014). These writings identified the duty of nurses to support social and healthcare justice, equity, health as a human right, and moral communities of care. In advocating for the protection of population health and social justice, relationships remain at the center of nursing care, even though the "relationship" is typically implied. For example, Ivanov and Oden (2013) described in some detail the actions that public health nurses need to take in advancing the ideals of healthy communities, many of which involve working with individuals and groups in communities to build capacity for social change. In this sense, nursing actions, and the decisions related to action in the community, still depend on the nature of the relationships that nurses form with other individuals, sometimes coming together as a group.

Bekemeier and Butterfield (2005) acknowledged the centrality of relationships in nursing, but provided an important insight related to how relationships contribute to nursing actions promoting social justice and health equity:

> Our often-intimate relationships with vulnerable populations, as well as our increasing knowledge of the science of social determinants of health, give us unique perspective and expertise regarding the complex structures that prevent many communities

and populations from achieving good health. As a result, we are more able—and compelled—to participate fully in collaboration with communities and individuals as we act upon the social and political contradictions in which we live together. (p. 160)

Austin offered an analysis at another level—the healthcare community as the relational grounding for ethics and morality. As Austin stated: "Ethical action takes place in community. A healthcare professional's response to the ethical question 'How should I act?' needs to be understood in relations with clients and colleagues" (Austin, 2007, p. 85). In essence, it appears that in fact the conceptualization of the "individual" emphasis in nursing, both ethically and theoretically, exists only at an ontological level, in the context of a larger social and political community. The interplay that we think of as "person-to-person" relationships and group dynamics are so closely intertwined that thinking of them as separate is in fact only a trick of the human mind—not a fact in reality. Grasping this complexity is not easy, but it is essential to move toward an ethic of caring in nursing that embraces the whole.

Returning to Cooper's (1991) analysis of the creative tension between principle-oriented ethics and the ethics of care, she made the point that moral action in nursing arises primarily from a relationship. Moral action is informed by rules and principles, but, from an ethic of caring, the right action is driven by the experience itself. The nature of experience, in nursing specifically of the health experience, is deeper, more complex, and in fact richer in meaning than any ethical code or principles. Cooper (1991) stated:

in the ethic of care, a priori rules and principles play a secondary role in informing and illuminating moral choice. Principles are not determinants of moral activity. Rather, **moral concern is with needs and corresponding responsibility as they arise within a relationship.** Interdependence is valued as the ideal moral position, reflecting not a helpless attachment but the acknowledgment that individuals are indeed naturally related to one another throughout life. (p. 23)

Narrative stories bring together the whole of the experience, which includes the moral responsiveness of the nurse, who, acting from an ethic of care, enters the experience with the intention of traveling within the experience of those cared for (Parker, 1990).

A MODEST PROPOSAL: A NURSING ETHIC OF CARE

This examination of the evolution of nursing's ethics of care has led to the possibility that a new model or framework is required. This new framework would be situated within the focus of nursing—caring in the human health experience—and also draw on the value threads that have historically defined the nature of caring in the human health experience. Such a framework would also prompt a mental structure that includes, but moves beyond, the individual person-to-person relationship so that individuals are experienced and valued within their own situation, their own life story. The nurse, moving into that experience, the "other" life story, does so with the intention of becoming a companion with the other, deriving direction for "right nursing action" from the shared experience that honors the shared humanity of all in the experience. Such a model would take into account the factors as described in Table 3.1.

TABLE 3.1 Elements of Caring in the Human Health Experience From Which Moral Action Arises

In an Encounter	In the Context
The experience of relationship—knowing the other(s) and being known by the other(s)—knowing the life story that is interrupted	The experience of the social and political context, knowing the social structure that is interrupted
The desire to diminish the possibility of dehumanization in the encounter	The desire to prevent dehumanizing conditions and to create humanizing environments—locally and beyond
The desire to flourish even in the context of human suffering	The desire for conditions that reduce human suffering, promote flourishing, and protect the environment and community
The experience of the struggle to find meaning, mutuality, and understanding	The experience of the struggle to create policies that benefit all in the shared human condition

The dimensions shown in the column labeled "In an encounter" are those dimensions that involve the "here and now" of the experience—what it is about the experience itself (with an individual or within a group) that informs "right action." The dimensions in the column labeled "In the context" require looking beyond the moment itself and how that context has shaped, and will shape, the moment of the caring encounter.

CONCLUSION

In conclusion, nursing has a rich history from which to draw in continuing to develop the ethics of caring. Despite the troubled nature of some of that history, nurses in all walks of nursing have persisted in exercising values that are consistent with a form of caring that promotes human flourishing, even in the most difficult of circumstances. Scholarship in nursing has been exemplary in addressing both troubles and triumphs of nursing, and in doing so has provided a ground from which a distinct ethic of caring arises. Our challenge in the coming decades is to continue to protect that heritage, in part by taking our values into the public sphere, with courage and conviction that what the world needs more than anything at this point in history is human caring.

NEXT ERA POSSIBILITIES

Education
- What teaching/learning experiences can I create to assure nursing's ethical commitment to human caring remains at the center?

Research

- How can I frame my research focus to reflect the whole of human experience?

Praxis

- How well do my actions reflect the fundamental values and ideals inherent in nursing's ethics of caring?

Theory and Knowledge Development

- How can my experience with moral decision making contribute to the dialogue and justification needed to develop ethical knowing in nursing?

 REFERENCES

Ashley, J. A. (1976). *Hospitals, paternalism, and the role of the nurse.* New York, NY: Teachers College Press.

Ashley, J. A. (1980). Power in structured misogyny: Implications for the politics of care. *Advances in Nursing Science, 2,* 3–22. doi:10.1097/00012272-198002030-00003

Austin, W. (2007). The ethics of everyday practice: Healthcare environments as moral communities. *Advances in Nursing Science, 30*(1), 81–88. doi:10.1097/00012272-200701000-00009

Bekemeier, B., & Butterfield, P. (2005). Unreconciled inconsistencies: A critical review of the concept of social justice in 3 national nursing documents. *Advances in Nursing Science, 28,* 152–162. doi:10.1097/00012272-200504000-00007

Bishop, A. H., & Scudder, J. R., Jr. (1987). Nursing ethics in an age of controversy. *Advances in Nursing Science, 9,* 34–43. doi:10.1097/00012272-198704000-00011

Bishop, A. H., & Scudder, J. R., Jr. (2003). Gadow's contribution to our philosophical interpretation of nursing. *Nursing Philosophy, 4*(2), 104–110. doi:10.1046/j.1466-769X.2003.00125.x

Carper, B. A. (1978). Fundamental patterns of knowing in nursing. *Advances in Nursing Science, 1,* 13–23. doi:10.1097/00012272-197810000-00004

Carper, B. A. (1979). The ethics of caring. *Advances in Nursing Science, 1,* 11–19. doi:10.1097/00012272-197904000-00004

Chinn, P. L., & Kramer, M. K. (2015). *Knowledge development in nursing: Theory and process* (9th ed.). St Louis, MO: Elsevier.

Clements, P. T., & Averill, J. A. (2006). Finding patterns of knowing in the work of Florence Nightingale. *Nursing Outlook, 54,* 268–274. doi:10.1016/j.outlook.2006.06.003

Cook, L. B., & Peden, A. (2017). Finding a focus for nursing: The caring concept. *Advances in Nursing Science, 40*(1), 12–23. doi:10.1097/ANS.0000000000000137

Cooper, M. C. (1988). Covenantal relationships: Grounding for the nursing ethic. *Advances in Nursing Science, 10*(4), 48–59. doi:10.1097/00012272-198807000-00008

Cooper, M. C. (1991). Principle-oriented ethics and the ethic of care: A creative tension. *Advances in Nursing Science, 14,* 22–31. doi:10.1097/00012272-199112000-00004

Curtin, L. L. (1979a). CPR policies in perspective. *Supervisor Nurse, 10*(8), 9. doi:10.1097/00006247-197908000-00001

Curtin, L. L. (1979b). The prostitution of CPR. *Supervisor Nurse, 10*(4), 7. doi:10.1097/00006247-197904000-00001

Easley, C. E., & Allen, C. E. (2007). A critical intersection: Human rights, public health nursing, and nursing ethics. *Advances in Nursing Science, 30*(4), 367–382. doi:10.1097/01.ANS.0000300185. 94595.6c

Falk-Rafael, A., & Betker, C. (2012). Witnessing social injustice downstream and advocating for health equity upstream: "The trombone slide" of nursing. *Advances in Nursing Science, 35*(2), 98–112. doi:10.1097/ANS.0b013e31824fe70f

Fowler, M. D. (2016). Heritage ethics: Toward a thicker account of nursing ethics. *Nursing Ethics, 23*(1), 7–21. doi:10.1177/0969733015608071

Fry, S. T. (1989). Toward a theory of nursing ethics. *Advances in Nursing Science, 11*, 9–22. doi:10.1097/00012272-198907000-00005

Greenleaf, N. P. (1980). Sex-segregated occupations: Relevance for nursing. *Advances in Nursing Science, 2*, 23–37. doi:10.1097/00012272-198002030-00004

Harmer, B., & Henderson, V. (1960). *Textbook of the principles and practice of nursing*. New York, NY: Macmillan.

Heide, W. S. (1973). Nursing and women's liberation: A parallel. *American Journal of Nursing, 73*, 824–827. doi:10.1097/00000446-197305000-00045

Hess, J. D. (1996). The ethics of compliance: A dialectic. *Advances in Nursing Science, 19*, 18–27. doi:10.1097/00012272-199609000-00004

Hess, J. D. (2003). Gadow's relational narrative: An elaboration. *Nursing Philosophy, 4*(2), 137–148. doi:10.1046/j.1466-769X.2003.00126.x

Hoyt, S. (2010). Florence Nightingale's contribution to contemporary nursing ethics. *Journal of Holistic Nursing, 28*(4), 331–332. doi:10.1177/0898010110383281

Ivanov, L. L., & Oden, T. L. (2013). Public health nursing, ethics and human rights. *Public Health Nursing, 30*(3), 231–238. doi:10.1111/phn.12022

Kagan, P. N. (2006). Jo Ann Ashley 30 years later: Legacy for practice. *Nursing Science Quarterly, 19*, 317–327. doi:10.1177/0894318406293121

Kagan, P. N., Smith, M. C., & Chinn, P. L. (2014). Philosophies and practices of emancipatory nursing: Social justice as praxis. New York, NY: Routledge Taylor & Francis.

Kangasniemi, M. (2010). Equality as a central concept of nursing ethics: A systematic literature review. *Scandinavian Journal of Caring Sciences, 24*(4), 824–832. doi:10.1111/j.1471-6712.2010.00781.x

Minicucci, D. S., Schmitt, M. H., Dombeck, M. T., & Williams, G. C. (2003). Actualizing Gadow's moral framework for nursing through research1. *Nursing Philosophy, 4*(2), 92–103. doi:10.1046/j.1466-769X .2003.00129.x

Newman, M. A., Sime, A. M., & Corcoran-Perry, S. A. (1991). The focus of the discipline of nursing. *Advances in Nursing Science, 14*, 1–6. doi:10.1097/00012272-199109000-00002

Newman, M. A., Smith, M. C., Pharris, M. D., & Jones, D. (2008). The focus of the discipline revisited. *Advances in Nursing Science, 31*, E16–E27. doi:10.1097/01.ANS.0000311533.65941.f1

Nightingale, F. (1969). *Notes on nursing: What it is and what it is not*. New York, NY: Dover. (Original work published 1860)

O'Connor, K. (2017). Nursing ethics and the 21st-century armed conflict: The example of Ciudad Juárez. *Journal of Transcultural Nursing, 28*(1), 6–14. doi:10.1177/1043659615620657

Packard, J. S., & Ferrara, M. (1988). In search of the moral foundation of nursing. *Advances in Nursing Science, 10*, 60–71. doi:10.1097/00012272-198807000-00009

Parker, R. S. (1990). Nurses' stories: The search for a relational ethic of care. *Advances in Nursing Science, 13*, 31–40. doi:10.1097/00012272-199009000-00005

Peplau, H. E. (1952). *Interpersonal relations in nursing*. New York, NY: G. P. Putnam's Sons.

Robb, I. H. (1900). *Nursing ethics: For hospital and private use*. Cleveland, OH: Kessinger.

Rogers, M. E. (1970). *An introduction to the theoretical basis of nursing*. Philadelphia, PA: F. A. Davis.

Schneider, D. G., & Ramos, F. R. (2012). Moral deliberation and nursing ethics cases: Elements of a methodological proposal. *Nursing Ethics, 19*(6), 764–776. doi:10.1177/0969733011420096

Sorrell, J. M. (2006). Listening in thin places: Ethics in the care of persons with Alzheimer's disease. *Advances in Nursing Science, 29*(2), 152–160. doi:10.1097/00012272-200604000-00008

The Isabel Hampton Robb Collection. (2002). Retrieved from http://www.medicalarchives.jhmi.edu/ papers/robb.html

Thompson, J. L. (2014). Discourses of social justice: Examining the ethics of democratic professionalism in nursing. *Advances in Nursing Science, 37*(3), E17–E34. doi:10.1097/ANS.0000000000000045

Twomey, J. G., Jr. (1989). Analysis of the claim to distinct nursing ethics: Normative and nonnormative approaches. *Advances in Nursing Science, 11*, 25–32. doi:10.1097/00012272-198904000-00007

Wolf, K. (1997). *Jo Ann Ashley: Selected readings*. New York, NY: National League for Nursing.

Yarling, R. R., & McElmurry, B. J. (1983). Rethinking the nurse's role in "do not resuscitate" orders: A clinical policy proposal in nursing ethics. *Advances in Nursing Science, 5*, 1–12. doi:10.1097/00012272-198307000-00004

Yarling, R. R., & McElmurry, B. J. (1986). The moral foundation of nursing. *Advances in Nursing Science, 8*, 63–73. doi:10.1097/00012272-198601000-00010

4

Caring as Emancipatory Nursing Praxis: The Theory of Relational-Caring Complexity*

Marilyn A. Ray and Marian C. Turkel

CARITAS LITERACIES

By the end of this chapter, the caring-healing nurse will be able to

1. Articulate the role of nursing practice within the framework of emancipatory nursing praxis.

2. Use the concepts of relational caring complexity as a guide for nursing leadership decision making.

3. Give authentic voice to social justice and human rights within nursing.

4. Identify the core values of social justice, human rights, and relational caring complexity.

5. Create praxis projects within their own system.

―

> *Peace power reflects a feminist ideal where the focus shifts to chosen values [caring ethics, love, human rights, and justice] that guide the exercise of power, and to considering what happens to people's relationships when power is used.*
> —(Chinn, 2013, p. 18)

*From Ray, M. A., & Turkel, M. C. (2014). Caring as emancipatory nursing praxis: The theory of relational caring complexity. *Advances in Nursing Science*, 37(2), 132–146. doi:10.1097/ANS.0000000000000024. Permission to reprint obtained from Netherlands: Wolters Kluwer Health.

Chinn's (2013) assertion of the importance of peace power is a call for respect for a feminist moral philosophy, related to power that energizes peace (praxis, empowerment, awareness, cooperation, and evolvement, and ensures human rights and justice; p. 10). The assertion reflects, in essence, a social caring ethic, a practice of how we think after identifying through critical reflection, dialogue, reasoned argumentation, beliefs and values of human dignity, human rights and justice (or fairness) that must be woven into the cultural fabric of daily life (Chinn, 2013; MacIntyre, 1996; Ray, 2010a, 2010b). As such, this social caring ethic is caring as emancipatory praxis. It is a science and art, "the simultaneous reflection and action directed towards transforming the world" (Kagan, Smith, Cowling, & Chinn, 2009, p. 67) and the subsequent understanding, through reasoned evaluation of meaning for participants in moral community life (Chinn, 2013; Ray, 1992, 1999). Overall, critical caring science or caring as emancipatory praxis (transformative practice) is reflective values-in-action (Chinn, 2013, p. 18) to improve and protect human rights and social justice by means of creative approaches to inquiry, critique, and praxis in the social world. The social world includes socioeconomic-political, transcultural knowledge development, and evaluation of and implementation of rules of law and systems to cocreate the meaning of critical human caring ethical action (Chinn, 2013; MacIntyre, 1996; Ray, 2010a, 2010b). [In this chapter, the use of hyphens orients the reader to the structure, process, and social action of reflective practice.]

In the postmodern era of professional nursing praxis, this moral way of life is a complex critical relational-caring science that calls for a renewal of our humanity, our spirituality, and the meaning of *being-in-relationship* by addressing ethical action-values-in-action in the complex nursing situation (Chinn, 2013; Davidson, Ray, & Turkel, 2011; Newman, Smith, Pharris, & Jones, 2008; Ray, 1992, 1999). The challenge to nursing today is seeking understanding of not only the language of social justice, human rights, and peace for self and others in current national or international sociopolitical systems, but also self-in-relation to environments that are complex, highly medicalized, and economically focused bureaucratic healthcare systems. To meet this test of caring-as-emancipation-as-praxis science and art of highly medicalized and bureaucratized healthcare systems, research was conducted over a decade-long period by Ray and Turkel (Davidson et al., 2011; Ray, Turkel, & Cohn, 2011) to facilitate awareness, understanding, and choice for transformation. A theory was discovered using both quantitative and qualitative research methods, including patient and professional tool development to study economically centered practices. The theory is *Relational Caring Complexity* and is the focus of this chapter (Davidson et al., 2011; Ray et al., 2011). It is a unique contribution to advancing our understanding of social justice and human rights and particularly the importance of the call for caring as emancipatory nursing praxis. The theory emphasizes socioeconomic-political communitarian spiritual and ethical caring in the world of nursing in complex healthcare organizations.

The Language of Social Justice and Human Rights

Both social justice and human rights are foundations for caring praxis and peace. Watson (2008b) advanced the idea that

> When we proceed with knowledge and practices [of caring] that others do not know or see, we then have responsibility to offer it to others ... In this line of thinking, there

is a connection between Caring (as connecting with, sustaining, and deepening our shared humanity) and Peace in the world. (p. 48)

Although social justice and human rights are articulated in society, there is opportunity for more clarity. For the purposes of this chapter, the concepts are shared in the following way. "Social justice" (the application of the ethical principle of equity—fairness or impartiality) is considered a central value of democratic societies and social institutions. Although not all scholars are in agreement, according to the theorist, Rawls (2007a, 2007b), justice as fairness or equity incorporates the following principles: (a) all persons have equal rights to basic liberty; (b) social and economic inequalities, for example, inequalities of wealth and authority are just only if they result in compensating benefits for everyone, in particular the least advantaged; (c) offices or positions are to be open to all; and (d) the system works to benefit the least advantaged as well as the advantaged (distributive justice). Moral reasoning by treating each person *as* a moral person is required to deal with the ideas of fairness and equality of opportunity. Social justice thus relates to both reward and punishment. As such, impartiality or fairness is concerned with everyone whose welfare might be affected by what we do, for good or evil, within moral and legal frameworks. Impartiality not only affects individual fairness or rights but also embraces the whole moral community or humanity across space and time (in all cultures, organizations, and nations) with no boundaries of race, religion, class, or sexual orientation (Chinn, 2013; Nussbaum, 1997; Rawls, 2007a, 2007b; Sandel, 2007, 2009).

The concept of "human rights" incorporates a foundational social goal of respect for human dignity. All human beings are born with equal and inalienable rights and fundamental freedoms (Nussbaum, 1997; Sandel, 2007, 2009). Freedoms consist of thought, conscience, and religion or belief (United Nations, 1948). In juxtaposition to social justice, human rights underpin the ethical principle of equity by moral participation and the rule of law highlighting "doing the right thing." Commitment to human rights reinforces respect for initiating and protecting civil rights for all people, including cultural rights, the rights of women, men, children, the elderly, immigrants, refugees, stigmatized groups, animals, and the environment. Moreover, the concept of human rights incorporates the right to information, determining economic rights, seeking understanding of social, economic, and environmental sustainability (outcome of the United Nations Millennium Development Goals Mandate; United Nations, 2015). Protection of individual autonomy, doing no harm, and doing good (beneficence) also includes the provision of healthcare for all, a goal of the World Health Organization (2006) and other international organizations, especially nursing (American Nurses Association [ANA], 2003; Cowling & Chinn, 2001; International Council of Nurses [ICN], 2009; Kagan et al., 2009; Miller et al., 2008). In a globalized and digital world, challenges of social justice and human rights face all leaders of nations and corporations in terms of issues of interpretation and meaning. How the domain of human rights and imparting justice are interpreted or complied with is both a test and a challenge in sovereign nations. National, cultural, or religious "rules of law" put side by side with international "rules of law and goals" often increase apprehension for leaders and citizens of the world (United Nations, 1948). The goal of the United Nations Declaration of Human Rights Charter (1948), however, is human rights for *all* people of the world no matter what national or religious interpretations may be articulated.

THE VOICE OF SOCIAL JUSTICE IN NURSING

In their examination and analysis of a nursing manifesto, Kagan et al. (2009) identified ideas to engage nurses to be more cognizant of the meaning of the values of social justice by turning to the meaning of emancipation in nursing research, practice, and education and leadership. The nursing manifesto highlighted ways to facilitate "raising the voice of nursing" to assume "ethical responsibility to work towards humanizing health care practices and promoting the ideals of social justice" (Kagan et al., 2009, p. 68). Moreover, ideas from books and position statements, such as the book *Peace and Power: New Directions for Building Community* (Chinn, 2013; Cowling & Chin, 2001), the *Transcultural Nursing Society Position Statement on Human Rights* (Miller et al., 2008), the *Standards for Culturally Competent Nursing Care: 2011 Update* (Douglas et al., 2011), and the conceptualization *Social Justice: A Framework for Culturally Competent* Care (Clingerman, 2011), examined and reinforced nursing's commitment to social justice and human rights. Competent caring, seeking understanding of and transforming healthcare organizations by setting up ethical standards and policies for the workplace, bring awareness and support to nursing's social responsibility around the world (Davidson et al., 2011; Ray, 2010a, 2010b).

SOCIAL RESPONSIBILITY IN NURSING

Historically, social responsibility has been a rallying cry for nursing since the time of Nightingale (1859/1992). Human rights and social justice were advanced since that time and in the United States by scholars and nurse activists, such as Dock, Nutting, Wald, Lloyd and others (Davidson et al., 2011; Kalisch & Kalisch, 2003; Lloyd, 1931), until the present time. The principles of social responsibility have been situated in scholarship (see, for example, *Advances in Nursing Science* and the *Journal of Advanced Nursing*), codes of ethics (ANA, 2003; Bekemeier & Butterfield, 2005), diverse schools of nursing university curricula, and national and international nursing organizations (ICN, 2009). Nursing science in general and as it relates to the tenets of contemporary social justice and human rights have been advanced and strengthened locally and globally over the past 40 years. Scholarship and the call for sociocultural action in nursing practice has concentrated attention on the following:

- The nursing manifesto as emancipatory praxis (Kagan et al., 2009)

- Peace and power for community building, empowerment, and transformational leadership (Chinn, 2013)

- Critical theoretical interpretation (Kirkham & Browne, 2006)

- Cultural healthcare rights, for example, via the Transcultural Nursing Society Position Statement on Human Rights (Miller et al., 2008), a model of cultural competence and advocacy (Pacquiao, 2008)

- A moral construct of caring as communicative action (Sumner, 2010; Sumner & Fisher, 2008)

- A model of Caring Science as a sacred and hopeful paradigm (Watson, 2005, 2008a)

- Communitarian/transcultural ethical caring (Ray, 1989a, 1994a, 1999, 2010a, 2010b)

- Critical caring theory advocating health equity (Falk-Rafael & Betker, 2012).

Ray (1981, 1987, 1989b), Turkel (1992, 2001), Turkel and Ray (2000, 2001, 2004), Ray and Turkel (2010), Ray, Turkel, and Marino (2002), and Davidson et al. (2011) began advancing ideas and conducted research of complex sociocultural, political, legal, technological, and economic dimensions in relation to relational, spiritual, and ethical caring in bureaucratic healthcare organizations over the past three decades. The research reflects the dialectic of the emergence of relational-caring complexity and how structures or patterns emerge and are synthesized from the study of the meaning of relational-caring actions in complex healthcare organizations.

COMPLEXITY SCIENCES AND RELATIONAL-CARING COMPLEXITY SCIENCE

Complexity science—or now the more comprehensive term complexity sciences—is/are the science/s of wholeness and quality incorporating theories of change. Complexity sciences are also known as "complex adaptive systems" (CAS) that emerge from nonlinear interactivity (Davidson et al., 2011; Smith, 2011). Complexity scientists state fundamentally that all things in nature are interconnected, integral with the environment, interrelated, nonlinear, structurally similar, holonomic, organized into patterns, and self-organizing (Davidson et al., 2011; Peat, 2003). Complexity science applications in nursing revealed that the idea of self-organization is a *relational* self-organizing process by virtue of caring, the action of love (Davidson et al., 2011). After Einstein's theory of relativity, quantum theorists and complexity scientists developed theories, such as quantum theory, nonlinear systems theory, particle theory, string theory, fractal theory, chaos theory, and so forth. In nursing, the science of unitary human beings (SUHB; Ray, 1994b), holographic theory (Ray & Turkel, 2010), and Relational-Caring Complexity Theory have reflected some (but not all) of these selected concepts (Davidson et al., 2011; Ray, 2011; Ray & Turkel, 2010, 2012; Rogers, 1970; Smith, 2011; Turkel & Ray, 2000, 2001). Within the sciences, the discovery of constructs, such as interconnectedness, belongingness, uncertainty, patterning, hysteresis (patterns reflect their past history), and pattern transformation facilitate understanding of change over time. These patterns reveal, for the most part, no rational predictable behavior, but the emergence of new, more complex structures known as "nonlinear emergent properties" (Peat, 2003). In this process, the observer cannot be separated from the observed (Heisenberg's Principle of Uncertainty); the future is always open, self-organizing yet always changing (emerging). Rather than a view of science earlier established as mechanistic, controllable, objective, and predictable there is now acknowledgment of views like spontaneous activity, uncertainty, and unpredictability that are dynamic, holistic, and complex within complexity sciences (Peat, 2003). The ontology and epistemology of nursing science as interconnected and relational is congruent with some of the principles of complexity sciences.

The simultaneity and unitary-transformative paradigms highlight some confluence (albeit not all) between the scientific worldview of nursing and complexity sciences (Newman et al., 2008). Four decades ago, Rogers's (1970) conceptual system of the SUHB illuminated the integrality of the human and environment. Her ideas highlighted the view that human beings are patterned energy fields without boundaries and are continually changing and creatively emerging. As such, Rogers's conceptual system of mutual patterning of the human-environmental field characterizes the human life and complex whole systems (known by their patterns that reflect wholeness). Rogers (1970) claimed that "[t]he capacity of life to transcend itself, for new forms to emerge, for new levels of complexity to evolve, predicates a future that cannot be foretold" (p. 57). Rogers rejected the notion of self-organization in preference for the coevolving, integral nature of the mutual process, which is also supported by the research of Ray and Turkel (Ray, 1981, 1987, 1989a, 1989b, 1994b; Ray & Turkel, 2010, 2012; Ray et al., 2002; Turkel, 1992, 2001; Turkel & Ray, 2000, 2001, 2004) and Davidson, Ray, and Turkel (2011). In the treatise on the contemporary state of nursing science grounded particularly on the SUHB followed by related theories, relationship emerged as the central focus of the discipline (Newman et al., 2008). Relationship in this view incorporates notions of a patterned energy field, the undivided whole of the mutually unfolding human-environmental field. Leininger (1977), Newman et al., (2008), Roach (1987/2002), Watson (1979, 1985, 2005, 2008a, 2008b), Ray (1981, 1989a, 2010a, 2010b), and Ray and Turkel (Davidson et al., 2011; Ray & Turkel, 2010; Turkel & Ray, 2000, 2001, 2004) to name a few nursing scholars envisioned this energy in the universe and in nursing as a caring relationship—an ethic of caring and love and a spiritual force, for example, immanent (relational process within the world) and transcendent (spiritual, inspired, intuitive, -eternal) energy forces wherein inspired value-based ethical choices in networks of relationship unfold. This process secures conscience in critical self-reflection within the moral tradition (Ray, 2010a). Relationalcaring complexity thus is a power that binds by definition and frees by spiritual and ethical choices so that creativity and "values-in-action" (Chinn, 2013) can continually emerge, flourish, and transform.

THE THEORY OF RELATIONAL-CARING COMPLEXITY IN NURSING LEADERSHIP

Nursing practice and healthcare leadership are driven by a complex system of humanistic-, spiritual-, and ethical-caring dimensions, economics, technology, legal regulations, and politics in local, national, and international organizations. Ray advanced a grounded Theory of Bureaucratic Caring (BCT) that emerged from a study in the complex organization of a hospital and identified these phenomena with *differential caring* discovered as a quality of caring in diverse clinical and administrative units. Use of Hegelian philosophy components of thesis, antithesis, and synthesis fostered the emergence of the formal BCT (structure in the complex organization) that became apparent in the study of the hospital organizational culture. The thesis of caring as humanistic, spiritual, ethical, and social in relation to the antithesis of the bureaucracy (political, legal, economic, and technological) was discerned as a new synthesis—the BCT (Davidson et al., 2011; Ray, 1981, 1987, 1989a, 1989b, 2010a, 2011; Ray & Turkel, 2010). "By researching and understanding the meaning of caring as an expression of the complex human-environment mutual process," (Davidson et al., 2011, p. xxxii) insight about the complexity of caring in nursing and organizations as holographic was revealed showing the *relational* self-organizing quality of the interrelationship of parts and wholes (holism) in the complexity of nursing as caring in organizational cultures. Caring, therefore, is a complex, transcultural, relational process, grounded in an ethical and spiritual complex organizational context of sociopolitical, economic, and technological patterning. Right action and justice or fairness in terms of the social-cultural and relational-caring dynamics were reflected upon, debated, and/or enacted within the complex dynamical structure of the organizational moral community.

Following the discovery the BCT, Ray and Turkel studied the "economics/business" of caring in nursing and healthcare organizations for two decades (Davidson et al., 2011; Ray, 1981, 1987, 1989a, 1989b; Ray & Turkel, 2010, 2012; Ray et al., 2002; Turkel, 2001; Turkel & Ray, 2000, 2001). Subsequently, they discovered the theory of Relational-Caring Complexity (economic-caring theory; Davidson et al., 2011; Ray & Turkel, 2012; Turkel & Ray, 2000, 2001). This theory is grounded in the BCT and additional research and theory development, such as Turkel's "Struggling to find a balance: A grounded theory of the nurse-patient relationship within an economic context." (1992, 2003). With both the knowledge gained from this research on economic caring and ideas inspired by the theorist, Foa (1971), on the relationship among goods, money, services, and interpersonal resources such as love (caring), status, and communication, the Relational Caring Complexity Theory highlighted how important it is for administrators and practicing nurse leaders to invest in human capital and social justice. From two decades of research and the transtheoretical evolution of the study of economic caring within complex healthcare organizations, Ray and Turkel's (2012) Relational Caring Complexity Theory illuminates the enfolding of an organizational community as a living organism where patterns and processes of nursing and caring in the contemporary organizational culture of healthcare systems unfold to influence, improve, and transform nurse and patient outcomes. The source of life in these organizations is the critical dimension of reflective dialogue, ethical values, action, and choice-making within networks of relationships (Ray, 1994b, 2011; Ray & Turkel, 2012). The what, why, when, where, and how of choice-making by the moral community affect the lives and well-being of the members of the community (patients and families, nursing and healthcare staff, physicians, and administrators), and ultimately the social system at large. Thus, the meaning of an organizational moral community unfolds as spiritual and ethical to protect human rights and enact social justice within the structure of relationships—a communitarian caring ethic (Ray, 2010b; Ray & Turkel, 2012).

THE MORAL CARING COMMUNITY AND CHAOS THEORY

The *phenomenon of dialogue, values, choice-making, and transformative action in the moral caring community* in healthcare organizations can be explained by Chaos Theory and its metaphors (the paradoxical science of wholeness), a theory within the Sciences of Complexity, principally from the work of the physicists, Poincarê and Lorenz; and in this presentation, Relational-Caring Complexity Theory that emerged from the study of caring in complex healthcare organizations. In Chaos Theory, patterns are interconnected in a network of relationships; how they are linked correspond to principles of order, a creative reordering or self-organization at the "edge of chaos," a communication and information-process that feeds back on itself (Peat, 2003). In this work and previous research in the Theory of Relational-Caring Complexity, self-organization is considered *relational* self-organization by virtue of the focus on the nature of caring as relational—a magnetic attractor for transformation to health, healing, and well-being (Davidson et al., 2011; Ray, 2011; Ray & Turkel, 2012). In all evolving human and material systems including healthcare systems, there is a tension between order and disorder at a margin that drives change. Systems considered inflexible and unyielding are actually turbulent (witness the state of nursing and healthcare today). There is dynamic turbulent activity that takes place at this margin or boundary called the "edge of chaos" where forces of reciprocity between order and disorder occur. Small changes can produce similar or sometimes different huge-patterned results. At this boundary, there is a bifurcation point where change takes place, where something new emerges or disintegration occurs (Peat, 2003; Ray, 2011). At this bifurcation point, a phase space (the edge of chaos between order and disorder), the system encounters a future that is wide open.

As an example of this process, one fluctuation or change in the system will become dominant and a new pattern forms with greater order, or self-organization. In this chapter, we equate this process to economic repatterning and ethical-caring action where new arrangements for order are activated. As such, the phase space is a place for potential entropy (disintegration, decay, or equilibrium) or transformation. At the potential point of decay (entropy or equilibrium state) in the phase space, a "magnetic appeal" of a system is exerted that pulls the system toward it. The system hesitates and is seemingly offered a choice among various possible directions in evolution. Through the intertwining of iterations or feedback loops in the phase space, the chaotic state (disorder and order) contain the possibilities for "self-organization"—structure, processes, patterns. The system is now free to seek out its own solution to the current situation; it chooses one possible future leaving the others behind. Chaos, rather than being a mindless movement has awareness; it seeks out and chooses its own subtle form of order. Bifurcation points constitute a living history of the choices made in living systems from primordial beginnings to complex cellular and sociocultural forms of today (Peat, 2003; Ray, 1994b, 2011). As such, systems self-organize through choice-making. The processes in human sociocultural systems reflect the mutual human-environment relationship. These processes are inseparable, representing an intricate holism within chaos (disorder and order) in the networks of relationship that are continually emerging (Peat, 2003; Ray, 1994b, 2011; Ray & Turkel, 2012). (To reiterate, self-organizing or self-organization in nursing is *relational* self-organization because of the magnetic appeal or attractor of relational caring [the action of love and ethical reflection] in the network of relationships [Foa, 1971; Turkel, 2003].)

Relational-Caring Complexity Theory is a dynamic model of nursing, caring, inquiry, and spiritual and ethical choice-making discovered through our research on organizational caring within networks of the caring relationship that emerges in holistic systems in nursing and healthcare. The magnetic appeal in the "phase space" was identified and validated as caring and the spiritual and ethical processes for transformation and again as reinforced throughout this paper, is referred to as "relational self-organization" (Davidson et al., 2011; Foa, 1971; Ray, 2011; Turkel, 2003). As such, order cocreated is that of choices made in relationship and is associated with patterns of spiritual and ethical caring. Patterns of the mutual human-environment caring relationship continually enfold and unfold in complex moral healthcare communities. The theory calls for new ways of continually seeking understanding of systems as living organisms and moral communities—as places where social justice and human rights within the complexity of political-economic-legal-technological BCT systems unfold by the choices made. New ideas, new ways of relating, new ways of leading, and new ways of managing organizations make possible reasoned economic and caring responses to the challenge of systems at the edge of chaos. The "call" within and outside of the profession of nursing is caring transformation (Davidson et al., 2011). The call to nurses is valuing and putting into practice relational-caring science and art within highly medicalized and bureaucratic economic systems. In studies related to the emergence of the Theory of Relational-Caring Complexity, relational human caring, not cost alone, was the predictor of the *value* of nursing and healthy outcomes for patients (Ray, 2011; Ray & Turkel, 2012; Ray et al., 2002, 2011; Turkel & Ray, 2000, 2001).

The following section presents examples of how starting small in organizations makes a huge difference in nursing practice and healthcare systems. A critical reflective action-learning framework has been identified to initiate change in select healthcare organizations (Ray et al., 2011). With relational spiritual and ethical caring at the center of choice-making, nurses are translating the Theory of Relational-Caring Complexity in practice and facilitating *relational* self-organization to emancipate nurses, patients, administrators, and others from many organizational issues, especially economic or bottom line and political issues. Relational-Caring Complexity Theory provides a framework to help nurses understand human rights and justice and the complexity of healthcare organizations in terms of how meaning and choices are made within the context of these complex organizations. The theory addresses how new *meanings* of knowledge are generated through dialogue, participation, and critical reflexive and reflective interpretation (the *emancipatory interest*; Ray, 2011; Ray & Turkel, 2012; Ray et al., 2002) can support or evaluate the choices made to transform the moral community.

The Praxis Environment of Nursing in the Complex System of Healthcare Networks

Social justice, caring values, and economic realities of nursing practice and healthcare policy, as we have learned, are not new challenges or concerns for the discipline and profession of nursing. Registered nurses have contributed to the scholarly discourse on and practice of the principles of social justice and human rights within economic healthcare systems for over 75 years. Nursing has been committed to a moral ideal of protecting, preserving, and enhancing human dignity and translating this ethical ideal and right into practice by integrating the language of human caring into moral action (caring values-in-action) from a theoretical and philosophical perspective (Davidson et al., 2011; Leininger, 1977; Ray, 1981, 1987, 1994b, 2010a, 2010b; Roach, 1987/2002; Sumner & Fisher, 2008; Watson, 1985). Within large healthcare organizations, registered nurses value integrating caring into practice but often leaders and administrators do not value caring as a practice framework nor empower nurses to implement their values throughout the organization. Hospital leaders focus on customer service approaches to care and patient satisfaction scores instead of valuing theory-guided professional nursing practice models. Concepts related to human caring in the past have not been dominant aspects of educational curricula for the majority of registered nurses. Baccalaureate education continues to focus on the medical paradigm, the disease process, and empirical knowledge; however, change is emerging with attention in university education to the identification of caring, culture, and complexity within the Essentials of Nursing of the American Association of Colleges of Nursing. With these changes in the area of nursing scholarship, the authors trust that new knowledge development will focus on not only clinical interventions, disease prevention, and the response to disease from the perspective of pathology and traditional empirical science but also the human caring perspective. Funding from the National Institute for Nursing Research (NINR) is focused primarily on scientific research related to symptom management, disease prevention, or response to disease. But change is occurring too with funding; for example, consideration is being given to palliative and end-of-life care. One can question, however, whether concepts such as relationships, peace, social justice, caring, humanity, morality, and consciousness will become central to the discipline of nursing and funding sources overall or will these concepts remain the core values and areas of discourse for a small select group of scholars? The bigger question is how will the traditional and nontraditional outcomes of aesthetic praxis, caring-healing modalities, and social justice be studied and disseminated if there is insufficient funding for scholars to pursue in-depth systematic research?

PRAXIS EMERGING FROM HISTORICAL CONSTRAINTS

Moral conflict ensues primarily because of issues related to healthcare economics and human caring (Davidson et al., 2011; Ray, 1987, 1989b), which have been either neglected or not reconciled by the majority of leaders in healthcare. For example, in 1929, Fox wrote about the concerns related to the economics of nursing when private nursing was a luxury that only 10% to 15% of the public could afford. Fox questioned whether (private) nursing care should be based on the patient's need for care rather than income. She expressed concerns related to inequality in the distribution of nursing services and the high cost of care within the current system. Fox (1929) concluded that the healthcare system of the future must "conduct the entire undertaking according to the most enlightened economic, social, and professional standards" (p. 1044).

Historically, before Fox's vision became a reality in terms of social justice within the economics of nursing, the Great Depression of the 1930s significantly influenced healthcare financing as hospital and physician organizations struggled with the growing inability of patients to pay their hospital bills. Nurses' passion for social justice prevailed, not as forcefully within the hospital setting, but more with public health/community nursing. When public health began to expand during the 1930s and 1940s, registered nurses proved themselves to be capable and courageous just as they had during World War I, in the 1930s and 1940s, as during the period of World War I and beyond. The irony of the era was that the nurses in practice continually faced social injustice from hospital administrators. Hospitals maintained control over nursing practice and education for a long period of time (L. Y. Kelly, 1985). Salaries for registered nurses were inadequate and nursing students provided the labor. Administrators made no attempt to identify the real cost-value of nursing care. As always, the focus of nursing care was doing for the patients even though nursing practice was dominated by the medical model and physicians' orders.

THE PARADOX BETWEEN CARING AND HEALTHCARE ECONOMICS

In 1965, Congress passed two healthcare programs, Medicare and Medicaid, both of which were amendments to the Social Security Act (Williams & Torrens, 1993). During the era of retrospective cost-based reimbursement from 1965 to 1983, hospitals were reimbursed according to their costs. This meant hospitals were paid their costs, whatever they were, plus 2% resulting in a net income and cash flow greater than anything hospitals had ever had before (Feldstein, 1988). In the 1950s and 1960s, nursing practice was influenced by the writings of Peplau (1952) and Orlando (1961), two theorists focused on the nurse–patient relationship. The concept, caring, was not specifically integral to their theories, but relationship was. During that time, social injustice within the practice of nursing continued; nursing was never costed out as a revenue source to hospitals or reimbursed as such. Instead, nursing costs continued to be included with room and board on a flat rate basis, regardless of what care or caring nurses were provided. This meant that the economic value of nursing care or caring could not be determined or reimbursed (Shaffer, 1985).

The unregulated year-after-year growth in healthcare costs served as the catalyst for the prospective payment system for Medicare reimbursement based on diagnostic-related groups (DRGs) in 1983 (Gapenski, 1993; Shaffer, 1985). As hospitals were reimbursed a flat fee for the entire hospitalization regardless of associated costs, hospital administrators concentrated on the salary and role of the registered nurses (Feldstein, 1988; Shaffer, 1985; Turkel, 2001). This emphasis on cost and productivity over values and caring practices of registered nurses created a dialectical tension among hospitals, administrators, and registered nurses. In some cases, this tension continues to exist today; in other cases, nurses have found their strength by committing to practicing their own caring values.

EXAMPLES OF PRAXIS PROJECTS: CARING AS EMANCIPATORY NURSING PRAXIS

The conflict of human rights and social justice *for nurses* in healthcare organizations ensues. But registered nurses are recognizing these issues as they reflect upon the state of affairs and what is needed for their patients and themselves. Nurses have been accustomed to this parallel universe in healthcare organizations, but now they are determined to give voice to their own anguish. They are committed to finding new ways to understand Caring Science, and to implement caring into their practice. The following are exemplars of caring in action being used within hospitals that reflect caring as emancipatory caring praxis:

- Creating caring-healing rooms on the nursing unit, integrating caring-healing modalities such as aromatherapy, art therapy, or music therapy into patient care

- Having self-care part of the evaluation and the traditional "skills day"

- Calling a "Code Lavender" when a colleague needs emotional support after dealing with a patient exhibiting aggressive or violent behavior

- Placing poems written by staff nurses within the unit and lounge to serve as a reminder to take a moment to center and reflect when providing care

- Initiating the language of caring including words such as "centering," "authentic presence," and "listening" as part of electronic documentation resulting in caring being visible and tangible. The choice to include such language is significant and is emancipatory. Nurses have discovered that hospital administrators cannot control caring practices!

- Organizing caring closets for patients who have no clean clothes to wear home upon discharge

- Partnering with a school to have students create cards for patients who are forgotten on the holidays

- Having unit-based bake sales to purchase bus passes for family members to visit more often than once or twice a week

- Adopting a school in the community and buying warm sweaters for the children in need.

As one nurse stated,

We open up our hearts and sometimes our wallets to do what we need to do. It is out of love; our patients are so vulnerable and have complex social and economic needs. We just do it; we don't ask permission and the feeling of giving to those in need is priceless. It reaffirms why we are in nursing.

The above exemplars are tangible expressions of caring values (values-in-action; Chinn, 2013) in practice. However, in some organizations, caring is not valued even among colleagues so one nurse practices what she referred to as the "caritas or caring conspiracy." She shared the following:

I practice caring in interactions with patients, colleagues, and physicians without labeling the behaviors as such or asking others to participate. I move forward one nurse at a time and honor small changes. I am going beyond the traditions while creating a vision for the future. I use the analogy of being the 'lone nut' and before I know it transformation begins and colleagues and physicians were commenting 'something is different, what's going on?' To me, this is an example of how as an "N of one" I created a caring movement.

RESEARCH AND NEW EMERGENCES

Turkel's (1992, 2001, 2003) research with nurse managers illuminated a dichotomy in practice between caring values and economics. In her research, the interpretive themes of nurses' way of being, reciprocal caring, and caring moment as transcendence reflected leadership practice grounded in caring values. Two direct quotes, "[i]t is frustrating being trapped in a bureaucracy that values money instead of caring," and "sometimes I find it so frustrating—I do battle in the name of caring every day" describe practice environments where caring values do not inform the philosophy and practice of leaders within complex organizations.

Watson (1979, 1985, 2005, 2008a) acknowledged human care to be the basic core value of nursing and developed a philosophy and human science of caring. Watson made explicit that human caring in nursing is a moral ideal with the intention of illuminating the nurse–patient relationship as a transpersonal caring moment. Ray (1987, 1989a, 1989b) reminded nurses that although caring may be expressed in various ways, nurses have a social covenant to society to preserve human caring in an increasing economically driven healthcare system. Ray encouraged members of the nursing profession to value interpersonal resources such as love and caring, communication, and education as a way out of the conflict in healthcare by legitimizing and expanding traditional economic models to include interpersonal resources (Ray, 1987). Ongoing research on the economics of caring showed that the preservation of caring values expressed within the nurse–patient relationship and humanistic caring were growing despite the heavy emphasis by administrators and insurance companies on cost control (Ray et al., 2002; Turkel & Ray, 2000, 2001).

With the emergence of the American Nurses Credentialing Center's (ANCC) Magnet Recognition Program® (Magnet), nursing theory moved from academia and research to practice. With new emergence and visions come discourse and at times critical critique. From a scholarly perspective, one research study demonstrated that although Magnet hospitals have greater nurse retention, enhanced nurse autonomy, and shared decision making there was no difference between Magnet and non-Magnet hospitals in terms of working conditions including nursing practice environment, patient safety culture, and overall job satisfaction (Trinkoff et al., 2010). Nursing unions such as the California Nurses Association and the Massachusetts Nurses Association have been highly critical of Magnet in terms of Magnet being a health promotion tool for hospitals while only superficially implementing key Magnet principles (Gordon, 2005) and questioned if Magnet offered only an illusion of nurse empowerment. On the web-based blog, "The Nurse Unchained," nurses have voiced concern that after Magnet is obtained, short-staffing and being excluded from decision-making returns, and that unsafe practices are in place in Magnet facilities.

However, the majority of scholarly research findings related to Magnet consistently demonstrate increased nurse empowerment, increased nurse satisfaction, increased patient satisfaction, and improved quality indicators (Goode, Blegen, Park, Vaughn, & Spetz, 2011; Hess, Desroches, Donelan, Norman, & Buerhaus, 2011; L. A. Kelly, McHugh, & Aiken, 2012). One important outcome is the integration of theory-guided practice within Magnet hospitals. Integration of caring theory into contemporary nursing practice allows for the creation of caring environments for nurses, patients, and families within today's complex healthcare organizations, a means for registered nurses to restore caring values that inform their practice (Davidson et al., 2011; Ray & Turkel, 2012; Turkel & Ray, 2004). Theory-guided practice advances both discipline and the profession of nursing. Ray and Turkel's research on organizational caring, and subsequently the Theory of Relational-Caring Complexity (Davidson et al., 2011; Ray & Turkel, 2010, 2012; Ray et al., 2002, 2011; Turkel & Ray, 2000, 2001, 2004) helps nurses begin to appreciate the complexity of caring in organizations, translate the theory into practice, and transform their knowledge and skill of spiritual and ethical choice-making to cocreate caring-healing environments at all levels. Practice outcomes demonstrate that the creation of caring-healing environments through spiritual-ethical caring action facilitates both human and environmental well-being (Chinn, 2013; DiNapoli, Nelson, Turkel, & Watson, 2010; Ray, 2011; Ray & Turkel, 2012; Ray, Turkel, & Cohn, 2011; Turkel & Ray, 2004).

By continually giving voice to the value of caring in nursing and focusing on the intentionality of creating caring interactions within complex organizations, cultural transformations become a reality. Caring theory is manifested in many practice environments through the intentionality of nurses engaging in caring interactions promoting positive outcomes of improved health and well-being for patients, families, and employees. As registered nurses are acknowledging the humanness of nursing through caring practices, new visions for the future are being cocreated. As new ways of practice emerge, traditional linear outcome measures, such as alleviation of physical symptoms for patients or traditional quality improvement appraisals, are no longer the *only* measures of success within an organization. Practicing from a caring as emancipatory nursing framework in complex organizations provides a unifying structure that guides moral choice making and allows for creative solutions of *human flourishing (transformation)* in organizations to emerge. For example, in organizations designated as Caring Science Affiliates by the Watson Caring Science Institute, the following strategies are in place: starting a board meeting with a caring reflection, initiating practices such as deep breathing and intentional focusing before entering a patient's room, acknowledging and valuing caring moments as part of nurse evaluations, and using nurse–patient relational stories and narrative for quality improvement. These examples reflect *human flourishing* (DiNapoli et al., 2010) and allow nurses and administrators to change the conversation of conflict over "bottom-line" issues toward the *valuation* of caring resources, and to move from disorder to order within the complexity sciences chaos theory framework. Moreover, attention to human flourishing as transformation provides an opportunity to think about issues from another way of knowing. Fundamentally, these caring-as-emancipation-as-praxis activities highlight the depth of the ways of knowing of Carper's (1978) empirical, ethical, aesthetic, personal knowing; Ray's (1981, 1989a, 1989b) and White's (1995) sociopolitical and economic knowing; and Chinn and Kramer's (2011) emancipatory knowing. At the same time, new approaches to the intricacies of the ways of knowing underscore the meaning of the interconnectedness of the human-environment relationship and also reenergizes the meaning of the moral community in an organization as a "living" organization.

Another example of a conceptual finding in nurse caring practice from the research leading to the discovery of the substantive Theory of Relational-Caring Complexity was *losing trust* (Ray & Turkel, 2012; Ray et al., 2002). Guided by a recent leadership practice approach within a complex healthcare system, the nursing leader Kingston (2011) noted that the trust between nursing administration and nursing staff was broken and the situation causing the loss of trust was the result of an extremely complex issue. As a consequence, negative energy ensued and impacted everyone, including patients. Each individual in the nursing situation carried within him or herself, and conveyed to each other and patients, the conflict, struggle, suffering, and pain of the complex issue. In this instance, in an example of "caring from the heart," the nurse leader helped to resolve the ethical issues and heal the moral community by initiating a caring-healing practice grounded in Caring Science. Practices or praxis of "caring from the heart" included open forums for dialogue to occur between leaders and staff, increased visibility and presence of leaders on all shifts, an intentional focus on nursing leadership to create a caring-healing environment, and practice of authentic presence and listening with staff. As D'Alfonso (2011) reminds us,

> Leaders at all levels of the healthcare organization must awaken to new ways of leading lasting change, remaining continually aware of and seeking to balance the fiscal and often dehumanizing aspects of the healthcare business debate with the

ethical-moral demands to care for the whole person (bodymindspirit) which remains central to our "raison d'être." (p. 186)

CONCLUSION

Nurses, including nurse leaders in hospitals and other complex healthcare systems, are calling for renewal to deal with critical socioeconomic-political issues in today's contemporary praxis environments. This call has been voiced for most of the "life" of professional nursing. We are between the past and future. Now is the time for continuing to illuminate this call as critical "Caring-as Emancipatory Praxis," spiritual and ethical caring science and action (values-in-action and emancipatory praxis). Delmar and Johns (2008) state, "caring ethics presupposes ethical mindfulness and the development of a perceptual, contextually bound attention" (p. 22). Thus, "the simultaneous reflection and values-in-action directed towards transforming the world" (Kagan et al., 2009, p. 67) must include significant assessment and engagement in what is critical to the well-being of both nurses and patients. The call for a dialogue about human rights and social justice, not only in academia but also and most important in practice, must be greeted with a commitment to caring action. Beginning to resolve the economic, political, and human-caring conflicts within the moral communal life of nurses and others in complex healthcare organizations *is* a necessity. This chapter sought to explicate the feminist philosophy of peace and power (Chinn, 2013) and explicate the processes of social justice and human rights using the history of the BCT, Complexity Sciences, and the Theory of Relational-Caring Complexity. The process captured the ideas of persons in the mutual human-environment process, the metaphor of chaos theory in complexity sciences, choice making in networks of relationship, and putting a theoretical name, Relational-Caring Complexity, to caring as emancipatory nursing praxis. It explored new ways to seek truth and understanding, especially to understanding human rights and justice at the direct level of praxis and how nurses can change the nature of their own practices and organizations. Moreover, the knowledge of spiritual and ethical human caring facilitated articulation of the difficulties, challenges, hopes, and transformations related to economic caring in current complex healthcare organizations. Knowledge can allow leaders of nursing to appreciate the moral voice of the community (now the moral voice of the nurse for the well-being of patients, other professionals, and themselves). Answering the call of Chinn (2013) that shows how the feminist ideal of love, ethics, human rights, and justice can guide our exercise of power is to be the advocates for these ideals within the practice of professional nursing at all levels.

Renewal is a transformative process. It is complex, human, and spiritual as well as a byword of history and complexity sciences. The renewal of cultivating humanity (Nussbaum, 1997) for human flourishing is necessary for all nurses. From the perspectives outlined in this chapter, we can see that the new sciences of complexity, the SUHB, theories of Caring Science, ideas from the study of complex healthcare organizations and economics, the BCTs and Relational-Caring Complexity, and the reflective art of leadership and practice have enlightened the meaning of nursing practice. Within the past 40 years, this unfolding of a critically oriented Caring Science illuminating complexity sciences and incorporating ideas of social justice and human rights is caring as *emancipatory praxis*. On the one hand, nursing has to demand from healthcare administrators, economists, politicians, and educators moral caring action, and on the other hand, demand from itself, ethical knowledge, caring wisdom, and prudence (values-in-action) to permit the moral voice of all to be heard. Voices that arise out of cultivating humanity (Nussbaum, 1997) and human caring amidst knowledge of history and culture, complex science, and complex organizations will encourage and support the unfolding of right ethical principles of justice and human rights to guide moral social behaviors and human flourishing in organizations and communities. The plea to enact feminist principles through the genuine power of love and peace building and emancipation is a challenging order. But it can be accomplished. It is based on the philosophical basis of social justice and human rights regarding fairness, equity, and protection of all people and an understanding of the historical evolution of what it means to be human in *all* socioeconomic-political contexts. The communal mode of relationship as creative love, ethics, and caring and healing is not sentimental but a dynamic spiritual power unfolding within each of us as persons who believe in the transformative power to cocreate something important. We have to grant to the other a share in our being through loving communion and communication (Ray, 2010b). If nurses demand human rights and social justice in the workplace, nurses have the obligation to understand social contexts, promote moral mindfulness, seek ethical knowledge, exercise ethical evaluation and judgment, and promote caring as emancipatory praxis within the moral community. Respect for persons, cultivating humanity through a commitment to peace, power, justice, and caring are uncompromising.

NEXT ERA POSSIBILITIES

Education
- How can we integrate concepts of social justice, human rights, and Relational-Caring Complexity into nursing curricula at all levels?
- How can we expand nursing curricula at all levels to allow for creation of praxis projects?

Research
- What future research studies can we develop using Relational-Caring Complexity as the nursing theoretical framework?
- How we can expand the traditional research paradigm to include social justice and human rights as a funding priority?

Praxis
- How can we reframe the language of emancipatory nursing praxis for nursing leadership?
- How can we assist registered nurses in practice and educational settings to use the concepts from social justice and human rights to enhance empowerment?

Theory and Knowledge Development
- What middle-range theory could we create grounded in social justice and Unitary Caring Science?
- How can we use emancipatory nursing praxis to advance disciplinary specific knowledge?

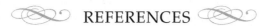 **REFERENCES**

American Nurses Association. (2003). *Code of ethics for nurses with interpretive statements*. Washington, DC: American Nurses Publishing.

Bekemeier, B., & Butterfield, P. (2005). Unreconciled inconsistencies: A critical review of the concept of social justice in 3 national nursing documents. *Advances in Nursing Science, 28*(2), 152–162. doi:10.1097/00012272-200504000-00007

Carper, B. (1978). Fundamental patterns of knowing in nursing. *Advances in Nursing Science, 1*(1), 13–23. doi:10.1097/00012272-197810000-00004

Chinn, P. L. (2013). *Peace and power: New directions for building community* (8th ed.). Burlington, MA: Jones & Bartlett.

Chinn, P. L., & Kramer, M. (2011). *Integrated theory and knowledge development in nursing* (8th ed.). St. Louis, MO: Elsevier Mosby.

Clingerman, E. (2011). Social justice: A framework for culturally competent care. *Journal of Transcultural Nursing, 22*(4), 334–341. doi:10.1177/1043659611414185

Cowling, W. R., & Chinn, P. L. (2001). Conversation across paradigms: Unitary-transformative and critical feminist perspectives. *Scholarly Inquiry for Nursing Practice, 15*, 347–370.

D'Alfonso, J. (2011). Economics, caring and complexity. In A. W. Davidson, M. A. Ray, & M. C. Turkel (Eds.), *Nursing, caring, and complexity science: For human-environment well-being* (pp. 186–189). New York, NY: Springer Publishing.

Davidson, A., Ray, M., & Turkel, M. (2011). *Nursing, caring, and complexity science: For human-environment well-being*. New York, NY: Springer Publishing.

Delmar, C., & Johns, C. (Eds.). (2008). *The good, the wise and the right clinical nursing practice*. Aalborg, Denmark: Aalborg Hospital, Arhus University Hospital.

DiNapoli, P., Nelson, J., Turkel, M., & Watson, J. (2010). Measuring the caritas processes: Caring factor survey. *International Journal for Human Caring, 14*(3), 16–21.

Douglas, M. K., Pierce, J. U., Rosenkoetter, M., Pacquiao, D., Callister, L. C., Hattar-Pollara, M., … Purnell, L. (2011). Standards of practice for culturally competent nursing care: 2011 Update. *Journal of Transcultural Nursing, 22*(4), 317–333. doi:10.1177/1043659611412965

Falk-Rafael, A., & Betker, C. (2012). Witnessing social injustice downstream and advocating for health equity upstream: "The trombone slide" of nursing. *Advances in Nursing Science, 35*(2), 98–112. doi:10.1097/ANS.0b013e31824fe70f

Feldstein, P. J. (1988). The politics of health legislation: An economic perspective. Ann Arbor, MI: Health Administration Press.

Foa, U. G. (1971). Interpersonal and economic resources. *Science, 171*(3969), 345–351. doi:10.1126/science.171.3969.345

Fox, E. (1929). The economics of nursing. *American Journal of Nursing, 29*(9), 1037–1044. doi:10.1097/00000446-192909000-00002

Gapenski, L. C. (1993). *Understanding healthcare financial management: Text, cases, and models*. Ann Arbor, MI: Health Administration Press.

Goode, C. J., Blegen, M. A., Park, S. H., Vaughn, T., & Spetz, J. (2011). Comparison of patient outcomes in Magnet® and non-Magnet hospitals. *Journal of Nursing Administration, 41*(12), 517–523. doi:10.1097/NNA.0b013e3182378b7c

Gordon, S. (2005). *Nursing against the odds: How health care cost cutting, media stereotypes, and medical hubris undermine nursing and patient care*. Ithaca, NY: Cornell University Press.

Hess, R., Desroches, C., Donelan, K., Norman, L., & Buerhaus, P. I. (2011). Perceptions of nurses in Magnet® hospitals, non-Magnet hospitals, and hospitals pursuing Magnet status. *Journal of Nursing Administration, 41*(7-8), 315–323. doi:10.1097/NNA.0b013e31822509e2

International Council of Nurses. (2009). *Nursing matters: ICN on health and human rights* [Fact Sheet]. Retrieved from http://www.icn.ch/images/stories/documents/publications/fact_sheets/10b_FS-Health_Human_Rights.pdf

Kagan, P. N., Smith, M. C., Cowling, W. R., & Chinn, P. L. (2009). A nursing manifesto: An emancipatory call for knowledge development, conscience, and praxis. *Nursing Philosophy, 11*, 67–84. doi:10.1111/j.1466-769X.2009.00422.x

Kalisch, P. A. & Kalisch, B. J. (2003). *American nursing: A history* (4th ed.). Philadelphia, PA: Lippincott Williams & Wilkins.

Kelly, L. A., McHugh, M. D., & Aiken, L. H. (2012). Nursing outcomes in Magnet® and non-Magnet hospitals. *Journal of Nursing Administration, 42*(Suppl. 10), S44–S49. doi:10.1097/01.NNA.0000420394.18284.4f

Kelly, L. Y. (1985). *Dimensions of professional nursing* (5th ed.). New York, NY: Macmillan.

Kingston, M. (2011). *When trust is broken: Let the healing begin.* Poster abstract and poster session at the International Caritas Consortium, Woodland, TX.

Kirkham, S. R., & Browne, A. J. (2006). Toward a critical theoretical interpretation of social justice discourse in nursing. *Advances in Nursing Science, 29*(4), 324–339. doi:10.1097/00012272-200610000-00006

Leininger, M. (1977, March). The phenomenon of caring. Part V caring: The essence and central focus of nursing. *Nursing Research Report, 12*(1), 2–14.

Lloyd, A. (1931). Social responsibility: An aim in nursing education. *American Journal of Nursing, 31*(8), 907–911. doi:10.1097/00000446-193108000-00002

MacIntyre, A. (1996). *A short history of ethics.* New York, NY: Simon & Schuster.

Miller, J. E., Leininger, M., Leuning, C., Pacquiao, D., Andrews, M., Ludwig-Beymer, P., & Papadopoulos, I. (2008). Transcultural nursing society position statement on human rights. *Journal of Transcultural Nursing, 19*(1), 5–7. doi:10.1177/1043659607309147

Newman, M. A., Smith, M. C., Pharris, M. D., & Jones, D. (2008). The focus of the discipline revisited. *Advances in Nursing Science, 31*(1), E16–E27. doi:10.1097/01.ANS.0000311533.65941.f1

Nightingale, F. (1992). *Notes on nursing.* Philadelphia, PA: J. B. Lippincott. (Original work published 1859)

Nussbaum, M. C. (1997). *Cultivating humanity.* Cambridge, MA: Harvard University Press.

Orlando, I. J. (1961). *The dynamic nurse-patient relationship.* New York, NY: G. P. Putman.

Pacquiao, D. F. (2008). Nursing care of vulnerable populations using a framework of cultural competence, social justice and human rights. *Contemporary Nurse, 28*(1-2), 189–197. doi:10.5172/conu.673.28.1-2.189

Peat, F. D. (2003). *From certainty to uncertainty: The story of science and ideas in the twentieth century.* Washington, DC: Joseph Henry Press.

Peplau, H. E. (1952). *Interpersonal relations in nursing.* New York, NY: G. P. Putman.

Rawls, J. (2007a). Distributive justice: Equality, entitlement and merit. In M. J. Sandel (Ed.), *Justice: A reader* (pp. 223–226). Oxford, NY: Oxford University Press.

Rawls, J. (2007b). Justice as fairness. In M. J. Sandel (Ed.), *Justice: A reader* (pp. 203–221). Oxford, UK: Oxford University Press.

Ray, M. A. (1981). *A study of caring within an institutional culture* (PhD Dissertation). Salt Lake City: University of Utah.

Ray, M. A. (1987). Healthcare economics and human caring in nursing: Why the moral conflict must be resolved. *Family & Community Health, 10*(1), 35–43. doi:10.1097/00003727-198705000-00007

Ray, M. A. (1989a). The theory of bureaucratic caring for nursing practice in the organizational culture. *Nursing Administration Quarterly, 13*(2), 31–42. doi:10.1097/00006216-198901320-00007

Ray, M. A. (1989b). Transcultural caring: Political and economic visions. *Journal of Transcultural Nursing, 1*(1), 17–21. doi:10.1177/104365968900100104

Ray, M. A. (1992). Critical theory as a framework to enhance nursing science. *Nursing Science Quarterly, 5*(3), 98–101. doi:10.1177/089431849200500302

Ray, M. A. (1994a). Communal moral experience as the starting point for research in health care ethics. *Nursing Outlook, 42*(3), 104–109. doi:10.1016/0029-6554(94)90085-X

Ray, M. A. (1994b). Complex caring dynamics: A unifying model of nursing inquiry. *Theoretic and Applied Chaos in Nursing, 1*(1), 23–32.

Ray, M. A. (1999). Critical theory as a framework to enhance nursing science. In E. C. Polifroni & M. Welch (Eds.), *Perspectives on philosophy of science in nursing: An historical and contemporary anthology* (pp. 382–386). Philadelphia, PA: Lippincott Williams Wilkins.

Ray, M. A. (2010a). *Transcultural caring dynamics in nursing and health care.* Philadelphia, PA: F. A. Davis.

Ray, M. A. (2010b). Creating caring organizations and cultures through communitarian ethics. *Journal of the World Universities Forum, 3*(5), 41–52.

Ray, M. A. (2011). Complex caring dynamics: A unifying model of nursing inquiry. In A. Davidson, M. Ray, & M. Turkel (Eds.), *Nursing, caring, and complexity science: For human-environment well-being* (pp. 31–52). New York, NY: Springer Publishing. (Reprinted from *Theoretic and Applied Chaos in Nursing, pp. 23–32,* with revisions from original article in *Theoretic and Applied Chaos in Nursing;* 1994, *1*[1], 23–32).

Ray, M. A., & Turkel, M. C. (2010). Marilyn Anne Ray's theory of bureaucratic caring. In M. E. Parker & M. C. Smith (Eds.), *Nursing theories & nursing practice* (3rd ed., pp. 472–494). Philadelphia, PA: F. A. Davis.

Ray, M. A., & Turkel, M. C. (2012). A transtheoretical evolution of caring science within complex systems. *International Journal for Human Caring, 16*(2), 28–49.

Ray, M. A., & Turkel, M. C. (2014). Caring as emancipatory nursing praxis: The theory of relational caring complexity. *Advances in Nursing Science, 37*(2), 132–146. doi:10.1097/ANS.0000000000000024

Ray, M. A., Turkel, M. C., & Cohn, J. (2011). Relational caring complexity: The study of caring and complexity in health care hospital organization. In A. Davidson, M. Ray, & M. C. Turkel (Eds.), *Nursing, caring, and complexity science: For human-environment well-being* (pp. 95–117). New York, NY: Springer Publishing.

Ray, M. A., Turkel, M. C., & Marino, F. (2002). The transformative process for nursing in workforce redevelopment. *Nursing Administration Quarterly, 26*(2), 1–14. doi:10.1097/00006216-200201000-00003

Roach, M. (2002). *Caring, the human mode of being* (2nd Rev. ed.). Ottawa, ON: Canadian Hospital Association. (Original work published 1987)

Rogers, M. E. (1970). *An introduction to the theoretical basis of nursing.* Philadelphia, PA: F. A. Davis.

Sandel, M. J. (2007). *Justice: A reader.* Oxford, UK: Oxford University Press.

Sandel, M. J. (2009). *Justice: What's the right thing to do?* New York, NY: Farrar, Straus and Giroux.

Shaffer, F. A. (1985). *Costing out nursing: Pricing our product.* New York, NY: National League for Nursing.

Smith, M. (2011). Philosophical and theoretical perspectives related to complexity science in nursing. In A. W. Davidson, M. A. Ray, & M. C. Turkel (Eds.), *Nursing, caring, and complexity science: For human-environment well-being* (pp. 1–20). New York, NY: Springer Publishing.

Sumner, J. F. (2008). *The moral construct of caring in nursing as communicative action: A theory for nursing practice.* Saarbrücken, Germany: VDM Verlag.

Sumner, J. (2010). A critical lens on the instrumentation of caring in nursing theory. *Advances in Nursing Science, 33*(1), E17–E26. doi:10.1097/ANS.0b013e3181cd8396

Trinkoff, A. M., Johantgen, M., Storr, C. L., Han, K., Liang, Y., Gurses, A. P., & Hopkinson, S. A. (2010). Comparison of working conditions among nurses in Magnet® and non-Magnet® hospitals. *Journal of Nursing Administration, 40*(7-8), 309–315. doi:10.1097/NNA.0b013e3181e93719

Turkel, M. C. (1992). *A journey into caring as experienced by nurse managers* (MS Thesis). Boca Raton: Florida Atlantic University, College of Nursing.

Turkel, M. C. (2001). Struggling to find a balance: The paradox between caring and economics. *Nursing Administration Quarterly, 26*(1), 67–82. doi:10.1097/00006216-200110000-00016

Turkel, M. C. (2003). A journey into caring as experienced by nurse managers. *International Journal for Human Caring, 7*(1), 20–26.

Turkel, M. C., & Ray M. A. (2000). Relational complexity: A theory of the nurse-patient relationship within an economic context. *Nursing Science Quarterly, 13*(4), 307–313. doi:10.1177/08943180022107843

Turkel, M. C., & Ray, M. A. (2001). Relational complexity: From grounded theory to instrument development and theoretical testing. *Nursing Science Quarterly, 14*(4), 281–287. doi:10.1177/08943180122108571

Turkel, M. C., & Ray, M. A. (2004). Creating a caring practice environment through self-renewal. *Nursing Administration Quarterly, 28*(4), 259–254. doi:10.1097/00006216-200410000-00004

United Nations. (1948, December 10). Universal declaration of human rights. Retrieved from http://www.un.org/en/universal-declaration-human-rights

United Nations. (2015, July 1). *The Millennium Development Goals Report 2015*. New York, NY. Retrieved from http://www.un.org/millenniumgoals/2015_MDG_Report/pdf/MDG%202015%20rev%20(July%201).pdf

Watson, J. (1979). *Nursing: The philosophy and science of caring*. Boston, MA: Little, Brown.

Watson, J. (1985). *Nursing: Human science and human care: A Theory of Nursing*. Norwalk, CT: Appleton-Century-Croft.

Watson, J. (2005). *Caring science as sacred science*. Philadelphia, PA: F. A. Davis.

Watson, J. (2008a). Social justice and human caring: A model of caring science as a hopeful paradigm for moral justice for humanity. *Creative Nursing, 14*(2), 54–61.

Watson, J. (2008b). *The philosophy and science of caring* (2nd Rev. ed.). Boulder: University Press of Colorado.

White, J. (1995). Patterns of knowing: Review, critique, and update. *Advances in Nursing Science, 17*(4), 73–86. doi:10.1097/00012272-199506000-00007

Williams, S. J., & Torrens, P. R. (1993). *Introduction to health services* (4th ed.). Albany, NY: Delmar.

World Health Organization. (2006, October). *Constitution of the World Health Organization: Basic Documents* (45th ed.). Retrieved from http://www.who.int/governance/eb/who_constitution_en.pdf

5

Caring in African Ontology—Ubuntu

Anna Nolte and Charlene Downing

CARITAS LITERACIES

By the end of this chapter, the caring-healing nurse will be able to

1. Describe the main characteristics of ubuntu.

2. Compare the main concepts of ubuntu with that of Watson's Caritas Theory.

3. Develop an individualized plan for caring based on ubuntu and Watson's Caritas Theory.

Caring is a universal principle. Along the journey of life, everybody needs people to care for them. The question is, What is the African concept of caring? Moreover, how does it differ from the Western concept of caring? Traditionally, the African concept of caring involved all the members of the village or community, family, relatives, tribe, and ancestors (Masango, 2006). In the African village, the principle of ubuntu introduces the concept of belonging. Meyer, Nel, and Downing (2016) support the shaping and manifestation of caring; caring happens very subtly, comes from the heart, and is manifested as love. According to Downing and Hastings-Tolsma (2016), ubuntu serves as a platform for intricate relationships between the persons and the community. Ubuntu epitomizes the promotion of standards of moral behavior while living the central philosophy of interaction between people and how relationships are manifested. Ubuntu philosophy intertwined with Watson's Caring Science is used as a theoretical lens to extend the application within the South African context.

Many sub-Saharan languages have different versions of the word "ubuntu" in their languages (Bell & Metz, 2011; Dolamo, 2013; Metz & Gaie, 2010; Prinsloo, 2001). The word means roughly "humanness" or "a person is a person through other persons." Ubuntu is seen as a tradition that is passed down from generation to generation, and through practices inherited from the past (Mohale, 2013; Murove, 2014). Moreover, ubuntu has moral values and indigenous culture codes and is often described as an indigenous philosophy (Letseka, 2012).

The newly elected postapartheid government of South Africa in 1994 adopted ubuntu as a concept to foster a stronger sense of unity. The policy of ubuntu is explained in the White Paper (Parliament of the Republic of South Africa, 1994) where it is used as a principle of "caring for each other's well-being, respect for human rights and responsibilities in promoting the well-being of the individuals and societal well-being" (Mbaya, 2010, p. 373). As an outcome of this White Paper, the concept of ubuntu was adopted in many other spheres in South Africa such as the law, the media, business, management, philosophy, and theology (Nolte & Downing, 2017). The popularity of the concept also owes much to Archbishop Desmond Tutu who developed an ubuntu philosophy embedded in Christian theology that sought to restore the oppressor's humanity by releasing and enabling the oppressed to see the oppressors as peers under God (McAllister, 2009). The extensive and important role of Desmond Tutu can be further explored at www.tutufoundationusa.org/mission-vision

In a concept analysis of ubuntu (Nolte & Downing, 2017), the authors found that ubuntu reflects an open and welcoming attitude in a person who is willing to share, to be generous and caring, and full of compassion. The community provides the relational context and support through which individuals develop and live (Whitworth & Wilkinson, 2013). Ubuntu emphasizes the values that are related to building relationships, namely sharing, compassion, understanding, reciprocity, kindness, solidarity, and sensitivity (Whitworth & Wilkinson, 2013). As a philosophy it focuses on human relations, attending to the consciousness of what it means to be human and to be in a relationship with one another (Swanson, 2007). From the concept analysis (Nolte & Downing, 2017) it became clear that caring in nursing and ubuntu are complementary because both emphasize caring.

The influence of colonization of nursing in South Africa cannot be ignored. Nursing knowledge is still largely based on apolitical, marginalizing, and racializing discourses. The process of knowledge production favors worldviews and paradigms over other views. The favoring is related to superiority of Western knowledge (Bhattacharya, 2016). The importance of building a foundation incorporating all cultural aspects into nursing care, nursing research, and nursing policy is imperative to move forward (Kirkham & Anderson, 2002). There is very little integration of postcolonial concepts and ideas into the current nursing discourse in the South African literature (McGibbon, Mulaudzi, Didham, Barton, & Sochan, 2013). The decolonization process involves affirming and activating paradigms of indigenous knowledge to reveal the wealth and richness of indigenous languages, worldviews, teachings, and experiences, all of which have been systematically excluded from history, contemporary educational institutions, and Eurocentric knowledge systems (Battiste & Young-Blood Henderson, 2012). There is almost no known nursing literature in South Africa where postcolonial-feminist concepts and ideas are integrated. Aspects that need to be addressed in such a South African caring theory might be an African philosophy, indigenous cultural aspects, social justice, and other feminist and ethical aspects of decolonization.

A question in this connection that must be answered is the following: Is there an existing middle range or grand theory in nursing related to caring that can be integrated with an African philosophy and within a postcolonialized theory? Watson's Caring Theory (WCT) has been selected to determine this. The purpose of this chapter is to look at WCT through an African lens and an African ontology, namely ubuntu, and to compare the values and ethics of ubuntu with those of WCT to show how the principles of ubuntu can be integrated with WCT to develop an African ontology of caring. This is done through a critical discussion and critique of the general concepts, values, and ethics of WCT compared with ubuntu.

THE CONCEPTS OF CARITAS THEORY COMPARED WITH UBUNTU

Nolte and Downing (2017) found some similarities between WCT and ubuntu in a concept analysis of ubuntu. First, Watson conceptualized caring as an interpersonal process between two people with transpersonal dimensions, which corresponds to the main attribute of ubuntu, namely that a person is who he or she is because of the existence and relationship with others and because of coexistence with them (Watson, 2012). Second, the caring moment, another main concept of Watson, is when the nurse and person come together in such a way that an occasion for human caring can happen. The occasion provides both parties with an opportunity to decide how to be in the relationship and what to do with the moment (Watson, 2012). The third main concept in Watson's theory relates to the Caritas Processes®. The practices of loving-kindness and compassion, and sustaining a loving trusting and caring relationship are embedded in these processes (Watson, 2012). These concepts within Watson's theory relate to the attributes of interrelatedness, reciprocity, mutuality, affinity, and kinship.

The previously discussed concepts in Watson's theory are focused to a large extent on the unique relationship between two people, whereas in ubuntu the emphasis is largely on the community which provides the relational context and support through which individuals develop. According to Watson (2012), caring requires a personal, social, moral, and spiritual engagement of the nurse and a commitment to self and other human beings. In the case of ubuntu, these requirements have to be fulfilled by the individual within a community (Watson, 2012). Watson's theory and ubuntu further share the concepts of respect, the protection and enhancement of human dignity, and the will and commitment to care (Watson, 2012). The authors recommended that future research could explore the similarities and differences between ubuntu and WCT.

Watson's Caritas Processes

Watson (1979) identified 10 carative factors in 1979 as core factors in professional nursing. The values of Watson's theory were blended with the 10 carative factors. The Caritas Processes evolved from this as a more meaningful concept. The core principles of caritas are the following (Watson, 2012):

- Practice of loving-kindness and equanimity

- Authentic presence: enabling deep belief of other

- Cultivation of one's own spiritual practice—beyond ego

- Being the caring healing environment

- Allowing for miracles

The Caritas Processes are the attributes of caring that characterize the transpersonal caring relationship. In the first five Caritas Processes, Watson focuses on the preparation of the nurse for caring and the development of a transpersonal caring relationship. Human caring requires the nurse to have a caring consciousness, an intentionality, and a healing presence (Watson, 2012). This is formed in the first five processes. The remaining five factors address those aspects of caring that involve assessing the client's health priorities and needs, the planning to address those needs, and evaluating the effectiveness of the caring processes (Rafael, 2000).

Ubuntu strongly resonates with the values of caritas in that it is grounded in concrete relationships. The values of ubuntu are based on basic respect for others, compassion, empathy, caring, and sharing. The cornerstone of ubuntu is the community. Our humanness can be enhanced only in the context of a community with other humans (Dolamo, 2013). The communal rootedness is emphasized but just as important is the interdependence of persons and the importance of human relationships (Waghid & Smeyers, 2012).

However, urbanization and industrialization have uprooted the close traditional relationships of people (Dolamo, 2013). Scott (2010) argues that the community in which ubuntu is lived is no longer the small, localized, and homogenous community, but has expanded to a larger, multicultural, international community. Ubuntu encourages a way of life that involves concern for others within an ever-widening community (Scott, 2010). The values of ubuntu can therefore also be generalized to situations in which people exist near one another, as in nursing. Ubuntu plays a universal role in the transformation of being a living phenomenon of transcending all past beliefs and understandings of a living world to embrace a living world for all humankind. Some of the most important characteristics of Watson's 10 Caritas Processes (Watson, 2008) will be compared with those of ubuntu.

Watson's Caritas Processes and Ubuntu

Caritas Process 1 is cultivating the practice of loving-kindness and equanimity toward self and other as foundational to caritas consciousness. This process is to a large extent about the personal preparation to practice and cultivate loving-kindness and equanimity toward self and other. It is a touchstone for setting intentions and developing the consciousness for caring and healing. Equanimity refers to an inner state of balance, allowing whatever there is to be observed without interference—without judging it. A practice of gratitude and forgiveness should also be cultivated. A humanistic-altruistic value system begins early in life and is influenced through interactions with others. Loving-kindness is an attitude, an intention, a stance that arises from a deeply held desire to love and to care. Centering is a way to enter into or prepare for and begin a more formal cultivation of loving-kindness and equanimity, and this can be achieved through mindfulness meditation. It can further be developed through consciousness-raising and introspection.

Personal preparation and caritas consciousness in ubuntu occur in people who grow up in a community where the phrase "I am because we are" encapsulates the interconnections between people (Poovan, Du Toit, & Engelbrecht, 2006). Ubuntu is also strengthened by a person's previous experiences in the shared spaces (Waghid & Smeyers, 2012). The formation of humanness comes through socialization. According to Mulaudzi, Libster, and Phiri (2009), a nurse can be born into and nurtured in an ubuntu community where he or she can develop a sense of belonging, commitment, and compassion. These identities of ubuntu are formed through relations in the living world: A person is who he or she is because of the existence and relationship with others and because of a coexistence with them. The living world thus provides the relational context and support through which individuals develop and live (Whitworth & Wilkinson, 2013). Humans are thus interdependently bound to each other in an ethic of care and respect (Schreiber & Tomm-Bonde, 2015).

Caritas Process 2 is being authentically present, enabling, sustaining, and honoring the faith, hope, and deep belief system and the inner-subjective life world of self or other. Everybody has a need for faith and hope. The presence of a nurse might become a beacon of hope for somebody who is alone, ill, or in despair. By being sensitive to her or his own presence and caritas consciousness, the nurse can enable the other person to access his or her own belief system. The presence of a caring professional may ignite another person's belief system and source of hope. In caritas consciousness, the nurse honors and tries to find out what is meaningful and important to the person and has respect for it. The therapeutic effects of faith and hope have through history taken on many different forms. Many of these forms are modalities grounded in diverse worldviews with spiritual-religious dimensions.

In ubuntu, spirituality lies in a person's connection to other people and the universe, as well as in a strong personal faith that drives each individual (Schreiber & Tomm-Bonde, 2015). The ubuntu view is holistic in its approach toward the human person, and it situates the well-being of a person within a web of relationships, and the source of the web is the Supreme Being. Whatever is out of balance in the human will cause spiritual, physical, and mental disease (Dolamo, 2013). Faith and a deep belief system are therefore very important in ubuntu and are realized through interpersonal relationships.

Caritas Processes 3, 4, and 5 are often combined (Watson, 2012) and are discussed together. These processes refer to the aspects of the nurse's development of self to be in caritas consciousness to practice caritas nursing. Caritas Process 3 is the cultivation of one's own spiritual practices and transpersonal self, going beyond ego-self. Nurses have to evolve and honor their own inner needs first. They have to accept themselves before they can work with the humanity of others. Nurses have to attend to their own spiritual growth, insight, mindfulness, and spiritual dimension of life to be sensitive to self and others. This process involves values clarification regarding personal and cultural beliefs that might pose barriers to transpersonal caring. Sensitivity to self can be developed by paying attention to one's own feelings and thoughts, and by being mindful of internal scripts. This process ultimately becomes transpersonal, that is, it connects the self with spirit and Source and that which is greater than ego. Caritas Process 4 is developing and sustaining a helping-trusting-caring relationship; a person becomes a person in the encounter with other persons (Jolley, 2010). In nursing, there are different types or layers of relationships: relationship to self, to the patient, to the community, and practitioner to practitioner. Authenticity and genuineness of human connection and responses are necessary for caring. Authentic caring relationship-building is concerned with the deepening of humanity, which involves a process of becoming more humane, compassionate, aware, and awake to our own and another's human dilemma. Self-awareness, sensitivity, and loving consciousness should be translated into informed moral practice in relation to self and other. A relationship is healing and is thus an intervention in itself. Nurses should be aware of how their presence and consciousness toward self and others can affect relationships with others. Caritas Process 5 is being present to and supportive of the expression of positive and negative feelings. In this process, there is attention toward feeling and expressing feelings with the assumption that this opens the door to healing. Being with another in a nonjudgmental way as the other expresses his or her feelings generates mutual trust and understanding. It sustains the authenticity of a caring relationship and affirms the shared humanity of both individuals.

Forming relationships is at the core of ubuntu and speaks to the human relational aspects of the nurse's development of self to be in caritas consciousness as reflected in Caritas Processes 3, 4, and 5. According to Nolte and Downing (2017), the main attribute of ubuntu is that identities are formed through relationships in the community, that is, a person is who he or she is because of the existence and relationship with others and because of a coexistence with them. Moreover, an ethic of care and respect binds people interdependently to each other (Schreiber & Tomm-Bonde, 2015). Humanity is thus shaped by the interaction with others (Letseka, 2012). Thus, according to ubuntu, all this implies that people cannot be human by themselves as individuals (du Plooy, 2014). In ubuntu, relations are paramount. Mutuality arises as a result of a relationship with others, and the relations are characterized by a spirit of mutual trust (Mbaya, 2010; Ncube, 2010; Ngcoya, 2015). Via ubuntu, people are thus bound together in an ethic of care and respect (Ngcoya, 2015). In ubuntu, relationships are characterized by compassion, humanness, kindness, care, loving-kindness, acceptance, empathy, friendliness, and helpfulness (Murove, 2014). Compassion is a key value in ubuntu and reflects a human quality of understanding others and wanting to help them (Nussbaum, 2003; Poovan et al., 2006).

Caritas Processes 6, 7, 8, and 9 describe the extent to which the foundational values of caritas are relevant to practice dimensions of nursing. These Caritas Processes occur within a context of mutuality in which the patient and nurse together decide not only which caring processes will be used but also the role each person will assume (Rafael, 2000). These skills are based on the practice of heart-centered loving-kindness, compassion, and equanimity. There are an intentionality and concern for the preservation of humanity, dignity, integrity, and wholeness of self and others (Watson, 2012).

Caritas Process 6 is the creative use of self and all ways of knowing as part of the caring process: engage in the artistry of caritas nursing. This Caritas Process honors creative, individualized caring that goes beyond a problem-solving process. It draws on all ways of knowing and is informed by all sources of knowing including but not limited to empirical evidence. Caritas Process 7 is engaging in genuine teaching-learning experience that attends to the unity of being and subjective meaning, that is, attempting to stay within the other's frame of reference. The intersubjective, relational aspect of teaching and giving health information is emphasized in this process. Aspects that are important here are a meaningful, trusting relationship, the readiness of the person to receive the information, and the meaning of the information for the person. It is a transpersonal process in that the experience, relationship, meaning, and significance of the experience affect both parties. Caritas Process 8 addresses creating a healing environment at all levels. This includes providing an environment of comfort, safety, beauty, and privacy where human dignity and the spirit is nurtured. The nurse's higher consciousness, including thoughts of loving-kindness, caring, healing, and forgiveness, affects the entire environment. The nurse becomes the healing environment for the other. Caritas Process 9 is administering sacred nursing acts of caring-healing by tending to human needs. Caritas nursing is a sacred act and not a physical task alone and takes place when persons are being cared for in a loving, kind way in which they feel safe and protected. The nurse thus creates a space for healing.

There are no processes and skills on how to practice ubuntu in nursing. In ubuntu, the emphasis is on belonging to a community. The patient is the center of the relationship. Both nurse and patient form part of the community. One of the characteristics of ubuntu, namely solidarity, is demonstrated through mutual responsibility and recognition (Nolte & Downing, 2017). There is a moral obligation to help the other. Relations are paramount in ubuntu. Mutuality is also very important in these relationships where the values of mutual trust, caring, support, responsibility, and recognition are pivotal (Chinouya & O'Keefe, 2006). Mutuality arises as a result of a relationship with the other, that is, a person is a person through other people. This holds for both nurse and patient. This reciprocal relationship between the nurse and patient is also built on trust and the other values of ubuntu, namely sharing, compassion, kindness, sensitivity, acceptance, and helpfulness (Ngcoya, 2015; Nolte & Downing, 2017).

Caritas Process 10 describes opening and attending to spiritual/mysterious and existential unknowns of life-death. This process makes provision for the mysteries of life and miracles that might happen as well as other deeper orders of life's phenomenological aspects that cannot be understood by the mind.

The traditional African religious view, and therefore that of ubuntu, is made up of different assumptions, namely that God is the Creator and sustainer of life and there are spirit beings in nature, and in long-departed humans, animals, and plants and objects (Dolamo, 2013). Ubuntu is about creating harmonious relationships in a community through a relationship with God (Dolamo, 2013). The whole community formulates the individual's spirituality. Faith and spirituality are communal (Masango, 2006).

CARING MOMENTS AND THE MUSIC OF UBUNTU

The dance between **ubuntu and caring moments** refers to a happening and is cherished by all the participants whereby they find a deeper and more meaningful interpretation of the moment of connectedness. Ubuntu is lived in the expression of the self and is formed in relation to the sense of belonging to the community. The individual and the community share an interconnectedness and together a greater sense of kinship and togetherness is formed. The dance of caring occurs between the individual and the moment of the happening of caring (Downing & Hastings-Tolsma, 2016).

Watson (2012) defined caring moments as an event or a happening where the nurse and patient come together in a moment of caring. In the moment of caring, a part of the person is relinquished and at the same time the persons in the interaction become more whole after the moment of connectedness. The connection is based on a position of equality and being loved and being conscious of the connection between individuals and the community. Being a partner in the dancing and the love that emanates from this connection can be compared to music that rises from the heart and where the song is written by both persons and community.

The connectedness is thus accompanied by a sense of respect and dignity for the equal needs of the persons involved in the engagement. Moreover, the nurse and patient arrive at a point where the growing of the moment will be encapsulated by both. The caring moments lead to the fittingness between the nurse and patient and set the scene for an evolution of caring that contributes to the wholeness of the nurse and patient.

Nurturing and connection is thus lived within the moment of caring (Sarpong, Bi, & Amankwah-Amoah, 2016). Intuition and openness to the needs of both patient and nurse allow for caring to be defined beyond the goal of cure and they promote caring with love within the connectedness. Listening to the heartsong, a person's needs are the platform for a deeper connection. This connection and enjoyment of the caring moment are not related to illness, but rather to the wholeness of the partnership (Downing & Hastings-Tolsma, 2016).

A caring moment forms the epicenter of the interaction; therefore, it is the center of the relationship and the cornerstone on which the relationship is b uilt (Walker & Gleaves, 2016). In the caring moment "I" becomes "we," and this unity affirms the power of caring (Watson, 2012).

A deep connectedness is found in the beating of the heart and through the art of sharing your heartspace with transpersonal caring is lived (Watson, 2012). Thus, there is movement from an unaffected position to a position of true change and radical transformation within an engagement. The connection has the potential to create unity and to be a place where greater transformation can take place, where also meaning in one's own life can be found (Watson, 2012).

Dossey and Keegan (2013) describe the whole self of the patient and professional nurse as primary ingredients within the caring relationship. The critical component is the meeting of the whole self of the patient and that of the professional nurse (Dossey & Keegan, 2013). The living with soul and deep meaning during the interactions with others and the environment thus reflects a complex connection. The interest of the nurse thus must go beyond the physical component or what is represented at the moment of initial contact. One of Watson's original definitions of the transpersonal is: "Transpersonal refers to an inter-subjective human-human relationship in which the person of the nurse affects and is affected by the person of the other ..." (Watson, 1985, p. 58).

The engagement of the authentic self and the "full use of self" in the caring moment reflects a higher consciousness (Dossey & Keegan, 2013). The sharing of the sacred space between the patient and nurse elevates the communication to a broader and deeper level of full understanding. It involves two persons meeting as one, exploring the authentic presence, providing caring, and finding meaning and purpose in the interaction (Dossey & Keegan, 2013). The relationship is thus at the center of a relational world (Walker & Gleaves, 2016). Parker in Lukose (2011, p. 29) defines transpersonal caring relationships as the connection with and embrace of the spirit and soul of the other through the process of caring, healing, and being authentic in the relationship within the specific moment.

Deep-rooted connectedness to the person in caring, the intent to bring about change, and willingness to move from curing to a caring phase are important in transpersonal caring. Subjective meaning and shared humanity serve the person and community (Clark, 2016). Transpersonal caring involves human-to-human caring with an acknowledgment that the caring outcome is healing (Watson, 2012). Moreover, according to Dossey, Selanders, Beck, and Attewell (2005), fostering and maintaining relationships is the collective call to maintain caring in a broader spectrum to support all.

Transpersonal caring involves striving to be with and to cooperate with others rather than polarizing each other. The intentionality is toward living the consciousness of love and acceptance and moving toward influencing the individual and collective well-being (Watson, 2012). Interdependence with yourself, other persons, and the wider community is a key component in living caring in terms of ubuntu. According to Chuwa (2014), "ubuntu is both a state of being and of becoming, both of which are anchored in reciprocity of care, thus as a process of self-realization through others, Ubuntu enhances the self-realization of others" (p. 39). According to Clark (2016), interdependence guides transpersonal human caring practices. Transpersonal caring is a concept supported by Nightingale (Dossey et al., 2005); she acknowledged that the care of the body and soul made nursing the finest of arts. The interwoven principle of nursing as an art and science is lived in the happening of transpersonal caring.

The capacity to extend warmth and show an awareness for other people with a level of mindfulness is a mark of transpersonal caring (Clark, 2016). A person living according to the principles of ubuntu finds that the coming together is more reflected in the collective "we" than in the individual "I." The sense of shared community is rooted deeply in a sense of belonging to a collective rather than a sense of individuality.

CONCLUSION

Living with the heartfelt moments of reflection and engagement with caring moments in life, and being part of a greater connectedness in the world is fundamental in ubuntu. We have an opportunity to cocreate and establish a caring practice in nursing that can be boundless and unique for each moment that occurs in our practice.

NEXT ERA POSSIBILITIES

Education
- How can I become and be a caring nurse educator?
- In what ways do nursing curricula reflect ubuntu?
- How do I role-model caring and ubuntu?

Research
- How can I study the outcomes of nursing practice grounded in caring and ubuntu?
- What are patients' perceptions of those practicing from a philosophy of caring and ubuntu?

Praxis
- Which dimensions of caring practice and ubuntu am I living?
- How does my current work relate to caring and ubuntu?
- What is the sound of my heart?

- How do I practice caring moments in my daily living?
- What does love sound like in the caring practice for my patients?

Theory and Knowledge Development
- What specific contributions to theory development can I make to caring and ubuntu as a nurse?
- How do I conceptualize the similarities and differences between Watson's theory and ubuntu?

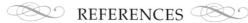 REFERENCES

Battiste, M., & Young-Blood Henderson, S. (2012). Oppression and the health of indigenous peoples. In E. A. McGibbon (Ed.), *Oppression: A social determinant of health* (pp. 89–96). Halifax, UK: Fernwood.

Bell, D. A., & Metz, T. (2011). Confucianism and ubuntu: Reflections on a dialogue between Chinese and African traditions. *Journal of Chinese Philosophy, 38*(Suppl. 1), 78–95. doi:10.1111/j.1540-6253.2012.01690.x

Bhattacharya, K. (2016). The vulnerable academic: Personal narratives and strategic de/colonizing of academic structures. *Qualitative Inquiry, 22*(5) doi:10.1177/1077800415615619

Chinouya, M., & O'Keefe, E. (2006). Zimbabwean cultural traditions in England: UbuntuHunhu as a human rights tool. *Diversity in Health and Social Care, 3,* 89–98.

Chuwa, L. (2014). *African indigenous ethics in global bioethics interpreting ubuntu.* New York, NY: Springer.

Clark, C. S. (2016). Watson's human caring theory: Pertinent transpersonal and humanities concepts for educators. *Humanities, 5,* 21. doi:10.3390/h5020021

Dolamo, R. (2013). Botho/Ubuntu: The heart of African ethics. *Scriptura, 112*(1), 1–10.

Dossey, B. M., & Keegan, L. (2013). *Holistic nursing: A handbook for practice* (6th ed.). Burlington. MA: Jones & Bartlett.

Dossey, B. M., Selanders, L. C., Beck, D. M., & Attewell, A. (2005). *Florence Nightingale today: Healing, leadership, global action.* Silver Spring, MD: American Nurses Association.

Downing, C., & Hastings-Tolsma, M. (2016). An integrative review of Albertina Sisulu and ubuntu: Relevance to caring and nursing. *Health SA Gesondheid, 21,* 214–227. doi:10.1016/j.hsag.2016.04.002

du Plooy, B. (2014). Ubuntu and the recent phenomenon of the charter for compassion. *South African Review of Sociology, 45*(1), 83–100. doi:10.1080/21528586.2014.887916

Jolley, D. R. (2010). *Ubuntu. (Master's thesis).* Cedar City: Southern Utah University.

Kirkham, S. R., & Anderson, J. M. (2002). Postcolonial nursing scholarship: From epistemology to method. *Advances in Nursing Science, 25*(1), 1–17. doi:10.1097/00012272-200209000-00004

Letseka, M. (2012). In defense of ubuntu. *Studies in Philosophy and Education, 31*(1), 47–60. doi:10.1007/s11217-011-9267-2

Lukose, A. (2011). Developing a practice model for Watsons's theory of caring. *Nursing Science Quarterly, 24*(1), 27–30. doi:10.1177/0894318410389073

Masango, M. J. S. (2006). African spirituality that shapes the concept of ubuntu. *Verbum et Ecclesia, 27*(3), 930–943. doi:10.4102/ve.v27i3.195

Mbaya, H. (2010). Social capital and the imperatives of the concept and life of ubuntu in the South African context. *Scriptura, 104,* 367–376. doi:10.7833/104-0-177

McAllister, P. (2009). Ubuntu: Beyond belief in Southern Africa. *Sites: New Series, 6*(1), 1–10. doi:10.11157/sites-vol6iss1id94

McGibbon, E., Mulaudzi, F. M., Didham, P., Barton, S., & Sochan, A. (2013). Towards decolonizing nursing: The colonization of nursing strategies for increasing the counter-narrative. *Nursing Inquiry, 21*(3), 179–191. doi:10.1111/nin.12042

Metz, T., & Gaie, B. R. (2010). The African ethic of ubuntu/botho: Implications for research on morality. *Journal of Moral Education, 39*(3), 273–290. doi:10.1080/03057240.2010.497609

Meyer, G. M., Nel, E., & Downing, C. (2016). Basic student nurse perceptions about clinical instructor caring. *Health SA Gesondheid, 21*, 444–452. doi:10.1016/j.hsag.2016.09.004

Mohale, G. (2013). What does ubuntu solve? Thoughts on the rhetoric used in the making of the Heritage Transformation Charter. *Social Dynamics, 39*(3), 481–495. doi:10.1080/02533952.2013.850813

Mulaudzi, F. M., Libster, M. M., & Phiri, S. (2009). Suggestions for creating a welcoming nursing community: Ubuntu, cultural diplomacy and mentoring. *International Journal for Human Caring, 13*(2), 45–51.

Murove, M. F. (2014). Ubuntu. *Diogenes, 59*(3-4), 36–47. doi:10.1177/0392192113493737

Ncube, L. B. (2010). Ubuntu: A transformative leadership philosophy. *Journal of Leadership Studies, 4*(3), 77–82. doi:10.1002/jls.20182

Ngcoya, M. (2015). Ubuntu: Toward an emancipatory cosmopolitanism. *International Political Sociology, 9*, 248–262. doi:10.1111/ips.12095

Nolte, A. G. W., & Downing, C. (2017). *Ubuntu – The essence of caring and being: A concept analysis.* Unpublished article.

Nussbaum, M.C. (Winter, 2003). Compassion & terror. *Daedalus, 132*(1), 10–26. Retrieved from https://www.jstor.org/stable/20027819

Parliament of the Republic of South Africa (1994). White paper on reconstruction and development [White paper]. *Government Gazette, 353,* 1–82. Retrieved from http://www.gov.za/sites/www.gov.za/files/16085_0.pdf

Poovan, N., Du Toit, M. K., & Engelbrecht, A. S. (2006). The effect of the social values of ubuntu on team effectiveness. *South African Journal of Business Management, 37*(3), 17–27.

Prinsloo, E. D. (2001). A comparison between medicine from an African (ubuntu) and Western philosophy. *Curationis, 24*(1), 58–65. doi:10.4102/curationis.v24i1.802

Rafael, A. R. (2000). Watson's philosophy, science, and theory of human caring as a conceptual framework for guiding community health nursing practice. *Advances in Nursing Science, 23*(2), 34–49. doi:10.1097/00012272-200012000-00005

Sarpong, D., Bi, J., & Amankwah-Amoah, J. (2016). On the nurturing of strategic foresight: The ubuntu perspective. *Futures, 75*, 14–23. doi:10.1016/j.futures.2015.10.007

Schreiber, R., & Tomm-Bonde, L. (2015). Ubuntu and constructivist grounded theory: An Africa methodology package. *Journal of Research in Nursing, 20*(8), 655–664. doi:10.1177/1744987115619207

Scott, C. D. (2010). Beyond racism: Ubuntu and the other. Skills at work. *Theory and Practice Journal, 3,* 71–79.

Swanson, D. M. (2007). Ubuntu: An African contribution to (re)search for/with a 'humble togetherness'. *Journal of Contemporary Issues in Education, 2*(2), 53–67.

Waghid, Y., & Smeyers, P. (2012). Reconsidering ubuntu: On the educational potential of a particular ethic of care. *Educational Philosophy and Theory, 44*(Suppl. 2), 6–20. doi:10.1111/j.1469-5812.2011.00792.x

Walker, C., & Gleaves, A. (2016). Constructing the caring higher education teacher: A theoretical framework. *Teaching and Teacher Education, 54*, 65–76. doi:10.1016/j.tate.2015.11.013

Watson, J. (1979). *Nursing: The philosophy and science of caring.* Boston, MA: Little, Brown.

Watson, J. (1985). *Nursing: Human science and human care, a theory of nursing.* Norwalk, CT: Appleton-Century-Crofts.

Watson, J. (2008). *Nursing. The philosophy and science of caring* (Rev. ed.). Boulder: University Press of Colorado Boulder.

Watson, J. (2012). *Human caring science: A theory of nursing* (2nd ed.). Sudbury, MA: Jones & Bartlett.

Whitworth, A., & Wilkinson, K. (2013). Tackling child poverty in South Africa: Implications of ubuntu for the system of social grants. *Development Southern Africa, 30*(1), 121–134. doi:10.1080/0376835X.2013.756219

6

Caring Science–Native Science: Paving Pathways of Courageous Authenticity, Advocacy, and Agency

Shawna M. McDermott

CARITAS LITERACIES

By the end of this chapter, the caring-healing nurse will be able to

1. Define values and constructs that encapsulate a Native Science worldview.

2. Recognize the expansive power and possibilities that arise from within a Caring Science–Native Science sphere of consciousness.

3. Develop a broader sense of self that reinforces an intrinsic value of being in relationship with the people, places, and (living and inanimate) things that exist in the world.

4. Identify pathways of courageous authenticity, advocacy, and agency within a professional and personal context.

⁓

Caring Science is a sacred science, a way of knowing, doing, being, and becoming that recognizes the divine and embraces the vulnerability of self and other (Watson, 2005). It is an ethic of belonging that holds space for authentic presence, embodies compassionate action, and fosters heart-centered connection. As such, it provides the courageous capacity to embrace Caring and Love—*Caritas*—as a life-giving source of knowledge and wisdom. Emerging from a relational ontology, Caring Science is energetically attuned and responsive to and reflective of a Native worldview that holds relationship as a dynamic, reverent dance of reciprocity. Thus, inviting forward a deeper exploration of Native American values, beliefs, and behaviors, and the relationships that inform and give rise from them provides a new perspective on the expansiveness of Caring Science and active engagement of loving-caring consciousness. From a shared "ethical-moral-spiritual stance"

(Watson, 2008), Caring Science and "Native Science" pave pathways of courageous authenticity, advocacy, and agency between the individual and the collective, establishing a conduit for healing and transformation.

NATIVE SCIENCE

Literature and studies related to Native American culture and history[1] are as diverse and dynamic as the people themselves, encompassing anthropological and ethnographical accounts as much as philosophical and mystical explorations. The intended focus here is to hone in on the ideas, ideals, and identity within a Native worldview that are aligned with Caring Science. Deep rooted in Native American philosophy and practices are four core values—*Interconnectedness, Wholeness, Discovery*, and *Being in Right Relation*. These values weave together in a vibrant dance, shaping and reinforcing beliefs, behaviors, and relationships that form the basis of Native ethics and culture. This dynamic interplay captures the idea that "values are the way human beings pattern and use their energy. If there is not balance between our values concerning ourselves and our values concerning others, we cannot continue to develop our true potential as human beings" (Bopp, Bopp, Brown, & Lane, 1984, p. 18).

Interconnectedness is the premise that all things are related, giving rise to opportunity and obligation to understand the impact and influence each person has on the people, places, and (living and inanimate) things that exist in the world. Holding this awareness is an invitation to honor synergistic and symbiotic ways of engagement, exchange, and expression. *Wholeness* builds upon Interconnectedness by bringing attentiveness to how everything fits together, to the connections, cycles, and components that are intertwined and integral for each individual element to derive purpose, meaning, and value. Holding this awareness is an invitation to operate from an understanding that the whole is greater than the sum of its parts and that the capacity to flourish is immanent when wholeness is embraced. *Discovery* is the dynamic unfolding of insight, inquiry, and imagination that occurs in any given moment and over the course of time. Holding this awareness is an invitation to gain perspective that the journey and the destination are one and the same, that each step, pause, and turn has the capacity to transform knowledge into wisdom. *Being in Right Relation* encompasses the power and potential of living, learning, and loving from a place of Interconnectedness, Wholeness, and Discovery. Holding this awareness is an invitation to the sacred and spiritual dimensions of "Source," where the quest for Balance and Harmony—for Truth—becomes a regenerative and life-giving process.

Greg Cajete, Director of Native American Studies at the University of New Mexico, uses the term "Native Science" to capture the philosophical and ethical underpinnings of a Native worldview. In a talk given at the Banff Centre on September 4, 2014, as part of an event exploring Indigenous Knowledge and Western Science, Cajete posits that:

> The goal of indigenous science is about ... resonance, this ability to know how to resonate ... with yourself and yourself, yourself and your community and the place in

---

[1]As of January 2018, there were 567 federally-recognized tribal entities in the United States (www.gpo.gov/fdsys/pkg/FR-2018-01-30/pdf/2018-01907.pdf). While the intent of the author is to bring forward a sense of the universal truths that influence a shared ethic across these tribal entities, each has a unique history that manifests in robust and distinct expressions of knowing, doing, being and becoming.

which you live and the natural world that you are a part of, and then ultimately with the cosmos. And so knowledge systems and ways of knowing and ways of perspective begin to congregate around those different levels of knowing and coming to know. (BanffEvents, 2015, 11:58)

Going forward, the term "Native Science" will be used to succinctly encapsulate the intrinsic and extrinsic values of Interconnectedness, Wholeness, Discovery, and Being in Right Relation, as well as the myriad of ways in which these are expressed, honored, and embodied. Specifically, two themes will be explored to bring forward the vitality and dynamic interplay of these values within the lives of Native American people, past, present, and future: Beauty and Belonging, and Ceremonies and Cycles.

Beauty and Belonging

At the most fundamental level of identity, the name that most Native tribes, clans, and nations use for themselves translates to "the People" in their own language. In many cases, this is not the name commonly known within the broader population because many tribes have long been referred to by names given to them by the European settlers and that reflect variations of terms used to describe them by other tribes (see Table 6.1). These common names either had no direct translation or meaning for the people of the tribe or had negative connotations, such as Apache—"enemy"; Comanche—"they fight with us"; or Sioux—"snakes" ("Original Tribal Names," n.d.). Over the past several decades, however, tribal leaders and communities have been reclaiming and making their own names for themselves more visible as part of intentional efforts to be known and recognized for the integrity of who they are, now and in connection to their ancestors. These tribal names reflect a Native worldview that holds deep reverence for community identity, connection with the natural world, and sense of place.

First, let us delve further into the energetic underpinnings of communal identity. Across time, Native peoples have extended welcome, expressed gratitude, invited prayer, and initiated ceremony by recognizing "All My Relations." Whether spoken in a casual or sacred context, the phrase evokes a sense of belonging, trust, respect, and unity in mind-body-spirit. Interwoven within this recognition of "All My Relations" is a discipline that acknowledges the intersection and interdependency of past, present, and future generations. This integrative knowing and thinking are captured within the well-known Great Law of Peace—Gayanashagowa (Murphy, n.d.) of the Haudenosaunee (common name "Iroquois") Confederacy:

Your heart shall be filled with peace and good will and your mind filled with a yearning for the welfare of the people of the Confederacy. With endless patience you shall carry out your duty and your firmness shall be tempered with tenderness for your people. … return to the way of the Great Law which is just and right. Look and listen for the welfare of the whole people and have always in view not only the present but also the coming generations, even those whose faces are yet beneath the surface of the ground "the unborn of the future Nation." (Sec. 28, para. 3)

This guidance is often referred to as the "seventh-generation" principle and brings sincere attentiveness to the responsibility for considering the impact actions have on the

TABLE 6.1 Native American Tribal Names and Meaning

Original Tribal Name (Reflective of Tribal Language and Culture)	Former/Common Name (Given by Others)
Akimel O'odham/*River People*	Pima/*from the Akimel O'odham phrase for "I don't know"*
Tohono O'odham/*Desert People*	Papago/*from the Akimel O'odham word for "eating tepary beans"*
Diné/*The People*	Navajo/*from a Tewa word for "planted fields"*
Haudenosaunee/*People of the Long House*	Iroquois/*from an Algonquian word meaning "real snakes"*
Onandowaga/*People of the Mountain*	Seneca/*possibly corrupted version of an Onandowaga village name, Osininka*
Dakota/*The Allies* Band names include Sisseton/*Marsh Dwellers*; Wahpeton/*Forest Dwellers*; Lakota/*The Allies*; also known as Teton/*Prairie Dwellers*	Sioux/*from an Ojibwe word meaning "little snakes"*
Anishinaabe/*Original People*	Ojibway/Ojibwe/Chippewa/*from an Algonquian word meaning "puckered," referring to their moccasin style*
Hinonoeino/*Our People*	Arapaho/*probably from a Pawnee word for "traders"*
Ohkay Owingeh/*Place of the Strong People*	San Juan Pueblo/*from Spanish custom naming a people or village in reverence to St. John the Baptist*

Source: Native American Tribe Names. (n.d.). Retrieved from http://blog.nrcprograms.org/american -indiantribes-names; Pima People. (n.d.). In *Wikipedia*. Retrieved June 24, 2018, from https://en .wikipedia.org/w/index.php?title=Pima_people&oldid=762098728; Tohono O'odham. (n.d.). In *Wikipedia*. Retrieved June 24, 2018, from https://en.wikipedia.org/w/index.php?title=Tohono _O%27odham&oldid=776844218

seven generations yet to come, as well as to holding awe, appreciation, and insight for the acts of the ancestors seven generations ago. In doing so, a person is, at this moment, an embodied life force of those who gave rise to them and those who will flow forward from them. This understanding goes beyond the intellectual-emotional process of remembering past generations or envisioning future generations. Rather, it takes root as a belief system that fosters an expansive whole-person identity, and that creates a sacred trust and impetus for leadership advocacy, personal integrity, and courageous action. This perspective forms the basis of Native identity, where individuals seek their own truths in the context of a greater collective whole. A "determination" that Mankiller (2004) shares embraces the traditional Aniyunwiya (common name: "Cherokee") premise to "not let go of one another"

(p. 50) as "Cherokee traditional identify is tied to both an individual and a collective determination to follow a good path, be responsible and loving, and help one another" (p. 50). Cordova (Moore, Peters, Jojola, & Lacy, 2007), a philosopher of Jicarilla Nde (common name "Apache") d escent, poignantly captures the duality of this identity formation:

> *We are part of a whole*
> *The "I" is a unique combination*
> *of the group*
> *that brings the "I"*
> *into existence*
> *"I" am the sum*
> *of the memories*
> *of the group*
> *of its experiences*
> *its knowledge … (p. 141)*

Accordingly, Native American families, both past and present, rely on a collaborative, intergenerational, communal infrastructure that extends beyond biological affiliations. Native language further reinforces the value and meaning of family relationships. Exploring "holism in Diné language and culture" (Witherspoon, 1977; Witherspoon & Peterson, 1995) highlights how kinship terms are articulated from a possessive point of view. For example, "it is not possible in Navajo language to say 'mother'" (Witherspoon & Peterson, 1995, p. 11); rather, the language frames the relationship by making reference to "my mother" or "your mother," and reverting to reference of "someone's mother" when the identity is more general. Furthermore, he postulates that "Navajo ontology … leads toward synthesis and integration as a means of expressing the nature of existence" (p. 12). This intimate and communal way of relating, in turn, provides a foundational frame of reference for seeing linkages across multiple dimensions, for holding a simultaneously intrinsic and extrinsic understanding of family, kinship, and community.

This relational framing leads us to explore the intuitive and metaphysical connection that Native people have with the natural world, an intimate bond made beautifully vivid by the Hopi belief that the four elements—Water, Air, Fire, and Earth—serve as primal and sacred "foundations of life." Specifically, Water is the first foundation of life, for we are first suspended in the fluid of our mother's womb. On birth, we take our first breath, and, thus, Air serves as the second foundation of life. Reliant on caregivers to nurture us as infants, the love that manifests symbolizes Fire, the third foundation of life. Moreover, finally, as we gain the physical strength and curiosity to sit, crawl, and walk, we become grounded by Earth, the fourth foundation of life (Schaefer, 2006, pp. 146–147).

Reinforcing the intentionality and consciousness that reverence for nature cultivates, Chief Luther Standing Bear spoke of how Lakota elders honored the interrelationship between humans and the world around them:

> The world was a library and its books were the stones, leaves, grass, brooks, and the birds and animals that shared, alike with us, the storms and blessings of earth. We learned to do what only the student of nature ever learns, and that was to feel beauty. (Nerburn, 1999, p. 16)

As a core value, this deep connection with all that is of the universe is possible given that:

> [in] a Native American worldview there is no divinity that exists outside the universe—primarily, because there is no "outside." Whatever is, is an indivisible, infinite, and divine something. All things are perceived as either participating in this one thing or being manifestations of the one thing. (Moore et al., 2007, pp. 145–146)

Therefore, there is no separation between human beings and the animate, inanimate, and energetic fields and forces that coexist with us, for "consciousness, awareness, is assumed to be a characteristic of the universe" (Moore et al., 2007, p. 147). Rather, there is a myriad of symbiotic intersections, synergistic extensions, and stabilizing foundations that have an innate capacity to exist in harmony (although there is recognition that humans are also capable of interfering with or disrupting this harmony).

One of the most well-known teachings of Black Elk beautifully captures the profound possibilities of embracing and embodying a unitary consciousness, a way of being and belonging that reflects the intimate connection Native peoples cultivate with the natural world and all that is:

> The first peace … is that which comes within the souls of people when they realize their relationship, their oneness, with the universe and all its powers, and when they realize that at the center of the universe dwells Wakan-Tanka, and that this center … is within each of us. (Black Elk & Brown, 1989, p. 115)

Finally, let us consider how the sense of place contributes to the identity and worldview of Native people. Cordova (Moore et al., 2007) passionately outlines the premise that "all indigenous peoples have a very strong sense of identity and that identity includes a sense of belonging in a very specific space" (p. 194). Furthermore, she postulates that "to feel the sense of place, of a bounded and definite space, involves a sense of relationship with that place, of a very specific responsibility toward that place, as a unified whole—people and place together" (p. 192). Similarly, Mankiller (2004) expresses that "the very identity of traditional tribal people is derived from the natural world, the land, and the community" (p. 14). And thus, it becomes apparent that sense of place is an integral component in solidifying the understanding of who one is within a Native worldview, related to, but distinct from, the influence of nature connection, family, and kinship.

When we hold reverence for the reciprocity of the place(s) we inhabit, we are able to hold awe for the beauty and blessings inherent in nature and for the mystery and magnificence of the universe. From this physical and metaphysical space, it is possible to foster a sense of giving, receiving, and being that is rooted and introspective as much as expansive and collaborative.

CEREMONIES AND CYCLES

Ceremonies and rituals are interwoven into the lives of Native people. In times past, they were as intrinsic an expression of life as breathing, honoring transitions and transformations, and often occurring in rhythm with nature. Today, traditional ceremonies and rituals continue or have been transformed and revitalized by Native Americans with pride, conviction, and reverence, taking place within local tribal communities as much as within urban areas where Native people are now dispersed and diverse. The focus here is on the overarching meaning and motivation of these ceremonies and rituals rather than on trying to capture the complexity and myriad of spiritual practices, values, beliefs, and behaviors. At a broad and not necessarily mutually exclusive level, ceremonies tend to fall into two categories: (a) Individual-based ceremonies characterized by acts of inquiry, invocation, and introspection; and (b) Community-based ceremonies characterized by expressions of grace, gratitude, and generosity.

Although there are a multitude of ceremonies and rituals distinctive to specific tribal peoples that reflect nuances of lifestyle, social structure/relationships, geography, and habitat, "many ceremonies [are] similar, and the meanings behind the ceremonies [are] also closely related" (McGaa, 1990, p. 45) across Native American tribes. These similarities seem to stem from a shared value system that honors Interconnectedness, Wholeness, Discovery, and Being in Right Relation.

A well-known Individual-based ceremony is the vision quest, a coming of age rite that encourages youth on the threshold of adulthood roles and responsibilities to "make contact with the Higher Power that is out there, all around us or within … to realize the vastness of the universe and our oneness with it" (McGaa, 1990, p. 75). The solitary focus of this spiritual practice is believed to connect the individual to his or her sacred and unique gifts, purpose, and life path. Balancing inquiry and introspection allows vision quest rituals to seek to expand, deepen, and integrate mental, physical, emotional, and spiritual pathways of knowing, and invite individuals to immerse themselves in the wonder and awe of the natural world to recognize that the wisdom of the universe is within them. Thus, the heightened sense of self that arises through this process is held within the context of community and the individual's place in the world at large as described in the prior section.

Regarding Community-based ceremonies, the premise of "thanksgiving" rituals is familiar to many today; however, the frequency and diversity of these ceremonies are less well known and recognized. The Haudenosaunee have a deep-rooted tradition of offering a "Thanksgiving Address," a practice that people of the six nations are encouraged to conduct daily and that serves as an integral element of their ceremonies and gatherings. The actual words from within each distinct Haudenosaunee language for this thanksgiving address translate, in one way or another, to "the words that come before all else." In a very powerful way, the thanksgiving address fosters and facilitates attunement—with one another and in connection, recognition, and gratitude for the gifts of the natural world that unfold through the seasons. Accordingly, the Haudenosaunee practice of gathering community for ceremonial thanksgiving across the year begins with the Mid-Winter Festival held in late January/early February; is followed sequentially by the Maple Festival, Thunder Festival, Strawberry Festival, and Green Corn Festival; and then ends with the Harvest Festival held in October (National Museum of the American Indian [NMAI], 2009). The excerpt of the Thanksgiving

Address that follows, developed and published in 1993 by the Six Nations Indian Museum and the Tracking Project, captures a version used within the Mohawk nation. These words of introduction provide a sense of the all-encompassing expressions of gratitude extended, as well as how this simple practice cultivates a complex understanding of unitary consciousness by calling attention to our oneness:

> We have gathered, and we see that the cycles of life continue. We have been given the duty to live in balance and harmony with each other and all living things ... we give greetings and thanks to each other as people. Now our minds are one. (Stokes & Kanawahienton, 1993, p. 1)

Although the Haudenosaunee Thanksgiving festivals capture the essence of Community-based ceremonies of Native tribes, it is important to recognize that many ceremonies bring community together to honor a transition or desired transformation that is relevant to specific individuals—puberty, wedding, health and healing, death—and thus Community is called upon to hold sacred space and to act as witness, collaborator, mentor, and confidant. Similarly, many tribes have purification and cleansing rituals, such as the sweat lodge ceremony, that invite deep personal introspection while sitting beside and among other members of the Community with shared intent for healing and spiritual transformation. As a unifying element of Native culture, "ceremony ... [is] an experiencing realization of the spirituality that surrounds all" (McGaa, 1990, p. 47) for "ceremonies ... remind us of our place in the universe and our responsibilities as human beings" (Mankiller, 2004, p. 14). Through an exploration of the structure, sequence, stories, symbols, and songs that inform and inspire Native ceremonies, it is possible to gain a sense of the reverence held for synergistic and symbiotic relationships, between people and land, between individual and community, between actions and words, between spiritual forces and singing voices. As such, it reinforces a Native worldview that the livelihood, vitality, and whole-person identity of the people are nurtured through a covenant of being in right relation. This is as true today as it was hundreds of years ago. Although there are many situations and stimuli that sadly perpetuate broken connections and imbalances among Native communities today, the wisdom is unequivocal and Native leaders within and across all tribal people are successfully bridging the divide between generations by bringing their traditional ways of knowing, doing, and being back into focus within a contemporary frame of reference (Mankiller, 2004; Markstrom, 2008; McGaa, 1990; Sheridan & Parezo, 1996; Smith, 2005). The peaceful protest against the Dakota Access Pipeline initiated by elders of the Standing Rock Indian Reservation in 2016 (standwithstandingrock.net) is a current expression of the deep-rooted and powerful conviction held for being in right relation. Extending a call to serve as "water protectors" and keepers of ancestral stories, Native and Non-Native people responded in solidarity, honoring the resonance and reciprocity of connection.

Embedded in Native values and beliefs, and reflected in ceremonies, is a recognition and deep appreciation for circles and cycles. This awareness provides context for the Native construct of viewing life as a journey and for the integrative and iterative discovery and conviction associated with living a "good life" and pursuing a "good path" with a "good mind" that holds a broad construct of community. Although all tribes have their own unique ways of conveying these themes, the message is profoundly and inextricably linked to their value system and fundamentally shapes their worldview.

Tohono O'odham—Desert People

Deep-rooted within the oral stories and cultural identity of the Tohono O'odham people is a symbol that is referred to as the "Man in the Maze." In reality, the image is a labyrinth, with seven concentric circles that take shape and form in such a way as to invite a journey toward the center. At the entry point of the maze is I'itoi, or Elder Brother, who represents Creator as much as every individual on the journey of life in this world. Because of the oral tradition, there is no one "true" version of meaning attributed to the symbol. At its core essence, however, the labyrinth acknowledges the synchronicity of being and becoming.

The center of the labyrinth holds a circle that represents the mystical wonder inherent in the four directions, the hope inherent in the regenerative cycles of the four seasons, the nourishing power inherent in the four elements, the intuitive wisdom inherent in the four states of well-being, and the transformational energy inherent across the life cycle. Thus, the inner circle shapes and reinforces an understanding that one is "a part of it." Although the center of the labyrinth represents a place of transformation and ease, the labyrinth path provides perspective on the sometimes arduous steps along the journey. Navigating the twists and turns through this symbolic labyrinth of life makes evident and reinforces the need for sacred pause and for calling upon all powers of the universe (and within) to guide and orient before taking action. With each step forward, the strength of the past as well as of the future is held in the present moment, enabling one to respectfully embrace and embody the Tohono O'odham *himdag*—the wisdom, experience, relationships, and traditions of the ancestors.

Anishinaabe—Original People

Well-known environmentalist and activist Winona LaDuke (Mississippi Band Anishinaabeg) describes "Mino Bimaatisiiwin," which means "to live a good life" (Smith, 2005, p. 43). This way of life is characterized by respectful attentiveness to the impact and influence an individual has on the world and by receptive awareness of the impact and influence the world has on him or her.

> In our community what that means is that you reaffirm those spiritual teachings from your ancestors in how you live your life, in how you make your prayers, in how you make your songs, and how you treat your relatives, who, we are taught, are of all kinds. (Smith, 2005, p. 53)

Kanienkehaka—People of the Flint

Douglas George-Kanentiio is a Haudenosaunee leader known for his passionate advocacy related to land, language, and indigenous ways of life. He shares a story about a group of people within the Mohawk community who came together in recent times with the intent to reclaim the truth of their ancestors and cultural identity. Bringing focus on "Kanekenriio," which he translates roughly into "a good mind," the group held an individual and collective desire to model and mentor (Smith, 2005, p. 89) ways of living that would "actively use the powers of persuasion, patience, tolerance, and love to restore harmony to the community" (Smith, 2005, p. 89).

Diné—The People

Deeply embedded within the ontological focus that shapes the values, beliefs, and behaviors of the Diné (common name "Navajo"), and reflected within their ceremonies, songs, rituals, and aesthetic art forms, is the concept of "Hózhó." Although this concept is often simply translated to the term "beauty," the concept of hózhó is far more expansive, holistic, and inclusive. According to Gary Witherspoon, a professor of anthropology and American Indian Studies at the University of Washington who married into a Diné family, "Hózhó … is a term that means much more than beauty. For the Navajo, hózhó expresses the intellectual notion of order, the emotional state of happiness, the physical state of health, the moral condition of good, and the aesthetic dimension of harmony" (Witherspoon & Peterson, 1995, p. 15).

As such, "Hózhóójí" is the most sacred ceremonial of the Diné; known as the Blessingway, it more accurately translates linguistically to "Along the Pathway of Hózhó" (Witherspoon & Peterson, 1995). Accordingly, ceremonial songs and prayers express the premise of being on a journey, guided and nurtured by hózhó as much as recognizing self as inseparable from hózhó.

> *With beauty (hózhó) before me, I walk.*
> *With beauty behind me, I walk.*
> *With beauty above me, I walk.*
> *With beauty below me, I walk. (p. 15)*

From generation to generation, this intricate and intimate recognition and knowing of hózhó sustains, as captured in Lyla June Johnston's (2012) spoken word piece:

> *Hózhó is Undeniable Beauty*
> *Hózhó is in every breath that we give to the trees.*
> *And in every breath they give to us in return.*
> *Hózhó is reciprocity.*
> *… Hózhó is remembering your own beauty.*
> *… Hózhó is not something you can experience on your own.*
> *… Hózhó is interbeauty.*

Lakota—The Allies

In the 1930s, American John Neihardt spent time with Black Elk, a Lakota holy man revered for a vision he had as a youth that conveyed a powerful understanding of universal connection, harmony, and vitality. At a time when Native American tribes were being decimated and fragmented, Black Elk's vision as told by Neihardt speaks to the strength of community that once was whole and that he proclaimed would be yet again in the future.

> I was standing on the highest mountain of them all, and round about beneath me was the whole hoop of the world … I saw that the sacred hoop of my people was one of many hoops that made one circle, wide as daylight and as starlight …. (Black Elk & Neihardt, 1988, p. 43)

FOUR DIRECTIONS

Another way of contemplating the qualities that enable one to navigate a "good life" on the "good path/road" is to reflect on the characteristics associated with each of the four directions. Although there are nuances and complexities within the teachings of Native tribes, there are foundational beliefs. The East inspires one to harness courage, step into truth, and seek pathways of renewal in energetic alignment with the rising sun as well as the season of spring. In doing so, it becomes possible to recognize and facilitate connections, to gain insight through inquiry, and to embrace roles of leadership and mentorship with humility. As the East also represents the time of childhood, it invites individuals to remember the beauty, tranquility, and gratitude that arise when they are fully aware and attuned to the present moment, for "as young children, we knew instinctively how to do this" (Bopp et al., 1984, p. 45).

The South taps into the radiance of self and relationships held with others energetically inspired by the life-giving rays of the midday sun and the abundance of summer. One is called to cultivate empathy and compassion for "the South is also the place of the heart, of generosity, of sensitivity to the feelings of others, of loyalty, of noble passions and of love" (Bopp et al., 1984, p. 48). From this emotional frame of reference, intelligence, and expansiveness, the senses are activated and integrated, enabling one to give and receive from a place of wholeness.

In the West, dreams are invited for one to consider what is possible with conviction, and to stay open in the midst of transitions and unknowns. Informed by the courage of faithfulness and trust in renewal inherent in the season of fall, one is guided by perseverance and vision for the West is ignited by the energy of "the Thunder Beings … the bringers of power: Power to heal. Power to protect and defend. Power to see and to know" (Bopp et al., 1984, p. 53). Thus, bringing forward our greatest sense of self from this place of integrity requires us to align our hearts and minds, to acknowledge our oneness with the universe, and to fully embrace all dimensions of our being—physical, emotional, mental, and spiritual.

Moreover, finally, in the North, imagination is relied on as much as intellect to guide one on his or her journey, embodying the energy of one's elders for the North is "the dawning place of true wisdom" (Bopp et al., 1984, p. 62). It is at this stage of the journey that endurance and wholeness are recognized as the ability to hold "the past, the present and the future as one" (p. 66). Associated with winter, this is a time to take sacred pause, to detach from the shadow side of things, and to bear witness to the completion of cycles.

Within the context of Ceremonies and Cycles, an attentiveness and affinity for discovery evolves, bringing into focus the dynamic states of transition and transformation, regeneration and renewal, and healing and wholeness that give rise to Beauty and Belonging. This frame of reference underpins Native American worldview and is differentiated from the Western worldview:

> In Western world view and in classical science, the ontological focus has been on the fundamental and smallest building blocks of the universe that can be isolated … This dissection of the world into ever smaller and smaller pieces is intended to take us closer to the nature of existence, revealing to us the keys to understanding our universe and life within it … The focus of [Diné] ontology is not on the particle, the element, or the individual, but on the whole and the links, the connections and the relationships that unite the parts of a whole. From the [Diné] perspective, the

fundamental reality is the whole, not the part. In the Western ontological perspective, wholes are generally considered to be contingent and usually temporary arrangements of the parts. In [Diné] ontological perspective, the wholes are the primary reality, and the parts are contingent and temporal. (Witherspoon & Peterson, 1995, pp. 7–9)

CARING SCIENCE–NATIVE SCIENCE

There are parallel, intersecting, and extending themes between the core tenets of the Caring Science and the four values outlined here as intrinsic to Native Science. When held within a sphere of Caring Science–Native Science, the value of *Interconnectedness* broadens understanding and the propensity to recognize, pursue, and cocreate synergy—within and among the people, places, living organisms, and elemental forces of nature held in relationship—intimately as well as peripherally, directly as well as indirectly, locally as well as globally. It highlights the interdependencies that extend across relationships, making it evident that there is an intricate root system that needs to be nurtured. No one relationship can be held as distinct, separate, and immune to the energy being given (or not) to the others. Thus, all relationships need to be held as sacred, starting and ending with the relationship with self in a continuous loop of honoring attentiveness. In addition, viewing Interconnectedness from this more extensive and interrelated paradigm transcends time, giving voice to the responsibility and resilience shared across generations. At the most centric level, Jean Watson posits that "Caring Science ... has as its starting point a relational ontology that honors the fact that we are all connected and Belong to Source ... Caring Science makes more explicit that unity and connectedness exist among all things in the great circle of life" (Watson, 2008, pp. 16–17). Accordingly, the language, intentionality, and sacred covenant espoused by Caring Science serve as a foundational ethic for caring in any relationship (not solely a clinical one).

When held within a sphere of Caring Science–Native Science, the value of *Wholeness* harnesses the intuition and intelligence that arise from a unified heart and mind, tapping into all ways of knowing, doing, and being, and recognizing that the whole is always greater than the sum of its parts. It reflects the full-bodied and whole-hearted desire to not merely survive or excel in any one area of life but, rather, to thrive and flourish across the full spectrum of identity in the context of all that has influenced and inspired in the past as well as all that will unfold in the future. Wholeness is thus embodied by embracing and creating caring-healing rituals, modalities, environments, and interactions that evoke all the senses and integrate an internal/external sense of well-being. As such, it acknowledges and exhibits a living and breathing trust in the belief held by the Diné: beauty radiates from within.

When held within a sphere of Caring Science–Native Science, the value of *Discovery* is embodied through the cultivation and navigation of Caritas consciousness as a journey that holds sacred the reciprocity of teaching and learning. Discovery thus promotes a sense of awe and wonder, encourages open-ended curiosity and inquiry, fosters reverence for the dynamic cycles inherent in nature, acknowledges the essential interplay between art and science, reinforces an intuitive sense of belonging, and holds sacred space for being *and* becoming.

When held within a sphere of Caring Science–Native Science, the value of *Being in Right Relation* is embodied within the sincerity and grace of authentic presence, the gratitude and beauty of helping-trusting-caring relationships, and the alchemy of transpersonal caring moments. The deep reverence and integrative focus on caring and loving—"Caritas"—holds as its truth a relational ontology. Although Being in Right Relation can be held as an overarching ideal or pursuit, it also serves as a barometer that every moment presents an opportunity to live, learn, and love with heart-centered intentionality. It makes evident the dynamic interplay between action and interaction, process and outcome, thinking and feeling, discovery and certainty, seen and unseen, self and other—and calls forward unitary responses that are rooted in courage, integrity, and respect.

> Caring forces us as individuals and professions to Face our relation of infinite responsibility of Belonging to other human beings as well as to a unitary field of all-our-relations. Such an orientation becomes non-dualistic, relational, and unified, wherein there is a connectedness of all. (Watson, 2005, p. 63)

It reinforces the value inherent in everything, breaking down artificial barriers that stem from perceived differences or worth by acknowledging that each individual is a part of the universe as much as the universe is a part of each individual. Thus, the concept of environment becomes both more expansive and more intimate through recognition of concentric circles of influence.

COURAGEOUS AUTHENTICITY, AGENCY, AND ADVOCACY

Across philosophical, ethical, and sacred dimensions, Caring Science–Native Science conveys a phenomenally powerful and pivotal responsibility for action, for courageous authenticity that serves as a portal to vulnerability, heart-centered intentionality, and energetic coherence.

Specifically, within Caring Science, four restorative and regenerative core tenets emerge across the evocative expressions embodied and embraced by the 10 Caritas Processes® (see Table 6.2). An attentiveness of Caring Science to foster helping-trusting-caring relationships calls forward the essential requirement of active participation and engagement. The reliance of Caring Science on a dynamic process of discovery calls forward a learning process that is illuminated by iterative cycles of action and reflection, inquiry and insight, curiosity and creativity. The attunement of Caring Science to cocreate healing environments is reliant on a "reunion of science and metaphysics" (Watson, 2005, p. 55) and calls forward a realm of sacred science that resonates with and reflects the passionate stance of Peter Reason (1993) that "human inquiry must be grounded in a sense of the sacred, and its purpose must be to nurture the growth of love, beauty, wisdom and compassionate action" (p. 277). Finally, the intimate focus that Caring Science places on honoring the whole person calls forward deep recognition, appreciation, and promotion of human flourishing.

TABLE 6.2 Core Tenets of Caring Science

Core Tenets of Caring Science	Caritas Processes Embodied and Embraced
Attentiveness to helping-trusting-caring relationships	• Fostering helping-trusting-caring relationships (#4)
	• Offering loving-kindness and equanimity toward self and other (#1)
	• Tending to the (basic) needs of another human being (#9)
Reliance on dynamic processes of discovery	• Going beyond ego-self (#3)
	• Inviting all ways of knowing (#6)
	• Embracing the full spectrum of teaching–learning experiences (#7)
	• Attending to the mysteries of spirit (#10)
Attunement to healing environments	• Cocreate healing environments (#8)
Focus on honoring the whole person	• Attending to the inner-subjective life of self and other (#2)
	• Holding space for positive and negative feelings (#5)

Source: Watson, J. (2005). *Caring science as sacred science* (1st ed.). Philadelphia, PA: F. A. Davis.

Native Science brings further attentiveness to the importance of connection and collaboration, reinforcing the Native worldview that individual identity is magnified, not diminished, from within a cohesive context of community composed of the human, animate, and inanimate forces of the world we inhabit; thus:

Indigenous spirituality, [keeps] … in the minds of a community … understanding of being with life, seeking life or in some ways revitalizing, to revive or to bring life back to something. And so it also includes respect for all. Actions stem from respect for and celebration of community. (Cajete, 2007, 33:11)

This intricate interweaving between the individual and the collective, between the part and the whole, is integral to Native Science and conveys an inherent action-oriented praxis, a viewpoint further articulated by Native scholars:

Indigenous education … [is] based on a relational philosophy … When you teach for relationship, you're actually teaching for an understanding of how best to not only create relationship but extend it, maintain it and make it the foundation of all the things that you do. (Cajete, 2007, 35:26)

Although Greg Cajete explores the expansiveness of relationship, Robin Wall Kimmerer reinforces its inherent reciprocity:

Each person, human or no, is bound to every other in a reciprocal relationship. Just as all beings have a duty to me, I have a duty to them … An integral part of a human's education is to know those duties and how to perform them. (Kimmerer, 2013, p. 115)

Thus, Native Science is grounded in a courageous authenticity that activates all ways of knowing, invites and ignites leadership advocacy, and gives rise to a voice that reverberates with conviction and connection to all that is and will be.

CONCLUSION

At a level of universal consciousness, Native Science embodies an ethereal vastness as much as an intricate root system, whereas Caring Science embodies the energetic fields of connection that fill the spaces in between. Thus, an integrated sphere of Caring Science–Native Science invites forward a sacred sense of self that rests in the beauty and belonging of other and all that is the universe. This understanding of self is expansive, dynamic, and flowing, always already evolving, emerging, and converging. When held with reverence, Caring Science–Native Science reveals pathways of courageous authenticity, agency, and advocacy that emerge from within the souls of individuals with the capacity to generate a complex nexus of vibrant, flourishing communities.

NEXT ERA POSSIBILITIES

Education
- How does a broader sphere of Interconnectedness and Being in Right Relation impact and influence how professional practice is taught, modeled, and mentored?
- How can I integrate a broader sphere of Wholeness and Discovery into plan of care conversations with patients and their families?

Research
- How might I pursue research from an action-oriented, participatory framework (e.g., community-based participative research) in alignment with Caring Science–Native Science?
- When opportunities for collaborative inquiry arise, how can I serve to activate all ways of knowing at an individual and collective level?

Praxis
- How does an expansive understanding of beauty and belonging shape my understanding of whole person identity and well-being as I care for myself and others?
- Within an integrated sphere of Caring Science–Native Science, how do I pave pathways of courageous authenticity, advocacy, and agency in my daily practice? In my profession?

Theory and Knowledge Development

- How does an expansive understanding of cycles transform the way I pursue and evolve my own worldview?
- Within an integrated sphere of Caring Science–Native Science, how can I promote human flourishing within person-centered care and culturally responsive healthcare models?

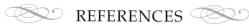 REFERENCES

BanffEvents. (2015, January 14). *Indigenous knowledge and western science: Dr. Gregory Cajete talk* [Video file]. Retrieved from https://www.youtube.com/watch?v=nFeNIOgIbzw

Black Elk, & Brown, J. E. (1989). *The sacred pipe: Black Elk's account of the seven rites of the Oglala Sioux* (Later Printing ed.). Norman: University of Oklahoma Press.

Black Elk, & Neihardt, J. G. (1988). *Black Elk speaks: Being the life story of a holy man of the Oglala Sioux.* Lincoln: University of Nebraska Press.

Bopp, J., Bopp, M., Brown, L., & Lane, P. (1984). *Sacred tree: Reflections on Native American spirituality.* Wilmot, WI: Lotus Press.

Cajete, Greg. (2007). Indigenous Paradigm: Building Sustainable Communities [Video]. Retrieved from https://nnigovernance.arizona.edu/greg-cajete-indigenous-paradigm-building-sustainable -communities

Johnston, L. J. (2012, September 29). Lyla June Johnston spoken word piece "Hozho" [Video file]. *As/Us: Literary Space for Women of the World.* Retrieved from https://asusjournal.org/issue-1/lyla -june-johnston-spoken-word

Kimmerer, R. W. (2013). *Braiding sweetgrass: Indigenous wisdom, scientific knowledge and the teachings of plants* (1st ed.). Minneapolis, MN: Milkweed Editions.

Mankiller, W. (2004). *Every day is a good day: Reflections of contemporary Indigenous women.* Golden, CO: Fulcrum.

Markstrom, C. A. (2008). *Empowerment of North American Indian girls: Ritual expressions at puberty.* Lincoln: University of Nebraska Press.

McGaa, E. (1990). *Mother Earth spirituality: Native American paths to healing ourselves and our world* (1st ed.). San Francisco, CA: Harper & Row.

Moore, K. D., Peters, K., Jojola, T., & Lacy, A. (Eds.). (2007). *How it is: The Native American philosophy of V. F. Cordova.* Tucson: University of Arizona Press.

Murphy, G. (n.d.). Great law of peace: The constitution of the Iroquois Nations: The great binding law, Gayanashagowa. Retrieved from https://www.pdx.edu/iroquois-democracy/great-law-of-peace

National Museum of the American Indian. (2009). Haudenosaunee guide for educators. Retrieved from http://nmai.si.edu/sites/1/files/pdf/education/HaudenosauneeGuide.pdf

Nerburn, K. (Ed.). (1999). *The wisdom of the Native Americans* (1st ed.). Novato, CA: New World Library.

Original Tribal Names of Native North American People. (n.d.). Retrieved from http://www.native -languages.org/original.htm

Pima People. (n.d.). In *Wikipedia*. Retrieved June 24, 2018, from https://en.wikipedia.org/w/index.php ?title=Pima_people&oldid=762098728

Reason, P. (1993). Reflections on sacred experience and sacred science. *Journal of Management Inquiry,* 2(3), 273–283. doi:10.1177/105649269323009

Schaefer, C. (2006). *Grandmothers counsel the world: Women elders offer their vision for our planet.* Boston, MA: Trumpeter.

Sheridan, T. E., & Parezo, N. J. (1996). *Paths of life: American Indians of the Southwest and northern Mexico.* Tucson: University of Arizona Press.

Smith, H. (2005). *A seat at the table: Huston Smith in conversation with Native Americans on religious freedom.* (P. Cousineau, Ed., 1st ed.). Berkeley: University of California Press.

Stokes, J., & Kanawahienton. (1993). Haudenosaunee thanksgiving address. Retrieved from http://nmai.si.edu/environment/pdf/01_02_Thanksgiving_Address.pdf

Tohono O'odham. (n.d.). In *Wikipedia.* Retrieved June 24, 2018, from https://en.wikipedia.org/w/index.php?title=Tohono_O%27odham&oldid=776844218

Watson, J. (2005). *Caring science as sacred science* (1st ed.). Philadelphia, PA: F. A. Davis.

Watson, J. (2008). *Nursing: The philosophy and science of caring* (Rev. ed.). Boulder: University Press of Colorado.

Witherspoon, G. (1977). *Language and art in the Navajo universe* (1st ed.). Ann Arbor: University of Michigan Press.

Witherspoon, G., & Peterson, G. (1995). *Dynamic Symmetry and Holistic Asymmetry.* New York, NY: Peter Lang.

7

Developing the Knowledge of Human Caring

Jacqueline Fawcett

CARITAS LITERACIES

By the end of this chapter, the caring-healing nurse will be able to

1. Describe the meaning of "nursology" and its relationship to developing knowledge of human caring.

2. Define nursology's metaparadigm and its relationship to human caring.

3. Identify several challenges in the development of the distinctive knowledge of human caring.

The purpose of this chapter is to discuss future directions in the development of nursology discipline–specific knowledge of human caring, which encompasses Human Caring Science and Unitary Caring Science. Two questions provide the structure for this chapter. The first question that must be answered when discussing the development of knowledge of nursology: What is nursology-distinctive knowledge of human caring? The second question: What are the challenges to use and in further development of nursology-distinctive knowledge of human caring?

I will answer the two questions from the perspective of more than 50 years as a registered nurse, of more than 40 years as a PhD-prepared nurse, and of my understanding of human caring science and unitary caring science. I have been thinking and writing about these questions and their answers since I began doctoral studies in 1972 at New York University (NYU). I have been greatly influenced by the faculty at NYU, including Martha E. Rogers, Florence S. Downs, and Margaret A. Newman—who taught me a great deal about knowledge development—as well as by Stephanie Edgerton—who taught me a great deal about philosophies of science and applied science. I also have been influenced by my colleagues and students, first at the University of Connecticut, then at the University of Pennsylvania, and now at the University of Massachusetts–Boston. Thus, paraphrasing Isaac Newton (1676), my thoughts flow from standing on the shoulders of these nurse stars and rising stars.

WHAT IS NURSOLOGY: DISTINCTIVE KNOWLEDGE OF HUMAN CARING?

I have been committed to the development, analysis, and evaluation of nursology-distinctive knowledge throughout my career. I now use the term, "nursology," as the name for our discipline, rather than "nursing," because nursology conveys more than nursing in that the focus of the discipline is the generation and testing of knowledge, dissemination of knowledge, and application of knowledge (Fawcett et al., 2015).

Regardless of the term used for the discipline, disciplinary knowledge encompasses the five components listed here (Fawcett & DeSanto-Madeya, 2013).

- A single **metaparadigm**, which identifies the distinctive global and perspective-neutral phenomena of interest to members of the discipline in the form of very abstract and general concepts and statements about the concepts.

- Multiple **philosophies**, which encompass various "ontological claims about the phenomena of central interest to a discipline, epistemic claims about how those phenomena come to be known, and ethical claims about what the members of a discipline value" (Fawcett & DeSanto-Madeya, 2013, p. 8).

- Multiple **conceptual models**, which are abstract and general concepts and statements about the concepts that address all the phenomena identified in the disciplinary metaparadigm and which reflect certain ontological, epistemic, and ethical claims.

- Multiple **theories**, which are relatively concrete and specific concepts and statements about the concepts. The concepts and statements of each theory are derived from a particular conceptual model.
    - Theories range in increasing levels of concreteness and specificity from grand theories, to middle-range theories, to situation-specific theories. My understanding is that *grand theories* are less abstract and general than conceptual models, but more abstract and general than middle-range theories and situation-specific theories. Grand theories include content addressing some, but not all of the metaparadigm concepts. *Middle-range theories* are less abstract and general than grand theories and address one or more concepts of a conceptual model or a grand theory. Middle-range theories are meant to be generalized to people with various health conditions and in various settings. *Situation-specific theories* are even less abstract and general than middle-range theories. Like middle-range theories, situation-specific theories address one or more concepts of a conceptual model or a grand theory. In contrast to middle-range theories, situation-specific theories address certain people (e.g., older adult females) with a particular health condition (e.g., myocardial infarction). Middle-range and situation-specific theories encompass

descriptions of a concept, *explanations* of the relations between two or more concepts, and *predictions* of the effects of one concept (e.g., an intervention) on one or more concepts that are outcomes.

- **Methods of scholarly inquiry**, which are very concrete and specific, approach the generation and testing of theories. Methods typically encompass the design of research or other scholarly inquiry; sources of data (observations, people, or documents); instruments used to collect data, including coding forms, interview guides, and questionnaires; and data analysis techniques. Data may be words or numbers or observations.

Nursology's Metaparadigm and Human Caring

Over the years, nurse scholars have argued for and against the inclusion of caring as a metaparadigm concept. I have never included caring in my version of the metaparadigm, arguing that caring is neither distinctive to our discipline nor perspective-neutral (Fawcett, 2005). Similarly, Cook and Peden (2017) pointed out that "Some wonder whether nursing can presume to lay claim over the entire domain of caring when so many other professions describe their function as also involving caring" (p. 12). After an extensive review of the literature, however, Cook and Peden (2017) concluded that "caring is [indeed] nursing's contribution to the knowledge base of the healthcare sciences" (p. 22). Thus, their work supports the inclusion of human caring in nursology's metaparadigm.

Philosophies and Human Caring

Philosophies evident in the works of nurse scholars range from positivism to postpositivism to interpretive philosophy to critical social theory to pragmatism (Weaver & Olson, 2006). Positivism is the philosophy least frequently used by contemporary nurse scholars, especially those nurse scholars who write about human caring science and not at all by nurse scholars who write about unitary caring science.

Human caring science typically reflects postpositivism, with its emphasis on theory-ladenness. In contrast, unitary caring science reflects interpretive philosophy. This philosophy and its variations (constructivism, transformative-emancipation, critical realism, and dialectics) emphasize lived (or living) experiences from the perspective of the participant (Creswell & Plano-Clark, 2011; Shannon-Baker, 2016; Weaver & Olson, 2006). Interpretive philosophy is evident in what Parse (1987) calls the "simultaneity worldview," what Newman (1992) calls the "unitary-transformative worldview," and what Fawcett and DeSanto-Madeya (2013) call the "simultaneous action worldview."

Conceptual Models and Theories of Human Caring

The distinction between human caring conceptual models and theories is admittedly difficult to discern. Various classification schemes about human caring that are used by authors and editors of widely used textbooks about nursing knowledge and a journal article about caring are listed in Table 7.1.

TABLE 7.1 Various Classification Schemes About Human Caring Used in Textbooks About Nursing Knowledge

Source of Classification	Classifications
Alligood (2014)	• Nursing philosophies • Nursing theories
Alligood (2018)	• Nursing philosophies • Nursing theories • Middle-range theories
Butts and Rich (2018)	• Models and theories focused on human existence • Theories focused on caring • Models and theories focused on culture
Cook and Peden (2017)	• Theories
Fawcett (2000a); Fawcett and DeSanto-Madeya (2013)	• Conceptual models • Grand theories • Middle-range theories
Fitzpatrick and McCarthy (2014)	• Theories applied to future research and practice
George (2002)	• Theories
McEwen and Wills (2014)	• Grand nursing theories based on human needs • Grand nursing theories based on interactive process • Middle-range nursing theories
Meleis (2012)	• Theories: On needs and self-care
Sitzman and Eichelberger (2017)	• Theories that define nursing or discuss nursing in a general sense (philosophies) • Theories about broad nursing practice areas (grand theories)
M. C. Smith and Parker (2015)	• Conceptual models and grand theories in the unitary-transformative paradigm • Grand theories about care or caring • Middle-range theories
M. J. Smith and Liehr (2014)	• Middle-range theories
Thornton (2013)	• Conceptual model

The diverse classifications of several nurses' perspectives of human caring are listed in Table 7.2. The perspectives listed in Table 7.2 are limited to those that include care or caring in the name and were included in the textbooks or the journal article that are in my personal library. Given the diversity of conceptual models and theories that include human caring as a concept, it is not surprising that the definition of "caring" varies (Cook & Peden,

TABLE 7.2 Classifications of Selected Nurses' Perspectives of Human Caring[a]

Name of Human Caring Perspective	Classification	Source of Classification
Benner's Theory of Caring, Clinical Wisdom, and Ethics in Nursing Practice	Philosophy	Alligood (2014, 2018)
Boykin and Schoenhofer's Theory of Nursing as Caring	Grand theory [b]Theory	M. C. Smith and Parker (2015) Alligood (2018); Butts and Rich (2018); George (2002)
Dorsey & Murdaught's Theory of Self-Care Management for Vulnerable Populations	Middle-range theory	M. J. Smith and Liehr (2014)
Duffy's Quality–Caring Model	[b]Theory Middle-range theory	Butts and Rich (2018) M. C. Smith and Parker (2015)
Eriksson's Theory of Caritative Caring	Philosophy [b]Theory	Alligood (2018) Cook and Peden (2017)
Gaut's Theory of Caring as Action	[b]Theory	Cook and Peden (2017)
Hall's Theory of Care, Core, and Cure	[b]Theory	George (2002) M. C. Smith and Parker (2015)
Leininger's Theory of Culture Care Diversity and Universality	Grand theory Middle-range theory [b]Theory Model and theory	Fawcett (2000a); Sitzman and Eichelberger (2017); M. C. Smith and Parker (2015) McEwen and Wills (2014) Alligood (2014, 2018); George (2002) Butts and Rich (2018)
Leenerts & Magilvy's Theory of Self-Care	Middle-range theory	M. J. Smith and Liehr (2014)
Locsin's Technological Competency as Caring in Nursing	Middle-range theory	M. C. Smith and Parker (2015)
Martinsen's Philosophy of Caring	Philosophy	Alligood (2018)
Orem's Self-Care Framework	Conceptual model Grand theory [b]Theory Theory: On needs and self-care	Alligood (2014, 2018); Fawcett and DeSanto-Madeya (2013) M. C. Smith and Parker (2015) McEwen and Wills (2014) George (2002) Meleis (2012)

(continued)

TABLE 7.2 Classifications of Selected Nurses' Perspectives of Human Caring[a] *(continued)*

Name of Human Caring Perspective	Classification	Source of Classification
Ray's Theory of Bureaucratic Caring	Philosophy [c]Middle-range theory	Alligood (2018) M. C. Smith and Parker (2015)
Riegel et al.'s Theory of Self-Care of Chronic Illness	[c]Middle-range theory	M. J. Smith and Liehr (2014)
Sanford's Theory of Caring Through Relation and Dialogue for Patient Education	[c]Middle-range theory	M. J. Smith and Liehr (2014)
Smith's Theory of Unitary Caring	Middle-range theory	M. C. Smith and Parker (2015)
Swanson's Theory of Caring	Middle-range theory	Alligood (2018); M. J. Smith and Liehr (2014); M. C. Smith and Parker (2015)
	[b]Theory	Butts and Rich (2018)
Thompson et al.'s Theory of Nurse Midwifery Care	[c]Middle-range theory	M. J. Smith and Liehr (2014)
Thornton's Model of Whole Person Caring	Conceptual model	Thornton (2013)
Watson's Theory of Human Caring	Philosophy	Alligood (2014, 2018); Sitzman and Eichelberger (2017)
	Grand theory	McEwen and Wills (2014); M. C. Smith and Parker (2015)
	Middle-range theory	Fawcett and DeSanto-Madeya (2013)
	[b]Theory	Butts and Rich (2018); Fitzpatrick and McCarthy (2014); George (2002)
Wuest's Theory of Precarious Ordering: Theory of Women's Caring	[c]Middle-range theory	M. J. Smith and Liehr (2014)

[a]See the source of classification references for and content about the perspectives.
[b]Type of theory (grand theory, middle-range theory) not specified.
[c]Could be classified as a situation-specific theory.

2017). More specifically, it is not surprising that each nursological conceptual model and theory about human caring might use a different definition of caring, as each is, per se, a different perspective (Fawcett & DeSanto-Madeya, 2013).

Five Types of Theories

Five types of theories—or fundamental patterns of knowing in nursology—have been identified. Carper (1978) identified empirical, aesthetic, ethical, and personal knowing theories. White (1995) added sociopolitical theories, which Chinn and Kramer (2015) refer to as "emancipatory theories." These theories may be middle-range theories or situation-specific theories.

Empirical theories constitute the science of nursology and encompass descriptive, explanatory, and predictive theories, all of which address "average" behavior of samples or entire populations. Empirical nursological theories abound—indeed, the product of nursological research always is theory (Fawcett & Garity, 2009), although the theory frequently is not explicitly labeled as such. Review of the content of the theories of human caring science and unitary caring science listed in Table 7.2 indicates that all of these are empirical, which is essentially a tautology, because science is empirical.

Aesthetic theories, which constitute the art of nursology, focus on understanding of each individual's behavior. Only one explicit aesthetic nursological theory could be located—Chinn's (2001/2006) theory of nursing. However, the theory does not address human caring per se.

Ethical theories constitute the ethics of nursology. Many ethical nursological theories are empirical theories. Those that are not empirical include ethical codes, practice standards, and philosophical essays about how nurses should behave. Tong (2018) presented a discussion of feminist ethics, and Rich (2018) presented a discussion of ethical theories and methods. Neither author, however, identified any explicit ethical nursological theories. An example of an explicit ethical nursological theory is the American Nurses Association's (2015) *Code of Ethics*. Although none of the nine provisions of the *Code* explicitly addresses human caring, all provisions reflect caring in some way.

Personal knowing theories focus on the interpersonal relationships of nursology in the non-empirical sense of the nurse knowing how to convey authenticity to patients, to convey that he or she cares about the patient. Nursological theories of personal knowing can be extracted from autobiographical stories and essays about nurses' experiences of their genuine, authentic selves. An example is Diers's (2005) autobiographical story of her work as a nurse. However, she did not explicitly address human caring. Although S. Nelson (2018) wrote about interpersonal relationships, she did not identify any theories that could be considered personal knowing.

Sociopolitical/emancipatory theories constitute the politics and policies of nursology. Fawcett and Garity (2009) explained that sociopolitical/emancipatory theories could be extracted from "documents and statements that indicate that the many voices involved in nursing practice are heard and acknowledged" (p. 18). For example, Browne's (2001) sociopolitical theory is a critique of nurses' "implicit [liberal] political allegiances" and the implications of these allegiances on the development of knowledge that "help us to understand whether our science disrupts or inadvertently helps to maintain social inequities" (p. 129). Although

Chinn (2018) presented a comprehensive discussion of emancipatory knowing, she did not identify any emancipatory nursological theories. The voices of nurse stakeholders who support human caring science or unitary caring science, translated into their written words, are, however, heard by the readers of this book.

METHODS OF SCHOLARLY INQUIRY FOR HUMAN CARING KNOWLEDGE DEVELOPMENT

Given the exclusive emphasis on human caring *empirical* theories, usual ways of generating and testing descriptive, explanatory, and predictive theories are relevant. Theories of *human caring science* typically are generated by qualitative methodologies used in various disciplines, such as simple description and phenomenology. These theories typically are tested by various widely used quantitative methodologies, such as correlational and experimental designs.

Watson's (2009) book includes several different instruments that were designed to measure "diverse concepts such as quality of care, patient/client/nurse perceptions of caring, caring behaviors, caring abilities, and caring efficacy" (p. xv). J. Nelson and Watson's (2012) book is "a collection of research that [explicitly] tests the construct of Caritas (caring and love) within the context of Caring Science and the Theory of Human Caring assembled over the last 30 years by Dr. Jean Watson" (p. xxi). J. Nelson and Watson (2012) pointed out that most of the tools used to collect data for the research reports included in the book were derived from the Caring Factor Survey (CFS). The CFS was explicitly designed to measure Watson's 10 Caritas Processes®; versions for providers and for recipients of the Caritas Processes have been developed (DiNapoli, Nelson, Turkel, & Watson, 2010; J. Nelson, Thiel, Hozak, & Thomas, 2016).

In contrast, most theories within the tradition of *unitary caring science* are generated using primarily qualitative nursology-specific methodologies. Leininger (2006), for example, offered ethnonursing as a way to develop what I regard as situation-specific theories of culture care diversity and universality. In addition, Smith (2015) described how the concepts of her theory can be translated into empirical indicators that constitute what I regard as a research methodology and a practice methodology (see Fawcett, 2018).

WHAT ARE THE CHALLENGES TO USE AND IN FURTHER DEVELOPMENT OF NURSOLOGY-DISTINCTIVE KNOWLEDGE OF HUMAN CARING?

Tapp and Lavoie (2017) joined others (e.g., Fawcett, 2000b; Nagle, 1999) in expressing pessimism about the use of nursology discipline-specific knowledge. They stated, "Discussions about theories and conceptual models seem to be losing their prominence with the nursing discipline" (p. 1).

In a more optimistic tone, they added, "However, some theorists remain very active and influential in academic circles" (p. 1). Some theorists' works are also evident in practice settings. For example, the Magnet® status for clinical agencies requirement for a professional practice model (American Nurses Credentialing Center, 2011) is sometimes interpreted as the use of a nursological conceptual model or theory (Fawcett & DeSanto-Madeya, 2013).

CHALLENGES: THE METAPARADIGM

A challenge for those nurse scholars who are interested in further formalization of the global perspective of the discipline is to determine the place of caring in the metaparadigm of nursology. Continuation of the debate about the need for caring—or human caring—as a metaparadigm concept is necessary, with dialogue focused on whether caring should replace nursing as a metaparadigm concept, be an additional metaparadigm concept, or be a dimension of the concept of nursing. My current preference is that human caring be considered a dimension of the metaparadigm concept of nursing.

CHALLENGES: PHILOSOPHIES

A challenge for those nurse scholars who are interested in philosophical issues is to determine the most relevant philosophy for human caring. A related challenge is to determine whether there should be different philosophies for human caring science and for unitary caring science.

CHALLENGES: CONCEPTUAL MODELS AND THEORIES

A major challenge about conceptual models and theories of human caring is to determine a specific classification of each one as a conceptual model, a grand theory, a middle-range theory, or a situation-specific theory. As can be seen in Table 7.2, very few of the perspectives of human caring have a single classification. Clearly, dialogue among the authors and editors of the numerous nursology knowledge textbooks is needed to reach consensus about classification. I believe that this is particularly important because classification determines how the perspective is used. For example, if a perspective is classified as a middle-range or situation-specific theory, users expect to be able to directly measure its concepts and apply those concepts and their connections directly in research and practice. If, however, a perspective is classified as a conceptual model or a grand theory, its concepts are not directly measurable and, therefore, middle-range and situation-specific theories must be derived from the conceptual model or grand theory so that the theories can be used for research and practice. Thus, the utility of a conceptual model or grand theory is a broad guide for research and practice (Fawcett & DeSanto-Madeya, 2013).

Another challenge is to better understand the limits of the use of descriptive and explanatory theories. The concepts of these theories can be used as the basis for the development of assessment tools (Fawcett & Garity, 2009). These theories do not, however, include content about the effects of interventions on outcomes; they are not predictive theories. Furthermore, any predictive theory about interventions and their outcomes is limited unless there is content that directs the user to know what should be assessed to determine what intervention to use.

Still another challenge is to expand thinking and theory development about who engages in caring and who are the participants in caring. Many of the perspectives listed in Table 7.2 focus on the behaviors of nurses as the ones who provide caring to others. A few perspectives focus on others' perceptions of the receipt of caring provided by nurses. Still fewer perspectives focus on caring provided by people who are not nurses.

A related challenge is to determine whether the vast literature about informal caregiving by family members and friends is relevant to human caring science or unitary caring science. The extensive amount of this literature was evident in an April 22, 2017, search of the Cumulative Index to Nursing and Allied Health Literature (CINAHL), using the search terms, "caregiving AND literature review," which yielded 239 references. As literature reviews, these 239 publications encompass references to many more publications about caregiving. The addition of the search term, "caring science," yielded one reference; inspection of the journal article indicated that the literature reviewed was not within the context of human caring science or unitary caring science.

The nurses who have developed human caring theories obviously support the use of nursology discipline-specific knowledge. That some researchers "regard caring ... as unnecessary or an unrealistic ideal that interferes with research goals" (Fawcett, 2013, p. 378) is, of course, a major challenge for scholars who have a vested interest in widespread use of human caring science and unitary caring science.

CHALLENGES: TYPES OF THEORIES

A major challenge is to greatly increase the number of explicit nursological aesthetic, ethical, personal knowing, and sociopolitical/emancipatory theories that address human caring. The current plethora of empirical human caring science and unitary caring science theories is an instance of what Chinn and Kramer (2015) call "patterns gone wild" (p. 18). They explained,

> When knowledge within any one pattern [type of theory] is not integrated within the whole of knowing, distortion—rather than understanding—is produced. Knowledge that is developed in isolation without the consideration of all patterns of knowing [i.e., types of theories] leads to uncritical acceptance, narrow interpretation, and partial use of knowledge. (p. 18)

It may be that development of other than empirical theories is hindered by the emphasis on human caring *science* and unitary caring *science*. Therefore, another challenge is to be very clear about what we mean by "science" when we refer to human caring science and unitary caring science.

Barrett (2002, 2017) defined nursing (i.e., nursological) science as "a basic science, [which] is the substantive discipline-specific knowledge that focuses on the human-universe-health process articulated in the [nursological] frameworks and theories" (2002, p. 51; 2017, p. 130). Might we then define nursological human caring science as a basic science that focuses on nurses' and others' perceptions and ratings of caring behaviors articulated in conceptual models and theories of human caring? Might we define nursological unitary caring science as a basic science that focuses on unitary human experiences of caring articulated in conceptual models and theories of unitary caring?

CHALLENGES: METHODS OF SCHOLARLY INQUIRY

A substantial challenge for nurse scholars who work within the context of human caring science or unitary caring science is to continue to create innovative methodologies for generation and testing of human caring science and unitary caring science nursological theories. It is important to understand that every instrument—forms to code data from documents and observations, interview guides used to collect word data, and question-naires used to collect number data—and every experimental condition are designed to measure some theory concept. Some reports of development of instruments that are pur-ported to measure some aspect of caring do not include an explicit theory concept that is measured by the instrument. Although Watson (2009) noted that these instruments are "atheoretically derived" (p. xv), it is more accurate to state that the theory is implicit. In as much as Popper (1970) maintained that "we approach everything in the light of a precon-ceived theory, we can conclude that atheoretical is an impossibility." (p. 52). Therefore, the challenge is to clearly and explicitly identify which concept of which theory is measured by which instrument, and which concept of which theory is operationalized by which experi-mental treatment.

CONCLUSION

The other chapters of this book attest to the many substantial and timely contributions to human caring science and unitary caring science by nurse scholars in many countries. Their work may already have overcome some of the challenges I identified in this chapter.

That unitary caring science is emphasized in this book signals considerable interest in a simultaneity/unitary-transformative/simultaneous action worldview. Acknowledging this worldview, Tapp and Lavoie (2017) commented that the more active and influential of con-temporary nurse theorists' work "converge[s] toward the 'simultaneity' paradigm associ-ated most often with the human sciences" (p. 2). Continuing, they explained, "Simultaneity paradigm scholars claim that their theories are more representative of, and connected to, a 'real' nursing knowledge, because of the originality of the nursing role promulgated and the knowledge put forward in their conceptualizations and methods" (p. 2).

This chapter was written with the dual goals of helping readers to better understand the structure of nursology knowledge that addresses human caring science and unitary caring science, and to stimulate thinking about how to overcome challenges to use and about fur-ther development of nurses' perspectives of human caring. Overcoming the challenges identified in this chapter requires the courage to march, as the "revolutionary creators of the nursing theory movement did" (Barrett, 2017, p. 132). The authors of the other chapters of this book have been marching in the footsteps of those revolutionary creators of the nurs-ing theory movement. I, too, have been marching in the footsteps of those revolutionary creators, even daring to add to the movement by working with colleagues to develop a con-ceptual model that addresses the intersection of nursology and health policy (Fawcett & Russell, 2001; Russell & Fawcett, 2005) and a conceptual model addressing the intersection of nursology and population health (Fawcett & Ellenbecker, 2015). My personal challenge now will be to think about how these two nursology discipline-specific conceptual models can be refined so that each addresses human caring and guides derivation of nursological human caring theories.

Finally, overcoming these challenges urgently requires, as Barrett (2017) maintained, a "discussion of philosophy, power, politics, and policy" (p. 132). I urge all readers of this chapter to engage in dialogue about these issues in their workplaces, at conferences, and in publications. If we are to survive as a discipline and if we really want to advance nursological knowledge of human caring, we *must* more fully understand what we believe and value (philosophy), how organizational structures and personal choices impede or advance work (power), and how stakeholders (politics) influence availability of resources (policies). Once understanding is enhanced, we must have the courage and motivation to act to advance the development of many more nursological conceptual models and theories that focus explicitly on human caring and to apply these perspectives in service to humankind.

NEXT ERA POSSIBILITIES

Education
- What are tangible steps toward creating a single classification schema for conceptual models, grand theories, middle-range theories, and situation-specific theories of human caring that may be widely accepted and taught to students?

Research
- How can Caring Science be integrated into nursing research initiatives toward the development of instruments that measure specific concepts of the theory?

Praxis
- In what ways can I identify practical uses of descriptive, explanatory, and predictive theories of human caring?

Theory and Knowledge Development
- Why is the evolution toward nursology a logical next step amid the progression of Caring Science theory and knowledge advancement?

 REFERENCES

Alligood, M. R. (Ed.). (2014). *Nursing theory: Utilization and application* (5th ed.). Maryland Heights, MO: Mosby Elsevier.

Alligood, M. R. (Ed.). (2018). *Nursing theorists and their work* (9th ed.). Maryland Heights, MO: Mosby Elsevier.

American Nurses Association. (2015). *Code of ethics for nurses with interpretive statements.* Silver Spring, MD: Author. Retrieved from http://www.nursingworld.org/MainMenuCategories/EthicsStandards/About/Tools-You-Need/Code-of-Ethics-For-Nurses.html

American Nurses Credentialing Center. (2011). ANCC Magnet Recognition Program®. Retrieved from https://www.nursingworld.org/organizational-programs/magnet

Barrett, E. A. M. (2002). What is nursing science? *Nursing Science Quarterly, 15,* 51–60. doi:10.1177/089431840201500109

Barrett, E. A. M. (2017). Again, what is nursing science? *Nursing Science Quarterly, 30,* 129–133. doi:10.1177/0894318417693313

Browne, A. J. (2001). The influence of liberal political ideology on nursing science. *Nursing Inquiry, 8,* 118–129. doi:10.1046/j.1440-1800.2001.00095.x

Butts, J. B., & Rich, K. L. (Eds.). (2018). *Philosophies and theories for advanced practice nursing* (3rd ed.). Burlington, MA: Jones & Bartlett.

Carper, B. (1978). Fundamental patterns of knowing in nursing. *Advances in Nursing Science, 1*(1), 13–23. doi:10.1097/00012272-197810000-00004

Chinn, P. L. (2001). Toward a theory of nursing art. In N. L. Chaska (Ed.), *The nursing profession: Tomorrow and beyond* (pp. 287–297). Thousand Oaks, CA: Sage. (Reprinted in Andrist, L. C., Nicholas, P. K., & Wolf, K. A. 2006. *A history of nursing ideas,* pp. 73–183. Boston, MA: Jones & Bartlett.)

Chinn, P. L. (2018). Critical theory and emancipatory knowing. In J. B. Butts & K. L. Rich (Eds.), *Philosophies and theories for advanced nursing practice* (3rd ed., pp. 143–162). Burlington, MA: Jones & Bartlett.

Chinn, P. L., & Kramer, M. K. (2015). *Knowledge development in nursing: Theory and process* (9th ed.). St. Louis, MO: Elsevier Mosby.

Cook, L. B., & Peden, A. (2017). Finding a focus for nursing: The caring concept. *Advances in Nursing Science, 40,* 12–23. doi:10.1097/ANS.0000000000000137

Creswell, J. W., & Plano-Clark, V. L. (2011). *Designing and conducting mixed methods research* (2nd ed.). Los Angeles, CA: Sage.

Diers, D. (2005). Am I a nurse?: I'm old but never former. *American Journal of Nursing, 105*(10), 39. Retrieved from https://journals.lww.com/ajnonline/Citation/2005/10000/Am_I_a_Nurse___I_m_old_but_never_former_.29.aspx

DiNapoli, P. P., Nelson, J., Turkel, M., & Watson, J. (2010). Measuring the caritas processes: Caring factor survey. *International Journal for Human Caring, 14*(3), 16–21.

Fawcett, J. (2000a). *Analysis and evaluation of contemporary nursing knowledge: Nursing models and theories.* Philadelphia, PA: F. A. Davis.

Fawcett, J. (2000b). The state of nursing science: Where is the nursing in the science? *Theoria: Journal of Nursing Theory, 9*(3), 3–10.

Fawcett, J. (2005). *Contemporary nursing knowledge: Analysis and evaluation of nursing models and theories* (2nd ed.). Philadelphia, PA: F. A. Davis.

Fawcett, J. (2013). Thoughts about multidisciplinary, interdisciplinary, and transdisciplinary research. *Nursing Science Quarterly, 26,* 376–379. doi:10.1177/0894318413500408

Fawcett, J. (2018). *Applying conceptual models of nursing: Quality improvement, research, and practice.* New York, NY: Springer Publishing.

Fawcett, J., Aronowitz, T., AbuFannouneh, A., Al Usta, M., Fraley, H. E., Howlett, M. S., … Zhang, Y. (2015). Thoughts about the name of our discipline. *Nursing Science Quarterly, 28,* 330–333. doi:10.1177/0894318415599224

Fawcett, J., & DeSanto-Madeya, S. (2013). *Contemporary nursing knowledge: Analysis and evaluation of nursing models and theories* (3rd ed.). Philadelphia, PA: F. A. Davis.

Fawcett, J., & Ellenbecker, C. H. (2015). A proposed conceptual model of nursing and population health. *Nursing Outlook, 63,* 288–298. doi:10.1016/j.outlook.2015.01.009

Fawcett, J., & Garity, J. (2009). *Evaluating research for evidence-based nursing practice.* Philadelphia, PA: F. A. Davis.

Fawcett, J., & Russell, G. (2001). A conceptual model of nursing and health policy. *Policy, Politics, and Nursing Practice, 2,* 108–116. doi:10.1177/152715440100200205

Fitzpatrick, J. J., & McCarthy, G. (Eds.). (2014). *Theories guiding nursing research and practice: Making nursing knowledge explicit.* New York, NY: Springer Publishing.

George, J. B. (Ed.). (2002). *Nursing theories: The base for professional nursing practice* (5th ed.). Upper Saddle River, NJ: Prentice Hall.

Leininger, M. M. (2006). Culture care diversity and universality theory and evolution of the ethnonursing method. In M. M. Leininger & M. R. McFarland (Eds.), *Culture care diversity and universality: A worldwide nursing theory* (2nd ed., pp. 1–41). Boston, MA: Jones & Bartlett.

McEwen, M., & Wills, E. M. (Eds.). (2014). *Theoretical basis for nursing* (4th ed.). Philadelphia, PA: Lippincott Williams & Wilkins.

Meleis, A. I. (2012). *Theoretical nursing: Development and progress* (5th ed.). Philadelphia, PA: Wolters Kluwer/Lippincott Williams & Wilkins.

Nagle, L. M. (1999). A matter of extinction or distinction. *Western Journal of Nursing Research, 21*, 71–82. doi:10.1177/01939459922043712

Nelson, J., Thiel, L., Hozak, M. A., & Thomas, T. (2016). Item reduction of the caring factor survey: Care provider version, an instrument specified to measure Watson's 10 processes of caring. *International Journal for Human Caring, 20*, 123–128. doi:10.20467/1091-5710-20.3.123

Nelson, J., & Watson, J. (Eds.). (2012). *Measuring caring: International research on caritas as healing.* New York, NY: Springer Publishing.

Nelson, S. (2018). Theories focused on interpersonal relationships. In J. B. Butts & K. L. Rich (Eds.), *Philosophies and theories for advanced nursing practice* (3rd ed., pp. 267–323). Burlington, MA: Jones & Bartlett.

Newman, M. A. (1992). Prevailing paradigms in nursing. *Nursing Outlook, 40*, 10–13, 32.

Newton, I. (1676, February 5). Letter to Robert Hooke. Retrieved from https://en.wikiquote.org/wiki/Isaac_Newton#A.E2.80.93F

Parse, R. R. (1987). *Nursing science: Major paradigms, theories, and critiques.* Philadelphia, PA: Saunders.

Popper, K. R. (1970). Normal science and its dangers. In I. Lakatos & A. Musgrave (Eds.), *Criticism and the growth of knowledge* (pp. 51–58). London, UK: Cambridge University Press.

Rich, K. L. (2018). Theories and methods in ethics. In J. B. Butts & K. L. Rich (Eds.), *Philosophies and theories for advanced nursing practice* (3rd ed., pp. 181–197). Burlington, MA: Jones & Bartlett.

Russell, G. E., & Fawcett, J. (2005). The conceptual model for nursing and health policy revisited. *Policy, Politics, and Nursing Practice, 6*, 319–326. doi:10.1177/1527154405283304

Shannon-Baker, P. (2016). Making paradigms meaningful in mixed methods research. *Journal of Mixed Methods Research, 10*, 319–334. doi:10.1177/1558689815575861

Sitzman, K., & Eichelberger, L. W. (2017). *Understanding the work of nurse theorists: A creative beginning* (3rd ed.). Sudbury, MA: Jones & Bartlett.

Smith, M. C. (2015). Marlaine Smith's theory of unitary caring. In M. C. Smith & M. E. Parker (Eds.). *Nursing theories and nursing practice* (4th ed., pp. 509–519). Philadelphia, PA: F. A. Davis.

Smith, M. C., & Parker, M. E. (Eds.). (2015). *Nursing theories and nursing practice* (4th ed.). Philadelphia, PA: F. A. Davis.

Smith, M. J., & Liehr, P. R. (Eds.). (2014). *Middle range theory for nursing* (3rd ed.). New York, NY: Springer Publishing.

Tapp, D., & Lavoie, M. (2017). The humanbecoming theory as a reinterpretation of the symbolic interactionism: A critique of its specific nature and scientific underpinnings. *Nursing Philosophy, 18*(2). doi:10.1111/nup.12123

Thornton, L. (2013). *Whole person caring: An interprofessional model for healing and wellness.* Indianapolis, IN: Sigma Theta Tau International.

Tong, R. (2018). Feminist ethics: Some applicable thoughts for advanced practice nurses. In J. B. Butts & K. L. Rich (Eds.), *Philosophies and theories for advanced nursing practice* (3rd ed., pp. 163–180). Burlington, MA: Jones & Bartlett.

Watson, J. (Ed.). (2009). *Assessing and measuring caring in nursing and health sciences* (2nd ed.). New York, NY: Springer Publishing.

Weaver, K., & Olson, J. K. (2006). Understanding paradigms used for nursing research. *Journal of Advanced Nursing, 53*, 459–469. doi:10.1111/j.1365-2648.2006.03740.x

White, J. (1995). Patterns of knowing: Review, critique, and update. *Advances in Nursing Science, 17*(4), 73–86. doi:10.1097/00012272-199506000-00007

II

Converging Paradigms: Constructing New Worldviews

II

8

Caring Science and Heart Science: A Guide to Heart-Centered Praxis*

Jean Watson and Robert Browning

CARITAS LITERACIES

By the end of this chapter, the caring-healing nurse will be able to

1. Develop an evidence-informed heart-centered praxis of Caritas, informed by a new synthesis of Heart Science–Caring Science, philosophy, and theory.

2. Explore CaritasHeart™ methodology as guide toward human caring/compassion renewal for self/other.

3. Examine CaritasHeart Praxis Protocols—Integrating Heart Science as guide to 10 Caritas Processes®.

∽

This chapter uncovers the synchrony of Caring Science theory with research and methods of Heart Science, as lived out through the shared philosophical, scientific, and integrative practices of human caring. Together these two foundational structures unite for human caring-healing practices, expanding and deepening our understanding of evidence-informed, authentic heart-centered caring and compassion. An evolved method of CaritasHeart Praxis is introduced as a foundational guide, unifying intellectual-experiential ways of Being and Becoming. *Caritas* is based on the Latin word for charity uniting divine

---

*Sections of this chapter are reprinted or adapted with permission from Watson, J., & Browning, R. (2012). Viewpoint: Caring science meets heart science: A guide to authentic caring practice. *American Nurse Today*, 7(8). Retrieved from https://www.americannursetoday.com/viewpoint-caring-science-meets-heart-science -a-guide-to-authentic-caring-practice

Love and caring. Through this unity of human caring theory and heart science, healthcare can be transformed, contributing to an evolved human consciousness for humanity itself.

CARING SCIENCE THEORY OF HUMAN CARING

The evolution of Caring Science and Heart Science has occurred over the past 10 years through the combined intellectual-theoretical and practical integration of the two fields by Robert Browning, master teacher of HeartMath, and Jean Watson, author of *Caring Science Theory of Human Caring* (Watson & Browning, 2012).

CARING SCIENCE—THEORY OF HUMAN CARING

Caring Science literature has evolved over the past three decades, now positing an evolved model of science with the "Ethic of Belonging" as the foundation (Levinas, 1996; Watson, 2006, 2008). The Theory of Human Caring Science consists of 10 Caritas Processes, defining and languaging the universals of the human caring phenomenon as the philosophical-theoretical-foundational guide to nursing and healthcare practices. At the core of Caring Science–Human Caring Theory is a Being-Becoming in the authentic living of caring theory in practice. The 10 Caritas Processes of the theory serve as guide. However, to authentically practice human caring requires *Becoming* the theory, living out the Caritas Processes in our personal/professional lifeworld. Sustaining authentic human caring and compassion requires evolved knowledge and skills beyond just theory.

Truly Being-Becoming the theory resides within our Being—in our thoughts, our consciousness, our intentionality, our feelings, and our movements, through informed moral actions, transforming practitioners into human instruments of healing and health. This evolved level of Being evokes, invites, and requires a depth of awareness, an awakening—to the oneness of our humanness and our heart-centered connections.

Caring Science is grounded in an evolved worldview and cosmology of infinite Universal Love. Watson (2006) considers the "Ethic of Belonging" (Levinas, 1996) as the first principle of Caring Science, that is, we all *belong* to the infinite source of Love, from which we all come and to which we all return. In Caring Science, the ultimate human-to-human–Source-earth connection is One World, One Humanity, One Heart, which aligns all humanity within the quantum Life Energy Field. This Life Energy Field is the source for sustaining our own and others' humanity—it becomes the breath of life itself.

We know at the primordial level that "what we carry in our heart matters" (Cowling, Smith, & Watson, 2008). Our heart is the core source of our life force for caring and compassion, for love, beauty, truth, the very source for sustaining our humanity. Without connecting through caring from our heart, the full manifestation of the theory is limited. Without authentically feeling from our heart, caring actually can be detrimental to ourselves and others, draining off our life energy in "trying to care."

This One-world, One-heart awakening takes us to the source of our caring and healing. We can now acknowledge that the core Caritas Processes, such as Caring, Compassion, Loving-Kindness, and authentic Presence, reside within our hearts, not our heads alone. It is the human-to-human heart energetic connection of infinite Love, in the moment, which unites us as one—humanity, one energetic field of unity, which transcends the moment, radiating into infinity.

TRANSPERSONAL CARING MOMENT

The essence of the theory of human caring is the caring moment. A caring moment is transpersonal in that it transcends time, space, and physicality. The actual moment of caring has a field of its own that is greater than the occasion itself, "as such the process can go beyond itself, yet arise from aspects of itself that becomes part of the life history of each person, as well as part of some larger, deeper complex pattern of life" (Watson, 2012, p. 72).

The "caring moment" is transpersonal, in that the presence of the *geist*, or spirit of both, creates a new field; it then expands the limits of openness; that moment has the ability to expand consciousness and human evolution (Watson, 2012, p. 72). Transpersonal connotes a spirit-to-spirit connection where the intersubjectivity of both persons is involved; transpersonal is beyond ego and invites authentic heart-to-heart consciousness (Watson, 2012, pp. 72–73).

To Be/Become the human transpersonal caring theory is simple, yet profoundly complicated at times. It takes a meaningful consciousness and intentionality at the heart level to authentically radiate transpersonal caring and loving and kindness in a caring moment. Caritas Process 1, Loving-Kindness, is not just soft-hearted idealism. It is a clinical, literal, and emotional state of being that can be manifested, can be chosen; it can be as is an existential-spiritual turning point, lived authentically and consciously.

We can think loving, kind thoughts; we can do loving, kind things; we can surround ourselves with loving, kind reminders and affirmations. However, if our *Being* does not inspire, express, "in the moment," an authentic inner feeling in our heart, which is the source of caring, caring becomes draining. It is not heart aligned with authentic human-to-human caring for self or other. Thus, the transpersonal moment can be biocidic or biogenic (Halldorsdottir, 1991), depending on consciousness, intentionality, and authentic heart presence of nurse and caregiver. The Caritas practitioner is called upon and challenged to carry out evidence-informed heart-centered caring practice knowledge and skills; this is where Caring Science meets Heart Science.

HEART SCIENCE

Again: "What we carry in our heart matters." The heart, the largest oscillating organ in the body, instantly reflects emotional states. Any human's emotional state can be determined with 75% accuracy by analyzing the heart's rhythmic patterns, which are radiated into the external environment in the heart's electromagnetic field. When we genuinely experience feelings such as loving-kindness in our heart, in a caring moment, the heart rhythm patterns instantly become harmonious and coherent. Any renewing emotion such as compassion, care, and appreciation will produce this signal. It is this simple (but authentic) shift in feeling that instantly changes our physiology. This in turn has a beneficial effect on our mental capacities, emotions, and overall well-being.

Likewise, when we are experiencing stressful emotions such as fear, frustration, or anxiety, our heart rhythm patterns, reflecting the state of our autonomic nervous system, instantly become chaotic (McCraty, 2001, 2015; McCraty, Atkinson, Tiller, Rein, & Watkins, 1995). Figure 8.1 illustrates chaotic and coherent heart rate variability difference between depleting (noncaring) and renewing (caring; see Figures 8.1 and 8.2).

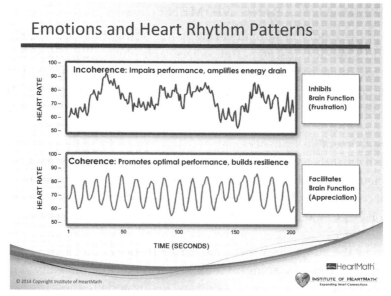

FIGURE 8.1 Heart rate variability and emotions.

Source: Courtesy of HeartMath, Inc. Used with permission.

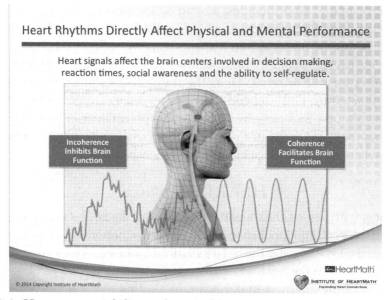

FIGURE 8.2 Heart rate variability and cortical function.

Source: Courtesy of HeartMath, Inc. Used with permission.

When our heart rhythms are chaotic, it is an inefficient use of energy, which can lead to burnout and inhibited brain function. We can maladapt and familiarize to this unhealthy pattern in our nervous system, and this strain can make it more challenging to appropriately care for ourselves and others. We are simply trying to survive. When we learn to generate coherent heart rhythms, it is an efficient use of energy and quickly builds resilience. These heart rhythms facilitate cortical function and our ability to choose appropriate behaviors and attitudes. This increases (with more ease) to be more genuinely loving and kind to ourselves and others. This literal and figurative "shift in heart" helps us "become the theory" (Box 8.1) from the inside out (McCraty, 2001, 2015).

BACKGROUND OF HEART RESEARCH PREMISES[1]

BOX 8.1

Heart Sciences Premises

- The heart is the source for caring, compassion, truth, beauty, and Love, the source for sustaining humanity and humanness.

- The heart is more than an organ that pumps blood and sustains life physically. New research has acknowledged that the heart has its own type of intelligence; it produces an electromagnetic field that can be detected several feet around an individual that communicates its energetic message nonverbally. The information in this field changes on the basis of our emotional state and has an impact on each other and our environment.

- The heart is now known to send more messages to the brain than the brain sends to the heart. These messages, whether biochemical, neurological, or energetic, help us make sense of our world and how to respond to it, both internally and externally. This evolving knowledge reminds us that "listening to our heart" may not be a figure of speech, and "what we carry in our hearts" may truly matter, for both old and new reasons, scientifically and otherwise.

- Love is a form of unitive Energy processed by the heart that brings all of life together, a "fifth force" as subtle energy, which is "vital" to our life force.

- Research on the heart at the Institute of HeartMath has been translated into concrete, heart-focused practices that manifest physiological and energetic coherence enabling us to be aligned with the optimal healing benefits of the heart, our love and deep care.

Source: Taken from Watson, J., & Browning, R. (2012). Viewpoint: Caring science meets heart science: A guide to authentic caring practice. *American Nurse Today*, 7(8). Retrieved from https://www.americannursetoday.com/viewpoint-caring-science-meets-heart-science-a -guide-to-authentic-caring-practice. Reprinted with permission from *American Nurse Today*.

CARITASHEART METHODOLOGY PRAXIS

On the basis of the theory and philosophy of Caring Science and research and premises of Heart Science, the CaritasHeart method has been developed as a method that translates theory to informed conscious human caring and healing. The core CaritasHeart

---

[1]This section is a partial reprint from Watson, J., & Browning, R. (2012). Viewpoint: Caring science meets heart science: A guide to authentic caring practice. *American Nurse Today*, 7(8). Retrieved from https://www.americannursetoday.com/viewpoint-caring-science-meets-heart-science-a-guide-to -authentic-caring-practice. Reprinted with permission from *American Nurse Today*.

methodology that we offer to clinical and educational partners was in part sourced from combining the philosophical-theoretical foundation of the Caritas Process with the HeartMath Institute (501c3; McCraty, 2001, 2015) method called a "Heart Lock-In®." The focus is on how to generate caring and compassion renewal, rather than stress, burnout, and compassion fatigue. The "Heart Lock-In" approach neutralizes stress, generating a renewing heart-centered emotion, which can authentically radiate to those for whom we are caring.

This HeartMath "Heart Lock-In" (McCraty, 2001, 2015) knowledge and method merges with Watson's Caritas Processes with the explicit intention of manifesting specifically Caritas Processes #1 and #8. However, the method and heart science underpin all the 10 Caritas Processes. For example, breathing and radiating heart-centered loving-kindness optimize the healing environment. This nurtures the potency, healing capacity of both the practitioner and the patient alike—optimizing healing for all. Every moment can then become an authentic caring-healing moment for both. This transpersonal moment results in an evolved heart-centered self-caring practice methodology.

CARITAS PRAXIS

Caritas Process (CP) 1: Sustaining Values Through Practice of Loving-Kindness and Equanimity. To manifest Caritas Process 1 is the umbrella and foundation to all the other Caritas Processes. When we step into loving-kindness, the other processes become more natural and easily manifested with ever-increasing creativity.

Caritas Process (CP) 8: Creating a Healing Environment at All Levels. The other core process that is central to the emergence of Caring Science and Heart Science is Caritas Process 8, creating a healing environment. The depth of this process at the advanced levels of the caring theory practice is to master the capability of being and becoming the healing environment, creating the environment on the physical plane, beyond the paint, plants, and beautiful fountains. Any hospital can build a new building, but if the hearts that beat within that new building remain in a chaotic and biocidic environmental field, practitioners and patients alike experience the energetic field environment as toxic and nonhealing. To realize we are part of the field and can affect the field calls for more personal responsibility, to breathe the attitudes that influence our energetic output. This is becoming the healing environment; thus, with the authentic heart practices of Caritas Processes, we indeed become the healing environment (Figure 8.3).

However, from a heart science perspective, any time we transform a depleting emotion into a renewing one (and stabilize this baseline of inner harmony), we further manifest and become the caring theory. Any feeling that is resilient building such as compassion, appreciation, love, care, forgiveness, and joy can instantly bring balance and harmony to our physiology and raise the overall vibration of the human system (McCraty, 2001, 2015). This shift inside is a profound first step into living the theory.

At the core, at the essence of the caring theory, is the creation, experience, and sharing of caring moments, which are transpersonal and transcendent. This first step into balancing ourselves and radiating more love is first a caring moment for ourselves, which

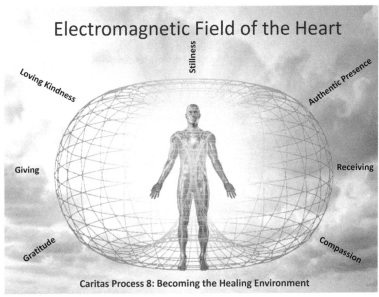

FIGURE 8.3 Electromagnetic field of the heart and Caritas Process 8.
Source: Courtesy of HeathMath, Inc. Used with permission.

then frees the energy needed to give it more fully to another, generating an energetic field beyond the two (Figure 8.4). This first step of being loving and kind to self (CP 1) gives us the energy to give love and create a more healing environment for another (CP 8). This is being and becoming. This is where we become a caring moment for another, and forever both of us are changed.

This broadens the definition of healing. Remembering the origins of the word "health": hale (the Anglo Saxon word for wholeness), to become whole, "holy" is the heart and essence of the Caring Science/Heart Science Praxis mode, to become whole.

The integration and convergence of Caring Science and Heart Science take us beyond the lower vibrating consciousness of "fixing the body physical," instead stepping into a method and informed moral and scientific praxis that guides us back to our hearts, to the heart of caring, of self, of our profession, back to soul care—returning to the essence of who we are. This combined CaritasHeart method leads to a higher energetic field of loving consciousness. It is not just *us* doing something to someone, or fixing anything. It is sharing a moment of loving presence, where "care is not a means to an end. It is an end unto itself," and perhaps the highest ethical commitment to humanity (Watson, 2008, 2012).

The added benefit in stepping into this deeper nature is that it creates an environment that optimizes healing on all levels: physical, mental, emotional, and spiritual. When the information in the electromagnetic field we broadcast is coherent and harmonious, it helps those in need to align with that coherence and balance within themselves. The resulting balance can affect the efficiency and effectiveness of their healing process as well (McCraty, 2001, 2015; McCraty, Atkinson, Tomasino, & Bradley, 2009).

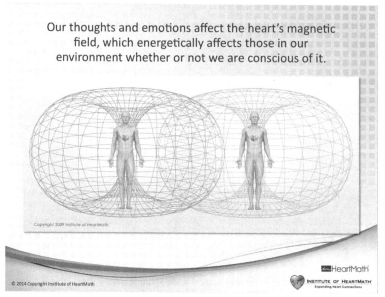

FIGURE 8.4 Heart electromagnetic fields intersecting.

Source: Courtesy of HeathMath, Inc. Used with permission.

CARITAS PRAXIS TEACHINGS CONGRUENT WITH HEARTMATH[2]

- "Authentic presence" is the starting point for practicing the caring theory; it is foundational for a "caring moment" (Watson, 1985, 2012) and human-to-human connection. Thus, an exercise of *"centering"*—emptying out and breathing—has been used as a Watson teaching/practice process over the years (Watson, 1985, 1999, 2003, 2005a, 2005b, 2006, 2008, 2009, 2011; Watson & Browning, 2009; Watson & Foster, 2003) to prepare nurses for authentic presence and connection. This concrete practice helps one to engage in the first Caritas Process: cultivation of loving-kindness and equanimity for self/other.

- These simple, concrete practices, emergent from the theory, are related to the nurse's capacity to sustain humanistic-altruistic values and caring-healing, authentic caring moments.

- The research on the heart affirms that one's heart-centered presence affects the entire field of practice and thus the authenticity of caring moments.

- The HeartMath method has specific research-based protocols that guide one through one's scientifically researched concrete heart-centered practices, thus facilitating

[2]This section is from Watson, J., & Browning, R. (2012). Viewpoint: Caring science meets heart science: A guide to authentic caring practice. *American Nurse Today, 7*(8). Retrieved from https://www.americannursetoday.com/viewpoint-caring-science-meets-heart-science-a-guide-to-authentic-caring-practice. Reprinted with permission from *American Nurse Today.*

authentic presence and capacity for genuine caring that is radiating from the heart. Thus, Caring Science Theory and its ethic and philosophical foundation for Caritas practices blend with the HeartMath protocols, resulting in a new methodology (McCraty, 2001, 2015).

TRANSLATING CARING SCIENCE THEORY TO AUTHENTIC HEART SCIENCE–INFORMED PRACTICES

Many believe that at the beginning of creation, there was an energetic impulse, a vibration that created all. Before there is matter, there is energy. Some models show how energy gives rise and manifestation to matter. Moreover, this notion underpins the ultimate emergence of the Caritas Processes in each human being. At the core of each process is energy, and as one aligns, creates, and manifests the core of that energy in one's heart and in one's feelings, it gives rise to all of the creative manifestations that each Caritas Process can become and give to the world. The key to truly living the theory is to become it (Tables 8.1 and 8.2). It is to be it. From here, our creative intuition can flow and manifest in appropriate ways that help each aspect of theory come alive in all contexts of our lives from home or work, with a family member, or patient or colleague.

CARITASHEART PRAXIS EXEMPLARS

TABLE 8.1 Ten Caritas Processes Guided by Caring Science/Heart Science

Caritas Processes	Guided by Caring Science/Heart Science
Caritas Process 1 Practice of loving-kindness	Feeling love and kindness for self and other in the heart—radiating within and without, affecting self/ other/field
Caritas Process 2 Authentically present	When we clear the stress and step into a more balanced heart, we become more present and able to care for ourselves and each other, enabling faith in hope
Caritas Process 3 Sensitivity to self/others	Nurturing individual beliefs and practices—as our heart rhythms are coherent, we become more sensitive to receiving and perceiving the needs of others and how to appropriately respond to the moment. As we become more sensitive and reflective of self, we are evolving in spiritual consciousness, closer to Source
Caritas Process 4 Trusting-caring relationships	As we are more coherent, through heart-centered feelings, we are able to connect to the heart rhythms of others, and the bonds of authenticity become more solid and real as opposed to scripted or artificial communication

(continued)

TABLE 8.1 Ten Caritas Processes Guided by Caring Science/Heart Science *(continued)*

Caritas Processes	Guided by Caring Science/Heart Science
Caritas Process 5 Allowing expression of positive–negative feelings	Holding compassion and neutrality, we have latitude to receive the polarity of all emotion, and this is healing. We offer authentic listening to another's story with discernment but no judgment
Caritas Process 6 Creative problem solving/ solution seeking	By being coherent, a signal is sent up the vagus nerve facilitating the higher centers of the brain, increasing the ratios of innovation, creativity, and access to our intuitive capabilities. When heart-centered and present, we access new approaches to difficulties, transforming them into creative challenges
Caritas Process 7 Transpersonal teaching–learning	When heart-centered, we have more discernment in how to meaningfully connect to another to share and connect, working from their frame of reference for authentic coaching and mutual sharing for learning
Caritas Process 8 Creating a healing environment	As we are coherent and feeling authentically caring emotions, the electromagnetic field of our heart radiates higher energy vibration into the field environment. This energetic field affects our authentic presence, and increases the chance of cultivating coherence in another. This optimizes healing and our energetic presence becomes the subtle healing environment
Caritas Process 9 Assistance with basic needs and sacred acts	As we are more centered and balanced in ourselves, we are more loving, kind, compassionate, and sensitive, and discerning how to practically handle and care for the basic needs for and with another. We touch another person as embodied spirit, offering soul care; CaritasHeart method becomes sacred Praxis
Caritas Process 10 Allowing for unknowns, mysteries, and miracles	As we are deep in our hearts, an inner alignment with our spirit and soul is created; this enables a greater awakened chance for nonlinear consciousness, opening to unknowns and phenomena that go beyond ordinary explanation; unexpected solutions to seemingly nonending problems can appear

Source: Taken from Watson, J., & Browning, R. (2012). Viewpoint: Caring science meets heart science: A guide to authentic caring practice. *American Nurse Today, 7*(8). Retrieved from https://www .americannursetoday.com/viewpoint-caring-science-meets-heart-science-a-guide-to-authentic-caring -practice. Reprinted with permission from *American Nurse Today.*

TABLE 8.2 Protocols and Praxis of CaritasHeart Methodology

Begin with "Centering–Authentic Presence" exercises, facilitating authentic heart-centered loving "presencing" to prepare for a "caring moment." These include Pausing, Silencing, and "Emptying out" before entering a patient's room; connecting with inner "still point"—breathing and releasing from heart-centered stillness; and welling up feelings of caring, loving-kindness, and compassion in one's consciousness and intentionality.

The next steps involve specific HeartMath "Heart Lock-In" exercises to engage and anchor in states of positive emotion. This method involves focusing in the area of the heart, imagining the breath flowing through the center of the chest, and activating positive heart feelings. These research-based approaches teach how to create and manifest coherence and the higher energetic caring field. This opens the heart to deep human-to-human caring feelings of gratitude, love, forgiveness, and compassion, thus experiencing and deepening the heart-centered feelings of Caritas.

The method then progresses by guiding participants through authentic personal and professional, individual, and collective self-caring, decision making, and deep heart-centered listening exercises, engaged dialogue, and feedback exchange.

Finally, the method asks participants to radiate the caring consciousness and heart-centered feelings to loved ones, colleagues, and all suffering in the world, and into the universe. The goal of radiating beyond self is to open to unitary field of universal Source for pure alignment, for renewal, to manifest a caring-healing environment, to "be/become" a healing environment of wholeness healing for self and others.

This completes the CaritasHeart methodology that integrates specific steps for theory-guided, evidence-based professional praxis.

The next step is for staff to translate this method to a caring-healing modality for patients/families—for example, inviting patients to pause, fall into their heart; breathe through their heart; experience heart feelings of love, gratitude, compassion, and forgiveness for self/other; and speak from their heart awareness and own inner wisdom as to what is most needed for their healing and caring this day.

Source: Taken from Watson, J., & Browning, R. (2012). Viewpoint: Caring science meets heart science: A guide to authentic caring practice. *American Nurse Today, 7*(8). Retrieved from https://www.americannursetoday.com/viewpoint-caring-science-meets-heart-science-a-guide-to-authentic-caring-practice. Reprinted with permission from *American Nurse Today*.

CONCLUSION

Evidence-informed, theory-guided nursing praxis is required for true healthcare reform. Caring Science Theory of Human Caring is deepened and extended by integration of heart-science healing practices. The CaritasHeart methodology generates a healing environment and contributes to person-center, caring-healing relationships; it is one-way forward toward evidence-informed Caritas Praxis (Watson & Browning, 2012). In addition, CaritasHeart methodology provides a Praxis Protocol for converging and translating Caring Science/Heart Science into exemplary, professional, authentic care, consistent with the public's desire for whole person healthcare (Watson & Browning, 2012).

NEXT ERA POSSIBILITIES

Education

- How does using CaritasHeart methodology promote energy and wholeness among nursing students? Nursing faculty?
- How can CaritasHeart methodology be used in nursing curricula to provide nursing students with strategies to promote wholeness in themselves and their patients?

Research

- What steps can I commit to in order to experience my deeper nature and true self, more often, especially in stressful situations?
- Is my heart desiring more authentic human-to-human caring moments?

Praxis

- How would Caring Science/Heart Science knowledge, combined with my personal practice of CaritasHeart methods, change the nature of nursing and healthcare reform?

Theory and Knowledge Development

- Can I envision implementing CaritasHeart methodology as a way to live the theory, in my personal/professional life?
- Do you know? Are you aware/awake to the fact that "what you carry in your heart matters?"

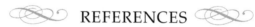 REFERENCES

Cowling, W. R., Smith, M. C., & Watson, J. (2008). The power of wholeness, consciousness, and caring a dialogue on nursing science, art, and healing. *Advances in Nursing Science, 3*(1), E41–E51. doi:10.1097/01.ANS.0000311535.11683.d1

Halldorsdottir, S. (1991). Five basic modes of being with another. In D.A. Gaut & M. M. Leininger (Eds.), *Caring: The compassionate healer* (pp. 37–49). New York, NY: National League for Nursing.

Levinas, E. (1996). *Totality and infinity*. Pittsburgh, PA: Duquesne University Press.

McCraty, R. (2001). Introduction to HeartMath. Retrieved from http://www.heartmath.org/research/science-of-the-heart/introduction.html

McCraty, R. (2015). *Science of the heart: Exploring the role of the heart in human performance*. Boulder Creek, CA: HeartMath Institute.

McCraty, R., Atkinson, M., Tiller, W. A., Rein, G., & Watkins, A. D. (1995). The effects of emotions on short-term power spectrum analysis of heart rate variability. *American Journal of Cardiology, 76*(14), 1089–1093. doi:10.1016/S0002-9149(99)80309-9

McCraty, R., Atkinson, M., Tomasino, D., & Bradley, R. T. (2009). The coherent heart: Heart-brain interactions, psychophysiological coherence, and the emergence of system-wide order. *Integral Review, 5*(2), 10–115.

Watson, J. (1985). *Nursing: The philosophy and science of caring*. Boston, MA: Little, Brown.

Watson, J. (1999). *Nursing: Human science and human care*. New York, NY: National League for Nursing.

Watson, J. (2003). Love and caring: Ethics of face and hand: An invitation to return to the heart and soul of nursing and our deep humanity. *Nursing Administration Quarterly, 27*(3), 197–202. doi:10.1097/00006216-200307000-00005

Watson, J. (2005a). *Caring science as sacred science*. Philadelphia, PA: F. A. Davis.

Watson, J. (2005b). Caring science: Belonging before being as ethical cosmology. *Nursing Science Quarterly, 18*(4), 304–305. doi:10.1177/0894318405280395

Watson, J. (2006). Caring theory as an ethical guide to administrative and clinical practices. *Nursing Administration Quarterly, 30*(1), 48–55. doi:10.1097/00006216-200601000-00008

Watson, J. (2008). *Nursing: The philosophy and science of caring.* Boulder: University Press of Colorado.

Watson, J. (2009). *Assessing and measuring caring in nursing and health sciences* (2nd ed.). New York, NY: Springer Publishing.

Watson, J. (2011). *Postmodern nursing and beyond.* Boulder, CO: Watson Caring Science Institute.

Watson, J. (2012). *Human caring science: A theory of nursing.* Sudbury, MA: Jones & Bartlett.

Watson, J., & Browning, R. (2009). *CaritasHeart methodology and practices.* Unpublished working papers.

Watson, J., & Browning, R. (2012). Viewpoint: Caring science meets heart science: A guide to authentic caring practice. *American Nurse Today, 7*(8). Retrieved from https://www.americannursetoday.com/viewpoint-caring-science-meets-heart-science-a-guide-to-authentic-caring-practice

Watson, J., & Foster, R. (2003). The Attending Nurse Caring Model: Integrating theory, evidence and advanced caring-healing therapeutics for transforming professional practice. *Journal of Clinical Nursing, 12,* 360–365. doi:10.1046/j.1365-2702.2003.00774.x

RESOURCES

HeartMath. www.HeartMath.com

HeartMath Institute. www.HeartMath.org

Watson Caring Science Institute. www.watsoncaringscience.org

Jean Watson's Facebook page. www.facebook.com/watsonjean

9

Expanding Global Reach Through a Massive Open Online Course in Mindfulness and Caring

Kathleen Sitzman

CARITAS LITERACIES

By the end of this chapter, the caring-healing nurse will be able to

1. Outline the nature and purpose of massive open online courses (MOOCs).

2. Discuss how professional collaboration enabled the creation of the first Caring Science, Mindful Practice (CSMP) MOOC.

3. Discuss key research findings related to the characteristics of global caring communities that emerged from CSMP MOOC course offerings.

4. Explain key research findings related to future caring intent after exposure to Caring Science and mindfulness content.

5. Describe how MOOCs can be used as a tool to enable the formation of multiple global caring communities when travel and face-to-face interaction across geographical distances are challenging.

The Internet is accessible to people all over the world. Emerging technologies have made Internet access possible via desktop and laptop computers, cell phones, tablets, and watches; "[an] ontological shift [beyond modern/postmodern thinking] invites us to recognize the evolving human potential that is emerging from the most recent 20th century [and now 21st century] phenomena whereby there now exists a symbiotic relationship between humankind-technology-nature and the universe" (Watson, 1999, p. 21). These resources provide expansive teaching/learning/sharing opportunities where geography, proximity, time, language, culture, and economics no longer present the formidable barriers they once did. The creation of a free MOOC, entitled "CSMP: Implementing Watson's Human Caring Theory," CSMP has enabled global caring/learning communities to emerge where trans-disciplinary, multicultural, diverse cohorts from all over the world periodically come together to learn about Watson's Caring Science and share unique perspectives about caring experiences and applications within their own disciplines, settings, and cultures.

The CSMP MOOC is taught annually in May and January in the Canvas Learning Management System. It is free of charge and open to anyone in the world with Internet access. Participants who complete 80% of the course content earn a certificate of completion. This has enabled a wide range of people in highly varied situations to benefit from the opportunity to learn, interact, and share in an academic setting that may not have been open to them earlier because of funding restraints or other limiting circumstances. The MOOC provides an opportunity to come together in an international 4-week long online asynchronous course to learn about Watson's Human Caring Theory and how to engage in simple mindfulness practices (Hanh, 2009) to support mindful, caring comportment in personal and professional life. The course is moderated by a volunteer team of Caring Science nurses and instructional designers from different regions in the United States. Learners review content, watch videos, and then participate in asynchronous discussion boards to share thoughts and experiences related to caring in their disciplines, agencies, regions, and cultures. A total of 2,630 individuals have interacted with the course content in varying degrees to date, and that number continues to grow with each new course session. Of the 2,630 people who have participated thus far, 413 (15.70%) have completed 80% of the course requirements and earned certificates of completion.

BACKGROUND INFORMATION ABOUT MOOCS

The first MOOC was offered in 2008 by Stephen Downes and George Siemens as an online course on connectivism and connective knowledge (Parr, 2013). More MOOCs with increasingly sophisticated content delivery designs followed (Mackness, 2013). Learning Management System companies that support MOOCs include Udacity, edX, Coursera, Udemy, Canvas Network, and FutureLearn.

Concerns related to offering free and open content to broad national and international audiences that have been considered by teaching professionals in higher education include the possibility of low-quality instruction, passive learning environments found in MOOCs, and low completion rates. Hew and Cheung (2014) found that the dropout rate in MOOCs could be as high as 90% because of low student motivation stemming from the absence of concrete incentives such as the opportunity to earn official academic credit on completion of the course. MOOCs, however, fill a different niche than high-stakes credit-earning academic courses. MOOCs represent a low-risk, no-cost opportunity to try online learning within and beyond academic settings. MOOC learners explore new topics and perspectives in open environments where exposure to new content and stimulation of interest, involvement, and thought development are more important than the end goal of completion. MOOC participant cohorts consist of participants from diverse disciplinary, geographical, racial, cultural, and socioeconomic backgrounds, which results in rich learning and sharing environments.

By December 2014, more than 400 colleges and universities offered more than 2,400 MOOCs, enrolling from 16 to 18 million students worldwide (Shah, 2014). According to

Sitzman, Jensen, and Chan (2016), "Humanities, computer science and programing, and business and management were the top MOOC subjects, accounting for 17 percent, 16 percent, and 12 percent of students, respectively. Health and medicine accounted for 10 percent, and education and teaching about 9.5 percent" (p. 269). MOOCs offering nursing content are rare, with only five offered between 2012 and 2015. Topics addressed in these nursing-related MOOCs included Rural Health Nursing, Impact of Nursing, Introduction to Nursing in Healthcare, Foundations of Evidence-Based Practice in Healthcare, and CSMP: Implementing Watson's Human Caring Theory (Sitzman et al., 2016).

ABOUT THE CSMP MOOC

The idea to create the CSMP MOOC came from a desire to create free and open opportunities for others to learn about ways that Caring Science and mindfulness could enrich personal and professional practices in interprofessional and transdisciplinary settings among nurses, allied health professionals, and beyond. The developer of this course created the requisite content but did not have the necessary infrastructure at her home institution to move forward. Colleagues at another institution had the needed infrastructure and were willing to partner in creating and offering the CSMP MOOC, so a fruitful cross-institutional collaboration was formed. The course content was created and provided by the course developer; instructional design and multimedia support were provided by colleagues at the second institution, and the Canvas Network provided the learning management system. Canvas Network manages the logistics of student enrollment and course access, allowing faculty and instructional designers to focus on course design, development, and facilitation. Two other organizations connected with Caring Science became supporting partners. A Memorandum of Understanding (MOU), outlining the responsibilities of all parties, was completed. The MOU clarified parameters related to faculty participation, copyright, intellectual property, supervision and evaluation of participants, technical support, accessibility, registration, records, continuing education units, marketing, and financial arrangements. After the content developer and instructional designers placed the course in the Canvas Network learning management system, nurses knowledgeable in Caring Science were invited to help facilitate the course sessions as volunteer faculty.

CSMP MOOC

This MOOC is offered every year in May and January. Each course session runs over a 4-week period. Learners who complete at least 80% of the overall course content earn a certificate of completion.

The overall purpose of the course is to facilitate basic conceptual understanding of caring and mindfulness and teach basic methods meant to facilitate mindfulness and caring practices in everyday work environments. Learners are introduced to Watson's Human Caring Theory and simple mindfulness practices in the tradition of Thich Nhat Hanh. Then they are asked to join asynchronous discussion boards twice a week to share caring insights, experiences, and practices through the use of reflective narrative and contemplative art. The discussion boards are actively moderated by a team of volunteer faculty members who provide encouragement, support, and feedback to each learner.

Topical areas covered during the 4-week period include the following:

- Overview of Watson's Theory
  a. Transpersonal Caring Moments
  b. Core and Trim of nursing practice
  c. The 10 Caritas Processes®

- Mindfulness in the tradition of Thich Nhat Hanh

- Caritas Consciousness Touchstones for Cultivating Love

Web links, video lectures, slide presentations, and instructional materials provide content that covers the course concepts. There is also a textbook available to accompany the course:

- Sitzman, K., & Watson, J. (2014). *Caring science, mindful practice: Implementing Watson's Human Caring Theory.* New York, NY: Springer Publishing.

PROCESS FOR ESTABLISHING INSTRUCTIONAL EXCELLENCE

Instructional success depended on multiple factors being collaboratively and proactively addressed by course developers (Sitzman et al., 2016), including the following:

- The course content was piloted with a small interprofessional group to determine needed adjustments to pacing and content.

- After the pilot, the course was developed into an MOOC in collaboration with seasoned instructional designers and technical support to assure aesthetic appeal and ease of navigation.

- MOOC design requires simplicity in content and process because of the diversity of learners who will likely participate. It is crucial to keep this in mind during the entire design process.

- Strong collaborative teamwork that includes expertise in the areas of content, instructional design, and the technical aspects of MOOC delivery is essential to support excellence.

- Flexibility in course administration is key in meeting unanticipated learner needs, for example, using Google Translate (translate.google.com), a free and open online translation service, to facilitate interacting, understanding, and learning when learners post in languages other than English in the discussion boards.

- The entire faculty team must be watchful on a daily basis for times when learners might need clarification or guidance so that stressful or difficult situations can be resolved quickly.

- Simple, carefully worded instructions to address specific concerns should appear in general announcements and be emailed to learners within 24 hours of a student or group of students indicating confusion or difficulty with processes or content.

- Frequent, open, and collaborative communication among faculty, designers, and learners will lead to a dynamic, learner-centered experience.

Two studies that explored multiple aspects of the first two CSMP MOOC sessions are presented in the following text. They provide further insight into the global caring communities that the CSMP MOOC enabled.

Two Studies Related to the CSMP MOOC

Sitzman et al. (2016) examined the first two CSMP MOOC sessions completed in 2015 and 2016 to determine demographics, learner satisfaction, course flow, and perceived usefulness of CSMP content for a broad international audience that included nurses, allied health professionals, and many others. The study was approved by an institutional review board and approved informed consent was obtained from participants. Course "Welcome" and "End-of-Course" surveys provided demographic information and ratings related to course satisfaction. Discussion board postings provided narrative data related to usefulness and applicability of caring and mindfulness content. These data were analyzed using descriptive statistics and content analysis of narrative data (Holloway & Freshwater, 2007). A combined summary of the findings (Sitzman et al., 2016) is shown in Table 9.1.

TABLE 9.1 Combined 2015 to 2016 CSMP MOOC Demographic Data

Gender (N = 234)	
Female	90.17% (n = 211)
Male	9.82% (n = 23)
Geographical Location (N = 234)	
North America	83.76% (n = 196)
Western Europe, Asia, Australia/South Pacific, Middle East, South America, and Central America	16.24% (n = 38)
Primary Language (N = 234)	
English	90.60% (n = 212)
Non-English	9.40% (n = 22)
Educational Level (N = 223)	
Master's degree or higher	43.94% (n = 98)
Undergraduate degree (4 years)	29.60% (n = 66)
Other educational experience	26.46% (n = 59)
Occupations (N = 222)	
Healthcare	85.14% (n = 189)
Non-Healthcare	14.86% (n = 33)

CSMP, Caring Science, Mindful Practice; MOOC, massive open online course.

TABLE 9.2 Course Ratings and Engagement Data

Registered Learners ($N = 996$)	
Learner engagement	
Reviewed Course Material	53.41% ($n = 532$)
Discussion Board Postings	5,534 postings
Certificates of Completion	16.66% ($n = 166$)
Course Ratings (0–5 stars, 0 being the lowest approval and 5 being the highest approval; $N = 136$)	
5 stars rating	69.85% ($n = 95$)
4 stars rating	25.74% ($n = 35$)
3 to 2 stars rating	4.41% ($n = 6$)
1 star rating	0% ($n = 0$)

Higher than expected learner activity levels were reflected in the number of registrants who took time to review the course materials and the number of learner and facilitator discussion board postings. The course completion rate, which is generally considered to be a success if above 4% to 6% (Margaryan, Bianco, & Littlejohn, 2015) for a MOOC, was 16.66% ($N = 166$) indicating an unusually high learner engagement for this MOOC. At the end of the course, participants were asked to provide an overall rating of the course, presented in Table 9.2. The rating scale ranged from 1 star (being the lowest approval rating) to 5 stars (being the highest approval rating). Of the total 136 participants, 130 (95.59%) rated the course at 4 to 5 stars, with only six participants rating the course at lower than 4 stars, confirming that content and delivery methods were effective for the course.

One hundred eighty-five learners, irrespective of whether they completed the course, communicated specific and detailed plans to implement mindfulness and Caritas practices at work and home after the course was over. Five themes emerged from these qualitative data (adapted and summarized from Sitzman et al., 2016, pp. 271 & 273)[1]:

1. **Pay attention to what is happening in the present moment with self, others, and surroundings.**
   - "I think one of the most beneficial things I did was to include the mindfulness bell as an app on my phone. I have it set to go off randomly throughout the day. When I hear it, I take a moment to reflect on what is going on at the time."

---

[1]This section has been adapted from Sitzman, K. L., Jensen, A., & Chan, S. (2016). Creating a global community of learners in nursing and beyond: Caring science, mindful practice massive open online course (MOOC). *Nursing Education Perspectives, 37*(5), 269–274. doi:10.1097/01.NEP.0000000000000062

- "For me, a big part of integrating the Caritas Processes into my daily practice is a commitment to creating the time and space to stop and pause and become centered … When things get hectic, and everyone is placing requests upon you, it is easy to get lost. Our work is not so much about what we do, but how we can 'be' and thus through our authentic presence, the enactment of the roles and tasks take on new meaning and new directions. This course has been a chance to stop and do that."

2. **Establish or reestablish a firm intent to care deeply for self, others, and surroundings.**
   - "The course has energized my commitment to reviving Caring Science at work …"
   - "This program has touched another layer of myself that I didn't know was what is was. … by tapping into this I appreciate me, my accomplishments and my dedication to myself, my family, my work and how I care. I love that I am a nurse and that I can make a difference in the lives I touch. What I didn't realize was that I wasn't always mindful of my surroundings, thoughts, actions, or feelings as it relates to the person I want to be. This has unshackled me again like times before and it gives me the confidence to grow in different directions and live again in the place most comfortable, nursing."

3. **Cultivate curiosity rather than judgment in relation to self and others.**
   - "By learning all of Jean Watson's Caritas (Processes), I can integrate all parts starting with myself then with my patients by realizing we all want the same things out of life and ourselves to be cared for with respect, dignity, and kindness."
   - "Well, I just had an experience at work yesterday where I was able to practice grounding, being mindful of myself and meditation on my immediate reaction to a situation …, as I was going towards the conference room I did some self-assessments and told myself 'just sit back and listen to what they have to say so you might get a better understanding of the decisions' … I am so glad that I have been in this class right now to remind me of this. I … listened, and I did come to a clearer understanding …"

4. **Unashamedly embrace caring as an ideal in nursing and in life.**
   - "I want to enmesh the 10 Caritas (Processes) into my whole existence, to help me become a better person to my family and friends as well as my patients."
   - "My goal is to help nurses rise above the current chaos and find the light offered by mindfulness and Caritas Consciousness touchstones."

5. **Create specific plans for undertaking visible, public projects in professional or home settings meant to teach or reinforce concepts related to mindfulness and caring.**
   - "This week I am meeting with my manager to plan to place a Caring Science bulletin board in our conference room, where shift huddles and meetings take place. It will be aesthetically beautiful and informative. I plan sections on the Caritas Processes, inspirations and reflections on caring and self-caring, resources, and upcoming events. At our next committee meeting, we will review our strategies for our quarterly classes and how we can incorporate a centering moment into shift huddles."

- "My immediate professional goal is to … create a healing environment for the physical and spiritual self who respects human dignity. … I am planning to establish [a] Caritas nursing workgroup that will target implementation of caring-healing environments in [my] units. We will meet every week, and we will introduce mindful practice to the group. I know we have many talents or stars among staff members and we want our patients to feel loved and cared for in the best environment possible. … I think this workgroup will [provide] a vehicle to express … creativity and uniqueness and will help foster teamwork as [our nurses] work together to transform their units."

Hebdon, Clayton, & Sitzman (2016) explored specific caring intentions of participants who completed the same CSMP MOOC that was examined in the study by Sitzman et al. (2016). The aim was to examine caring intention transformation among participants, specifically caring intentions of participants after completing the course. The data were in the form of posting board discussions where learners posted descriptions of what they planned to do to continue caring practice after the course was over. The content was analyzed for themes and consistencies. Five primary themes with accompanying subthemes emerged from the data (summarized and adapted from Hebdon et al., 2016)[2]:

1. **The ripple effect from caring and interconnection**
   - Those we serve need to know we care.
   - Caring is reciprocal.

2. **The importance of self-care to support the provision of optimal care for others**
   - Through self-care, we can heal.

3. **Validation of caring/mindfulness practices in varied settings**
   - Courage helps us continue to care.
   - Caring and mindfulness extend to all aspects of life.

4. **Infusion of Caring Science into mentoring relationships at work**
   - Caring and mindfulness are integral in any professional practice.
   - Cultivate collegiality in caring.
   - Caring Science must be integrated into nursing culture.

5. **Application of mindfulness and caring concepts**
   - Recentering and self-care are necessary in ongoing ways.
   - Continuing education is always needed.
   - Sharing and learning about caring and mindfulness supports empowerment, which facilitates the process of enacting caring concepts.

---

[2]This section has been adapted from Hebdon, M., Clayton, M., & Sitzman, K. (2016). Caring intention transformation in an interprofessional massive open online course. *International Journal for Human Caring*, 20(4), 185–192. doi:10.20467/1091-5710-20.4.185

Results from both Sitzman et al. (2016) and Hebdon et al. (2016) provided evidence that caring and mindfulness content resonated with learners and helped to strengthen commitment to establish and maintain a firm intent to care personally and professionally. Demographic data confirmed that the MOOC reached a widely varied group of individuals from diverse backgrounds; however, course ratings, level of satisfaction, and emergent themes indicated that the content resonated with learners despite identified differences. Participation of these diverse learners demonstrated a desire to learn about and practice professional caring that transcends boundaries, confirming the notion that mindfulness and caring can be effectively taught in international, transdisciplinary, free, and open, online teaching/learning environments. Anecdotally, participants consistently expressed gratitude for the opportunity to share and receive validation from others regarding experiences, practices, and perceptions related to mindfulness and caring. All of the MOOC sessions to date have demonstrated that establishing global caring online teaching-learning-sharing communities is possible and that there is an international population of learners ready and willing to share and participate.

CONCLUSION

In 2002, Watson provided a vision of the metaphysical dimensions of Caritas-based teaching, learning, and interacting that mirrors the tangible outcomes associated with the CSMP MOOC:

> The emerging metaphysics for both real and virtual caring learning transformation is one of wholeness, of unitary awareness of a universe that is alive, unfolding, saturated with many more hidden orders of harmony than people can imagine, opening us again to the mysterious order that is organic and integrated … Thus, within the new metaphysics of transpersonal caring and virtual caring communities, one of the key criteria is whether individual and collective learning is being pursued in a way that supports powerful, positive, and enduring life transformations in individuals and groups. (Watson, 2002, p. 44)

This vision affirms the importance of creating global Caritas communities in the digital world such as the CSMP MOOC and calls us to create additional openings and possibilities for furthering the reach of Caring Science in this limitless realm that we are only beginning to grasp.

The transcultural/global movement toward informed and rigorous caring in healthcare and beyond has begun according to Watson (1999):

> In this emancipatory clearing for nursing and all health care practitioners, there is another movement towards the making of some common world: a world in which individuals and practice communities transcend traditional professional boundaries. (p. 19)

And according to Watson (1999), these individuals and practice communities:

come together to share unabashed love for caring and healing practices, integrating the human-nature-universe relationships in artful, aesthetic, healing practices and bringing together art, science, and spirituality to a new depth for those engaged in healing work. (p. 19)

Opportunities for collective connection, inspiration, and continuity—Cyber Communitas—are an integral component of establishing global caring consciousness (Sitzman & Watson, 2014).

Results of the two studies presented earlier suggest that well-designed MOOCs taught in the spirit of love, inclusiveness, collaboration, and mindful attentiveness can be an effective way to create global communities of learners where widely diverse nurses, healthcare professionals, and laypeople have opportunities to learn, connect, share, recount experiences, and facilitate understanding. Although MOOCs do not directly generate monetary income for those who offer them, they do offer exceptional service opportunities for those with a desire to share vital knowledge with a global audience who may otherwise be unable to participate because of geographical distance, socioeconomics, culture, and time constraints. Two of the most fundamental nursing functions, regardless of specialty area, are to care and to share knowledge that facilitates enhanced quality of life for self and others. MOOCs provide a platform for Caring Science professionals to fulfill these fundamental functions on an international scale, which will facilitate and sustain CyberCommunitas now and into the future.

NEXT ERA POSSIBILITIES

Education
- What Caring Science knowledge and practices could I share that would be helpful to a global audience?
- In what ways can I facilitate the expansion of nursing education to prepare nurses to work effectively within our deeply interconnected world and universe?
- How might I contribute to the creation of benchmarks that will model global caring within digital/cyberspace communities of patients, learners, colleagues, and beyond?
- What can I do to create openings for more MOOCs and other free and open educational offerings to meet the learning needs of all without regard to proximity and geosocial-political-economic boundaries?

Research
- What further Caring Science research is needed to form a solid theoretical and data-based foundation for purposeful and planned expansion into the digital world?
- What can Caring Science researchers do to expand and disseminate a cybercaring/digital caring lexicon that will aid the profession in engaging in meaningful dialogue related to best caring practices in cyberspace?

Praxis

- What aspects of my own practice can I infuse with Caring Science principles right now to support caring and loving-kindness for myself and others?
- What work-related projects and activities could be reimagined within a framework of Caring Science to support caring transformation at the institutional or organizational level and beyond?

Theory and Knowledge Development

- What further development is needed in educational settings to bring recognition to the need for creating and administering open educational opportunities that create openings for global sharing, fellowship, and dialogue?
- What must be done by organizations to ensure that nurses in clinical settings are encouraged and supported to reach out on a global scale to share knowledge and caring for others in free and open settings?

 REFERENCES

Hanh, T. N. (2009). New trainings for a new generation. *Mindfulness Bell, 52,* 14–15. Retrieved from https://www.mindfulnessbell.org/archive/2015/01/new-trainings-for-a-new-generation

Hebdon, M., Clayton, M., & Sitzman, K. (2016). Caring intention transformation in an interprofessional massive open online course. *International Journal for Human Caring, 20*(4), 185–192. doi:10.20467/1091-5710-20.4.185

Hew, K. F., & Cheung, W. S. (2014). *Using blended learning.* Berlin, Germany: Springer.

Holloway, I., & Freshwater, D. (2007). *Narrative research in nursing.* Oxford, UK: Blackwell.

Mackness, J. (2013, October 22). cMOOCs and xMOOCs: Key differences [Web log comment]. Retrieved from https://jennymackness.wordpress.com/2013/10/22/cmoocs-and-xmoocs-key-differences

Margaryan, A., Bianco, M., & Littlejohn, A. (2015). Instructional quality of massive open online courses (MOOCs). *Computers & Education, 80,* 77–83. doi:10.1016/j.compedu.2014.08.005

Parr, C. (2013, October 17). Mooc creators criticise courses' lack of creativity. *Times Higher Education.* Retrieved from http://www.timeshighereducation.co.uk/news/mooc-creators-criticise-courses-lack-of-creativity/2008180.article?page=0 percent2C0

Shah, D. (2014). Online courses raise their game: A review of MOOC stats and trends in 2014 [Web log comment]. Retrieved from http://www.class-central.com/report/moocs-stats-and-trends-2014

Sitzman, K. L., Jensen, A., & Chan, S. (2016). Creating a global community of learners in nursing and beyond: Caring science, mindful practice massive open online course (MOOC). *Nursing Education Perspectives, 37*(5), 269–274. doi:10.1097/01.NEP.0000000000000062

Sitzman, K., & Watson, J. (2014). *Caring science, mindful practice.* New York, NY: Springer Publishing.

Watson, J. (1999). *Postmodern nursing and beyond.* London, UK: CPI Anthony Rowe.

Watson, J. (2002). Metaphysics of virtual caring communities. *International Journal of Human Caring, 6*(1), 41–45.

Conscious Dying: Human Caring Amid Pain and Suffering*

William Rosa, Tarron Estes, Stephanie Hope, and Jean Watson

CARITAS LITERACIES

By the end of this chapter, the caring-healing nurse will be able to

1. Discuss Conscious Dying as a unique framework emerging from an ontology of Caring Science.

2. Embrace Conscious Dying principles amid complex pain and suffering.

3. Self-reflect on Caring Science, Conscious Dying, and self-transcendence as elements of creating a healing environment for the dying one.

Caring Science is an extant theory of human relationship, guiding the profession of nursing with the understanding and application of a moral-ethical praxis that promotes, protects, and provides human dignity throughout the life continuum (Watson, 2008, 2012). For more than 30 years, Caring Science has transformed nursing by calling for a heightened ethos of human dignity in how nurses practice, educate, research, and evolve the profession. It continues to expand and adapt to the needs of patients, nurses, and health systems worldwide, being integrated into policies, and contributing to the emergence of additional nursing paradigms. Conscious Dying is a framework rooted in a human caring ontology, which strives to deepen the nurse healer's awareness in tending

*This chapter is adapted from two manuscripts with permission: Rosa, W., Estes, T., & Watson, J. (2017). Caring science conscious dying: An emerging meta-paradigm. *Nursing Science Quarterly, 30*(1), 58–64. doi:10.1177/0894318416680538; Rosa, W., & Hope, S. (2017). Pain and suffering at end of life: Birthing the sacred passage. *Beginnings, 37*(4), 10–13.

to a patient's dying and death, returning death to its sacred place in the cycle of life (Estes, 2013). These two paradigms share much in common, as they both call for an elevated and evolved human consciousness in the care of self and other, from both personal and global perspectives.

Reflective inventories are self-reflection tools that have been used to encourage nurses' personal growth and development, and may be employed in individual or group settings (Rosa, 2017; Rosa & Santos, 2016). They may be applied to aid nurses in self-renewal and self-care through individual reflection on the values of Caring Science (Rosa, 2014a), and to evaluate the heart-centered readiness of systems through a more collective approach to reflection, based on the ideals of Conscious Dying (Rosa, 2014b). Reflective inventories are provided in this article to illustrate the connections between Caring Science and Conscious Dying. The purpose herein is to introduce an emerging meta-paradigm that links self to system, interweaving and integrating the teachings of Caring Science and Conscious Dying through the use of reflective inventories for both the individual nurse and collective of nursing.

CARING SCIENCE PARADIGM (*DRAWS UPON PREVIOUS PUBLICATIONS)

Caring Science, as the disciplinary philosophical-ethical foundation in nursing and health-healing science has been quietly evolving for the past 25 years or so (Watson, 1979/1985, 1985/1999, 2008, 2012). As it has come of age, it has become more universal across cultures, countries, worldviews, and belief traditions. It is offered as an evolving view for science and for reverential, if not holy, professional caring-healing, living-dying practices, beyond the conventional, body-physical, biomedical, techno-cure science of medicine.

The discipline of nursing within a Caring Science context has a worldview in which ethics, caring relations, and an acknowledgment of our *Belonging* (connectedness with the infinite Universal field of consciousness of Spirit/energy/Source) becomes the ethical starting point. Therefore, our "Belonging" comes before our separate ontology of "Being" for itself alone. With that as ground of our Being/Belonging on the Earth plane, then Ethic of Belonging becomes the first principle of science—result: Caring Science (Levinas, 1969/2000; Watson, 2005a, 2008, 2012).

The European philosophy of Levinas (1969/2000) and his notions of totality and infinity remind us of our belonging and the human-cosmos-oneness. The Ethic of Belonging becomes the primordial source for sustaining our humanity and the source for all human evolution and the sacred circle of life, death–no death.

Therefore, a metaphysical relationship between our physical-scientific world and the universal infinity of the evolving human consciousness is reestablished (Watson, 2005a). This view helps to reunite the human spirit with the infinite source of cosmic Love. Once one has backed up to this level of consideration of life and human-cosmic relationship, as one of Belonging before Being, then we have a new cosmology for considering the human place in the universe, not separate from the universal field of infinite Love. This cosmology of Belonging becomes an ethic and moral foundation for how it guides and sustains our Being-in-the-world and how we engage in our living and dying on the physical plane (Watson, 2005b).

TRANSPERSONAL CARING MOMENT

The unitary relation with infinity of Universal Love opens us to a quantum world, or a quantum cosmology. That is, we now know from science and quantum thinking that the mere act of participating, or observing a system, causes a system to change its behavior. Caring Science, with nursing and transdisciplinary practices, grounds the expanded, quantum worldview by embracing the quantum field of the whole: Universal Consciousness.

For example, this thinking translates into: One's Caring-Healing consciousness in a given moment energetically can affect the quantum field. In Caring Science, which is referred to as Transpersonal Caring—which can happen in a given moment; and as such Transpersonal Caring acknowledges:

- Caring consciousness transcends time, space, and physicality.

- Caring consciousness can be joined—with infinite quantum universal field of Infinite Love.

- Caring Consciousness in a given moment transcends the moment and becomes part of the larger complex pattern of the life field.

- Consciousness can evolve to higher levels—Caring Loving consciousness—referred to as Caritas Consciousness (Watson, 2008).

Teilhard de Chardin reminded us that the human can continue to evolve to a higher level of consciousness, beyond physical—even to the Omega point—or closer to Godhead—that is Universal Love, that is, *Caritas* Consciousness (Watson, 2008)—Caring and Universal Love converge.

The work of David Hawkins (2002), spiritual teacher, scientist, psychiatrist, and mystic, highlighted the power of the Human Spirit and the evolution of consciousness. With his scientific and spiritual teaching, the subtle and not so subtle connections between consciousness (Caritas-Love) are connected with energetic healing in that the energy is radiating into the field of the whole.

Hawkins noted, if we really understood this basic knowledge, the world as we know it would be irrevocably changed—requiring all practices of politics, war, communications, media, economics, and other fields including medicine to transform their consciousness and patterns of practice (Watson, 2014).

Such transformation is part of the evolutionary, if not revolutionary, approach to living and dying caring-healing practices. For example, conventional practices of bodily physical death and dying associated with physical disease reside in a lower vibration field and do not allow for evolution of human consciousness to a higher vibrational field—for example, opening to conscious dying practices—living well/dying well at Universal Spirit field level—transcending and evolving even beyond death as we know it on a physical plane.

On the basis of this evolution of consciousness and the Ethic of Belonging to Universal consciousness of infinite Love, perhaps the next phase of the work in living and dying is to go beyond the dense lower vibrations of exclusive physicality and separation; therefore a moral imperative to systematically move toward higher vibrational field of Unitary Caritas consciousness for whole person health, healing, death, and conscious dying—taking our practices to another level of consciousness beyond physical. This includes the high-energy heart-healing practices of transitioning for a sacred passage allowing flow of gratitude, forgiveness, grace, caring, compassion, love combined with sacred rituals, prayers, practices that unify physical with nonphysical as one (Watson, 2013).

Caring Science, Transpersonal Caring-Healing, Caritas Consciousness have an entirely different meaning for affecting human living/dying and caring-healing for all living things to which we all Belong, reside, live, dwell, share, draw upon, come from, and return to in the sacred circle of birthing, living, dying, and rebirthing.

CONSCIOUS DYING PARADIGM

In the 1970s, Elisabeth Kübler-Ross became a powerful and leading voice urging better care for the dying. Kübler-Ross (1969), through her seminal work with the Five Stages of Grief, described the series of emotional processes experienced when faced with the impending death of self or a loved one. Kübler-Ross placed much emphasis on a direct, honest, and reflective style of patient/family interviewing throughout all five stages; denial, anger, bargaining, depression, and acceptance. This type of conversation includes a caring, confident, conscious, and open communication style that builds trusting-caring-healing relationships with patients, allowing them to go through a much wanted and needed life review as well and emotional completion process (Kübler-Ross, 1969). Furthermore, her work demonstrates that when a patient and care provider discuss dying courageously and candidly, anticipatory grief can be attended to in a more timely manner and, most importantly, a good death is possible (Kübler-Ross, 1969; Kübler-Ross & Kessler, 2005).

Kübler-Ross's model creates the opportunity for *healing*, as opposed to *curing*. *Healing care* is conscious care that springs courageously from our hearts and assumes our interconnectedness to each other and to all life (Watson, 2008). In a curative approach, the focus is the eradication of a disease's signs and symptoms, which does not necessarily diminish a patient's distress or disease, and may not always be possible, whereas healing can be multidimensional, occur on an emotional, mental, spiritual, or physical plane, and is *always* possible (Quinn, 2016). Death, itself, is included as a healing event and, often with the aid of supportive, courageous guides, healing in other nonphysical domains of life that the transformative portal surrounding end of life makes accessible is possible (Conscious Dying Institute [CDI], 2013). Offering healing (vs. curative) care depends on the use of emotional intelligence and empathic capacity and assumes that because human beings are capable of experiencing and expressing a full range of intimate, human-caring qualities through the five senses and in all domains of life, they are also capable of providing the full range of intimate, human-caring-healing offerings to others during vulnerable stages of life through death.

Healing care attempts to humanize both the Golden Rule, "Do unto others as you would have them do unto you," and the vital pledge of the Hippocratic Oath, "Do no harm." When one thinks of his or her dying time or being with others during his or her death in this way, one must imagine: What is it that *I*, as an individual, really want? What care do *I* want *now* and at end of life *beyond* medically curative care? If one is a nurse or other clinician: How can *I* serve *beyond* "Do no harm?" What would *I* want for myself and for my loved ones?

Just as Watson (2012) acknowledged the dehumanizing and bureaucratically dominated aspects of the healthcare crisis as an opportunity to bring healing care to patients, facilities, and providers, Kübler-Ross (1969) saw the dying process as an opportunity of healing, not only for patients and families but also for hospital staff and the systems they sustain as well. During the later years of her work, she talked about the imperative for a new model of end-of-life education for clinicians and caregivers. For without this new form of education, she believed, the fear-based culture of death and dying and restoration of human dignity for patients and families and their ultimate healing would not be addressed. Through her use of Conscious Dying Care and Communication, she improved the experience for the dying and was instrumental as a leader in the evolution of human consciousness.

CDI (2013) delivers conscious dying education and care that goes beyond the compassionate palliative and hospice team-based model, bringing a sacred, caring-healing philosophy and experience of wholeness back to caregivers who practice the call to awaken by serving at end of life, unifying the many nonmedical offerings of the team-based model under the scope and intentionality of a single individual caregiver. Conscious Dying views each caring professional as the *primary healing instrument* whose consciousness, presence, and love reach beyond, breathing humanity into the technical interventions associated with curative medical attention (Rosa & Estes, 2016). This level of care brings quality life moments to all during the dying time through caring-healing modality training in five domains of life: spirit, emotion, purpose, physical, and practical after-death care.

Conscious Dying work provides forums for caregivers to receive comforting and healing care, which increases their authentic caring-healing presence and uncovers their innate gifts and talents, gives time to inquire and uncover fears, hopes, and wishes related to end of life, connect personal views with the care they provide, and explore their relationship to death. This, in turn, increases self-knowledge, supports the realization and evolution of caring consciousness, and diminishes barriers between self and others. The work of Conscious Dying is directly tied to exploring feelings and thoughts about one's own death, allowing for direct contact with spiritual beliefs, life's purpose and soul's calling, unfinished business, what the body needs or wants, how one influences and is influenced by the environment and relationships. By becoming confident in discussing death, ultimately one may have more influence on how he or she and others die; one grows emboldened to advocate in the reduction of sometimes harsh, costly interventions that threaten what is most valuable: time to love and complete with those who are loved. There is a shift in awareness and attention toward love and realizing the spiritual life, as opposed to living at any cost. This sensitivity and education allows one to be more available to life's blessings, mysteries, miracles, and unexplainable events (CDI, 2013; Watson, 2008, 2012).

Conscious Dying teaches how to create a sacred container, holding both nurse and patient through the dissolution of physical form and providing support toward how to enter one's formless spiritual nature, exposing all involved to the pure state of consciousness from which all beings come and to which all return (Rosa & Estes, 2016). Conscious dying understands love as the healing element of life; the love that holds each being as he or she begins to pass from form to formlessness; the love enabling the dying to do the deep spiritual, invisible, mysterious work of leaving the body (Rosa & Estes, 2016). It is this love that enables one to remain whole and intact as he or she explores the naturally arising spiritual existential questions like:

- Who am I really?

- What is important now?

- What do I believe?

- Will I be remembered?

- Who will remember me?

- How will I face death?

- Who will stand with me on this journey into the mysterious, subtle realms of life-death?

PAIN AND SUFFERING AT END OF LIFE

The relationship between pain and suffering is endlessly complex and multifaceted. Pain is at once an isolating event, fully understood only by the individual bearing it, and yet, connects us through its power as a shared human experience. The textured edges and depths of suffering remain highly subjective and deeply personal, carrying with it implications at the physical, mental, emotional, and spiritual-existential levels. However, the suffering of humanity is also felt at the transpersonal level—the metaphysical space where we are privileged to share one consciousness and one mind, as explained by Larry Dossey (2013). Pain and suffering, and the way they are managed, become particularly complex in settings where patients may be unable to fully verbalize the hows, whats, and whys of their experience; these include advanced serious illnesses, acute medical events, and the dying process. At the end of the physical life, the human being walks a sacred passage that should be birthed with awareness, presence, and awe (Rosa & Estes, 2016). It is a time when pain and related suffering become frequent currencies of expression.

During this pivotal process of physical decline, the energetic spiritual-existential aspects of the patient are also in transition. Pain and suffering become signals often met with family concern, provider distress, and "evidence-based" treatment responses. But the pain and suffering expressed while walking the sacred passage are not always reflective of discomfort—they can also be a call for awakening and spiritual growth. They can be a gift too often masked with medications, interventions, and "fixes" that ease the sense of helplessness felt by lookers-on. Understanding the myriad qualities and expressions of pain, and its resultant suffering, is ultimately a whole-person experience—one that typically requires attending to by caregivers who are holistic in their assessment and evaluation of pain. These are healers who are whole in what they bring to the nurse–patient interaction, sojourning along the sacred passage in integrity and true partnership.

Nurses are entrusted companions along this sacred passage; we walk at the side of the dying, who may very well be facing their "dark night of the soul." And at this crossroad, with our support and caring presence, the dying one may possibly discover what Bennhold

(2006) describes as a transformation of letting go and surrendering into the unknown with an open heart:

> Hidden deep within the grief, the layers of desolation, the circles of despair, right in the center of [one's] sorrow, there lies the potential for deeper insight into the mystery of life and death. Anguish and distress hold deep within themselves the nascent promise of a new life, radically transformed and redeemed. (p. 350)

The pain and suffering of the dying one can be mysteries to lookers-on, and should be approached with humility before the holy "oneness" of life and death: the shadows, light, and unforeseeable potential for wisdom.

SUFFERING AS A RITE OF PASSAGE

The word "suffer" comes from the Latin *suffero*, with the root *fero* meaning "to bear." Suffering is a process of bearing what life offers us. Although it is usually used as a passive construct, "to suffer" can also be an active verb as in "to suffer an illness" rather than to suffer from one. In this active conception of suffering, it is not something that befalls us; it is something that we do. How we suffer an experience is our unique human expression.

All religious traditions speak to suffering, and many encourage its direct approach. The first of the Buddha's Four Noble Truths is that life involves suffering, or *dukkha*: the state of being unsatisfied, arising from clinging to pleasant, as well as recoiling from unpleasant phenomena. Internal suffering is the result of personal identification with temporary experiences. In the practice of meditation, a willingness to sit with this internal suffering allows it to be witnessed and ultimately transcended. Many traditions of indigenous American people require endurance of physical discomfort, such as the Lakota Sun Dance, which involves spiritual purification and sacrificing one's own flesh as an offering to the Creator. The ceremony culminates in four days of fasting and dance in which the dancers gaze at the sun, and their flesh is pierced and then tethered to a pole or heavy animal skulls until the piercings are torn free. In this tradition, what may look to some like suffering is conceptualized as sacrifice.

Indigenous people of the Amazon regions use sacred plants to engender healing. These "master teacher" plants administered by shamanic elders in night-long ceremonies or multiple-day fasts can induce deep discomfort, vivid, sometimes terrifying visions, and intense vomiting and diarrhea. These medicines induce "purging" of physical and spiritual ailments. Enduring such discomfort consciously is an essential part of the healing.

Nursing also speaks directly to human suffering. Within its definition of nursing, the American Nurses Association (2017) states that the art and science of the profession includes "alleviation of suffering through the diagnosis and treatment of human response." Although it is right and good to alleviate suffering when possible, there are times when there is no way around suffering—only a journey through it. Pharmacological means cannot reach the suffering that comes with the loss of identity, relationships, and attachments. Through witness, reflection, and service, nurses hold space as patients and families find their own human responses to these existential struggles. Together, we cocreate the potential for suffering to be experienced as a rite of passage.

THE LOTUS OF CONSCIOUS DYING

Estes (2011) proposes that many events occurring throughout the trajectory of the dying process are often indiscriminately labeled as "pain." If patients moan or appear restless—we rush to medicate; if they are talking to people who are not present in the physical sense—we reorient them to time and place; if their families are grieving—we fix them to look "better." But the theoretical framework of Conscious Dying asks holistic nurses to consider that the human being at the end of life is, in fact, moving through the crowning moment of his or her earthly journey (Rosa & Estes, 2016). What we perceive as "pain" may be the "pains" of spiritual growth. This means that the relationship with patients must be fostered and nurtured before they are unable to speak so we might know their values, wishes, fears, and expectations.

Figure 10.1 illustrates The Lotus of Conscious Dying. The lotus is a spiritual representation of unfolding consciousness with countless patterns and petals that spring forth from a muddy earth and awaken toward a sky of possibility. At the foundational level of the lotus, we find the subtle ways of being and knowing within the nurse–patient relationship;

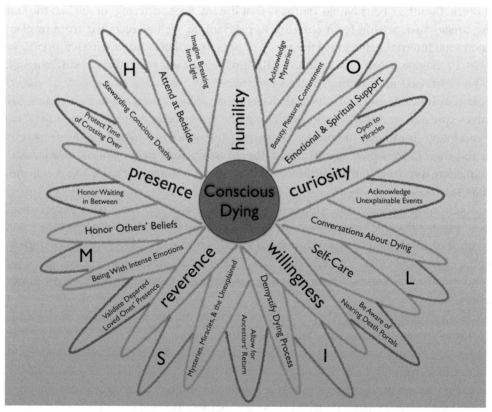

FIGURE 10.1 The Lotus of Conscious Dying.

these lay the groundwork for guiding a Conscious Dying experience and birthing a sacred passage for the patient, family, and nurse. It requires that, as healers, we remain

- Humble: Surrender ego and assumptions before rushing to label, judge, or bandage the event.

- Curious: Ask more questions, consider alternative rationales, and remain available.

- Willing: Be willing to risk self-imposed boundaries and limitations, and confront personal discomfort to provide a Conscious Dying experience.

- Reverent: Remember the passage is sacred; it is one we will all walk; embody expectation and hope as one does for a birth or other seminal event in life.

- Present: Never overlook the need for attentive and authentic presence; presence is a skill that needs refining on a moment-to-moment basis.

The next layer of the lotus represents the Conscious Dying Principles and Practices (Estes, 2011)—the moral and ethical guideposts that ensure a sacred passage. For example, demystifying the states of the dying process allows both the caregiver and the patient to arrive in a place of clarity where expectations can be explored in mutual process and shared humanness.

Beyond this layer of the lotus lies the Subtle Energy Realms (Estes, 2011)—the signs that represent a shift in consciousness and awareness for both patient and nurse. For instance, protecting the time of crossing over means to not only protect the patients' physical space in a respectful way but also create a healing environment that secures the energetic-spiritual field around them to be in alignment with their values (for more information on these principles, see Rosa & Estes, 2016).

Ultimately, the final layer of lotus petals represents HOLISM: a truly whole-person/whole-spectrum approach to pain and suffering at end of life. Holism encapsulates what Conscious Dying is all about: a truly human-centered approach to life, living, dying, and death. Conscious Dying is not really about death—it is about the vitality and preservation of the richness of life until the final breath and beyond. The bud of Conscious Dying is held at the center of holism and holistic and Caring Science principles.

NURSING'S ROLE IN LIVING AND DYING WELL

There are two inherent and fundamental aspects of the human life that require no evidence nor necessitate any reference. The first is that each person needs love and caring in order that he or she might sustain self and grow. The second is that each individual, regardless of wealth, stature, position, culture, religion, health, or age, will die. There is no morbidity intended or suggested; only a succinct exploration of truth. The former statement implies that every being has a period of physical, emotional, and spiritual maturation and the latter that there is a period of decline resulting in the eventual cessation of physiological processes.

Tolle (2005) elaborates that this sense of expansion and contraction, the outgoing into physicality and return to Source consciousness, summarizes the entire history of one's brief earthly existence. In Buddhist philosophy, the living and dying are parts of a greater and inseparable whole and, in fact, "Death is a mirror in which the entire meaning of life is reflected" (Rinpoche, 2003, p. 11). Implicit is the suggestion that learning *how* to die is accomplished by living consciously, whereas learning *how* to live is achieved by maintaining an ever-present awareness of death from moment to moment.

Caring Science facilitates the profession's goal of helping both self and other to proliferate this consciousness and nurture all aspects of both parties' self-relationship so they may experience a deeper sense of wholeness and well-being (Watson, 2012). In turn, Conscious Dying empowers healers and end-of-life care providers to hold others with love, the healing element of life and of the heart, as they move from form to formlessness, while allowing for the personal inquiry and development into one's own death. Both theoretical frameworks embrace an evolving and loving consciousness as paramount to the awakening and peaceful existence of humanity.

Integral to Rinpoche's (2003) aforementioned message is that one will not be able to die well if he or she is unable to learn how to live well. Humanity is urged by the ancients to engage intimately with every fleeting moment of life, to use the tangibles of the world to awaken and gradually enlighten, and to understand the core nature of life: that death is immanent and possible at any moment, without notice or explanation (Padmasambhava, 2005). With this knowledge, the miracle of life becomes both precious and coveted. In life, the charge is to learn how to progressively embody a *transpersonal* worldview; a humanized understanding that every person is the physical representation of body-mind-spirit-soul and that each being on the planet is inextricably interconnected to the other, the larger environment, and the cosmos or Source consciousness (Quinn, 2016). The striving for and cultivation of such a spiritually grounded comprehension is what may be here defined as "living well." The task as death is nearing is similar and may be here defined as "dying well." Dying well implies a peaceful transition for the patient, entailing the knowledge that his or her life was meaningful and the realization that he or she exists in transpersonal connection to others, a higher power, and Source consciousness (Keegan & Drick, 2016). A superficial assessment of the tasks of living and dying show they are identical; they call on human beings to consciously awaken and evolve, understand the meaning of their individual contributions, and discover within them their unitary wholeness and irrefutable connection to the Infinite.

Nurses are the procurers and protectors of both a human-caring environment and a conscious, reverential dying experience. In this role, the nurse is viewed as healer; embodying the sacred tenet of healing Nightingale identified as ethically core to the profession (B. M. Dossey, Selanders, Beck, & Attewell, 2005). The adept nurse-healer understands *healing* to be an emerging process, unifying the self, other, and bio-psycho-social-spiritual-cultural-environmental dimensions into balance and integration for a deeper level of knowing and harmony (B. M. Dossey, 2016). The possibility for healing is available at any moment along the life-death continuum and is the strived for, moral/ethical keystone of nursing praxis (B. M. Dossey, 2016; Watson, 2012).

Possibly the most crucial endeavor of the nurse-healer is to reconnect with the eternal connection to Source that is inherent in the embodied spirit-human being experience. He or she endeavors for this pinnacle experience for both the realization of self and continued emergence of other. The "Bhagavad Gita" describes a common theme among many of the world's religions, which describes the inherent truth of this remembrance: "It is not born and it does not die. Unborn, eternal and ancient, the Self is not killed when the body is killed" (Satchidananda, 1988, p. 15). Resting in this knowledge, the nurse-healer continues his or her own spiritual endeavors so he or she may engage with and support self and other in a journey conducive to self-actualization; a process imbued with Caring Science; a sacredness defined by Conscious Dying; the nurturing and sustaining of integrity throughout both the expansion and contraction. In this highest expression of caring- healing, the nurse *becomes* the primary healing instrument (Rosa & Estes, 2016).

SELF-TRANSCENDENCE AND THE NURSE'S ROLE

In Reed's (2013) Theory of Self-Transcendence, suffering can be an opportunity for human development. Experiences that confront us with our human vulnerability also offer the opportunity to expand our boundaries of who we think we are. Reed argues that self-transcendence is "a developmental imperative, meaning that it is a human resource that demands expression, much like other developmental processes .... These resources are a part of being human and of realizing one's potential for well-being ... and nursing has a role in facilitating this process" (p. 111).

How can a nurse engender the possibility of self-transcendence in a patient who appears to be suffering? How can a nurse honor a patient's suffering as his or her sacred rite of passage?

The first step is to recognize when suffering is present, and allow it to be. This is difficult. Suffering often holds a negative connotation, an indication that something has gone wrong. Not only compassion but self-compassion is required to be a witness to suffering. Self-compassion theorist Neff (2003) writes that this "involves being touched by and open to one's own suffering, not avoiding or disconnecting from it ... offering nonjudgmental understanding to one's pain, inadequacies and failures, so that one's experience is seen as part of the larger human experience" (p. 87). Especially important is to recognize that a suffering patient does not reflect a failure of the nurse.

Even while administering medication to alleviate physical symptoms, a nurse must recognize that the patient's unique experience and expression of suffering cannot be reduced to a 1 to 10 rating on a pain scale. It is in this more open and curious space, when suffering is observed as a natural and integral part of the human experience, that it holds the potential as a catalyst for growth. It is here that consciousness awakens.

CARING SCIENCE CONSCIOUS DYING: AN EMERGING META-PARADIGM

Caring Science Conscious Dying is an exploratory framework for the betterment of both self and system; a model integrating fundamental aspects of two theoretical frameworks for the realized pinnacle of nursing praxis. Caring Science Conscious Dying provides opportunity for nursing to actualize the core tenets of the profession identified by Nightingale: healing, leadership, and advocacy (B. M. Dossey et al., 2005). As this model evolves from self to other, through system to Source, the nurse rediscovers shared humanity as the very starting point for being-doing-knowing and reinstates the Nightingalean vision as quintessential to the dignity of nurses and nursing throughout the life-death continuum.

MATURATION OF SELF AND SYSTEM

The singular evolutionary journey of self will not exact the change required to provide ethically sound, humanistic care at a global level. The continued growth and reflective practice of the system currently being sustained is a necessary component. It is a joint effort: an evolutionary and ethical maturation of both self and system for the betterment of human and humane care. *Emergence* is a theme of this meta-paradigm and can be defined as *the continued self/system-actualization of an engaged, conscious, altruistic, and dignified living-dying relationship*. There is partnership between the emergence of both self and system; a collaboration fundamental to the realization of this work.

Table 10.1 shows Watson's 10 Caritas Processes® paired with questions for personalized self-reflection (Rosa, 2014a). Originally created for the nurse experiencing compassion fatigue, the reflective inventory is applicable to any clinician seeking to procure an expansive conscious awareness. It provides nurses the opportunity to operationalize the value system of Caring Science, helping to translate theory into practice. Teaching individuals self-care strategies and methods for engaging in self-reverent practices is essential to procuring a professional community with a moral/ethical foundation (Rosa, 2014c). Through the reflective process, nurses are supported in exploring their own individual story of human caring; the very story that connects them to the collective of shared humanity (Rosa, 2014c). Reflective inventories have also been used in nursing as a tool for preceptor development and in guiding nurses to become agents of meaningful and effective change (Rosa, 2017; Rosa & Santos, 2016).

From self to system, the reflective inventory expands in Table 10.2 to include the nurse–patient relationship, the living-dying experience, and the personal to global impact of nursing practice (Rosa, 2014b). In the table, the 10 Conscious Dying Principles© paired with reflective questions for the expanded consciousness of system-wide awareness are listed. Although the prior inventory focused on the individual processes of self-healing, Rosa (2014b) broadens the lens to include the global impact of system-healing. Through diligent, articulate, and honest reflection of the systems maintained and sustained by nursing, the profession may begin to rid itself of nursing-specific malignancies such as compassion fatigue, burnout, moral distress, and bullying, and refocus intentions on providing Human Caring-Conscious Dying, compassionate practices (Rosa, 2014b, 2014d).

The consciousness of the individual and system are linked; in fact, they are one and the same. One cannot consider him or herself to be aware, sensitive, and compassionate to another while facilitating the detached and inhumane message of a system that continues to miss the mark. Personal growth leads to system awareness and, in turn, system awareness leads to more conscious and caring living-dying. As this model evolves, reflective inventories that provide opportunities to actualize theoretical approaches to care will continue to emerge.

THE REALIZATION OF A VISIONARY PRAXIS

The merging of two substantial bodies of work requires a refocusing of intention and a clarifying of purpose. Although the inventories used above aid the nurse to link individual and systemic implications, professionals must return to the fundamentals of both Caring Science and Conscious Dying, aligning the paradigms' ethical presumptions and creating

TABLE 10.1 Translating the Global to the Personal: In Process With Self

10 Caritas Processes	Reflective Caritas Inventory for the Individual Processes of Self-Healing
1. Embrace altruistic values and Practice loving-kindness with self and others.	*Have I set an intention of self-caring and self-kindness today? Have I centered myself with an act of self-love so that I might be restored?*
2. Instill faith and hope and honor others.	*Am I clear about what I have faith in? Have I reminded myself of the people, places and spaces that give me hope?*
3. Be sensitive to self and others by nurturing individual beliefs and practices.	*Have I responded to my thoughts and feelings today with gentleness, knowing that my experience is unique and sacred?*
4. Develop helping-caring-trusting relationships.	*Have I empowered myself to release toxic relationships and embrace supportive connections in my life with truth and vulnerability? Just for today, can I trust myself to be there for me?*
5. Promote and accept positive and negative feelings as you authentically listen to another's story.	*Have I authentically accepted my own story? Do I fully embrace all aspects of who I am; the positive and the negative, the light and the dark?*
6. Use creative scientific problem-solving methods for caring decision making.	*Do I recognize how creative I am? Have I celebrated my "me-ness" in how I approach, interact with, and inspire this world around me?*
7. Share teaching and learning that addresses the individual needs and comprehension styles.	*Am I forthcoming about my needs at work and at home? Do I remain flexible and energized or easily tire with my old patterns of rigidity?*
8. Create a healing environment for the physical and spiritual self which respects human dignity.	*Have I physically or energetically touched my heart today? Have I connected with my own heartbeat; the same heartbeat shared by all of humanity? Have I admitted to myself that my healing starts within?*
9. Assist with basic physical, emotional, and spiritual human needs.	*Have I paused to attend to my own hunger? My anxiety? My worries? My frustrations? Do I recognize my individual needs as valid?*
10. Open to the mystery and Allow miracles to enter.	*Can I release the need to be certain, to explain, defend, protect, and define? Can I surrender to the moment and allow life to unfold as it will?*

Note: Jean Watson's 10 Caritas Processes (Watson Caring Science Institute, 2018) are paired with questions for personalized self- reflection.

Source: Adapted with permission from Rosa, W. (2014a). Caring science and compassion fatigue: Reflective inventory for the individual processes of self-healing. *Beginnings, 34*(4), 18–20.

TABLE 10.2 Translating the Personal to the Global: In Process With System

Conscious Dying Principles (Estes, 2013)	Reflective Systems Inventory for the Collective Processes of Global Healing (Rosa, 2014b)
1. Increase beauty, pleasure, contentment.	*Does the system provide space for beauty? Do I see patients having time to value and partake in pleasure?*
2. Provide emotional and spiritual support.	*Have we as a system attended to the spiritual needs of the patient today? Has the patient been emotionally seen, heard, and acknowledged today?*
3. Initiate conversations about dying process.	*Are my colleagues and I comfortable talking about death and dying? Is the patient aware that death is a process?*
4. Practice self-care to prevent burnout and emotional fatigue.	*Are the connections clear between my own self-care and the care I provide for my patient? Can I coidentify with the vulnerability of my patient and gently attend to my own self-care needs?*
5. Demystify the stages of the dying process.	*Am I clear about the mental-emotional-spiritual stages of the dying process? Is the patient attended to throughout the spectrum? Is there a dissonance between my knowledge, system-wide protocols and patient needs?*
6. Acknowledge mysteries, miracles, and unexplained events.	*Are systems willing to bear witness to the mystical? If yes, am I able to validate and share the patient's subjective experiences within this realm despite my personal discomfort?*
7. Learn how to be with intense emotions.	*Do systems "lean into" the difficult emotions? Can we guide providers to invest in and engage with the actual, moment-to-moment story of our patients and families?*
8. Honor other's beliefs without them threatening your own.	*Are systems able to release agendas selflessly to support the patient's beliefs with flexibility? How can we facilitate and empower individualism through compassionate advocacy and empathy?*
9. Be a steward of conscious deaths.	*Do we see systems pave the path for peaceful transitions of integrity? How can we humanize dying by creating an environment of dignity and adequate, anticipatory preparation?*
10. Attend at bedside—no one dies alone.	*Does the infrastructure of the system allow for sustained human presencing? How can we systematically prepare in meeting the undeniable need to bear witness?*

Note: Tarron Estes's Conscious Dying Principles (Estes, 2013) are paired with questions for the collective processes of global healing.

Source: Reprinted with permission from Rosa, W. (2014b). Conscious dying and cultural emergence: Reflective systems inventory for the collective processes of global healing. *Beginnings, 34*(5), 20–22.

new possibilities for theoretical-practical applications. In addition to the reflective inventories provided herein, these assumptions guide the practitioner in creating new self and system guidelines in the delivery of human-centered care.

Caring Science Conscious Dying is a meta-paradigm concerned with the evolution of human consciousness, in elevating how nurses and nursing can influence both living and dying well. Through the use of reflective inventories, individuals and systems have the potential to grow past current limitations and embrace human caring in a sacred and profound way. The use and integration of the Caring Science Conscious Dying assumptions into theoretical frameworks and practice may aid in broadening perspectives and embracing a more holistic way of being-doing-knowing.

NEXT ERA POSSIBILITIES

Education
- In what ways can Conscious Dying be integrated into current educational models pertaining to care for the dying?
- How do I, as a healer, use my experiential wisdom of Conscious Dying to inform the understanding of others?

Research
- How can research be rehumanized to include principles of Conscious Dying?

Praxis
- What practice evolutions can be cocreated and implemented to aid in the embodiment of this framework?

Theory and Knowledge Development
- What opportunities exist to further develop Caring Science Conscious Dying as an emerging meta-paradigm?
- How do we invite safe and supportive dialogue in the theory development surrounding Conscious Dying?

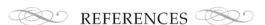 REFERENCES

American Nurses Association. (2017). *What is nursing?* Retrieved from https://www.nursingworld .org/practice-policy/workforce/what-is-nursing

Bennhold, C. (2006). Transformation and redemption through the dark night of the soul. In C. M. Puchalski (Ed.), *A time for listening and caring: Spirituality and the care of the chronically ill and dying* (pp. 345–352). New York, NY: Oxford University Press.

Conscious Dying Institute. (2013). *About the Conscious Dying Institute.* Retrieved from http://www .consciousdyinginstitute.com/about-the-conscious-dying-institute-and-related-links

Dossey, B. M. (2016). Nursing: Holistic, integral, and integrative – local to global. In B. M. Dossey & L. Keegan (Eds.), *Holistic nursing: A handbook for practice* (7th ed., pp. 3–52). Burlington, MA: Jones & Bartlett.

Dossey, B. M., Selanders, L. C., Beck, D. M., & Attewell, A. (2005). *Florence Nightingale today: Healing, leadership, global action.* Silver Spring, MD: Nursesbooks.org.

Dossey, L. (2013). *One mind: How our individual mind is part of a greater consciousness and why it matters.* Carlsbad, CA: Hay House.

Estes, T. (2013). Breaking into light. *Natural Transitions, 3*(3), 14–16. Retrieved from https://static1 .squarespace.com/static/51c9e6b8e4b043b66a213762/t/54166196e4b05407cce5dead/1410752918929/ Natural+Transitions+Magazine+Article+-+Tarron+Estes.pdf

Hawkins, D. (2002). *Power vs. force.* Carlsbad, CA: Hay House.

Keegan, L., & Drick, C. A. (2016). Dying in peace. In B. M. Dossey & L. Keegan (Eds.), *Holistic nursing: A handbook for practice* (7th ed., pp. 415–438). Burlington, MA: Jones & Bartlett.

Kübler-Ross, E. (1969). *On death and dying: What the dying have to teach doctors, nurses, clergy, & their own families.* New York, NY: Scribner.

Kübler-Ross, E., & Kessler, D. (2005). *On grief and grieving: Finding the meaning of grief through the five stages of loss.* New York, NY: Scribner.

Levinas, E. (2000). *Totality and infinity.* Pittsburgh, PA: Duquesne University Press. (Original work published 1969)

Neff, K. (2003). Self-compassion: An alternative conceptualization of a healthy attitude toward one-self. *Self and Identity, 2,* 85–101. doi:10.1080/15298860390129863

Padmasambhava. (2005). *The Tibetan book of the dead.* New York, NY: Penguin Books.

Quinn, J. F. (2016). Transpersonal human caring and healing. In B. M. Dossey & L. Keegan (Eds.), *Holistic nursing: A handbook for practice* (7th ed., pp. 101–110). Burlington, MA: Jones & Bartlett.

Reed, P. G. (2013). Theory of self-transcendence. In M. J. Smith & P. R. Liehr (Eds.), *Middle range theory for nursing* (3rd ed., pp. 109–139). New York, NY: Springer Publishing.

Rinpoche, S. (2003). *The Tibetan book of living and dying* (Rev. ed.). New York, NY: HarperCollins.

Rosa, W. (2014a). Caring science and compassion fatigue: Reflective inventory for the individual processes of self-healing. *Beginnings, 34*(4), 18–20.

Rosa, W. (2014b). Conscious dying and cultural emergence: Reflective systems inventory for the collective processes of global healing. *Beginnings, 34*(5), 20–22.

Rosa, W. (2014c). Intertwined narratives of the human caring story. *Creative Nursing, 20*(3), 171–173. doi:10.1891/1078-4535.20.3.171

Rosa, W. (2014d). Reflections on self in relation to other: Core community values of a moral/ethical foundation. *Creative Nursing, 20*(4), 242–247. doi:10.1891/1078-4535.20.4.242

Rosa, W. (2017). Change agent. In P. Dickerson (Ed.), *Core curriculum for nursing professional development* (5th ed., pp. 230–241). Chicago, IL: Association for Nursing Professional Development.

Rosa, W., & Estes, T. (2016). What end-of-life care needs now: An emerging praxis of the sacred and subtle. *Advances in Nursing Science, 39*(4), 333–345. doi:10.1097/ANS.0000000000000136

Rosa, W., Estes, T., & Watson, J. (2017). Caring science conscious dying: An emerging metaparadigm. *Nursing Science Quarterly, 30*(1), 58–64. doi:10.1177/0894318416680538

Rosa, W., & Hope, S. (2017). Pain and suffering at end of life: Birthing the sacred passage. *Beginnings, 37*(4), 10–13.

Rosa, W., & Santos, S. (2016). Introduction of the Engaged Feedback Reflective Inventory during a preceptor training program. *Journal for Nurses in Professional Development, 32*(4), E1–E7. doi:10.1097/ NND.0000000000000280

Satchidananda, S. S. (1988). *The living Gita: The complete Bhagavad Gita.* Yogaville, VA: Integral Yoga®.

Tolle, E. (2005). *A new earth: Awakening to your life's purpose.* New York. NY: Penguin.

Watson, J. (1985). *Nursing: The philosophy and science of caring.* Boulder: Colorado Associated University Press. (Original work published 1979).

Watson, J. (1999). *Nursing: Human science and human care, a theory of nursing.* Sudbury, MA: Jones & Bartlett. (Original work published 1985).

Watson, J. (2005a). *Caring science as sacred science.* Philadelphia, PA: F. A. Davis.

Watson, J. (2005b). Caring Science: Belonging before Being as ethical cosmology. *Nursing Science Quarterly, 18*(4), 304–305. doi:10.1177/0894318405280395

Watson, J. (2008). *Nursing: The philosophy and science of caring* (Rev. ed.). Boulder: University Press of Colorado.

Watson, J. (2012). *Human caring science: A theory of nursing* (2nd ed.). Sudbury, MA: Jones & Bartlett.

Watson, J. (2014). Integrative nursing caring science, human caring, and peace. In M. J. Kreitzer & M. Koithan (Eds.), *Integrative nursing* (pp. 101–108). New York, NY: Oxford University Press.

Watson Caring Science Institute. (2018). Ten Caritas processes. Retrieved from https://www.watsoncaringscience.org/jean-bio/caring-science-theory/10-caritas-processes

11

Reflective Practice and Caring Science*

Sara Horton-Deutsch and William Rosa

CARITAS LITERACIES

By the end of this chapter, the caring-healing nurse will be able to

1. Identify the relationship between reflective practice and Caring Science.

2. Explain various methods of reflection for working with self, partners, groups, organizations, and communities.

3. Apply reflective practice and Caring Science principles to one's personal–professional life as a method of self-care and self-renewal.

4. Understand the role of reflective practice and Caring Science in creating systems and societies that flourish in caring, healing, health, and well-being.

⁂

Reflective practice as a concept has been around since ancient times. The origins of reflection evolved many centuries ago from Eastern and Western philosophers, including Buddha, Plato, and Lao Tzu. They all emphasized human self-reflection as a willingness to learn more about one's fundamental nature, purpose, and essence. Self-reflection leads to inquiry of the human condition and the philosophical consideration of consciousness and awareness.

---

*Parts of this chapter have been reprinted from Rosa, W., & Horton-Deutsch, S. (2017). The role of reflective practice in creating the world we want. In W. Rosa (Ed.), *A new era in global health: Nursing and the United Nations 2030 Sustainable Development Agenda* (pp. 461–474). New York, NY: Springer Publishing.

The values and principles of Caring Science are essentially sustained through an ongoing relationship with reflection and reflective practice. The commitment of reflective peoples, practitioners, and populations imply a society furthered by an emergence in consciousness, embodied by an ethical gravity that grounds the human spirit in awareness, authenticity, vulnerability, and compassion. In this thread, reflection becomes a mode of caring—a vehicle to connect with the currents of intention. It is an entryway toward the dissolution of stagnated ways of seeing that keep one fixed in limiting polarities of hate–love, resistance–acceptance, anger–forgiveness, and fragmentation–wholeness. Reflective practice brings one into communion with the widest range of contemplative thought and emotion available amid the daily practices of living and caring.

Reflective practice is an art of being with, digesting, assimilating, integrating that which serves and releasing that which does not. It is a dynamic process of mental-emotional-spiritual growth and provides the space and opportunity to know deeply the root level impediments that prevent self and systems from realizing a desired state of balanced function. As the paradigm of Caring Science continues to expand, so does the opportunity to reflect on the past-present and present-future with a hope to discover the healing needs of humanity, and respond with a renewed commitment to preserving its dignity.

REFLECTIVE PRACTICE: A GUIDE FOR THE BETTERMENT OF SELF AND SOCIETY

The views of reflection and its use in more practical contexts originated from John Dewey, an influential 20th century educational philosopher. He defined "reflection" as the active, persistent, and careful consideration of beliefs supported by knowledge. He emphasized not just rigor in practice, but the importance of incorporating scientific knowledge into reflection (Dewey, 1933). He equally valued external knowledge from research and internal knowledge that emerged when practitioners mindfully examine the impact of their practice. Building on these ideas, Schön (1983, 1987), an expert in the field of organizational learning, identified learning as the foundation of individual and organizational improvement. His work authenticated both what was directly taught (explicit learning) and what was learned through experience (implicit learning), including observation and modeling. He emphasized that humans learn best when tapping into both internal and external resources to inform decisions. Concisely, these bodies of work characterize reflective practice as an active thought process intended to aid in understanding current truths of practice and at the same time seeing multiple possibilities for improvement. The fundamental importance is that reflective practice leads to informed action.

Christopher Johns, the leading nurse expert on reflective practice, has published widely on the topic for decades. Johns (2017) describes "reflective practice" as a mindful way of being within practice and a process to reflect-on-experience to appreciate and resolve contradiction with the intent of realizing one's own vision for practice as a lived reality. This definition grounds the practitioner in who they are as a learner and a practitioner. More broadly, Taylor (2000) describes "reflection" as a focused way of discerning practice and includes any attentive consideration such as thinking, contemplation, or meditation that helps clarify sense and leads to contextually appropriate changes. Freshwater (2008) extends this definition to not just discerning current practice but also questioning the underlying political, ethical, historical, and cultural traditions. More recently, reflection has been linked to the vital nursing skill and human attribute of self-awareness and authentic presence (Horton-Deutsch & Sherwood, 2008, 2017; Lombard & Horton-Deutsch, 2012).

Reflective practice contributes to working from our deeper sense of mission and purpose, where we consider what we know, believe, and value within the context of a particular situation in our work and/or life. It helps us to develop spiritual resources as we are encouraged to ponder meaning and our own way of being in the world. Being a reflective practitioner is an intentional strategy for professional development and expands our capacity for leadership. It supports and advances values clarification, an important reflective endeavor, and guides us to act and do the right thing, in our own leadership journey (Young, Pardue, & Horton-Deutsch, 2015).

WAYS OF REFLECTING

There is neither one universal definition of "reflection" nor one universal way to reflect. No one person, group, or organization integrates reflective practice in precisely the same way. It is an active, iterative process that continually seeks to assess, understand, and adjust practices. Thus, it is often framed as a cyclical or spiraling process—cycling forward and backward to challenge thinking and produce deeper practice knowledge (Gibbs, 1988; York-Barr, Sommers, Ghere, & Montie, 2016). The Gibbs reflective cycle (1988) includes six stages, and at each stage, a question or cue is provided to aid in reflection. The model is wide-ranging and can be applied to numerous situations. The six stages are as follows:

1. Describe what happened.

2. If it happened again what would you do?

3. What were you thinking/feeling?

4. What else could have been done?

5. What was good and bad about the experience?

6. What sense can you make of the situation?

Another example, the Reflective Practice Cycle, developed by educational scholars York-Barr et al. (2016) can be used in group settings and starts with being grounded in *purpose*, followed by being actively *present* to observe and learn, being open and partaking in the *inquiry*, acquiring *insights* from the learning and adding to the dialogue so others gain new insights, taking informed *action* based on the knowledge that is generated, and concludes with continually asking "Are we seeing the results we want to see?" If yes, the group asks "Now what?" And, if no, then the group asks "Now what?" This cycle is a continual back and forth to challenge thinking and harvest deeper knowledge and understanding. Contained between the purpose and the results are thought and regulatory cycles that circle back to previous steps to assess, challenge, and fine-tune the cycle. This iterative process helps to ensure that the process recycles and it remains rooted in the purpose. The Reflective Practice Cycle is available for download at resources.corwin.com/YorkBarrReflective.

A less prescriptive, more qualitative mode of reflection is offered by nursing scholar Christopher Johns (2006). The Model for Structured Reflection offers cues to assess the depth of reflection for learning through experience. The cues become internalized through time and can be continuously refined. The cues correspond to Carper's (1978) four fundamental ways of knowing: aesthetic, ethical, empirical, and personal. The map can be viewed in Johns (2006) and guides learners to frame learning through reflection. At the center of the map is the aesthetic response that encompasses four key processes:

1.   Appreciating the pattern of the particular situation

2.   Making judgments based on care needs

3.   Responding in a particular way within the situation

4.   Making judgments about the efficacy of response in meeting care needs

Next, asking the following three questions which are outlined in the periphery of the map respond to the other components of Carper's (1978) ways of knowing from ethical, empirical, and personal perspectives:

1.   Did I act for the best?

2.   What knowledge informed my practice? And, what knowledge should have informed my practice?

3.   What were personal factors influencing me?

In addition to the ways of knowing proposed by Carper (1978) and addressed by Johns (2006) in his Model for Structured Reflection, other patterns of knowing have been proposed that may be incorporated into this model. For example, Munhall (1993) proposed a pattern of knowing titled "unknowing" while White (1995) added sociopolitical knowing. More recently, Chinn and Kramer (2008) added emancipatory knowing to address issues of equity, justice, and transformation in all areas of practice. Inclusively, the seven patterns of knowing inform areas of nursing praxis including those that encompass informed moral action. Additional reflective questions related to these ways of knowing are as follows:

1.   What else could it be?

2.   What are the sociopolitical aspects of this situation?

3.   Are there issues related to equity, justice, and transformation that I need to consider? If yes, what are they and how can they be addressed?

These three models for reflective practice are a representative sample; many others exist. However, they have particular value for both self-reflection and reflecting with others and represent contributions from nursing and educational scholars alike. The next three sections offer strategies for individual reflective practice, reflective practice with partners/ groups, and reflective practice with organizations.

INDIVIDUAL REFLECTIVE PRACTICE

Reflective practice is about tapping into the deepest part of ourselves, our compassion for ourselves, for others, and humanity. Put into action, it is reflected in how we continuously learn, grow, contribute, serve, and "be" in the community. As an individual practice, it is often triggered by a negative or uncomfortable experience projected into our conscious thought. As we become more self-aware, more of our experiences become available for reflection. Over time, individual reflection supports being a good listener, observing one's own and others' practices, viewing circumstances from multiple perspectives, thoughtfully interpreting events, and seeing possibilities for improvement. The value of individual reflection is that it (Johns, 2006; York-Barr et al., 2016)

- Supports access to and builds on experiential learning and other forms of knowledge

- Expands awareness and insights that can lead to behavioral change

- Resolves contradictions among actions and behaviors

- Increases knowledge and skills that lead to personal and professional development

- Restores balance and perspective by creating space for thoughtful consideration and learning

- Renews clarity of personal and professional purpose by helping to align practice with intentions

Likely, the most important consideration for individual reflection is creating time and space in our lives to be fully present. Presencing is not easy but is essential for reflection to occur. Obstacles to creating space in our lives to be fully present include our fear of vulnerability and going against social norms, our primitive stress reactions, and our challenge with not knowing how to nurture ourselves or honor vulnerability. By practicing compassion for ourselves and others, we open ourselves to our own fear and vulnerability. This practice creates more space, which helps to develop a greater presence with ourselves and others (Lombard & Horton-Deutsch, 2012).

To be a reflective practitioner, individually, we must choose to be reflective in our work and life. It is in the quiet and solitude that insights from life take on meaning and form. There are multiple ways to reflect alone including journaling, poetry, reading literature, exercising, or walking in nature to clear our minds, meditation, contemplation, creating a piece of art, noticing, and witnessing our own practice through video or webinars. Engaging in one of the many forms of reflection available is a commitment to our own growth and development. It is how we develop the expertise and insights that accumulate into wisdom. Becoming more reflective heightens awareness of the yearning to make sense of the world and to become the best one can be (York-Barr et al., 2016).

REFLECTIVE PRACTICE WITH PARTNERS AND GROUPS

As we learn and grow as reflective practitioners, we increase our capacity to effectively engage, support, and facilitate others' personal-professional development. According to Johns (2006), working together demands a culture of mutual respect for each one's role and requires group learning. Group learning begins with dialogue and the capacity of individuals to suspend their assumptions and create space to think together. Through this process, we recognize patterns of interaction in groups that may undermine learning. Reflection opens a space for individuals to express and nurture their voices so that they can be heard and respected. It also helps us to deliver our messages in a thoughtful and considerate manner. It is often said what we say is not as important as how it is said. Through reflection, we learn to carefully craft how we say something, so it is likely to be received in the intended manner. The value of reflecting with partners or groups (Johns, 2006; York-Barr et al., 2016) includes the following:

- Enhances learning from varied experiences and expertise

- Increases professional and social support

- Supports the development of more effective interventions given shared purpose, responsibility, and expertise among partners and/or members

- Produces a sense of hope and encouragement for meaningful, sustained improvements

- Increases collegiality and connections among partners/members through greater understanding of one's own and others' experiences, expertise, and perspectives

There are multiple ways to reflect with partners or in groups including traditional study groups and/or research projects, as well as less conventional ways to improve processes. Liberating Structures (LS) are a nonhierarchical collection of methods based on complexity science for thinking, relating, and working together (Lipmanowicz & McCandless, 2014). Reflection is an integral part of LS in a backward way. The idea is that we can act our way into thinking through LS to quickly make changes in our patterns of interaction, leading to reflection (Swenson & Sims, 2012). Changing the way we interact is about changing our culture, which is about changing our habits and behaviors. The goal of LS is to unleash the collective wisdom and creativity of everyone in the group. Through reflection, we notice how much our relationships have changed through the use of LS. To learn more about LS and how ordinary people can use these methods based on complexity science visit www.liberatingstructures.com

REFLECTIVE PRACTICE WITH ORGANIZATIONS AND COMMUNITIES

Growing a reflective practice community means that at each level of a system, members listen and observe practice. Moving reflective practices to organizational and community levels can be challenging because of the complexity of working with entire systems and the complexity and particularity of different communities (Sherwood & Horton-Deutsch, 2015).

However, when reflection becomes part of an overall way of doing and being, the value can result in (Johns, 2006; York-Barr et al., 2016) the following:

- Greater coherence of the entire organization and/or community through a sense of common purpose and shared responsibility

- Alignment of resources for achieving system/community advances aimed at equitable outcomes for all

- Shared knowledge and planning so issues are deeply understood, and insights gained to guide next steps

- Coordination and collaboration across partners/groups within the organization or community to align work and development

- Increased support for the expanding network of relationships and sharing expertise with the larger organization or community

Similar to working with partners or groups, LS are methods that can be used with entire organizations. Again, on the basis of complexity science, LS can unleash the power of everyone to think and act in new ways. Participants focus on letting go to foster cycles of self-organization versus control to foster a culture of dependence. When letting go is ascendant, the culture engages in interdependent work and shared accountability. Common behaviors in these reflective systems include listening, asking for help, removing barriers to innovation, taking more responsibility, seeking full participation, information sharing, and taking risks (Swenson & Sims, 2012). LS can be scaled up or down depending on the size of the organization/community and the nature of the work to be done. The key is they are open, inclusive, and thoughtful, and value all points of view.

THE DEEPER RELATIONSHIP BETWEEN REFLECTIVE PRACTICE AND CARING SCIENCE

As we asserted throughout this chapter, reflective practice is about tapping into things profoundly human; our own experience, knowledge, understanding, and wisdom as well as others'. This form of learning is transformative, occurs from the inside out, and emphasizes the development of a deeper understanding of ourselves as the foundation for how we meaningfully connect with and understand others (Horton-Deutsch & Sherwood, 2017). As a result, when interacting with others, reflective practitioners have a built-in process for how to remain open, listen, reevaluate beliefs and behaviors, and respond in a wise, compassionate, and honorable manner. Similarly, Caring Science emphasizes the importance of building on self-knowledge, self-discovery, and shared human experiences, combined with the study of human emotions and relations that reveal our shared humanity through a process of reflection (Watson, 2008).

Vitally important, both reflective practice and Caring Science highlight the importance of the words we use and how we use them. Words carry considerable power to influence others (Bache, 2001; Watson, 2017) and can be used to oppress and dominate or to convey the desire to continually evolve in understanding and consciousness that includes honoring self and other. Thus, reflective practice and Caring Science begin with an ontology that is open, loving, caring, and compassionate. Reflective practitioners embody Caring Science by being sensitive to the need and responsibility for morale efficacy and see this process as a lifelong journey of being/becoming, self-awareness, self-healing, self-growth, mindful, and deliberate spiritual practices and actions.

CONCLUSION

Combined, reflective practice and Caring Science provide a foundation for and direction on how nurses and other healthcare professionals can more deeply reflect on their own practice, including the language they use, and how they use it to meaningfully connect with self and others. This includes the capacity to deepen one's understanding of culture, ethical and humane social views and policies that honor what it means to be human (Watson, 2017). Ultimately, Caring Science deepens reflective practice by connecting reflection and caring with love as the basis for practice in a way that supports healing, health, and wholeness for humanity.

NEXT ERA POSSIBILITIES

Education
- What are the needs of educational systems to promote reflection and Caring Science in learning and teaching?
- How can I be a part of leading educational progress that promotes learner engagement with reflective practice as a part of professional development?

Research
- How would research change if it were approached from a lens of reflective practice?
- What potential studies could be created to explore the interplay between Caring Science and reflective practice?

Praxis
- How is my own practice of Caring Science influenced by an ongoing commitment to reflective practice?
- In what ways do I already practice reflectively? How can I deepen a practice-based relationship with reflection?

Theory and Knowledge Development
- What emerging aspects of theory development call for an integration of Caring Science and reflective practice?
- When in an environment that promotes reflective practice, how does my understanding of the knowledge at hand change and evolve?

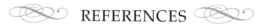 REFERENCES

Bache, C. (2001). *Transformative learning*. Sausalito, CA: Noetic Sciences Institute.

Carper, B. (1978). Fundamental patterns of knowing in nursing. *Advances in Nursing Science, 1*(1), 13–23. doi:10.1097/00012272-197810000-00004

Chinn, P. L., & Kramer, M. K. (2008). *Integrated theory and knowledge development in nursing* (7th ed.). St. Louis, MO: Mosby/Elsevier.

Dewey, J. (1933). *How we think: A restatement of the relation of reflective thinking to the educative process.* Boston, MA: D.C. Heath.

Freshwater, D. (2008). Reflective practice: The state of the art. In D. Freshwater, B. J. Taylor, & G. Sherwood (Eds.), *International textbook of reflective practice in nursing* (pp. 1–18). Oxford, UK: Blackwell.

Gibbs, G. (1988). *Learning by doing: A guide to teaching and learning methods.* Oxford, UK: Further Education Unit. Retrieved from https://thoughtsmostlyaboutlearning.files.wordpress.com/2015/12/learning-by-doing-graham-gibbs.pdf

Horton-Deutsch, S., & Sherwood, G., (2008). Reflection: An educational strategy to develop emotionally-competent nurse leaders. *Journal of Nursing Management, 16*(8), 946–954. doi:10.1111/j.1365-2834.2008.00957.x

Horton-Deutsch, S., & Sherwood, G. (2017). *Reflective practice: Transforming education and improving outcomes* (2nd ed.). Indianapolis, IN: Sigma Theta Tau International.

Johns, C. (2006). *Engaging reflection in practice: A narrative approach.* Oxford, UK: Blackwell.

Johns, C. (Ed.). (2017). *Becoming a reflective practitioner* (5th ed.). Hoboken, NJ: John Wiley & Sons.

Lipmanowicz, H., & McCandless, K. (2014). *The surprising power of liberating structures.* Seattle, WA: Liberating Structures Press.

Lombard, K., & Horton-Deutsch, S. (2012). Creating space for reflection: The importance of presence in the teaching-learning process. In G. Sherwood & S. Horton-Deutsch (Eds.), *Reflective practice: Transforming education and improving outcomes* (pp. 43–61). Indianapolis, IN: Sigma Theta Tau International.

Munhall, P. L. (1993). 'Unknowing': Toward another pattern of knowing in nursing. *Nursing Outlook, 41*(3), 125–128.

Rosa, W., & Horton-Deutsch, S. (2017). The role of reflective practice in creating the world we want. In W. Rosa (Ed.), *A new era in global health: Nursing and the United Nations 2030 Sustainable Development Agenda* (pp. 461–474). New York, NY: Springer Publishing.

Schön, D. A. (1983). *The reflective practitioner. How professionals think in action.* New York, NY: Basic Books.

Schön, D. A. (1987). *Educating the reflective practitioner: Toward a new design for teaching and learning in the professions.* San Francisco, CA: Jossey-Bass.

Sherwood, G., & Horton-Deutsch, S. (2015). *Reflective organizations: On the frontlines of QSEN and reflective practice implementation.* Indianapolis, IN: Sigma Theta Tau International.

Swenson, M., & Sims, S. (2012). Reflective ways of working together: Using liberating structures. In G. Sherwood & S. Horton-Deutsch (Eds.), *Reflective practice: Transforming education and improving outcomes* (pp. 229–244). Indianapolis, IN: Sigma Theta Tau International.

Taylor, B. J. (2000). *Reflective practice: A guide for nurses and midwives.* Buckingham, UK: Open University Press.

Watson, J. (2008). *Nursing: The philosophy and science of caring* (Rev. ed.). Boulder: University of Colorado Press.

Watson, J. (2017). Human caring literacy. In S. Lee, P. Palmieri, & J. Watson (Eds.), *Global advances in human caring literacy.* New York, NY: Springer Publishing.

White, J. (1995). Patterns of knowing: Review, critique, and update. *Advances in Nursing Science, 17*(4), 73–86. doi:10.1097/00012272-199506000-00007

York-Barr, J., Sommers, W. A., Ghere, G. S., & Montie, J. K. (2016). *Reflective practice for renewing schools: An action guide for educators* (3rd ed.). Thousand Oaks, CA: Corwin.

Young, P., Pardue, K., & Horton-Deutsch, S. (2015). Practices of reflective leaders. In G. Sherwood & S. Horton-Deutsch (Eds.), *Reflective organizations: On the frontlines of QSEN and reflective practice implementation* (pp. 49–67). Indianapolis, IN: Sigma Theta Tau International.

12

*Linking the Unitary Paradigm to Policy Through a Synthesis of Caring Science and Integrative Nursing**

Mary Koithan, Mary Jo Kreitzer, and Jean Watson

CARITAS LITERACIES

By the end of this chapter, the caring-healing nurse will be able to

1. Link the principles of integrative nursing to the Caritas Processes®.

2. Align the tenets of the unitary paradigm with integrative nursing and Caring Science.

3. Identify nursing interventions for a Caritas Nursing practice plan.

4. Define a policy agenda that promotes a healthcare system that embodies Caring Science and integrative nursing.

5. Commit to a healthcare policy action plan that supports Caritas Nursing values and integrative nursing principles.

In 2014, the American Academy of Nursing became a founding member of the Nurses on Boards Coalition, a group of national nursing organizations working together to increase nurses' presence on corporate and nonprofit health-related boards of directors throughout

*From Koithan M. S., Kreitzer M. J., & Watson J. (2017). Linking the unitary paradigm to policy through a synthesis of Caring Science and Integrative Nursing. *Nursing Science Quarterly*, *30*(3), 262–268. doi:10.1177/0894318417708415. Copyright © 2017. Permission to reprint obtained from Thousand Oaks, CA: SAGE Publications.

the country. The Academy did this, citing the need and potential contribution that nursing's expertise and authority on the patient experience, quality of care, and patient safety would bring to ensure the nation's health. With the goal of placing 10,000 nurses on boards of directors by 2020 and the incredible opportunities that we have to positively impact the healthcare system, we are left to ponder whether there is a guiding framework for these policy endeavors. What policy wisdom can be found within nursing's paradigmatic perspectives? Can our discipline's beliefs and values guide not only our clinical care but also the policies that could create a healthcare system that provides care that is culturally safe, personalized, and meaningful in a way that is financially responsible and responsive?

This article addresses these questions from a unitary perspective of nursing, which originated with the visions of Nightingale and Rogers. Many scholars have since elaborated on this unitary view for nursing. Here, we use principles from integrative nursing and Caring Science to articulate a unitary perspective for recommending policy for contemporary nursing practice.

NURSING'S UNITARY PARADIGM

From its earliest beginnings, nursing has been a discipline focused on caring and healing from a holistic perspective, consistent with what we today refer to as the "unitary paradigm." Florence Nightingale (1859/1946), often referred to as the founder of modern nursing, noted in the late 1800s that the role of the nurse was to put the patient in the best possible condition so that nature could act and healing occur.

The unitary perspective was originally articulated by Rogers (1970) in her science of unitary human beings, elaborated as the unitary-transformative paradigm (Newman, Sime, & Corcoran-Perry, 1991), and applied to progressive practices such as unitary appreciative inquiry (Cowling & Repede, 2010) and emancipatory practice (Kagan, Smith, Cowling, & Chinn, 2009). Some scholars have aligned the unitary perspective specifically with a Rogerian view of holism (Cowling, 1994; Reed, 1997; Rogers, 1990). A unitary ontology refers to a holistic view of human beings as more than the sum of parts, and that is integral to the environment in the process of ongoing and innovative change. This view incorporates an emphasis on human patterning and living systems' inherent wholeness and potential for organization amidst increasing complexity. Nursing theorists have interpreted the unitary paradigm in distinct ways, for example, as Rogers's person-environment process, Parse's human universe connectedness, Watson's bodymindspirit, as well as other nursing theorists' biopsychosocial view of holism. Also, concepts such as relationship-based care, caring, health-as-wholeness, and healing-as-transformative are congruent with unitary views in nursing.

Although the essence of nursing has long been theorized from these unitary paradigmatic views, the contemporary practice of nursing in many settings around the globe has become increasingly fragmented and destabilized. Nursing shortages in many parts of the world are significant, yet administrative bureaucracies often remove nurses from the point of care, be that the bedside, home, or clinic, replacing them with less skilled workers, shifting nursing responsibilities toward documentation and other administrative tasks. Technology, although lifesaving, also has the potential of creating distance between the nurse and the patient, particularly if the nurse attends more to the "machine" than the patient.

Patients tell this story from a different point of view. Many experience a long parade of "care providers" who are too busy to actually care. Alternatively, they encounter different nurses on every shift day after day, making it very difficult to establish a relationship that builds trust and confidence. In many settings, care has become so fragmented that care coordinators or care managers are required to maintain some semblance of order.

We propose that together the principles of integrative nursing and Caring Science align with the unitary paradigm in a way that can practically shape nursing knowledge to inform the delivery of care across patient populations and clinical settings. Moreover, we posit that it is time to transform our healthcare system through policy initiatives that support praxes that honor nursing's unitary paradigm, clearly recognizing that it is challenging to change nursing practice until all relevant systems (legal/regulatory, financial, scientific, professional, ethical) re-envision health and well-being and the actions that support its attainment. This call to action provides a distinct and hopeful perspective in the ongoing throes of the national healthcare policy debate and offers nurses the opportunity to lead from a position of shared vision and common purpose.

CARING SCIENCE: DEFINING THE MORAL AND ETHICAL BASIS OF PATIENT-CENTERED INTEGRATIVE NURSING

As noted by Donaldson and Crowley (1978), nursing has a responsibility to evolve its moral and ethical commitment to humanity continuously. Since the 1970s, care and caring have been identified as foundational to nursing's covenant with society (Leininger, 1980; Watson, 1979). The American Nurses Association (ANA), American Association of Colleges of Nursing, and National League for Nursing have identified caring as a foundational value for nursing. ANA (2015) describes caring as the "moral ideal of nursing, consisting of human-to-human attempts to protect, enhance, and preserve humanity and human dignity, integrity, and wholeness by assisting a person to find meaning in illness, suffering, pain, and existence" (p. 11). Caring, from a unitary perspective, is differentiated from emotion and benevolent wishes; rather, caring is knowledge manifested as competent, sensitive, mature, skilled action that is grounded in science.

First described by Watson in 1979, Caring Science is based on the Ethic of Belonging and the Ethic of Face, developed by Emmanuel Levinas (1969), a French philosopher, who posited that our ethical worldview is the first principle of science. An Ethic of Belonging acknowledges that we all belong to the infinite field of universal cosmic love; we come from this source and will all ultimately return to it, manifesting the sacred circle of life-death. Thus, the following ideas apply:

- The universal whole (belonging) precedes our separate being.

- The human spirit is infinite.

- Consciousness—that awareness of the infinite source—is unified and nonlocal.

- Our belonging ties us morally to the unfolding and continuous evolution of consciousness toward infinity.

Translated, we conclude that an ethic grounded in caring means that we should act in such a way never to treat the other person as a means to an end, but rather as an end in him or herself.

In the Ethic of Face, Levinas (1969) reminds us that our presence with "the other" in any caring-healing relationship is not merely physical or aesthetic. The face we encounter is authentic, raw, and vulnerable and is viewed as irreducible and without bounds, one in which we glimpse our own humanity. The "face" is not relegated to abstractions or ideations but is instead experienced "as-lived" in its totality. In person-centered, relationship-based care, we are "invited" to "demand more of ourselves," accept our "obligation to demand justice" for the whole, and "commit ourselves to ensuring a meaningful world for the other" (Levinas, 1969, pp. 66, 198, 201, 219). Therefore, when we see self as other and other as self, we acknowledge the depth of our shared humanity and "establish the primordial basis for our caring" and the unitary nature of our existence (Watson, 2008, p. 57). Through *caritas*, nursing commits to a practice that is precious and deeply meaningful; caring that is life-giving and life-receiving, affirming the discipline's unitary perspective

CARITAS PROCESSES: FOUNDATION OF PERSON-CENTERED, RELATIONSHIP-BASED CARE

The 10 Caritas Processes, informed by the values of Caring Science, operationalize nursing's moral-ethical commitment to person-centered, relationship-based care. Together, these processes convey how we nurses enter into transpersonal caring moments with patients, families, and communities, and how we hold ourselves accountable to care that sustains the human body-mind-spirit and supports the evolution of consciousness, locally and globally. They form the foundation of our practice.

Therefore, nurses define person-centered care as heart-centered; honoring and protecting the human dignity of the other and believing in the other's intrinsic value and worth. It is a relationship that is deeply respectful; we meet the other authentically and intentionally—human to human. We hold the space within which we build this relationship as sacred, reflective of the greater whole and the compassionate love that we all merit.

INTEGRATIVE NURSING: A PRACTICE MODEL FOR CONTEMPORARY HEALTHCARE SYSTEMS

Although Caring Science provides the moral-ethical foundations of nursing practice, integrative nursing offers direction that can inform and shape both practice and policy. At a time when nurses individually and nursing departments collectively are adopting Caring Science as their professional practice model, the principles of integrative nursing offer additional clarity about nursing's role in the delivery of care across patient populations and clinical settings to promote health and well-being.

Integrative nursing is described as a whole person/whole system way of being-knowing-doing that advances the health and well-being of persons, families, and communities through caring/healing relationships (Kreitzer & Koithan, 2014). Six principles guide the practice of integrative nursing (see Table 12.1). These are aligned with the unitary nature of human beings and healing, particularly as expressed in Watson's Caring Science. The

TABLE 12.1 The Principles of Integrative Nursing

1. Human beings are whole systems, inseparable from their environments.
2. Human beings have the innate capacity for health and well-being.
3. Nature has healing and restorative properties that contribute to health and well-being.
4. Integrative nursing is person-centered and relationship-based.
5. Integrative nursing practice is informed by evidence and uses the full range of therapeutic modalities to support/augment the healing process, moving from least intensive/invasive to more, depending on need and context.
6. Integrative nursing focuses on the health and well-being of caregivers as well as those they serve.

Source: Kreitzer, M. J., & Koithan, M. (2014). *Integrative nursing.* New York, NY: Oxford University Press. Used with permission.

Ethics of Belonging and Face inform integrative nursing's moral and ethical foundations (Principle 1), whereas the Caritas Processes describe the nature of person-centered, relationship-based care (Principles 2 and 4) and provide behavioral guidelines for the integrative nurse. Similarly, integrative nursing (Principles 3, 5, and 6) extends Caring Science and informs nursing action and policy in the current healthcare delivery system. Therefore, Caring Science encompasses the universals of human caring, whereas integrative nursing encompasses the universals of human healing providing a paradigm for 21st-century nursing and healthcare.

THE FOUNDATIONS OF INTEGRATIVE NURSING

Three principles of integrative nursing are grounded in the unitary paradigm and are aligned with Caring Science and the Caritas Processes. Clinical manifestations associated with each principle correspond with policy implications for practice.

HUMAN BEINGS ARE WHOLE SYSTEMS INSEPARABLE FROM THEIR ENVIRONMENTS

People are dynamic, individualistic, and complex, and as such cannot be reduced to diagnoses, symptoms, and deviations from norms. Caring for the "whole person" requires attentiveness to the indivisible nature of the person (body-mind-spirit) and the inseparability of person from environment. The Ethic of Belonging situates this principle—morally and ethically. Integrative nurses view their patients and families as a reflection of self; rendering care with loving-kindness (Caritas Process 1) and reverentially and respectfully assisting the patient to sustain human dignity (Caritas Process 9). Human beings are complex adaptive systems, so integrative nurses are open to the mystery of unfolding futures; they expect that outcomes can be unexpected, miracles do occur, and that local interventions often create change that is unanticipated (Caritas Process 10).

Clinical manifestations of these beliefs and values include the following:

- Comprehensive assessment focused on body-mind-spirit of the person as well as his or her environments and contexts

- Personalized care that reflects the patient's and family's unique needs, strengths, and preferences

- A personalized care environment that is conducive to healing

- Recognition that the nursing attitudes, actions, and body language are part of the healing environment

Practicing nursing from a whole person/whole systems perspective begins with the recognition that the healthcare system must work for all people, regardless of socioeconomic, developmental, cultural, or physician needs and limitations. As such, ensuring health equity and adequate access to high-quality, culturally safe, and affordable care becomes one of nursing's policy imperatives. In addition, the profession is called to create a system that is reflective of the whole population and to create educational programs that admit not only the brightest students but also those who can contribute to the well-being of our emerging social identity.

HUMAN BEINGS HAVE THE INNATE CAPACITY FOR HEALTH AND WELL-BEING

The roots of this principle can be found across nursing theory, beginning with Nightingale (1859/1946) who encouraged nurses to "assist the reparative process which Nature has instituted" (p. 6). Likewise, Parse (2015) claimed that health is a process of human enfolding/unfolding coconstituted with human-universe process. The tenets of Caring Science propose that healing is a transformative process that occurs as the person recognizes the essential connectedness between self and universal consciousness.

Integrative nursing recognizes that the body has healing and restorative capacities on many levels. When the integrity of the skin is damaged by a cut, scrape, or deeper wound, the body automatically begins a process of inflammation, cell proliferation, and ultimately cellular repair. Although neurons do not divide and are not capable of mitosis after injury, surviving nerve cells, appropriately supported and reorganized, establish new neural connections. Neuroplasticity, an intrinsic capacity of the brain that occurs as a result of experiences and mental activities and thought, results in changes of structure and function, creating new neural pathways to heal and restore. Positive emotions flood our brains with dopamine and serotonin, enhance immune system functioning, diminish the inflammatory response to stress, and change the scope and boundaries of the brain.

Although recognizing that the capacity to heal is innate, integrative nurses also recognize that change is unpredictable and emergent. For example, the inflammatory response is helpful over a short period of time but, when present over several weeks or months, this same inflammatory process can produce a host of negative physiological changes. Integrative nursing practice seeks to reduce negative effects by providing the degree of support that is necessary to facilitate the innate healing process. For some patients, healing is supported by being authentically present and enabling faith/hope/belief (Caritas Process 2), clearly adopting the stance that the locus of healing is within the individual and not externally controlled. In other cases, support may require more intensive treatments that include hydration and medication administration. Always, integrative nurses are open to possibilities and embrace the mystery of the unknown to unfold and manifest (Caritas Process 10).

Clinical manifestations of these beliefs and values include the following:

- A focused intention for healing and wholeness during care procedures

- A nurturing and empowering presence with hope and belief in the agency of the patient/family/community

- A focus on strengths, resources, and opportunities rather than problems and weaknesses

When guided by the principle that healing is an innate capacity of the person, the healthcare system becomes supportive rather than directive. Consumers become active participants in their health rather than passive recipients of care. With this shift in focus, providers must have adequate time to coach and support an active patient and caregiving system. The primary care team will expand to include coaches, RN care coordinators, and other disciplines that can provide services that include stress reduction techniques, nutritional support, and lifestyle enhancement. Providers partner with individuals, families, and communities with their roles and accountabilities greatly expanded. Health-related interventions move from prescription of medication to social interventions and societal transformation (e.g., transportation, housing, nutrition) as a first line of support. Integrative nursing invites policy that recognizes the particular context (social, relational, temporal, cultural) and supports interventions that are affordable, feasible, and actively engage patients as partners.

INTEGRATIVE NURSING IS PERSON-CENTERED AND RELATIONSHIP-BASED

Caring-healing relationships, characterized by empathy, caring, love, warmth, trust, confidence, credibility, honesty, kindness, respect, and authentic communication provide the context for integrative nursing. Person-centered care focuses on care of the whole person—body-mind-spirit. Relationship-based care is built on continuity over time and calls upon the nurse to be fully present (Caritas Process 2), to listen deeply (Caritas Process 5), and to establish an authentic connection with the patient and family (Caritas Process 4). Providing care of this nature requires a deep knowledge and connection with those whom the nurse serves, which is cultivated by listening to the other person's story (Caritas Process 5), staying within the other's frame of reference (Caritas Process 7), and creatively seeking solutions that honors the other (Caritas Process 6). Relationship-based care requires the integrative nurse to cultivate self-understanding and sensitivity to self in relationship through reflective practices. Reflection allows the nurse to discern when care is ego-centric and facilitates adoption of a more transpersonal, heart-centered, and emergent approach (Caritas Process 3).

Clinical manifestations of these beliefs and values include the following:

- Staff that knows the patients' stories, contexts, and aspirations

- Care that is individualized, anticipatory, and based on patient/family needs and preferences

- Staff that listens deeply: listens to learn, uses silence, and suspends judgment

- Staff and administration that value and practice reflectively

- Staff members who are concerned about each other, recognizing the whole persons with whom they are working

Integrative nursing invites us to embrace the moral commitment that we live in right with each other, our communities, with the earth and its creatures, and with ourselves. Therefore, policy implications are wide-ranging: from organizational staff/scheduling patterns that lead to continuity of nurse/patient relationships to support for a robust and active public health system that employs community health workers who can establish meaningful relationships within the sociocultural environments of diverse populations. Integrative nurses are activists—recognizing that whole person well-being is intimately tied to the food security, safety of our communities, respect and personal freedom for individuals as well as the sovereign rights of indigenous nations, and our sense of space and place. Integrative nurses are committed to creating systems that are responsive, compassionate, and caring at both individual and global levels of scale.

NURSING PRACTICE AND CARE DELIVERY: PARADIGM-BASED POLICY RECOMMENDATIONS

Three additional principles, derived from foundational principles consistent with Caring Science, provide the basis for developing policy that facilitates the nursing praxis within contemporary healthcare systems. These principles extend our understanding of nursing interventions, nursing care delivery, and health policy, aligning with current safety and quality initiatives including the Quadruple Aim, Magnet Recognition Program®, and Beacon Award for Excellence. They also reflect the public's interest in self-care, prevention, and less invasive therapeutic interventions and an increasing evidence base for a broad range of therapies and healing practices including mind-body techniques, body-based therapies, and natural products.

NATURE HAS HEALING AND RESTORATIVE PROPERTIES THAT CONTRIBUTE TO HEALTH AND WELL-BEING

According to the biophilia hypothesis, human beings are innately drawn to nature and the natural world, and nature has properties that are healing and restorative (Wilson, 1984). Recent systematic literature reviews support the growing evidence that being in nature is associated with reduction in blood pressure as well as reduced heart rate and respiratory distress/shortness of breath, with preliminary evidence pointing to changes in biological markers associated with the stress response and changes in neurological activity and brain activation (Devlin & Arneill, 2003; Ulrich et al., 2008). Recognizing the healing power of nature, evidence-based design of healthcare facilities is incorporating elements of biophilic design, including the use of natural light, color, art, and architectural features, such as curves, that mimic nature. There is significant growth in nature-based therapeutics, including the use of labyrinths, healing gardens, animal-assisted interactions, and facilitated green exercise.

Clinical manifestations of these beliefs and values include the following:

- Clinical settings that provide access to natural light

- Clinical settings that integrate intentional use of color, art, and music that connect patients, families, and staff to nature-based environments

- Interventions (e.g., guided imagery, meditations, movement therapies) that draw upon nature

- Clinical settings that use labyrinths and healing gardens and spaces

Once again, nurses are called to extend their policy commitments and activism beyond what has historically been considered mainstream health-related policy to those that protect our natural resources, ensure biodiversity, and guarantee that our food supplies are devoid of chemicals and harmful modifications that challenge human and animal systems. We remember that our well-being is intricately linked to the multitude of systems that surround us and that all of us thrive when we have access to natural light, green environs, and adequate whole foods. Local policy implications include advocacy for the arts in schools, support for public art, and promotion of responsive rather than functional architecture (Beesley, Hirosue, Ruxton, Trankle, & Turner, 2006).

INTEGRATIVE NURSING IS INFORMED BY EVIDENCE AND USES THE FULL RANGE OF THERAPEUTIC MODALITIES TO SUPPORT/AUGMENT THE HEALING PROCESS, MOVING FROM LEAST INTENSIVE AND INVASIVE TO MORE, DEPENDING ON NEED AND CONTEXT

Over the past 20 years, there has been significant growth in the use of integrative therapies and healing practices (Nguyen, Davis, Kaptchuk, & Phillips, 2011; Okoro, Zhao, Li, & Balluz, 2013). The drivers of these global phenomena are many and include the limitations of Western medical approaches in managing symptoms, particularly of chronic disease, and the desire of people to use nonpharmacological approaches to improve their health and well-being. Many of the so-called integrative therapies fall within the scope of nursing practice, and in the United States, some state nurse-licensing boards have developed specific statements that acknowledge the use of integrative therapies.

Clinical manifestations of these beliefs and values include the following:

- Interventions are based on a patient's condition (depth of distress and dysfunction), needs, wants, and preferences

- Providers (nurses, physicians, therapists, ancillary staff) use a full range of therapeutics and healing practices to manage symptoms, improve clinical outcomes, and quality of life

A major focus in integrative nursing is the effective management of symptoms, acknowledging the role of the nurse as supportive of the innate healing process, aligning nursing's science and philosophical beliefs and values with their practice. Conventional biomedical management of symptoms frequently begins with a pharmacological intervention intended to suppress symptoms and "fix" the problem, with the locus of healing often on the provider of care. Integrative nursing shifts the focus from curing to healing, thus changing the nature of problem solving and prioritizing. This does not imply that biomedical interventions are discarded. Rather they are introduced when that level of intervention is warranted, and the system condition requires more intensive support. Nurses practicing from an integrative perspective are not merely "adding on" integrative therapies; integrative therapies become *core* to their practice.

Cutshall and Van Getson (2014) describe the evidence base underlying the use of integrative therapies for the management of nausea that includes dietary interventions, aromatherapy oils (ginger and peppermint), mind–body approaches (guided imagery, relaxation, hypnosis, and deep breathing), acupressure (P6 acupressure point), and energy healing such as Reiki. Nonpharmacological pain management approaches include mind–body interventions such as the relaxation response, guided imagery, and mindfulness-based stress reduction as well as acupressure and acupuncture, yoga and movement therapies, massage, and access to nature (Wagner & Thompson, 2014). Integrative approaches are also described for the management of stress, sleep, anxiety, depressed mood, fatigue, cognitive impairment, and care of the human spirit.

Policy implications suggested by this principle are wide-ranging to include agency-based protocols that facilitate the use of the full range of therapeutics, delineating methods of integrative assessment, and clinical decision making that allows a broad range of providers to practice to the full scope of their education, licensure, and certification. Our healthcare team and our definitions of interprofessional practice would expand when considering the full policy implications of this principle; professional credentialing and privileging would be extended to include Traditional Chinese Medicine providers, massage therapists, healing touch practitioners, and others. Reform would stretch across the insurance and reimbursement systems to appropriately pay for therapies that have been deemed both effective and safe by an expanded definition of evidence that includes multiple ways of knowing.

Consider for one moment the potential impact of policy reforms suggested by this single principle alone. How many iatrogenic conditions could we prevent if we could simply teach children to treat pain using hot/cold before reaching for medication? What might be the long-term, downstream financial, social, and physiological effects when an entire generation believes in and expects to be able to address common symptoms through self-care and low-cost therapies rather than a neighborhood pharmacy and a pill? How much could we save if we tried manipulative, body-based therapies for recurrent headaches before we demanded an MRI and extensive neurological testing? What impact would we have on cost, quality of life, and productivity if we encouraged people to participate in stress-reduction activities rather than asking for the latest prescription advertised on television? This is what integrative nursing invites us to do—return to a system grounded in our roots—a system focused on "putting the patient in the best condition for nature to act," a system that is accessible, patient/family-centered, and culturally safe; a system that embraces health for all—including its caregivers.

INTEGRATIVE NURSING FOCUSES ON THE HEALTH AND WELL-BEING OF CAREGIVERS AS WELL AS THOSE THEY SERVE

Nurses work in intense, high-stress environments and are vulnerable to stress and burnout that impact their own health and well-being as well as the care of patients. Caring Science emphasizes that nursing is essentially a reciprocal process where nurse and patient are in mutual relationship. This reciprocity requires that the nurse attend to his or her own needs; the nurse needs to take care of self to be able to care for others (Watson, 2001).

Self-awareness and self-care are core practices that are foundational to integrative nursing. Self-awareness allows the nurse to notice inner experiences as he or she engages in caring for patients. Self-reflection, a form of ongoing inquiry, can lead to deeper learning and insights. Self-care is the most sustainable healthcare practice and comprises attentiveness to lifestyle behaviors (including healthy eating, exercise, sleep and stress management) and may include the use of integrative therapies such as meditation, yoga, energy therapies, and massage.

Clinical and policy implications of these beliefs and values include the following:

- Staffing patterns reflect a value of provider self-care, allowing for adequate break times, staffing support, and reflective practice.

- Staff development and on-boarding processes provide for reflective practice skill development.

- Work environments incorporate self-care settings and services that are available for staff and public use (e.g., wellness centers, mind-body and movement classes, spas).

- A personal plan for health and well-being is developed and implemented.

- Clinical policies include clinical ladders and promotion/tenure criteria that reward engagement in self-care and lifestyle change.

CONCLUSION

Consistent with the historic call for nursing to come of age as a mature discipline and profession of caring, healing, and health, the convergence of Caring Science and integrative nursing advances our understanding of nursing's metaparadigm and provides a blueprint for a practice that is grounded in the unitary paradigm and reflective of our emphasis on caring presence during the human health experience. By aligning the moral-ethical foundations provided by Caring Science and the Caritas Processes with an integrative practice model, we provide a practical approach for nursing in the 21st century. This unified approach honors nursing's unitary paradigm while clearly charting the course for the discipline's policy agenda.

NEXT ERA POSSIBILITIES

Education

- How can I transform the educational programs with which I am associated to embrace Caring Science and integrative nursing practice?
- What additional literacies do nursing faculty need to transform education to reflect a healing-caring perspective and integrative nursing praxis?

Research

- What methodological innovations are required to expand Caring Science and knowledge about impact of integrative nursing practice?
- What role do Caritas nurse scientists play in developing an expanded evidence base for interventions based on the unitary perspective?

Praxis

- What specific nursing intervention can I immediately adopt to better align my practice with caring-integrative nursing praxis?
- How can I reframe my nursing interventions with increased understanding of caring-integrative nursing praxis?
- What healthcare policy innovation that aligns with caring-integrative nursing praxis can I commit to actively supporting?

Theory and Knowledge Development

- What knowledge expansion is essential to support caring-integrative nursing praxis?
- How does my specialty practice align with caring-integrative nursing values and principles?
- How does caring-integrative nursing praxis challenge my beliefs, assumptions, and theoretical perspectives?

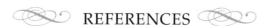 REFERENCES

American Nurses Association. (2015). *Nursing: Scope and standards of practice* (3rd ed.). Silver Spring, MD: Author.

Beesley, P, Hirosue, S, Ruxton, J, Trankle, M., & Turner, C. (Eds.). (2006). *Responsive architectures: Subtle technologies*. Riverside, CA: Riverside Architectural Press.

Cowling, W. R. (1994). Unitary knowing in nursing practice. *Nursing Science Quarterly, 6*(4), 201–207. doi:10.1177/089431849300600409

Cowling, W. R., & Repede, E. (2010). Unitary appreciative inquiry: Evolution and refinement. *Advances in Nursing Science, 33*, 64–77. doi:10.1097/ANS.0b013e3181ce6bdd

Cutshall, S., & Van Getson, L. (2014). Integrative nursing management of nausea. In M. J. Kreitzer & M. Koithan (Eds.), *Integrative Nursing* (pp. 221–236). New York, NY: Oxford University Press.

Devlin, A. S., & Arneill, A. B. (2003). Health care environments and patient outcomes. A review of the literature. *Environment and Behavior, 35*(5), 665–694. doi:10.1177/0013916503255102

Donaldson, S. K., & Crowley, D. M. (1978). The discipline of nursing. *Nursing Outlook, 26*(2), 113–120.

Kagan, P. N., Smith, M. C., Cowling, W. R., & Chinn, P. L. (2009). A nursing manifesto: An emancipatory call for knowledge development, conscience, and praxis. *Nursing Philosophy, 11*, 67–84. doi:10.1111/j.1466-769X.2009.00422.x

Kreitzer, M. J., & Koithan, M. (Eds.). (2014). *Integrative nursing*. New York, NY: Oxford University Press.

Leininger, M. (1980). Caring: A central focus for nursing and health care services. *Nursing and Health Care, 1*(3), 135–143, 176.

Levinas, E. (1969). *Totality and infinity: An essay on exteriority* (A. Lingis, Trans.) Pittsburgh, PA: Duquesne University Press.

Newman, M. A., Sime, A. W., & Corcoran-Perry, S. A. (1991). The focus of the discipline of nursing. *Advances in Nursing Science, 14*(1), 1–6. doi:10.1097/00012272-199109000-00002

Nguyen, L. T., Davis, R. B., Kaptchuk, T. J., & Phillips, R. S. (2011). Use of complementary and alternative medicine and self-rated health status: Results from a national survey. *Journal of General Internal Medicine, 26*(4), 399–404. doi:10.1007/s11606-010-1542-3

Nightingale, F. (1946). *Notes on nursing*. London, UK: Harrison and Sons. (Original work published 1859)

Okoro, C. A., Zhao, G., Li, C., & Balluz, L. S. (2013). Has the use of complementary and alternative medicine therapies by U.S. adults with chronic disease-related functional limitations changed from 2002 to 2007? *Journal of Alternative and Complementary Medicine, 19*(3), 217–223. doi:10.1089/acm.2012.0009

Parse, R. R. (2015). Rosemarie Rizzo Parse's humanbecoming paradigm. In M. C. Smith & M. E. Parker (Eds.), *Nursing theories & nursing practice* (4th ed., pp. 263–277). Philadelphia, PA: F. A. Davis.

Reed, P. G. (1997). Nursing: The ontology of the discipline. *Nursing Science Quarterly, 10*(2), 76–79. doi:10.1177/089431849701000207

Rogers, M. E. (1970). *An introduction to the theoretical basis of nursing*. Philadelphia, PA: F. A Davis.

Rogers, M. E. (1990). Nursing: Science of unitary, irreducible human beings: Update 1990. In E. A. M. Barrett (Ed.), *Vision of Rogers' science-based nursing* (pp. 5–11). New York, NY: National League for Nursing.

Ulrich, R. S., Zimring, C., Zhu, X., DuBose, J., Seo, H. B., Choi, Y. S., … Joseph, A. (2008). A review of the research literature on evidence-based healthcare design. *Health Environments Research and Design Journal, 1*(3), 61–125. doi:10.1177/193758670800100306

Wagner, J., & Thompson, S. (2014). Integrative nursing management of pain. In M. J. Kreitzer & M. Koithan (Eds.), *Integrative nursing* (pp. 292–306). New York, NY: Oxford University Press.

Watson, J. (1979). *Nursing: The philosophy and science of caring*. Boston, MA: Little, Brown.

Watson, J. (2001). Post-hospital nursing: Shortages, shifts, and scripts. *Nursing Administration Quarterly, 25*(3), 77–82. doi:10.1097/00006216-200104000-00012

Watson, J. (2008). *Nursing: The philosophy and science of caring*. Boulder: University of Colorado Press.

Wilson, E. O. (1984). *Biophilia: The human bond with other species*. Cambridge, MA: Harvard University Press.

III

Caring Science Literacy: From Caritas to Global Communitas

13

Ways of Being/Knowing/Becoming

Jean Watson and Sara Horton-Deutsch

CARITAS LITERACIES

By the end of this chapter, the caring-healing nurse will be able to

1. Understand Caritas ways of Being, Knowing, and Becoming with Caritas Processes® as guide.

2. Integrate the concept of Unitary-Cosmic-Infinite Love as vision for humanity's evolution.

3. Connect with global *Communitas*—an evolved vision for a moral community for human-Planet survival.

This chapter addresses "Ways of Being/Knowing/Becoming" within Unitary Caring Science Consciousness and Caring Literacy. As we explore the evolution of Human Caring Science and the concept of Caring Literacy and Caritas (Universal Love), we bring forth new dimensions of our Ways of Being/Doing/Becoming (Watson, 2017). We also discover how the 10 Caritas Processes (Watson, 2008) serve as a guide for engaging in this journey of Being/Knowing/Becoming within Unitary Caring Science—ever-evolving in Caring Literacy:

While the meaning of literacy is associated with the abilities to read and write, the notion of having fluency in caring at both personal and professional levels introduces new meaning to deepen our ways of attending to and cultivating how to *Be* deeply human/humane, and how to *Be-caring* ... Such literacy includes an evolved and continually evolving emotional heart intelligence, consciousness and intentionality and level of sensitivity and efficacy, followed by a continuing lifelong process and journey of self-growth and self-awareness. (modified from Watson, 2017, p. 3)

Whole person literacy for professional practices of caring-healing and health requires maturity and self-reflection (Sherwood & Horton-Deutsch, 2012; Freshwater, 2008; Johns, 2009). As one becomes more reflective, an evolved awareness reveals Unitary Caring Science as one of the most advanced guides for living out our humane ways of Being/Knowing/Becoming—more evolved, more conscious, more literate in our ways of *Being* human. Caritas consciousness and Caritas Ways of Being/Knowing/Becoming … invite one to whole person presence, with an evolved consciousness that opens to the higher level, energetic, infinite spiritual field of one's humanity. (Watson, 2017)

CARITAS-WAYS-OF-BEING

Caritas-Ways-of-Being were identified as educational materials for the Watson Caring Science Caritas Coach Educational Program. They include the following ways of Being—Human-Being/Caritas (www.watsoncaringscience.org). They include the following Ways-of-Being-Human-Being/Caritas:

- Being Loving-Kindness

- Having Heart-Center Authentic Presence

- Offering Compassionate Forgiveness

- Living Gratitude-Appreciation

- Practicing Energetic Caritas Consciousness evolution—personal spiritual practices

- Opening to Giving-Receiving

- Being Still—Silence—Holding the Still Point

- Connecting with infinite Cosmic field of Universal Love

- Manifesting Caritas field (to sustain caring and our humanity)

- Listening-Hearing

- Reflecting-Awakening

- Holding heart space for mystery, awe, wonder

- Honoring the Infinite

To cultivate and live out these Caritas Ways-of-Being, the 10 Caritas Processes of the *Theory of transpersonal caring* (Watson, 1985, 2008, 2012) can serve as both a theoretical and practical guide for personal/professional Being/Knowing/Becoming Caritas. This next section explores the 10 Caritas Processes with guiding consciousness steps toward Caritas Literacy. The exemplars in Table 13.1 can serve as a guide to Being/Knowing/Becoming more literate.

TABLE 13.1 A Guide to Caritas Literacy in Being/Knowing/Becoming

---

Caritas Process 1: Practicing loving-kindness and equanimity within the context of caring consciousness

By having loving-kindness and compassion for self, I am more able to have compassion and loving kindness for others.

Caritas Process 2: Being authentically present and enabling and sustaining faith and a deep belief system of self and one being cared for

Through my awareness of the oneness of all, honoring diverse beliefs, I am able to respect and support all others' diverse practices of faith-hope.

Caritas Process 3: Cultivating one's own spiritual practices and transpersonal self, going beyond ego-self

By being more accountable for my own self-growth and spiritual practices, I am more able to be authentically present and open to transpersonal caring moments, potentiating healing for self-other.

Caritas Process 4: Developing and sustaining loving, trusting, caring relationships

I create heart-to-heart, human-to-human relations that allow authentic connections for helping-trusting caring relationships with all others.

Caritas Process 5: Being present to, and supportive of, the expression of positive and negative feelings—authentically listening to another person's story

I cocreate safe space for authentic listening, giving permission for others to express their true feelings.

Caritas Process 6: Creative solution seeking through full use of self and artistry of caring-healing practices

I draw upon expressive, creative arts—the artistry of being, and all ways of knowing/being/becoming as potential caring-healing modalities—accessing inner energetic healing possibilities.

Caritas Process 7: Engaging in transpersonal teaching-learning within the context of a caring relationship

I stay within the other's subjective frame of reference, allowing for deep personal learning that supports healing, wholeness, and well-being/becoming.

Caritas Process 8: Creating a healing environment at all levels

I maintain an energetic, authentic, caring-healing human presence as the environmental healing field.

Caritas Process 9: Reverently assisting with basic needs as sacred acts

In touching and assisting physical needs with dignity, I am practicing "caring science as sacred science," touching the life force and body/mind/spirit of the other.

Caritas Process 10: Opening to spiritual mystery and unknowns

I allow for miracles—opening to, and trusting in, unknowns of the infinite field of the universe.

CARITAS WAYS OF KNOWING

Epistemology is the study of knowledge, what counts as knowledge, and how we develop knowledge and honor ways of knowing. Epistemology is influenced and informed by our philosophy of science, our worldview or ontology, of what is valued as knowledge, whether we understand knowledge as something "out there" or whether we coparticipate in creating knowledge, working from within as well as from without. Epistemology and ontology inform our thinking and consciousness about what we consider knowledge that is trustworthy. In Caritas Science, one's philosophy of science view of knowledge guides one's consciousness toward critiquing issues of epistemology and what counts as knowledge, transcending conventional ways of knowing and what counts as knowledge.

The classic publication of Carper (1978) first raised the consciousness of nurses and nursing scientists by critiquing and identifying multiple ways of knowing, beyond empirical, technical, objective knowledge. She brought forth whole person ways of knowing embraced by nursing that go beyond the knowledge that medical and nursing science hold as supreme. For example, Carper acknowledged multiple ways of knowing in nursing practice, such as personal, aesthetic, intuitive, and ethical knowing. All ways of knowing are valued and incorporate into clinical decision making for the nurse and for the patient and medical team.

Other scholars added to the Carper discourse. For example, Jill White (1995) raised the issue about "knowing policy" and politics as another area of knowing and knowledge for nursing. Still others such as Munhall (1989) suggested that we have a category of unknowing or "not knowing"—acknowledging that we have to unlearn and unravel the dominant paradigm, away from the objective/empirical as the primary form of knowledge. Later, Smith (1992) raised the ante by positing that no knowledge exists outside personal knowledge; personal knowing, that is, ultimately all knowledge is personal knowledge.

The discourse on knowledge within Caring Science and unitary-transformative thinking continues to expand and deepen. More current research and theories have incorporated and broadened the field, for example, emotional knowing, caring literacy, intelligent heart, aesthetic knowing, mystical-spiritual knowing, wisdom—beyond knowledge, and psychic, psychedelic knowing. All of these emerging areas of "knowing" are valued as part of the infinity of the human mind and spirit to higher and deeper levels of consciousness, for example, mythical knowing, unconscious knowing, believing—trust and faith as an inner form of knowing.

Ken Wilber (2001) makes a case for direct experience as a legitimate knowing, acknowledging that the world's great yogis, saints, and sages have reported that direct spiritual experiences are a living reality, including direct experience with Spirit, when in deep introspective, transpersonal experiences. These evolving forms of knowing can be considered "Caritas ways of Knowing"—all considered higher domains of knowing—acknowledging a human's ability to have direct experiences with universal consciousness, infinite field of universal Love.

Thus, Unitary Caring Science honors and celebrates *all* ways of knowing that can be identified, and yet are still emerging/evolving with humanity's evolving. Diverse and "All-ways-of-Knowing," including Caritas/Love, all become openings to the infinite field of unitary consciousness. They are all honored as reflective of the universality of human becoming; all these ways of knowing are honored as legitimate areas of inquiry and scholarship within Caring Science.

CARITAS WAYS-OF-BECOMING

Here in exploring Caritas-Ways-of-Becoming, we embrace and honor all nonconventional-knowing, nonscientific, metaphysical, mystical, psychic, spiritual, direct experience-knowing that do not conform to the conventional Western science separatist world view. However, these dimensions open us to new levels of the expanding evolution of humanity, connecting with both physical and nonphysical forms of knowledge. Exploring Ways-of-Becoming welcomes all the vicissitudes of humanity and multiple, diverse complexi-ties of human experiences; they all count as knowing and ways of Becoming—more humane, more evolving toward higher/deeper levels of universal global conscious-ness. When bringing all the Caritas Ways-of-Being/Knowing/Becoming together— personally and globally—we can now acknowledge these expanded forms of knowledge and ways of knowing; they are unlimited and continuous with the evolution of human consciousness.

CARITAS WAYS-OF-BEING/KNOWING/BECOMING: EVOLVING TO OMEGA POINT—UNIVERSAL LOVE

Caritas Ways-of-Being flow into Caritas Ways-of-Becoming, through deeper inner transfor-mative awakening, connecting with Infinite Source, Higher self, Infinite Love. Teilhard de Chardin (1955) noted that humans have evolved as much as they are going to evolve, biologically. The next evolution of human kind is the evolution of consciousness: evolving to the "Omega Point"—Universal Love—Godhead.

As we live out Caritas Ways-of-Being and experience the Caritas Processes for our self-other, we are *Becoming Caritas—Becoming Love*. If love is the highest level of consciousness, then we meditate from the heart center above, in the energetic body system. We become closer in our connection with the Divine, the Beloved—the Cosmic Infinite Universal LOVE. The Cosmic Love to which we all belong and to which we can come closer is what Levinas (1996) describes as an Ethic and the first principle of science.

The ancient teachings and art of Hildegard of Bingen, a 12th-century German nun and healer, artist, visionary, musician, writer, and mystic, manifest her vision of humans "resid-ing in a unitary field of consciousness" and coincide today with contemporary physicists and scientists; that is, the body resides within a unitary field of consciousness, inverting the paradigm. Our conventional worldview is that consciousness resides within the body/mind/brain. The emerging ancient and contemporary worldviews of consciousness acknowledge and affirm the concept of "nonlocal consciousness." The writings and research of Dossey (2014), van Lommel (2011), Alexander (2012), and Wilber (2001) attest to this new explanatory model.

In other words, new models of consciousness go beyond the physical body and open up a new reality so that we can access a higher consciousness. This ancient/new thinking is leading to new explanatory models for such phenomena as prayer, distant healing, direct spiritual experiences, near death and altered states of consciousness, and psychic experiences. Caritas

Ways-of-Being-Knowing-Becoming awaken humanity to wonder, awe, and oneness, and the beauty of all.

CONCLUSION

Global Unitary Consciousness One World–One Heart

In exploring Caritas Ways-of-Being/Knowing/Becoming, we move from Personal Caritas to Global Communitas. Once we expand our worldview from a separatist world/universe to a Unitary worldview of oneness, we awaken to a new reality that everything in the universe is connected with everything else. Once we have this awakening for humanity/Planet Earth/ universe, we are called to be more intentional, more committed to personal/global awakening to new realities.

What we do to self/we do to others/Planet. What we do to others, we do to self/Planet. As we evolve closer to the consciousness of universal Love, which holds us all together, we are closer to cocreating moral Caritas Communitas/Community for our world; our planet/our evolving universe, spinning into infinity. One Heart/One World, making new connections between human caring/caritas and peace in our hearts and our humanity. In closing— Coleman Barks, who translated Rumi's poetry, told the story about a question he asked his teacher, Bawa, before his death December 8, 1986 (Barks, 1999, xix).

"Will what I see in your eyes ever come up behind mine and look out through me?"
His teacher answered
"When the **I** (eye) becomes a **We**."

Finally, the beauty and wisdom of Global Caritas Communitas awakens us to The Great *I AM*.
We are all ONE.

NEXT ERA POSSIBILITIES

Education
- How am I expanding my ways of knowing-unknowing in order to learn and evolve toward whole person knowing?
- Is there a way that opens me to all ways of knowing and being receptive to new forms of knowledge?

Research
- How do Caritas ways of Being, Knowing, and Becoming with Caritas Processes lead to new questions, and to new, creative, emergent methodologies for Caring Science inquiry and research?

Praxis
- How am I continually nurturing and cultivating my ways of being human? How congruent are my practices with the theoretical basis of Unitary Caring Science?
- In what ways do I connect with deep self and infinite field to access a higher consciousness and awaken my humanity to wonder and to the unity of all?

Theory and Knowledge Development

- What new theories are needed to expand and complement the Unitary-Infinite Love and Global Communitas field and through their evolution and synthesis expand ways of knowing, being, becoming more human?

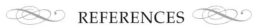 REFERENCES

Alexander, E. (2012). *Proof of heaven*. New York, NY: Simon & Schuster.

Barks, C. (1999). *The glance. Songs of soul meeting*. New York, NY: Penguin Putman.

Carper, B. (1978). Fundamental patterns of knowing in nursing. *Advances in Nursing Science, 1*(1), 13–23. doi:10.1097/00012272-197810000-00004

de Chardin, P. T. (1955). *The phenomenon of man*. New York, NY: Collins.

Dossey, L. (2014). *One mind. How our individual mind is part of a greater consciousness and why it matters*. Carlsbad, CA: Hay House.

Freshwater, D. (2008). Reflective practice: The state of the art. In D. Freshwater, B. J. Taylor, & G. Sherwood (Eds.), *International textbook of reflective practice in nursing* (pp. 1–18). Oxford, UK: Blackwell.

Johns, C. (2009). *Becoming a reflective practitioner* (3rd ed.). West Sussex, UK: Wiley-Blackwell.

Levinas, E. (1996). *Basic philosophical writings*. Bloomington: Indiana University Press.

Munhall, P. L. (1989). Philosophical ponderings on qualitative research methods in nursing. *Nursing Science Quarterly, 2*, 20–28. doi:10.1177/089431848900200109

Sherwood, G. D., & Horton-Deutsch, S. (2012). *Reflective Practice. Transforming education and improving outcomes*. Indianapolis, IN: Sigma Theta Tau International.

Smith, M. C. (1992). Is all knowing personal knowing? *Nursing Science Quarterly, 5*(1), 2–3. doi:10.1177/089431849200500102

Teilhard de Chardin, P. (1959). *The phenomenon of man*. New York, NY: Harper & Row.

Van Lommel, P. (2011). *Consciousness beyond life: The science of near death experience*. New York, NY: Harper Collins.

Watson, J. (1985). *Nursing: The philosophy and science of caring*. Boston, MA: Little, Brown.

Watson, J. (2008). *Nursing: The philosophy and science of caring* (pp. 3–12). Boulder: University of Colorado Press.

Watson, J. (2012). *Human caring science: A theory of nursing*. Sudbury, MA: Jones & Bartlett.

Watson, J. (2017). Global advances in human caring literacy. In S. Lee, P. Palmieri, & J. Watson (Eds.), *Global advances in human caring literacy*. New York, NY: Springer Publishing.

White, J. (1995). Patterns of knowing: Review, critique, and update. *Advances in Nursing Science, 17*(4), 73–86. doi:10.1097/00012272-199506000-00007

Wilber, K. (2001). *Quantum questions. Mystical writing of the world's great physicists*. Boston, MA: Shambhala.

14

Curriculum Development Processes and Pedagogical Practices for Advancing Caring Science Literacy

Marcia Hills and Chantal Cara

CARITAS LITERACIES

By the end of this chapter, the caring-healing nurse will be able to

1. Identify different trends in Caring Science pedagogy and curriculum development illustrating growth in Caring Science literacy.

2. Describe how Caring Science literacy is being used to advance pedagogy and curriculum development in nursing education.

3. Identify different approaches to promoting Caring Science literacy in a nursing curriculum.

When most nurse educators discuss curriculum, they are usually referring to a program of studies or a sequence of courses that leads toward specific learning outcomes (Bevis & Watson, 1989; Gagné, 1970; Tyler, 1949). This understanding of curriculum was redefined by Bevis and Watson (1989), to be "the interactions and transactions that occur between and among students and teachers with the intent that learning occur" (p. 5). This reorientation highlighted the centrality of pedagogy within the curriculum process, underscoring the significance of *how* nursing educators teach, being as important, if not more important, than *what* they teach. In nursing education, this emphasis on *how* to teach needs to be understood at the deepest philosophical level to guide the design of nursing education programs. Curriculum is entirely and fundamentally about teachers' relationships with their students

(Bevis & Watson, 1989; Hills & Watson, 2011). The purpose of this chapter is to articulate current trends in Caring Science pedagogy and curriculum development processes that promote Caring Science literacy. Exemplars are provided to demonstrate ways Caring Science is used to develop curriculum in nursing education.

CARING SCIENCE LITERACY—WHAT IS IT?

The word "literacy" is generally associated with the abilities to read and write but, in the Caring Science context, it has a more expansive meaning. Watson (2008) states that Caring Science literacy "deepen[s] our ways of attending to and cultivating how to *Be-deeply Human* (...) and *Be-Caring* and Having a Healing presence. This form of Being is a form of human literacy, human artistry" (p. 23). She goes on to say that "Being literate extends to the ability to incorporate concrete experience, experiential learning, context, and situations into one's life field. Thus, the term *literacy* has evolved to reflect the fact that there are multiple literacies" (Watson, 2017, p. 5). Furthermore, thinking of literacy in this way requires one to understand the ontological meanings of being and becoming (Watson, 2017).

This chapter explores significant curriculum processes and pedagogical practices that promote Caring Science literacy. Watson's work (2017) gives rise to the following questions in nursing curriculum and pedagogy:

- What does it mean to be/become a caring teacher?

- How could Caring Science help teachers to be in relationships with their students?

- How can teachers evaluate their students while being informed by Caring Science?

CARING SCIENCE PEDAGOGY—WHAT IS IT?

Most dictionary definitions of "pedagogy" focus on teaching—referring to the art, the science, the profession, the methods, and the discipline ... of teaching only. However, Dewey (1933), Combs (1982), Rogers (1969), and Freire (1972) argue that defining pedagogy in terms of teaching alone, without a consideration of learning, limits the true meaning of pedagogy. Hills and Watson's (2011) definition of pedagogy as "a relational inquiry process that facilitates the transformation of consciousness through which learning and deeper insight occurs" (p. 53) broadens the understanding of pedagogy beyond teaching alone, to focus on learning, as well as the relationships among teachers, students, and learning.

Learning can also be viewed from different perspectives. The dominant perspective in nursing education to this day is behaviorism (Hills, 2016). In the behaviorist perspective, a banking concept of learning is used, recognizing the teacher as the "holder" of information, whereas the student is the "recipient" of that information (Freire, 1972). From this perspective, the teacher's responsibility is to give information to the students, usually by lecturing to them. The students' responsibility is to receive the information and to regurgitate that information back to the teacher, usually through standardized testing such as multiple-choice exams. Student progress is evaluated using measureable behavioral objectives. Although this way of teaching may be useful in "giving information," it also creates passive learners who learn only what their teachers think is important (Bevis & Watson, 1989; Freire, 1972; Hills & Watson, 2011).

At this point, it is important to acknowledge the contribution that the Tylerian behaviorist model (Tyler, 1949) has made to nursing more generally. Nursing has made significant progress in becoming a recognized independent healthcare profession in part because of its embracing a Tylerian behaviorist educational model that provided a highly organized, measureable, evaluation-oriented structure that lifted up the profession (Bevis, 1989a). It can be stated that behaviorism assisted nursing to move its educational programs from training programs to colleges and universities (Bevis, 1989a). However, our adherence to this strictly behaviorist model has made nursing become only what can be measured. As Kliebard (1968, as cited in Bevis, 1989a) eloquently states: "From a moral point of view, the emphasis on behavioral goals, ... still borders on brainwashing or at least indoctrination rather than education. We begin with ... how we want a person to behave and then we try to manipulate him ... so as to get him to behave as we want" (p. 246).

There are many aspects of nursing that are not measureable such as caring, compassion, alleviating suffering, kindness, presence, hope, to name a few (Bevis & Watson, 1989; Cara, 2017; Hills, 2017; Watson, 2008). Over the years, this adherence to strict behaviorism has made many critical aspects of nursing, such as those just mentioned, invisible. As nursing evolves its disciplinary foundation, it is time to stand in this base and claim those invisible aspects of nursing as core to our practice and therefore to nursing education (Hills, 2017).

In contrast to the behaviorist perspective, a Caring Science perspective views learning as the transformation of consciousness (Cara & Girard, 2013; Hills, 2016; Hills & Watson, 2011). In other words, a student's learning takes place within the teacher–student caring relationship, and the teacher and student together cocreate knowledge (Cara & Girard, 2013; Hills & Watson, 2011).

Inspired by several works (Hills, 1992, 2016, 2017; Hills & Lindsey, 1994; Hills & Watson, 2011; Watson & Smith, 2002), pedagogy and curriculum, from this Caring Science perspective, require the following characteristics:

- A commitment to Caring as the moral imperative of nursing

- A primary focus on people and their experiences

- A perspective that is informed by a philosophy of phenomenology and critical social theory

- An orientation that reflects a health/health promotion/healing perspective

- The course content organized according to Caring Science and nursing rather than medical concepts and ideologies

- An orientation to teaching/learning that is interactive, dialogic, and challenging; and which encourages the development of personal meaning

- A recognition of multiple ways of knowing such as intuitive, aesthetic, empirical, constructed, and emancipatory

- A student–teacher caring relationship that is authentic, egalitarian, respectful, and humanistic

Building on these characteristics, five curriculum processes and pedagogical practices are proposed to advance Caring Science literacy.

FIVE CARING SCIENCE CURRICULUM PROCESSES AND PEDAGOGICAL PRACTICES

Based on the authors' previous work and experiences in Caring Science curriculum development and nursing education, the following components are relevant in nursing education to advance Caring Science literacy:

1. Claiming Caring Science as the moral, theoretical, and philosophical foundation of the discipline of nursing and, therefore, nursing education

2. Using Caring Science language to articulate nursing education and practice

3. Teaching and learning in caring collaborative relationship

4. Creating Caring Science curriculum design and structure

5. Evaluating students' clinical practice on the basis of Caring Science rather than behavioral objectives

CLAIMING CARING SCIENCE AS THE MORAL, THEORETICAL, AND PHILOSOPHICAL FOUNDATION OF THE DISCIPLINE OF NURSING AND, THEREFORE, NURSING EDUCATION

Understanding Caring Science as the foundation of the nursing discipline and consequently, nursing education, is not a new concept. Its origins can be traced back to the days of Nightingale (1860/1969), the founder of modern nursing. More recent roots are in the curriculum revolution, a noteworthy and influential event in the evolution of nursing education (National League for Nursing [NLN], 1988) that continues to set the context for nursing education to this day (France & Ray, 2014; Hills, 2017; Hills & Watson, 2011; NLN, 2003).

This curriculum revolution had two interrelated and significant goals: (a) to gain freedom from nursing's ambivalent and tormented relationship with medicine by basing nursing education on Caring as the moral, theoretical, and philosophical foundation of nursing (Bevis & Watson, 1989; Hills & Watson, 2011; NLN, 1988, 2003); and (b) to transcend the Tylerian behavioral, educational, theoretical framework in which nursing had been entrenched for decades (Bevis & Watson, 1989; Hills & Watson, 2011; NLN, 1988, 2003).

Although many advances have been made in nursing education particularly as a result of this historic time in nursing education (Bevis & Watson, 1989; NLN, 1988, 2003), these two goals remain mostly unmet and continue to challenge nursing education programs throughout the world (Hills, 2017; Hills & Watson, 2011; NLN, 2003). And the question arises: If you are not going to use behavioral objectives and principles to organize, teach, and evaluate nursing student's learning and progress, what will you use?

To realize the first curriculum revolution goal, we have to explore and understand the differences and similarities between nursing's and medicine's domains of practice. Nursing has people and their experiences with health, health promotion, and healing at the center of its domain along with Caring as the focus of its practice (Cara, 2017; Cara et al., 2016; Hills, 2016; Hills & Watson, 2011; Watson, 2012; Watson & Smith, 2002). In contrast, medicine focuses on curing with a knowledge base of etiology, pathology, diagnosis, and/or treatment of diseases (Hills & Watson, 2011). Of course, there is an area of overlap between nursing and medicine but their respective domains of practice are unique and complementary (Hills & Watson, 2011). All too often, nurse educators teach from a medical science perspective rather than a nursing science one (Hills et al., 1994; Hills & Watson, 2011; Watson, 1999).

Nurse educators must be able to articulate nursing's domain of practice so that they can teach clearly from that perspective. Consequently, it is recommended that all Caring Science nursing education programs should be based on a clearly articulated, moral, theoretical, and philosophical underpinning that embraces a humanistic caring perspective (Bevis & Watson, 1989; Hills, 2017; Hills & Watson, 2011). For example, this means understanding people's (patients, families, and communities) perspectives and their experiences of health and healing, as well as the importance of relationships (Cara, 2017; Cara et al., 2016; Hills, 2017; Hills & Lindsey, 1994; Hills et al., 1994).

The second goal of the curriculum revolution (NLN, 1988) was to transcend the Tylerian behaviorist educational model in which nursing had been entrenched for over 40 years, now 70 years (NLN, 2003). Some progress has been made toward attaining this goal (Hills & Lindsey, 1994; Hills et al., 1994; Hills & Watson, 2011; Iwasiw, Goldenberg, & Andrusyszyn, 2008; NLN, 2003; Young, 2007). However, for many schools of nursing throughout the world, most curriculum planning, student learning, and evaluation continues to be based on behavioral objectives (Hills & Watson, 2011; NLN, 2003). Even if nursing schools are successful in using a Caring Science pedagogy, many continue to use behavioral objectives to standardize programs and evaluate students' performance and progress (Hill, 2017). On the basis of the works of Hills et al. (1994) as well as Hills (2017), the difficulty with this situation is that the behaviorist educational model assumes the following:

- Given the same or similar experiences, all students learn the same or similar things.

- Learning always manifests itself in behavioral changes.

- What the teacher identifies as desirable behaviors are the only ones worth evaluating and grading.

- Students will take on faith that the prescribed behaviors are the desirable ones and strive to attain them.

- Everything worth learning is in the curriculum and is reflected in the behavioral objectives.

To move toward a Caring Science educational model, nurse educators need to align themselves with the students and move from a place of control and domination to one of empowerment and emancipation (Hills & Watson, 2011). As Bevis (1989c) explained "[w]ithout emancipation, education is an oppressive tool ... an assembly-line industry producing nurse-workers who ... follow the status quo. They may make waves, but they stay within the rules while living lives ... circumscribed by the inflexibility of large medical empire-bureaucracies and bear the inevitable stamp of banality and mediocrity" (pp. 162–163). In other words, emancipatory education encourages learners to ask the unaskable, confront injustices and oppression, and be active agents in their lives and in their work.

There are many ways for nursing education to overcome its love affair with behaviorism; some of these strategies are described subsequently. The authors of this chapter like to conceptualize the current state of affairs in nursing education as a move from revolution to renaissance. The word "renaissance," taken from the French, means "rebirth", which means conceiving a rebirth of nursing's historical claim to caring for people and their health and healing experiences as its foremost contribution to healthcare in our current society.

Transcending both a medical science perspective and a behaviorist educational model matters because, until nurses are able to do so, nursing education cannot reach its full potential. To be an independent discipline, to meet its ethical commitment to society, nursing must be guided by its own theories and philosophies with caring as its moral compass (Boykin, Touhy, & Smith, 2011; Hills & Watson, 2011; Watson, 1999, 2008, 2017). To develop into such a discipline, nursing educators need to engage in "industrious [...] self-development efforts so that [*our societal*] trust will be steadfastly and excellently honored" (Bevis, 1989c, p. 153).

USING CARING SCIENCE LANGUAGE TO ARTICULATE NURSES' EDUCATION AND PRACTICE

Language is powerful; it reveals one's thinking, one's worldview, and one's awareness. Being inspired by Watson (1999), the authors believe that words carry energy and impact all interactions and transactions between and among teachers and students. As Zukav (1990) suggested, negative emotions such as anger or fear create a lower energy frequency compared to positive emotions such as kindness, compassion, or love. Turkel (2014) states, "When emotions are expressed through words, the negative energy drains our own system and negatively radiates to others while positive energy expressed through words is uplifting to our systems and radiates peaceful, calm, or soothing energy to others" (p. 176). In nursing education, the power of language is relevant as it relates to teaching and learning situations. When educators convey loving-kindness, they are working at a higher level of consciousness.

Similarly, the language nurse educators use to describe and articulate their understanding of what nursing is, reflects nurses' perspective, and reveals what they think is important. Consequently, being conscious of the words used to describe nursing's domain of practice becomes a critical aspect of nursing education. So, when using language that *emphasizes* the biomedical, physiological, technical, and skills aspects of nursing, there is the risk of making the compassionate, caring, relational, and spiritual aspects of the discipline of nursing less important and, often, invisible. If nurse educators continue to describe nursing using medical language of diseases, diagnoses, and treatments, nursing risks remaining trapped in the medical paradigm. On the contrary, when nurse educators use the language of health, healing, people's experiences, suffering, caring, being with, being present, or authentically listening, they are allowing the invisible work of nursing to emerge ontologically for nursing students.

TEACHING AND LEARNING IN CARING COLLABORATIVE RELATIONSHIP

Currently, many nursing programs refer to the concept of "student-centered learning" (Young & Paterson, 2007). Although this is an important concept, it falls short of describing the importance of the student–teacher relationship as a critical aspect in the learning process. As Cara and Girard (2013), Hills and Watson (2011), and Noddings (2012) claim, student–teacher relationships are ontologically fundamental to students' learning. Many nurse educators contend that learning occurs at the juncture where the teacher and student are in a caring relationship and are cocreating knowledge leading to new insights and deeper understandings that culminates in the transformation of consciousness (Hills, 2016; Hills & Watson, 2011). Furthermore, caring relationships allow teachers to affirm, encourage, follow up, and celebrate students' successes, thereby inviting personal growth of both students and teachers (Watson, 2008).

Consequently, it is not enough to simply focus on the student as in the "student-centered learning" perspective since in that situation, teachers can be student-centered but remain aloof. From a Caring Science perspective with its emancipatory pedagogy, "students and teachers must be partners in the learning process" (Hills & Watson, 2011, p. 74). They are critical agents in the act of knowing and both, the student and the teacher, are simultaneously teaching and learning (Hills & Watson, 2011). It is not possible to "be aloof" when fully engaged in a caring relationship, as commitment is to the student, not to the content per se. The teacher–student relationship is crucial in order for learning to occur (Cara & Girard, 2013; Hills & Watson, 2011; Noddings, 2012, 2013). As Freire (1972) contends, if teachers and students were to seize the power available to them in the classroom, they could remake society. Hence, an emancipatory pedagogy invites a discussion of power (Hills & Watson, 2011). Indeed, the concept of "being in relationship" is closely linked to the concept of "power" within the student–teacher relationship. "Power dynamics exist in all teaching/ learning situations" yet they are seldom acknowledged (Hills & Watson, 2011, p. 76).

There are many ways that power is expressed in teaching/learning situations (the way the classroom is organized; where the teacher stands; who gets to speak and when, etc.) and many are routinely "power over" situations. For example, the mere fact that nurse educators evaluate students' progress places them in a "power over" situation with their students (Hills & Watson, 2011).

But aspects of "power over" can be negotiated, and there is always a choice about how teachers use their power. The question to be considered is: Do teachers want to have "power over" their students or "power with" their students (Hills & Watson, 2011; Labonté, 1990)? Watson (2008) states that her "*Caritas Process* of teaching-learning is more relational, trusting, exploratory, engaging … It involves power and control with, not over, the learner" (p. 126). To be informed by a Caring Science perspective, nurse educators must choose "power with" strategies to create the emancipation necessary to cultivate a graduate who will be an independent, self-reliant, and confident nurse who also demonstrates critical thinking and lifelong learning.

CREATING CARING SCIENCE CURRICULUM DESIGN AND STRUCTURE

As mentioned earlier, when most nurse educators hear the words "curriculum development," their initial thoughts are about the design and structure of a program (Bevis, 1989b). Hills and Watson (2011) suggest that nurse educators typically consider the "program of studies" and the sequencing and "leveling of courses" that make up the program as curriculum design and structure. Because, even if nurse educators redefine curriculum to focus on pedagogical practices, they still need to consider how to organize the content to be taught. And the same question explored throughout this chapter remains: *If you don't use a behavioral education model, what will you use to organize content?*

There are numerous ways to use transformational Caring Science frameworks to organize content and learning experiences over the duration of the nursing program—a critical aspect of nursing education. According to Hills and Watson (2011), "Caring Science provides this deep underpinning for a scientific-philosophical-moral context from which to explore, describe, and research human caring–healing phenomena as integral to our humanity. As the disciplinary foundation for nursing, Caring Science clarifies for the profession, and the professional, the question of ontology . . ." (p. 12). Therefore, having a Caring Science lens, acknowledges students' control over their apprenticeship and joint involvement in the learning process, "[S]tudents also have authority in their own knowing and experiences that can be shared and jointly critiqued for deeper knowledge, understanding, integrative insights and wisdom, ultimately, resulting in transformation of consciousness" (Hills & Watson, 2011, p. 17).

Two exemplars are provided to guide nurse educators' thinking about how to create a Caring Science curriculum design and structure within the context of different schools' circumstances.

In the first exemplar from the Collaborative Nursing Program of British Columbia, Hills, along with her colleagues (1994), used focus groups to ascertain stakeholders' (nurse educators, administrators, former students, practicing nurses, nurses' union, Provincial College of Nursing leaders, et al.) perceptions of nursing in the future. The following questions were asked: What will nurses need to *know* to practice nursing in the 21st century? What will nurses need to be able to *do* to practice nursing in the 21st century? and How will nurses need to *be* to practice nursing in the 21st century? (Hills et al., 1994). They also conducted a Delphi study with stakeholders throughout that province (Beddome et al., 1995). A thematic analysis was conducted that resulted in all nursing content being organized under the following four content themes: people's experiences of health, people's experiences of healing, people's experiences of self and others, and finally, people's experiences of professional growth. In addition, two meta-themes were integrated throughout the curriculum, which were an ethic of caring and health promotion. Also, four critical constructs, (a) ways of knowing, (b) personal meaning, (c) time/transitions, and (d) context, were woven into every course throughout the program (Hills et al., 1994).

Moreover, for each of the semesters, the themes were used to develop courses, and the level of complexity was increased sequentially across all semesters (Hills et al., 1994). This allowed students to learn gradually and progressively throughout their program. For example, in the first semester, year 1, the content focused on health as a resource for everyday living while the students also learned how to be "in relationship" with others. In the second semester of year 1, the content focused on chronic health challenges while the students learned how to have people tell their stories about that experience. In the first semester of the second year, the course content focused on episodic health challenges of the students' learning about caring relationships with patients experiencing acute health conditions. And in the next semester, the content focused on complex episodic health challenges while students learned to engage in a caring relationship with their patients. In a similar fashion, the entire curriculum was developed integrating people's experiences while being in caring relationships. In all semesters, students had to complete a 78-hour practicum, in addition to a consolidated clinical experience. The entire curriculum was informed by the concept of praxis (Freire, 1972; Grundy, 1987). Praxis is the dialectical movement of theory and practice (Freire, 1972). It is like a dance with theory and practice both informing each other: a reflexive relationship in which both action and reflection build on one another. As Freire (1972) states: "The act of knowing involves a dialectical movement which goes from action to reflection and from reflection to new action" (p. 31).

In the second exemplar, the Université de Montréal grounded its work on the competency approach (Tardif, 2006), the cognitive learning model, including research results obtained within the school (Boyer, 2013; Goudreau, Boyer, & Létourneau, 2014; Pepin, Dubois, Girard, Tardif, & Ha, 2011), as well as the Humanistic model of care (Cara & Girard, 2013; Cara et al., 2015; Cara et al., 2016) developed within the faculty, related to Caring Science. The vice dean of the baccalaureate program was acting as the leader for this project (Faculté des sciences infirmières, 2015). Initially, eight working groups, composed mostly of faculty members, clarified each competence, its definition, its elements, and its indicators. For example, the first competence was to "Act with humanism according to a disciplinary perspective" (Faculté des sciences infirmières, 2015, p. 7). After that initial work, additional focus groups were held over a period of 2 years. These focus groups included 30 individuals (nurse educators, nurse lecturers, clinical supervisors, doctoral students, directors of nursing, and practicing clinical nurse specialists, et al.) who met to validate the work that was originally done. This process aimed to ensure the congruence among the eight competencies in regards to their descriptions as well as their indicators, while being synchronized with the Humanistic model of care (Faculté des sciences infirmières, 2015). Also, the focus groups worked to confirm that there was an increase in complexity over the 3-year program (Faculté des sciences infirmières, 2015). Baccalaureate students, at the end of the first year, were sensitive to the caring values, attitudes, and behaviors involved in the nurse–patient relationship. Students were also interested in understanding the patient's situation and concerns (Faculté des sciences infirmières, 2015). At the end of the second year, students were able to recognize the importance of caring values in their relationships with patients and families. Students also sought strategies to humanize practices and promote health (Faculté des sciences infirmières, 2015). At the end of the third year, students engaged in a caring relationship to accompany patients in their health experiences. From a disciplinary perspective, students pursued various solutions to promote patients' health, to support their power to act, and to humanize practices (Faculté des sciences infirmières, 2015).

These exemplars are not the only ways to create a coherent Caring Science curriculum framework, but are provided as guidance and suggestions about ways to begin this process. There are many possibilities, and the authors of this chapter invite readers to be creative!

Evaluating Students' Clinical Practice Based on Caring Science Rather Than Behavioral Objectives

One can create an exquisite Caring Science curriculum and use innovative emancipatory pedagogical practices and then undermine all the advances by making inappropriate choices about methods of evaluating students' practice and progress. If the evaluation methods used do not embrace and are not congruent with Caring Science, the previous work will be eroded.

Typically, setting behavioral objectives and testing for their achievement remain the single most popular method for evaluating students' performance and progress particularly in relation to clinical experiences (Hills & Watson, 2011). Evaluation sends a powerful message about what is really important and valued in nursing education (Benner, Sutphen, Leonard, & Day, 2010; Hills & Watson, 2011). For students to be successful in a Caring Science curriculum, Hills and Watson recommend that nurse educators create evaluation strategies that do not reduce evaluation of nursing students' practice to merely a measurement of observable behaviors. So many aspects of nursing practice—compassion, empathy, thoughtfulness, consideration, perceptual awareness, discretionary decision making, touch, listening for understanding, warmth, respect, authenticity, and others—are not easily measured. Nevertheless, they are critical aspects of caring for people and they are essential to Caring Science curriculum and pedagogy.

The following is an alternative approach to evaluating student's clinical experiences that is consistent with Caring Science. Again, this is presented as an exemplar, not as "the answer." It is intended to guide the development of Caring Science evaluation strategies that will work in a particular nursing school's context.

This exemplar also comes from the Collaborative Nursing Program of British Columbia (Hills et al., 1994). When nurse educators were developing this program, they were aware of their need to choose and use appropriate evaluation methods. They learned of colleagues in Britain who were using Benner's (1984) work to evaluate students' clinical practice that set them on a path of exploring this theorist's seven domains of practice. Benner's work was inspirational because it was based on research and nurses' experiences in clinical practice that uncovered much of nursing's work that was otherwise invisible. The educators "adapted" Benner's (1984) work to suit their context and created five domains of practice: the "Health/healing Domain," the "Teaching/learning Domain," the "Clinical Judgment Domain," the "Professional Responsibility Domain," and the "Collaborative Leadership Domain" (Hills, 1992, 2016; Hills & Watson, 2011). These domains of practice remain constant throughout the nursing program with competencies that were developed for each domain to "level" expectations of students' performance across the program. Each domain has quality indicators for each semester, which also "levels" students' expectations of progress during clinical experiences. Students recorded stories in their journals and used the quality indicators as criteria to analyze their clinical experiences that provided evidence for the teacher of how the students were meeting the competencies within a semester (Hills, 1992, 2001, 2016; Hills & Watson, 2011).

CONCLUSION

This chapter explored significant curriculum processes and pedagogical practices that uphold Caring Science literacy in nursing education. The authors highlighted that *how* the nurse educators teach is as important as the content they provide. They also specified that the students-educator caring relationship is essential to the students' apprenticeship of nursing. Moreover, they emphasized how this orientation can be understood at the deepest philosophical level; shifting everything in nursing education and offering guidance at the most basic level to redesign nursing education programs. In addition, this chapter demonstrated curriculum as being entirely and fundamentally about teachers' relationships with their students, focusing on the meaning of being/becoming a caring teacher.

NEXT ERA POSSIBILITIES

Education
- What is the underpinning of the nurse educator's teaching practice? Is it based on Caring Science or on a biomedical model?
- What is the meaning of being a caring teacher?
- How can "being a caring teacher" support, facilitate, and empower students' learning toward becoming professional nurses?
- How does being in a relationship with students influence their learning? What does the nurse educator learn from those experiences?
- How does the nurse educator's relationship with students nurture and foster them to become caring nurses?

Research
- Using phenomenology as a research methodology, how can nurse educators describe and understand the meaning of being a caring teacher with undergraduate students?
- Using Collaborative Action Research and Evaluation (CARE) methodology, how can nurse educators change pedagogical practices to be more caring on the basis of evidence from their daily practice?
- Using phenomenology as a research methodology, how can nurse educators describe and understand the meaning, from graduate students' perspectives, of being in a caring relationship with their teacher and how it contributes to their thesis realization?

Praxis
- What strategies can nurse educators use to teach from a Caring Science perspective— to be inspiring to students?
- How will being informed by Caring Science literacy change nurse educators' teaching practice?
- How can nurse educators use a Caring Science–based approach in various educational settings (both course work and clinical) to facilitate students' learning?

- In what ways does a caring teacher contribute to the transformation of students' consciousness to include caring as their moral imperative in nursing?
- How can a caring ontology inform the evaluation process to have power with students?

Theory and Knowledge Development

- What nursing education theory would be needed to integrate Caring Science literacies?
- How can a Caring nursing education theory assist nurse educators to develop caring relationships with students and promote their apprenticeship of caring?

 REFERENCES

Beddome, G., Budgen, C., Hills, M. D., Lindsey, A. E., Duval, P. M., & Szalay, L. (1995). Nursing Faculty, Okanagan University College, Kelowna, BC, Canada. *Journal of Nursing Education*, *34*(1), 11–15.

Benner, P. (1984). *From novice to expert: Excellence and power in clinical nursing practice*. Menlo Park, CA: Addison-Wesley.

Benner, P., Sutphen, M., Leonard, V., & Day, L. (2010). *Educating nurses: A call for radical transformation*. Stanford, CA: Jossey-Bass.

Bevis, E. O. (1989a). Illuminating the issues: Probing the past, a history of nursing curriculum development: The past shapes the present. In E. O. Bevis & J. Watson (Eds.), *Toward a caring curriculum. A new pedagogy for nursing* (pp. 13–35). New York, NY: National League for Nursing.

Bevis, E. O. (1989b). Nursing curriculum as professional education: Some underlying theoretical models. In E. O. Bevis & J. Watson (Eds.), *Toward a caring curriculum. A new pedagogy for nursing* (pp. 67–106). New York, NY: National League for Nursing.

Bevis, E. O. (1989c). Teaching and Learning: The key to education and professionalism. In E. O. Bevis & J. Watson (Eds.), *Toward a caring curriculum. A new pedagogy for nursing* (pp. 153–188). New York, NY: National League for Nursing.

Bevis, E. O., & Watson, J. (1989). *Toward a caring curriculum. A new pedagogy for nursing*. New York, NY: National League for Nursing.

Boyer, L. (2013). *Coconstruction d'un modèle cognitif de l'apprentissage d'une compétence en vue d'assurer la validité et l'équité de son évaluation : le cas de la compétence « Exercer un jugement clinique infirmier »* (Thèse de doctorat) [Co-constructing a cognitive model of learning a competency to ensure the validity and fairness of its evaluation: The case of the competence "To exercise a clinical judgment" (Doctoral dissertation)], Université de Montréal, QC, Canada. Retrieved from ProQuest Dissertations & Theses. (UMI No. NR94425)

Boykin, A., Touhy, T., & Smith, M. (2011). Evolution of a Caring-based college of nursing. In M. Hills & J. Watson (Eds.), *Creating a caring science curriculum: An emancipatory pedagogy for nursing* (pp. 157–184). New York, NY: Springer Publishing.

Cara, C. (2017, June). *Rediscovering love, compassion, and caring to alleviate dehumanization*. Keynote at the 38th annual conference of the International Association for Human Caring, Rediscovering Love and Compassion: In Caring Practice and in Caring Science, Edmonton, AB, Canada.

Cara, C., Gauvin-Lepage, J., Lefebvre, H., Létourneau, D., Alderson, M., Larue, C., ... Mathieu, C. (2016, June). Le Modèle humaniste des soins infirmiers – UdeM: Perspective novatrice et pragmatique [The Humanist Model of Nursing—UofM: Innovative and pragmatic perspective]. *Recherche en soins infirmiers*, *125*, 20–31. doi:10.3917/rsi.125.0020

Cara, C., & Girard, F. (2013, May). *The humanist model of nursing care: A driving force for nursing education*. Poster session presented at the 34th International Association for Human Caring Conference. Lake Buena Vista, FL.

Cara, C., Roy, M., Thibault, L., Alderson, M., Beauchamp, J., Casimir, M., … Robinette, L. (2015). *Modèle humaniste des Soins Infirmiers - UdeM: Synopsis du Modèle pour son opérationnalisation* [Humanistic Model of Nursing - UofM: Synopsis of the Model for its operationalization]. Montréal, QC, Canada: Faculté des sciences infirmières de l'Université de Montréal.

Combs, A. W. (1982). *Personal approach to teaching: Beliefs that make a difference.* Boston, MA: Allyn & Bacon.

Dewey, J. (1933). *How we think* (Rev. ed.). Boston, MA: D. C. Health.

Faculté des Sciences Infirmières de l'Université de Montréal. (2015). *Référentiel de compétences: Baccalauréat en sciences infirmières* [Repository of competencies: Bachelor of Nursing Science] (2nd. éd.). Montréal, QC, Canada: Université de Montréal.

France, N., & Ray, M. (2014). *Studying caring science in nursing: The foundation of the discipline and profession of nursing at Florida Atlantic University, USA.* Boca Raton: The Christine E. Lynn College of Nursing Florida Atlantic University.

Freire, P. (1972). *Pedagogy of the oppressed.* London, UK: Penguin Books.

Gagné, R. M. (1970). *The conditions of learning* (2nd ed.). New York, NY: Holt, Rinehart & Winston.

Goudreau, J., Boyer, L., & Létourneau, D. (2014). Clinical reasoning in nursing practice: A cognitive learning model based on a think aloud methodology. *Quality Advancement in Nursing Education – Avancées en formation infirmière, 1*(1), 1–20. Retrieved from http://qane-afi.casn.ca/journal/vol1/iss1/4

Grundy, S. (1987). *Curriculum: Product or praxis.* Lewes, UK: Falmer Press.

Hills, M. D. (1992). *Collaborative nursing program of BC. Development of a generic integrated nursing curriculum with four partner colleges.* Report to Ministry of Advanced education. Centre for Curriculum and Professional Development.

Hills, M. D. (2001). Using cooperative inquiry to transform evaluation of nursing student's clinical practice. In P. Reason & H. Bradbury (Eds.), *Handbook of action research, participatory inquiry and practice* (pp. 340–347). London, UK: Sage.

Hills, M. D. (2016). Emancipation and collaboration: Leading from beside. In W. Rosa (Ed.), *Nurses as leaders: Evolutionary visions of leadership* (pp. 293–309). New York, NY: Springer Publishing.

Hills, M. D. (2017, November). *Creating a Caring Science curriculum: Transcending the bio-medical & behaviorist paradigms.* Unpublished Keynote address. Global Human Caring Congress, Santiago, Chile.

Hills, M. D., & Lindsey, A. E. (1994). Health promotion: A viable curriculum framework for nursing education. *Nursing Outlook, 42*(4), 158–162. doi:10.1016/0029-6554(94)90003-5

Hills, M. D., Lindsey, A. E., Chisamore, M., Bassett-Smith, J., Abbott, K., & Fournier-Chalmers, J. (1994). University-college collaboration: Rethinking curriculum development in nursing education. *Journal of Nursing Education, 33*(5), 220–225.

Hills, M. D., & Watson, J. (2011). *Creating a caring science curriculum: An emancipatory pedagogy for nursing.* New York, NY: Springer Publishing.

Iwasiw, C. L., Goldenberg, D., & Andrusyszyn, M.-A. (2008). *Curriculum development in nursing education.* Boston, MA: Jones & Bartlett.

Labonté, R. (1990). *Empowerment practices for health professionals.* Toronto, ON, Canada: ParticipACTION.

National League for Nursing. (1988). *Curriculum revolution: Mandate for change.* New York, NY: National League for Nursing.

National League for Nursing. (2003). *Position statement. Innovation in nursing education: A call to reform.* Retrieved from http://www.nln.org/docs/default-source/about/archived-position-statements/innovation-in-nursing-education-a-call-to-reform-pdf.pdf?sfvrsn=4

Nightingale, F. (1969). *Notes on nursing: What it is and what it is not.* New York, NY: Dover. (Original work published 1860)

Noddings, N. (2012). The caring relation in teaching. *Oxford Review of Education, 38*(6), 771–781. doi:10.1080/03054985.2012.745047

Noddings, N. (2013). *Caring: A relational approach to ethics and moral education.* Berkeley: University of California Press.

Pepin, J., Dubois, S., Girard, F., Tardif, J., & Ha, L. (2011). A cognitive learning model of clinical nursing leadership. *Nurse Education Today, 31*, 268–273. doi:10.1016/j.nedt.2010.11.009

Rogers, C. R. (1969). *Freedom to Learn*. Columbus, OH: Charles E. Merrill.

Tardif, J. (2006). *L'évaluation des compétences: Documenter le parcours de développement*. Montréal, QC, Canada: Chenelière Éducation.

Turkel, M. C. (2014). Leading from the heart: Caring, love, peace, and values guiding leadership. *Nursing Science Quarterly, 27*(2), 172–177. doi:10.1177/0894318414522663

Tyler, R. W. (1949). *Basic principles of curriculum and instruction*. Chicago, IL: University of Chicago.

Watson, J. (1999). *Postmodern nursing and beyond*. Toronto, ON, Canada: Churchill Livingstone.

Watson, J. (2008). *Nursing. The philosophy and science of caring* (Rev. ed.). Boulder: University Press of Colorado.

Watson, J. (2012). *Human caring science: A theory of nursing* (2nd ed.). Sudbury, MA: Jones & Bartlett.

Watson, J. (2017). Global advances in human caring literacy. In S. Lee, P. Palmieri, & J. Watson (Eds.), *Global advances in human caring literacy* (pp. 3–11). New York, NY: Springer Publishing.

Watson, J., & Smith, M. C. (2002). Caring science and the science of unitary human beings: A transtheoretical discourse for nursing knowledge development. *Journal of Advanced Nursing, 37*(5), 452–461. doi:10.1046/j.1365-2648.2002.02112.x

Young, L. E. (2007). Story-based learning: Blending content and process to learn nursing. In L. E. Young & B. L. Paterson (Eds.), *Teaching nursing: Developing a student centered learning environment* (pp. 164–188). Philadelphia, PA: Lippincott Williams & Wilkins.

Young, L. E., & Paterson, B. L. (Eds.). (2007). *Teaching nursing: Developing a student-centered learning environment*. Philadelphia, PA: Lippincott Williams & Wilkins.

Zukav, G. (1990). *The seat of the soul*. New York, NY: Fireside, Simon & Schuster.

15

Loving-Kindness and Equanimity: Illuminating the Nursing Literature Through a Caring Lens

Zane Robinson Wolf and Marian C. Turkel

CARITAS LITERACIES

By the end of this chapter, the caring-healing nurse will be able to

1. Describe the foundations of loving-kindness and equanimity in humanistic altruistic values as noted in nursing literature.

2. Reflect on the meaning of the Caritas Process® of Cultivating the Practice of Loving-Kindness and Equanimity Toward Self and Other.

3. Compare exemplars of loving-kindness and equanimity practices across nursing, patient, and organizational systems.

This chapter examines the roots and major influences of the first of Watson's Caritas Processes (Watson, 2008), Caritas Process 1—*Cultivating the practice of loving-kindness and equanimity within the context of caring consciousness,* and follows with examples of its dissemination in the literature of nursing. Examples serve as Caring Science evidence for the diffusion of loving-kindness and equanimity into nursing practice. Watson (2005) states, "It is when we include caring and love in our science we discover our caring healing professions and disciplines are much more than a detached scientific endeavor, but a life-giving and life-receiving endeavor for humanity" (p. 3). The following databases were searched to locate exemplars: Cumulative Index to Nursing and Allied Health Literature (CINAHL), Essential Nursing, PubMed, Proquest Dissertations and Theses, and Summon. The search terms, "loving-kindness," "humanistic altruistic values," "staff nurse," and "nursing" were used alone or in combination. Only English-language articles were accessed and reviewed. The personal collections of the authors were also reviewed.

The first Caritas Process has permeated professional nursing practice, chiefly because of the influences of Jean Watson's numerous publications, Watson's Caring Science Institute, the Caritas Coach Education Program®, Magnet®-certification initiatives, and professional meetings, during which this and other Caritas Processes (Watson, 2008) have been examined and related activities implemented in healthcare institutions. No doubt Watson's (2008) conceptualizations of the first Caritas Process and the altruistic-humanistic values orienting it matched implicit and explicit norms, beliefs, and practices of nursing. However, naming and describing it has shed light on an essential nursing activity.

Loving relationships have the potential of transforming healthcare (Jackson, 2010), according to scholars, and have been incorporated into clinicians' daily practice. Nurses and other providers have been internalizing and cultivating the practice of loving-kindness and equanimity by reflection, journaling, and other methods. In addition, the practice of mindfulness meditation to achieve loving-kindness, literature and workshops of many professions on loving-kindness (Boellinghaus, Jones, & Hutton, 2014; Moody et al., 2013), and operationalized clinical actions have helped to influence caring outcomes. The achievement of positive patient outcomes has been attributed specifically to changes in nursing staff's caring practices.

Researchers have asserted that nurse–patient relationships, shaped by caring interactions, affect patient health and healing (Brewer & Watson, 2015; Persky, Nelson, Watson, & Bent, 2008). The nurse–patient relationship, the center of the nursing universe, incorporates the lived dialogue of the nursing act and is demonstrated when the needs of the patient are paramount (McCamant, 2006). In this unique space, the activities of loving-kindness are carried out.

An early assumption by Watson (1988) related to human caring was "Caring and Love are the most universal, the most tremendous and the most mysterious of cosmic forces; they comprise the primal and universal psychic energy" (Watson, 1988, p. 32). Watson (2003) suggested that individuals benefit from a shared humanity, and that nursing work as a calling is motivated by love. She claimed that love is within us and, if latent, needs to be uncovered. A framework of caring and love helps us to heal by "returning to our own inner light and inner self-love" (Watson, 2003, p. 199) and by making love available to self and patients. Love benefits nurses and those cared for. Both are helped to heal. As nurses and patients interact in the "magnetic field" (Watson, 2003, p. 200) of a caring moment, the power, beauty, and energy of love radiates and connects to the universe. Given such propositions, it is not surprising that the transformation of the Carative Factors to Caritas Processes (Watson, 2008) showed loving-kindness and equanimity to be the first.

LOVING-KINDNESS AND EQUANIMITY FOR SELF AND OTHERS: ROOTS

Altruism. An altruistic-humanistic system of values, at the root of the healthcare profession, is espoused by many cultural groups and members of these professions (Lee & Wang, 2014; Sasser & Puchalski, 2010). Altruism, an other-directed value, is witnessed in clinical actions according to Burks and Kobus (2012). These authors proposed that one assumption of the helping professions is that the norms of altruistic and humanistic actions on behalf of others are promoted during the socialization of novice healthcare professionals. Another widespread assumption is that both altruistic persons and those cared for benefit from caring for others. Burks and Kobus also suggested that although members of the helping professions struggle to keep engagement and objectivity in balance as they care for people, altruism prevails. Even so, healthcare providers' prosocial, altruistic behavior is often taken for granted by them.

Burks and Kobus (2012) observed that the literature of the helping professions shows that when healthcare professionals are mindful of their thoughts and emotions, benefits result. Proponents of mindfulness have espoused practicing self-reflection, cultivating empathy, and modeling the behaviors of empathetic providers. Burks and Kobus also acknowledged the need to include mindfulness training in the regular curriculums of the health professions, at the same time emphasizing the need for mindfulness practice. Caring acts, oriented in altruism and humanism and carried out mindfully, result in personal gains for healthcare providers and benefit those being cared for.

Watson (1979, 1985) described Carative Factors when explaining her theory of caring; the first factor was the formation of a humanistic-altruistic values system and was presented as foundational to nurse caring. She noted that caring was based on kindness, concern, and love of self and others (Watson, 1979). According to Watson (1985), "Altruistic values and behavior bring meaning to one's life through relationships with other people" (p.11). She noted that the satisfaction humans experience through giving and values-oriented behaviors might be developed through "consciousness raising and careful examination of views, beliefs, and values" (Watson, 1985, p. 11). Her propositions correspond to other nurse theorists, such as Paterson and Zderad (1976) and McCamant (2006).

Mindfulness: Understanding the first Caritas Process of *cultivating the practice of loving-kindness and equanimity within the context of caring consciousness* (Watson, 2008) requires touching base with Buddhist principles and guidelines. Buddhist traditions have emphasized the importance of cultivating connection and love toward others. Compassion is emphasized. Initially, comprehending and applying the Buddhist principles of interbeing helps individuals to be in touch with, continue, realize, and make it in the *here and now* (Hanh, 1993). Being present and mindful are paramount for self-awareness and offer knowledge of the beauty and suffering in the world. Framed by Hanh's (1993) Order of Interbeing, ethical values, conscientiousness, and compassionate living result from being present and mindful.

According to Hanh (1993), understanding and compassion follow when humans are aware of the processes of inner life. First, by rediscovering our true minds and by being aware of inner life processes, individuals get in touch with the reality of the world. Their appreciation of the world is followed by understanding and recognition of suffering, joy, and the world's beauty. Next, as getting in touch with our inner lives is practiced, enlightenment continues. As individuals are transformed by getting in touch with the sources of understanding and compassion, through the inner self and the world, joy, happiness, calmness, and serenity can be shared with others.

Hanh (1993) shared that connection with the present moment needs to be practiced and helps individuals make it in the here and now. Enlightened individuals are mindful of all activities and practice and engage in them mindfully and peacefully. Although nurses and other healthcare providers may not practice the life of interbeing as Buddhists, they might have or already have found the value of mindfulness and a present orientation as important contributors to peace and joy in their personal and professional lives as they care for people who suffer and are joyful.

Love: Loving-kindness and equanimity are oriented in Buddhist sublime states of mind (Jormsri, Kunaviktikul, Ketefian, & Chaowalit, 2005, p. 585). They help nurses get in touch with self and realize peace and joy found through the intimate interconnections between ourselves and those for whom we care as we interact with them (Hanh, 1993). By *cultivating the practice of loving-kindness and equanimity within the context of caring consciousness* (Watson, 2010), nurses and other providers could realize peace and joy daily in professional and personal areas of life. Hanh (2011) proclaimed that understanding another is the essence of LOVE. He further defined the four key aspects of love grounded in the Buddhist tradition as *maitri* or loving-kindness, *karuna* or compassion, *mudita* or joy, and *upeksha as* equanimity or freedom. Essential to being able to express love to self and others is bringing a person's true presence when entering into the relationship with the other. True presence is enhanced by mindfulness, mindful breathing, reciting mantras, and meditation.

According to Hawkins (2013), love is uplifting, holistic, and gracious; he defines "love" as "a way of being" and "a way in which individuals light up the world" (p. 172). Love is an energetic force radiating from the heart and has the potential to facilitate healing (Hawkins). His perspective is congruent with the energy system of the body or the Chakra system; as a person's consciousness toward love as energy rises, the energy moves up to the heart chakra. The heart chakra is the center for love and compassion (Myss, 1996). The heart chakra is closely aligned with the first Caritas Process, *Cultivating the practice of loving-kindness and equanimity within the context of caring consciousness.* A nurse practicing from heart-centered consciousness contributes to the energetic field of love, caring, and healing.

Chapman (2009), as a hospital administrator, implemented the idea of radical loving care, expressed as a continuous chain of loving care and a means of creating the healing hospital. The focus in such hospitals is healing of patients, not curing. In a radical, loving care institution, all employees in all roles are caregivers who provide loving service; when called and needed, they step out of their role functions to care for patients. According to Chapman, it is through the inverted invitation that hospital staff are guests of patients requiring care. To accomplish the change from curing to caring, the culture of the hospital needs to change. Chapman shared the process of culture change. He emphasized important symbols. For example, as symbolized by faith in God, represented as the *Golden Thread*, organizations that commit to radical loving care live the meaning of the symbol. Two additional symbols denote healing: a pair of *Intersecting Circles* that signify the merging of love, need, and hope during Sacred Encounters, and the *Red Heart*, indicating the nature of the Servant's Heart. Chapman's approach converges with Watson's (2010) caring moment. During a caring moment, the nurse practices loving-kindness and creates sacred space when caring for a patient while being authentically present with him or her.

Intentionality: The words "intention" and "intentionality" are often used interchangeably within the caring nursing literature. Dossey (2016) defined "intention" as "being in the present moment with a conscious heart" (p. 24). Next, Mariano (2016) saw intention as the conscious awareness of being in the present moment to help facilitate the healing process and a volitional act of love; conscious alignment of essence and purpose allowing the highest good to flow through a healing intervention. Shields and Wilson

(2016) considered intention as "choosing to act, think, or be in a certain way" (p. 188). Within the context of Caritas Processes, Watson (2008) expanded on such perspectives to include centering on the person in the moment, holding loving consciousness, approaching others with authentic presence, and being open to creative emergence and infinite possibilities.

Creating an intention to be present with another helps the nurse to be the caring-healing environment. Quinn's (1992) evolving view of the nurse as the environment and the patient–nurse field as one entity was grounded in the concept of universal love. Quinn reflected, "How can my heart-centered presence and the loving/caring consciousness help to align in this moment with energy/infinity of spirit/Universal Love?" (Quinn, as cited in Watson, 2005, p. 94). Smith (1999) expanded on this question by acknowledging the transformative potential of caring for self and other; "Caring is a way of inviting creative emergence by practitioner holding sacred/holy space through intentional use of heart energetics, consciousness of caring and love" (Smith, as cited in Watson, 2005, p. 94).

Intentionality is viewed by Dossey (2016) as "holding the heart-space with compassion in our knowing, being and doing while performing an action" (p. 24). According to Watson (2005), intentionality is not the same as intentions or having good intentions. She defined the construct of intentionality as "a more technical, philosophical meaning referring to a consciousness and awareness that are directed toward a mental object, with purpose and efficacy toward action, expectation, belief, volition and even the unconscious" (p. 191). Watson (2008) referred to intentionality as "a deep focus on a specific mental object of attention and awareness" (p. 94).

These perspectives on intentionality suggest that a personal commitment is needed for individuals to focus on the many opportunities to practice loving-kindness and equanimity daily. The cultivation of the practice of loving-kindness and equanimity requires healthcare providers to consider the opportunity and then to act purposefully with kindness and calmness in the moment, directed to self and others. Being open to the potential of a caring moment and intentional in bringing loving-kindness into that nurse–patient field provides nurses and patients situations in which transformation develops.

Loving-Kindness and Equanimity for Self

The need to achieve loving-kindness and equanimity for self, within the context of caring consciousness, is seen in nurses' daily encounters during patient care. Both nurse and patient are vulnerable as both face unknowns. For example, compassion fatigue has been attributed to the many stressful situations in which nurse's care for patients and families witnesses to their suffering (Lachman, 2016). Lachman advocated prevention and management of compassion fatigue and described studies in which low compassion satisfaction was related to high secondary traumatic stress scores. Lachman also highlighted the American Nurses Association (ANA) *Code of Ethics and Interpretative Statements* (ANA, 2015), noting that nurses owe the same duties to self as to others, including promoting health and safety, preserving wholeness of character and integrity, and maintaining competence and continued personal and professional growth. Although loving-kindness was mentioned as an uplifting, required attribute, Lachman did not suggest it as an approach to prevent nurse nonattachment. Equanimity was also advocated as a strategy to eliminate negative attitudes. Lachman identified mindfulness training as a strategy for nurses to prevent compassion fatigue, along with complementary therapies.

The potential for nurse leaders to practice loving-kindness activities for self was explored. Pipe (2008) emphasized the inner journey of nursing leaders as they applied Watson's theory of human caring to inform their own leadership approaches and ultimately to support the nursing workforce. By focusing on loving-kindness and equanimity in the context of caring consciousness, leaders might cultivate loving-kindness and compassion for self. Pipe proposed that practicing loving-kindness could take place during daily work-related opportunities; leaders could be conscious of caring while carrying out common functions, such as delivering presentations and answering the phone. Developing a trusting relationship with the self, Pipe suggested, fosters personal growth and development, so that nurse leaders increase stamina, ultimately applied to interactions at work so that nursing staff and others benefit.

Similarly, the need for nursing leaders to go on an inner journey of self-understanding was explored by Brown, Bishop, and Bar (2013). They emphasized that a healing environment could be created so that work days are balanced and time for quiet reflection is set aside. By listening to self and seeing what is needed to care for self, leaders develop awareness of the need to change to heal; this can be accomplished while recognizing personal and professional demands. Strategies such as yoga poses and walking were suggested in the context of mindful living. Brown et al. suggested that leaders need to envision their best self by acknowledging already internalized altruistic values and practicing loving-kindness with self and others. Consistent with the first Caritas Process, the author's emphasized self-forgiveness, self-compassion, giving thanks, and self-acceptance with resultant improved personal and professional effects. By continuing the journey of self-care, nursing leaders practice self-assessment to set self-care goals. To continue the inner journey, they seek spiritual advisers, time away from work, or other ways of achieving sustained changes that result in due course in continued self-care and support of others.

Following a literature review, a nursing task force in a hospital identified best practices for nurse preceptors so that new hires benefitted from their mentoring (Small & Good, 2013). Through consensus, the group decided that their preceptor program needed to promote care for self and peers among preceptors, so that a healing, trusting environment for staff was created. They supported preceptors, intending that caring could be practiced by preceptors and new hires during preceptorships in the hope that it was "hard-wired" into practice. The gap analysis helped the task force members frame the preceptor program in caring for self and in demonstrating loving-kindness to others. Meditation and centering practices were emphasized to facilitate stress reduction among new nurses. Other Caritas principles were incorporated into topics for the preceptor program. Preceptors and the chief nursing officer viewed the program positively. Ultimately, new hires might benefit during clinical days from interactions with their preceptors so that positive, caring relationships develop. In the two examples cited, the assumption is that seasoned nurse leaders and preceptors who incorporate loving-kindness strategies for self will have the effect of generating loving-kindness among others.

Next, Marks (2013) conducted a qualitative study to understand nurses' ($N = 8$) emancipatory experience, comportment, and self-agency as they participated in theory-guided practice in a Magnet-designated healthcare system. Narrative data were analyzed using critical narrative inquiry. Written and audio data from in-person interviews were analyzed. Nurses used Human Caring (Caritas Processes [Watson, 2008]) and *Integral Nursing* (multiparadigmatic framework in context of healthcare reform based on values and nurse advocacy [Marks, 2013]) concepts to inform practice. Nurses practiced self-care as shown in their stories. They exhibited loving-kindness as they created caring-healing environments by honoring patients' and families' wishes.

Turkel and Ray (2004) referred to the soul of nursing as seeking the good of self and others through compassionate caring. They noted that self-care and self-renewal are essential for caring and healing. A nurse sees personal and professional frameworks as holistic and engaging in self-care creates harmony with others though authentic presence in the caring moment. The authors discussed the value and importance of self-renewal through caring for self, which aligns with Watson's (2008) Caritas Process, *cultivating the practice of loving-kindness and equanimity toward self and other.* The authors offered exemplars for creating caring-healing environments. Examples included starting the work day with a centering experience, include caring-healing modalities such as mediation, aromatherapy, or human touch into yearly competency education for nursing staff, and creating a healing room for nurses.

Examples of ways to increase caring self-efficacy for students through self-care include having students practice a centering or meditation activity before starting the clinical day, integrating caring for self-modalities within the nursing curriculum, and allowing students to have a self-care break during clinical rotations. Turkel developed a mantra for undergraduate students for setting the intention to pass the NCLEX-RN® examination on the first attempt: "I commit to reading and studying; my mind is focused; I will pass NCLEX-RN on the first attempt."

Loving-Kindness and Equanimity for Others

Moral competence in professional practice has been described as an important nursing construct. It is not surprising that loving-kindness stands as an attribute of moral competence (Jormsri et al., 2005). For example, Thai nurses selected it as essential to a model of the nursing values system. Furthermore, in a qualitative study, investigators (Gallagher-Lepak & Kubsch, 2009) collected 126 stories to identify one story that best illustrated 10 Carative Factors. Carative Factor 1, the formation of a humanistic-altruistic system of values, matched an account whereby a developmentally disabled resident responded to nurses' intentional commitment to the resident by extending themselves to him and by ignoring his verbal assaults. The resident's verbal aggressiveness subsided. Nurses' caring activities were seen in their moral obligation to care for this resident. Humanistic values helped nurses center as they care for people, so that transpersonal caring is provided (Gallagher-Lepak & Kubsch, 2009).

Norman, Rutledge, Keefer-Lynch, and Albeg (2008) analyzed 18 clinical narratives to determine deductively how elements of Watson's theory, the Caritas Processes (Watson, 2008), were evident in the clinical stories. They compared the narratives to 10 clinical Caritas Processes (Watson, 2008) and found statements matching each. Specifically, *the practice of loving-kindness and equanimity within the context of caring consciousness* was translated into altruistic loving-kindness by the investigators at that hospital. They aligned statements from the narratives with the Caritas Process (Watson, 2008) of loving-kindness and equanimity. The following example was presented, "Considers patients as complete individuals, nurse shows that he or she is interested in more than a health problem… Accepts patient as he or she is without prejudice" (p. 327). The researchers also compared narratives across Benner's categories; many of the advanced beginners' narratives demonstrated loving-kindness behaviors. An excerpt follows:

> Her family realized she would die soon. I wanted to provide all the comfort measures. I held her and took her hand. I just let her cry and express her feelings. Every time an alarm sounded, they jumped…I spoke to him softly. (Norman, Rutledge, Keefer-Lynch, & Albeg, 2008, p. 332)

After identifying that the core principles and language of Watson's theory of caring matched their hospital's values, the Clinical Practice Council of a nursing department adopted Watson's theory (Norman, Rossillo, & Skelton, 2016). Their care framework recognized the interconnection of patients' bodies, minds, and spirits. This perspective is consistent with many clinicians who consider mind/body/spirit a framework for compassionate care that addresses suffering throughout the illness experience. The Council used educational approaches to teach the staff about the theory and found that the terminology was difficult for them to understand. Next, they sent nurses to the Caritas Coach Education Program for training that would ultimately help staff implement *Caritas* concepts into the daily practice of the work environment. The Caritas coaches (Caritas Coach Education Program) piloted the dissemination of Watson's theory at the hospital (Norman et al., 2016). Classes and experiential exercises addressed self-care and approaches to deepen spirituality and human connectedness. Other units were involved next in classes on the theory. Clinical educational staff were also mentored; they used exercises to guide experiential learning sessions in other departments. Registered nurses began to document caring interventions in the electronic medical record.

Although the nurses at that hospital focused on all of the Caritas Processes (Watson, 2008), cultivating the practice of loving-kindness and equanimity were emphasized (Norman et al., 2016). Consistent with a loving-kindness approach, the focus was on helping nurses form deep transpersonal connections with their patients. Patient feedback confirmed that loving-kindness was experienced through expressed gratitude for sincere, compassionate, efficient, and positive nursing care. Also, the Patient/Family Advisory Council designed a Compassionate Care Award to recognize staff members evidencing a depth of care valued by patients and families. Nurses also wrote narratives illustrating daily Caritas nursing practice. Staff meetings began with a reflection often based on Watson's theory; stories illustrating Caritas practices were published and shared with staff and the community.

Emphasizing the importance of authentic, professional, human-caring practices as compared to scripted communication, Brewer and Watson (2015) conducted a comparative descriptive study of 1,010 randomly selected, patient responses following administration of the Watson Caritas Patient Score (WCPS) instrument. The WCPS measures a patient's subjective experience of receiving caring. One of the five close-ended items on the WCPS is: "Deliver my care with loving kindness," a measure of the first Caritas Process. Additional items matched other Caritas Processes (Watson, 2008). Eight hospitals, affiliates or research partners of Watson Caring Science Institute, participated using data in quarterly, unit-aggregated, instrument responses entered into a database by trained data collectors. Hospitals and 10 unit types differed on WCPS scores (F = 3.042, p = .012), indicating overall influences of a caring professional practice model that shaped hospital environments. It is assumed that the research affiliates did not follow the caring professional practice model compared to the Caritas affiliates. Study findings also showed a weak relationship between selected items on the Hospital Consumer Assessment of Healthcare Providers and Systems instrument and specific WCPS items.

Nurse leaders' situations are opportunities whereby their incorporation of being mindful and cultivating loving-kindness can change organizational cultures. Watson (2000) used the four *Via* described by Fox (1991) as a framework for transformative leadership, grounded in intentional caring and healing. She emphasized the need for nurse leaders to practice authentic leadership to create and sustain caring and healing within healthcare systems. The *Via Negativa* acknowledges the dark shadow side of the work of nurse leaders. According to Watson (2000), as nurse leaders begin to see the darkness within the organization, they are able to shed light and reestablish balance between the lightness and darkness of systems allowing for human values, human flourishing, and caring to emerge. *Via Positiva* honors light and healing and serves as a reminder to fall in love at least three times a day (Fox, 1991). While on this path, the nurse leader becomes open to finding beauty and joy in the day, celebrating joy and Love, honoring caring moments, and creating healing environments. *Via Creativa* allows for visionary leadership, honoring of individuals' unique gifts, and leadership practices that flow from the heart. The final path on the journey is the *Via Transformativa* where the nurse leader is empowered, reflective, mindful, and open to new ways of being and becoming. Transformed leaders are visionary, value focused, mindful, practice with authentic presence, and create caring moments. Within the *Via* framework, transformative leaders foster loving-kindness and equanimity in nursing departments and across organizations. Consequently, staff and patients benefit.

CONCLUSION

Watson (2003) invited nurses to deepen their humanity and return to the heart and soul of nursing practice within a framework of caring and love offering light, love, and beauty for those served. Without caring and love from nurses, healing and wholeness for patients cannot occur. Watson (2003) reminded us, "It is our humanity that both wounds us and heals us, and those whom we serve, and in the end it is only love that matters" (p. 515). Cultivating the practice of loving-kindness, a self- and other-directed process, requires practice. Self-care is foundational to authentic caring between nurses and patients and the development of helping, trusting, caring relationships. The other-directed aspect of this Caritas Process is provided for patients and others for whom nurses care in the context of the nurse–patient interaction, a relationship that is transpersonal (Watson, 2008) and mutual. When nurses are exhausted and worn down, it is very difficult to care compassionately for others. Cultivating the practice of loving-kindness through daily self-care activities (Turkel, 2015) fosters calmness and helps nurses to gain energy for professional and personal lives.

NEXT ERA POSSIBILITIES

Education

- How could nurse educators encourage students to share their stories of cultivating the practice of loving-kindness with fellow students?
- What assignments could be created by faculty to enable students to develop equanimity as they experience stressful experiences with patients and families?
- How can faculty integrate self-care into the nursing curriculum for students at all levels?

Research

- What research designs could nurses implement to provide evidence that practicing loving-kindness and equanimity affected specific patient outcomes?
- How might a randomized controlled design study be implemented that incorporates practicing loving-kindness and equanimity strategies bundled into an intervention that affects patient satisfaction measures?
- What is the meaning of cultivating the practice of loving-kindness from the perspective of nurses, patients, and leaders?
- Ask patients one simple, Caring Science question: "Was your care provided with loving kindness?" "Yes" or "No." Please share an example.

Praxis

- How might nurse educators create programs that orient newly hired registered nurses to the daily practices that demonstrate loving-kindness and equanimity?
- How might staff development nurses foster implementation of self-care activities into staff educational sessions and throughout the organization?
- What self-care strategies could be implemented by nurse leaders that have a positive impact on the satisfaction of nursing staff with their leadership?

Theory and Knowledge Development

- How might middle-range theory be developed that tests nursing interventions incorporating the practice of loving-kindness and equanimity with patients' perception of Caritas as measured by the WCPS?
- What tests of Watson's Theory of Human Caring could be performed that connect interventions framed by specific Caritas Processes (Watson, 2008) on outcomes?

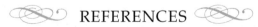 REFERENCES

American Nurses Association. (2015). *Code of ethics for nurses with interpretive statements.* Silver Spring, MD: Author.

Boellinghaus, I., Jones, F. W., & Hutton, J. (2014). The role of mindfulness and loving-kindness meditation in cultivating self-compassion and other-focused concern in health care professionals. *Mindfulness, 5,* 129–138. doi:10.1007/s12671-012-0158-6

Brewer, B. B., & Watson, J. (2015). Evaluation of authentic human caring professional practices. *Journal of Nursing Administration, 45,* 622–627. doi:10.1097/NNA.0000000000000275

Brown, C. J., Bishop, M., & Bar, B. B. (2013). Creating and sustaining peace within for the journey of nursing leadership. *Nursing Administration Quarterly, 37,* E1–E7. doi:10.1097/01.NAQ.0000434947.57388.b3

Burks, D. J., & Kobus, A. M. (2012). The legacy of altruism in health care: The promotion of empathy, prosociality and humanism. *Medical Education*, 46, 317–325. doi:10.1111/j.1365-2923.2011.04159.x

Chapman, E. (2009). *Radical loving care*. Nashville, TN: Baptist Healing Hospital Trust.

Dossey, B. M. (2016). Nursing: Holistic, integral, and integrative-local to global. In B. M. Dossey, & L. Keegan (Eds.), *Holistic nursing: A handbook for practice* (7th ed., pp. 3–52). Burlington, MA: Jones & Bartlett.

Fox, M. (1991). *Creation spirituality: Liberating gifts for the peoples of the Earth*. San Francisco, CA: Harper.

Gallagher-Lepak, S., & Kubsch, S. (2009). Transpersonal caring: A nursing practice guideline. *Holistic Nursing Practice*, 23, 171–182. doi:10.1097/HNP.0b013e3181a056d9

Hanh, T. N. (1993). *Interbeing: Fourteen guidelines for engaged Buddhism* (Rev. ed.). Berkeley, CA: Parallax Press.

Hanh, T. N. (2011). *True love: A practice for awakening the heart*. Boulder, CO: Shambhala Press.

Hawkins, D. (2013). *Letting go: The pathway of surrender*. Carlsbad, CA: Hay House.

Jackson, C. (2010). Using loving relationships to transform health care: A practical approach. *Holistic Nursing Practice*, 24, 181–186. doi:10.1097/HNP.0b013e3181e90319

Jormsri, P., Kunaviktikul, W., Ketefian, S., & Chaowalit, A. (2005). Moral competence in nursing practice. *Nursing Ethics*, 12, 582–594. doi:10.1191/0969733005ne828oa

Lachman, V. D. (2016). Compassion fatigue as a threat to ethical practice: Identification, personal and workplace prevention/management strategies. *MEDSURG Nursing*, 25, 275–278.

Lee, I., & Wang, H. H. (2014). Preliminary development of humanistic care indicators for residents in nursing homes: A Delphi technique. *Asian Nursing Research*, 8, 75–81. doi:10.1016/j.anr.2014.03.001

Mariano, C. (2016). Current trends and issues in holistic nursing. In B. M. Dossey & L. Keegan (Eds.), *Holistic nursing: A handbook for practice* (7th ed., pp. 77–100). Burlington, MA: Jones & Bartlett.

Marks, L. W. (2013). *The emancipatory praxis of integral nursing: The impact of human caring theory guided practice upon nursing qua nursing in an American Nurses Credentialing Center MagnetRTM re-designated healthcare system*. (unpublished doctoral dissertation). Retrieved from Proquest Dissertations and Theses. Albany, NY: Sage Colleges. (UMI Order #AA13591134)

McCamant, K. L. (2006). Humanistic nursing, interpersonal relations theory, and the empathy-altruism hypothesis. *Nursing Science Quarterly*, 19, 334–338. doi:10.1177/0894318406292823

Moody, K., Kramer, D., Santizo, R. O., Magro, L., Wyshogrod, D., Ambrosio, J., … Stein, J. (2013). Helping the helpers: Mindfulness training for burnout in pediatric oncology: A pilot program. *Journal of Pediatric Oncology Nursing*, 30, 275–284. doi:10.1177/1043454213504497

Myss, C. (1996). *Anatomy of the spirit: The seven stages of power and healing*. New York, NY: Harmony Books.

Norman, V., Rossillo, K., & Skelton, K. (2016). Creating healing environments through the theory of caring. *Association of periOperative Nurses Journal*, 104, 401–409. doi:10.1016/j.aorn.2016.09.006

Norman, V., Rutledge, D. N., Keefer-Lynch, A. M., & Albeg, G. (2008). Uncovering and recognizing nurse caring from clinical narratives. *Holistic Nursing Practice*, 22, 324–335. doi:10.1097/01.HNP.0000339344.18876.54

Paterson, J., & Zderad, L. T. (1976). *Humanistic nursing*. New York, NY: John Wiley & Sons.

Persky, G. J., Nelson, J. W., Watson, J., & Bent, K. (2008). Creating a profile of a nurse effective in caring. *Nursing Administration Quarterly*, 32, 15–20. doi:10.1097/01.NAQ.0000305943.46440.77

Pipe, T. B. (2008). Illuminating the inner leadership journey by engaging intention and mindfulness as guided by caring theory. *Nursing Administration Quarterly*, 32, 117–125. doi:10.1097/01.NAQ.0000314540.21618.c1

Quinn, J. F. (1992). Holding sacred space: The nurse as healing environment. *Holistic Nursing Practice*, 6(4), 26–36. doi:10.1097/00004650-199207000-00007

Sasser, C. G., & Puchalski, C. M. (2010). The humanistic clinician: Traversing the science and art of health care. *Journal of Pain and Symptom Management, 39*, 936–940. doi:10.1016/j.jpainsymman .2010.03.001

Shields, D., & Wilson, D. (2016). Energy healing. In B. M. Dossey & L. Keegan (Eds.), *Holistic nursing: A handbook for practice* (7th ed., pp. 187–220). Burlington, MA: Jones & Bartlett.

Small, G. E., & Good, P. (2013). Preceptorship: Embracing a culture of caring. *Journal for Nursing in Professional Development, 29*, 301–304. doi:10.1097/NND.0000000000000013

Smith, M. C. (1999). Caring and the science of unitary human beings. *Advances in Nursing Science, 21*(4), 14–28. doi:10.1097/00012272-199906000-00006

Turkel, M. C. (2015). Caring for self: Guest editorial. *Scandinavian Journal of Caring Sciences, 29*, 613–614. doi:10.1111/scs.12288

Turkel, M. C., & Ray, M. A. (2004). Creating a caring practice environment through self-renewal. *Nursing Administration Quarterly, 28*, 249–254. doi:10.1097/00006216-200410000-00004

Watson, J. (1979). *Nursing: The philosophy and science of caring.* Boston, MA: Little, Brown.

Watson, J. (1985). *Nursing: The philosophy and science of caring.* Niwot: University Press of Colorado.

Watson, J. (1988). *Human science and human care.* Boston, MA: Jones & Bartlett.

Watson, J. (2000). Leading via caring-healing: The fourfold way toward transformative leadership. *Nursing Administration Quarterly, 25*, 1–6. doi:10.1097/00006216-200010000-00009

Watson, J. (2003). Love and caring: Ethics of face and hand: An invitation to return to the heart and soul of nursing and our deep humanity. *Nursing Administration Quarterly, 27*, 197–202. doi:10.1097/ 00006216-200307000-00005

Watson, J. (2005). *Caring science as sacred science.* Philadelphia, PA: F. A. Davis.

Watson, J. (2008). *Nursing: The philosophy and science of caring* (Rev. ed.). Boulder: University Press of Colorado.

Watson, J. (2010). *Core concepts of Jean Watson's theory of human caring/caring science.* Boulder, CO: Watson Caring Science Institute. Retrieved from https://www.watsoncaringscience.org/files/PDF/ watsons-theory-of-human-caring-core-concepts-and-evolution-to-caritas-processes-handout.pdf

IV

Caritas Literacy as a Foundation for Nursing Education

16

Teaching From the Heart

Nancy Vitali

CARITAS LITERACIES

By the end of this chapter, the caring-healing nurse will be able to

1. Identify ways to be present to students that engage them in caring-healing relationships.

2. Recognize the connection between self-care and reflective practices and the ability to teach from the heart.

3. Choose reflective and aesthetic practices to include in nursing coursework.

4. Plan empowering and emancipatory activities for faculty and students that honor subjective experience and multiple ways of knowing.

5. Describe ways in which faculty and students can "hear the story of another" in an educational setting.

6. Understand that developing trusting/caring relationships with students is an essential aspect of teaching from the heart. As Watson (2008) states, these relationships between faculty and student are exemplars for the nurse–patient relationship.

7. Consider Watson's (2008) Caritas Process #10, "Opening and Attending to Spiritual/ Mysterious and Existential Unknowns of Life-Death" (p. 191), and its relation to teaching from the heart.

Teaching from the heart is a transpersonal caring experience. "Transpersonal caring relationships consist of connections that embrace the spirit or soul of the other through processes of full, authentic, caring/healing attention in the moment" (Hills & Watson, 2011, p. 249). These scholars invite us to consider and honor the richness of context of each person:

> Once again it is helpful to remind ourselves that everyone is situated in a personal, relational, historical, cultural deep phenomenal life experience context. This backdrop needs to be considered, as each context of self and other is deeply rooted in a personal inner life contextual phenomenal field of history and meaning. In a Caring Science framework, the basic tenet is that one person's level of humanity reflects on the other and at the deeply human level, we are all one and connected through our shared humanity. (Hills & Watson, 2011, p. 39)

BACKGROUND

The climate of nursing education in the United States in the second decade of the 21st century is one of constant change and enormous complexity. A nursing organization, funded by the Robert Wood Johnson Foundation, was formed following the convening of the Institute of Medicine (2001, 2003) Summits between 1999 and 2003 (Quality and Safety Education for Nurses [QSEN]) and is working to realign nursing practice and education, embracing a systems approach to healthcare that is intended to reduce error and fragmentation (Dalansky & Moore, 2013). Another systemic change is the ongoing implementation of the Affordable Care Act (Affordable Care Act, 2010) whose goal is the provision of affordable and accessible healthcare for all Americans, and whose failed repeal in 2017 has tipped the scales toward chaos. Those and other factors add up to a climate of unpredictable change, pressure, and complexity as multiple complex adaptive systems are dynamically influencing one another and challenging nursing educators "to prepare students for practice in complex environments … This formation requires the development of personhood and may involve the use of reflective and spiritual practices and aesthetic engagement" (Davidson & Topolski, 2011, p. 17).

Other researchers have made their life's work studying the dynamics within nursing education that create stress for faculty and students, often resulting in hostility and incivility (Clark, 2014; Clark & Springer, 2010; Luparell, 2011). Clark (2014) identified stress as a "collision course" for incivility, and defines "incivility" in nursing education as "… rude or disruptive behaviors that often result in psychological or physiological distress for the people involved, and may progress into threatening situations when left unaddressed" (Clark & Springer, 2010, p. 320).

Other writers and researchers have focused on the current curricular problems with nursing education. Benner, Sutphen, Leonard, and Day (2010), Ironside (2001), Dossey, (2009), Diekelmann and Diekelmann (2009), and Hills and Watson (2011) all investigated new pedagogies for advancing nursing education, empowering students, promoting apprenticeships, using multiple ways of knowing, and bringing theory and clinical practice in closer proximity to one another.

Why Teaching From the Heart?

Teaching from the heart means teaching from the depths of who we are with the hope that we will touch the hearts of those with whom we work.—Jerold Apps, *Teaching From the Heart*, 1996

Nurses are asked or "ordered to care" (Reverby, 1987) for persons experiencing challenging and life-threatening situations on a daily basis. Compassion and empathy compete with technological approaches in nursing curricula across the country, and the increasing focus on humanizing nursing curricula has led to changes in course requirements over the past half-century (Boykin, 1994; Bevis & Watson, 2000; Hills & Watson, 2011). It is incumbent on nursing faculty to not "model" but to be the nurse they are teaching students to be, which requires showing not only technical competence but also compassion, caring, and kindness to students. The motivation to understand how this happens and does not happen is the source of the following question: What is the experience of nursing faculty teaching compassionately and kindly, or "from the heart?"

Teaching From the Heart in the Literature

Education at its best ... is about healing and wholeness. It is about empowerment, liberation, transcendence, about renewing the vitality of life. It is about finding and claiming ourselves and our place in the world.—Parker Palmer, *The Heart of Learning: Spirituality in Education*, 1999

In searching Cumulative Index to Nursing and Allied Health Literature (CINAHL), Educational Resources Information Center (ERIC), and WorldCat, several dozen references were found for teaching from the heart. None were from nursing, and all but one were related to K–12 education. In this discussion of teaching from the heart, references are made to this author's research study that is the only known nursing research into that phenomenon (Vitali, 2017).

The 14th Dalai Lama (Tenzin Gyatzo, 1999) expressed that responsibility to community, ethics, and heart-based facets of education was traditionally an essential of the educational process when schooling was centered in church and religious-sponsored organizations, but over the centuries, this aspect of education has been displaced. He stated that compassion is much needed in education today, especially in fast-paced, materially focused cultures similar to that in the United States.

Noddings (1984, 1992), a lifelong educator, researcher, and educational philosopher, wrote that caring and attending to student needs are the ethical and moral responsibility of educators. She differentiated between "caring for" and "caring about" and emphasized that the latter, which requires more involvement and actual caring encounters between teachers and students, needs more attention in education.

English professor, philosopher, and author of over 30 books on education, spirituality, race, gender, power/oppression, and art, bell hooks (1999) expresses that love is a necessary force in education, that it "can bridge that sense of otherness. However, it is a practice to beam that love out. It takes work" (p. 118). She discusses the power of "communities love" to lift people out of suffering, and describes education as "the practice of freedom" (p. 113).

Parker Palmer (1987) wrote extensively about the heart of a teacher on the basis of his personal experience with depression:

> As good teachers weave the fabric that joins them with students and subjects, the heart is the loom on which the threads are tied: the tension is held, the shuttle flies, and the fabric is stretched tight. Small wonder, then, that teaching tugs at the heart, opens the heart, even breaks the heart—and the more one loves teaching, the more heartbreaking it can be. We became teachers for reasons of the heart, animated by a passion for some subject and for helping people to learn. But many of us lose heart as the years of teaching go by. (p. 11)

Watson (2008) sees human relationships and caring as the desired epicenter of nursing curricula, with all other knowledge and skills taking these central themes into account. Yet, in nursing curricula across the country, technology and technological skills are valued and emphasized (Benner et al. 2010). In an effort to focus on what nursing brings to the health-care setting, Hills and Watson (2011) and Watson and Smith (2002) define Caring Science as "an evolving ethical-epistemic field of study that is grounded in the discipline of nursing and informed by related fields" (p. 456). Hills and Watson (2011) describe Caring Science as being the disciplinary foundation of the nursing profession and emphasize its distinction from medical science as being focused on caring-healing, with medicine being focused on diagnosing-curing. They write of an emancipatory relational pedagogy that is interested in the cocreation of knowledge obtained by investigating understandings and meanings of world experiences.

Teaching from the heart, as a phenomenon, is grounded in Caring Science. In it, the caring relationship between faculty and student can be an exemplar for the caring relationship between nurse and patient. Heart-based teaching is not found in the nursing literature, and it seems ironic that a discipline that relies on empathy does not have more to say about the heart's role in education. Faculty who related stories of teaching from the heart saw their students as whole humans with wisdom and gifts to bring to their relationships rather than as blank slates to be written on or soldiers carrying out prescribed behaviors (Vitali, 2017). With the complexities described in nursing education and the demand that certain curricular features be distributed among students, nursing programs can take on an assembly-line quality if the ethics of honoring each student's individual gifts is not attended to. Faculty also acknowledged the reciprocal nature of teaching and learning. In all interactions, both faculty and student alternate between the roles of teacher and learner.

Topics of consciousness, intuition, spirituality, neuroscience, neurocardiology, noetic science, and educational philosophy were considered in a literature search as potential aspects of teaching from the heart. The following activities were selected as ways of teaching from the heart:

- Using a centering method including deep, focused breathing (J. Watson, personal communication, May 1, 2010; L. Wagner, personal communication, February 15, 2012)

- Focusing on the heart (use of HeartMath® tools has been researched to be effective; McCraty, 2001)

- Honoring the dignity and experiences of all participants (Palmer, 1987)

- Setting an intention to listen for understanding and clarity

- Acknowledging and accepting that all are teachers and all are learners (Freire, 1972; Sherwood & Horton-Deutsch, 2012; Hills & Watson, 2011)

- Providing for a supportive, protective, physical/emotional/spiritual environment (Watson, 2008)

- Using a ritual and/or prayer to prepare the classroom space before students' arrival (Watson, personal communication, 2010)

- Inviting behaviors/attitudes/speech toward all who gather

- Embodying Caritas/caring consciousness (Watson, 2008)

- Using art/aesthetics/music (Chinn & Watson, 1994)

- Observing for synchronous events

- Being aware that we teach in all of our relationships inside and outside of the classroom

Arts-Informed Narrative Inquiry

Art and Aesthetics in Nursing (Chinn & Watson, 1994) was written to advance the centrality and value of the artistic expression to the survival of nursing as a discipline of caring and concern for humanity. Energy devoted to empirical knowing technologies in the 20th and 21st centuries continued to expand at the expense of attention to healing modalities of art, music, poetry, theater, writing, and photography. According to Sherwood & Horton-Deutsch (2012, p. 205), "Sharing aesthetic ways of knowing helps us reach into our inner-most thoughts and feelings to surface values and attitudes that are so much a part of how we respond to others." It is this premise that art is central to the health of nursing as a discipline that guided the focus of the inquiry into teaching. The stories of master teachers, illuminated by their artistic representations, helped to create a community of faculty who were united in their focus on heart-based learning-in-relationship (Vitali, 2017).

Lindsay (2006, 2008, 2011) used a variety of arts-based approaches: an installation featuring found objects, collage, poetry, and journals in ongoing arts-informed narrative inquiry, "I learn how arts-based methods (objects, poems, scrapbooks, writing) facilitate multi-dimensional awareness before there are words to explore experience. I affirm that inquiry into autobiography is an important source of identity, knowledge, and curriculum construction" (Lindsay, 2006, p. 7).

On the basis of the studies presented (Butler-Kisber, 2010; Caine & Steeves, 2009; Carper, 1978; Casey, 2009; Chinn & Watson, 1994; Lakoff & Johnson, 1980; Lindsay, 2006, 2008, 2011; Simmons & Daley, 2013), and the researcher's personal experiences of facilitating arts activities with students, the arts-informed narrative inquiry was recognized as a way to use the creative process to "access the borderlands" (Caine & Steeves, 2009, p. 9) of nursing faculty's inner wisdom. It was found to bring about deep, soulful communication, to assist in formulating creative solutions, and to access paths to healing of self, other, and organizations. Collage was chosen as an art modality of potential value in evoking memories, thoughts, feelings, and subconscious and suppressed responses, and for inspiring the conscious use of metaphor for nursing faculty teaching from the heart. The transformational capacity of these processes will be realized after its continued use and study in the practices of nursing faculty and students.

HeartMath® Tools

Since the 1960s, research into the heart's intelligence and role in learning and consciousness has continued to grow (Pearsall, 1998; McCraty, 2001, 2015; McCraty, Bradley, & Tomasino, 2005; McCraty & Childre, 2010). The heart plays a central role in relationships, regulation of body systems and emotions, stress responses, and learning, and that information is not part of mainstream nursing education. HeartMath techniques have been part of the curriculum in the nursing program where I teach since I was trained in 2008. Before every exam and class, students and faculty meditate for 3 to 5 minutes, using a technique that helps to modulate heart rate variability, calm anxiety, and enable the communication of new information to the cerebral cortex.

Synchronicity in the Classroom

Several years ago, in an orientation day during one of these classes, I began to feel a nudge to tell a story of genuine caring about two babies who died about 30 years before as a result of a rare genetic condition that caused large blisters, and then sloughing of skin at the slightest bit of friction. The outcome of this condition was the equivalent of second-degree burns any place on the body that was exposed to friction: upper thighs on diapers, back of the head, shoulders, and back—literally everywhere on the body that rubbed against the surface of the bed. Repositioning them only caused friction in different areas, and more blisters. When the blisters broke, there was a loss of fluid, protein, and electrolytes from the babies' bodies. There was no cure, and the babies' lives were not sustainable. Both of them died from this illness. They were siblings, born 2 years apart. The parents, a couple from Asia, chose to have the second baby because they were counseled that there was only a 1-in-8 chance of it being present in other children.

I shared the babies' story, and I shared my story of caring for them over time, at a time when I was having my first child as well. As their primary nurse, I was involved with the other nurses in problem solving how to go about caring for them to prevent friction and infection, how to administer their pain medication, to comfort them, to try to meet their need for fluids and nutrition, and how to communicate respectfully with their parents. The father spoke English, but the mom did not. There were cultural barriers because they were Muslim. It proved a difficult and heart-breaking journey, especially with the hope they had that their second baby would be healthy. It strained the skills of the nursing staff who were so accustomed to premature infants with lung problems. During the telling of the story, a student raised her hand, but quickly withdrew it and declined to speak. After the class, she came up and shared with the faculty that she had the skin condition (epidermolysis bullosa) that the babies had. The other faculty and I were shocked and wondered how she was alive, and the babies died. She shared that she has a dominant form of the disease, and the babies had the recessive form.

What is unusual statistically is that the condition in any form occurs at the rate of 1 in every 20,000 live births (Dystrophic Epidermolysis Bullosa Research Association of America, 2017). It was baffling that I had these thoughts and memories that pushed me to tell the story connecting the babies with my student. The student was having a challenging time with commuting a long distance, with the strain of having a child who had a chronic health problem, and with the death of a parent later in the semester. Nevertheless, she persisted and was successful in graduating from the nursing program and passing the National Council Licensure Examination (NCLEX)®. Perhaps this event served to pull her out of the crowd and obtain support that she needed. This synchronous event seemed to be related to teaching from the heart in terms of connecting with the energetic field of that student during the meditation process.

FACULTY STORIES OF TEACHING FROM THE HEART

Faculty stories informed by artistic expression paint pictures of what teaching from the heart means to them. Because nursing, narrative inquiry, and qualitative research in general honor subjective experience as sources of data, these expert faculty offer significant knowledge to Caring Science. The following seven stories and collages illustrate what caring faculty experience as the phenomenon of teaching from the heart.

ANNIE'S STORY (Figure 16.1)

A student was designated by faculty in a previous course as not possessing the capability to be a nurse, and Annie was given the responsibility of failing the student. She felt pressured and was appalled that this would take place in a caring-focused nursing program. After she

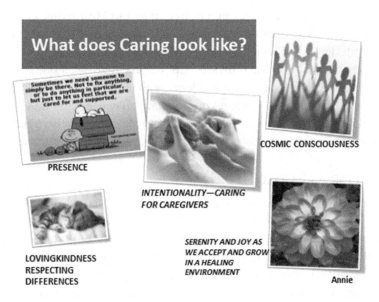

FIGURE 16.1 Annie's collage.

had noticed behaviors in the student she identified as problematic, she spoke with the student and asked what was going on. They identified anxiety as the problem, and Annie came up with a novel solution to decrease the anxiety that involved the whole class. Her approach was to allow the students to take over the class for 5 minutes every day and do whatever they wanted. Sometimes that meant telling off-color jokes to make the teacher blush.

The student did pass the course and the NCLEX and is now a registered nurse. Annie viewed these challenging situations with this statement of determination, "Arm in arm, lock-step, we will get through this together." Whether a student passed or failed, it was her determination not to abandon him or her, and to treat him or her with dignity and kindness. Referring to her collage, Annie reflects on what caring means to her:

> And so in putting the collage together, it's really not separate elements. It's actually a symphony of how it works, how everything works together. And I think for me, it all starts with the idea of presence—of being fully present in the moment with whoever you're with. Whether you're in a learning mode or you're in a teaching mode, or you're in both but most of the time we are.

Lark's Story (Figure 16.2)

Lark is the chair of Graduate Nursing Education and associate professor at a private university in the mid-southern United States. She is a pediatric nurse practitioner who has been nurse for a little over 40 years, and a faculty member for about half of that time. She has consciously chosen to teach in private universities because she feels that they do not have as many internal political struggles, that faculty "play well with others," and are more amenable to a caring nursing philosophy. In describing what "teaching from the heart" means to her, Lark points to the central image on her collage (Figure 16.2), a woman emerging from a heart, with the inscription, "She believed in a wide-open heart," and asserts:

> You could look at it as either being open or fractured, but I think that a lot of what you do when you are *teaching from the heart* is you are showing not only your love of sharing that with students, but you are also showing your vulnerability and the fact that there are moments that you have messed up. I think that helps one of the primary things that we want to get across to students is that we all make mistakes. But the important thing is if you do, or when you do, that you can step up and say, 'I made a mistake,' and rectify that before any harm hopefully is done. So also being wide open and then using everything that is given. So, you share your joys and your heartaches.

Grace's Story (Figure 16.3)

Grace describes a situation with a student who struggled with the process in a doctoral course:

> I don't know what her personal evaluation of the class was, but I did feel like it was a transformative moment for both of us; I opened my heart to her, and she agreed to stay in the class, accept where she was at. When we first got on the phone, she wanted to know immediately if she could withdraw and she wanted to know if there was another class she could take instead because the class was making her very uncomfortable.

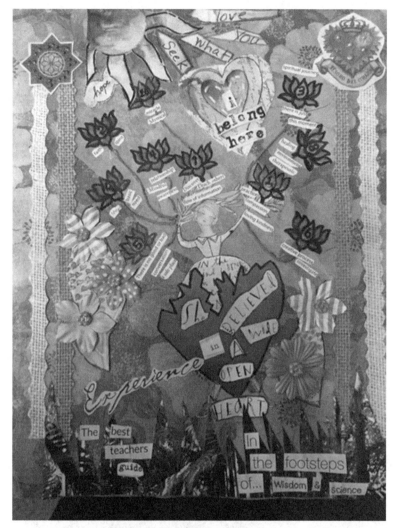

FIGURE 16.2 Lark's collage.

But we were able to move past that and come to a place that I was able to encourage her that she was safe to stay in class, and it was comfortable, and that she was comfortable enough to stay really warmed my heart. You know, sometimes we just plant seeds with students, and I just hope that I planted a seed for her; it's a gift for me when someone comes to me and shares something that is very personal and concerning to them, and I have an opportunity to be in dialogue with them around that in a heart-centered way.

SANDY'S STORY (Figure 16.4)

Sandy's collage, which is composed of Internet images, shows that life seems to be cyclical and that people revisit places they need to work on, always growing and expanding consciousness each time they return. Also, on her collage (Figure 16.4) is an image of a

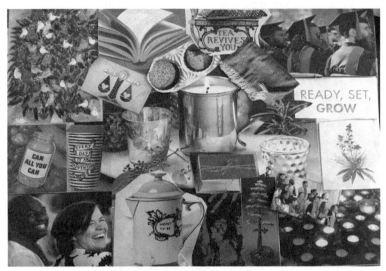

FIGURE 16.3 Grace's collage.

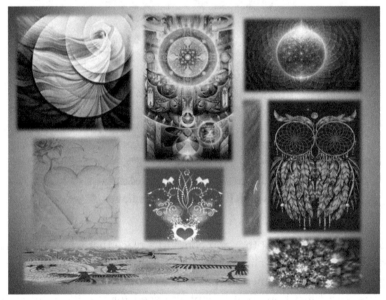

FIGURE 16.4 Sandy's collage.

water color of a dancing woman in a multicolored spiraling dress, which, she asserts, represents her true self, which she is on a continuous quest for. She emphasizes the higher consciousness level of most of the images compared with that of the first one she found of a heart with a rose growing from it. Unity of being, ancestral guidance, spirituality, cosmic consciousness, energetic fields, alone-ness (she stated that we were on the phone talking at that moment, but when we hung up, she would be by herself, as no one in the city where she lives shares the experience of teaching from the heart within a framework of human caring), wisdom, transformation (butterflies emerging from an open heart), helping people to "catch their dreams," and uniqueness and beauty of all persons are emphasized in the vibrant images on her collage.

She directed (the collage images had to be transferred to another [Word®] document) that the background was to be gradations of blue, honoring dark-to-light aspects of *teaching from the heart*. Sandy emphasized that multiple ways of knowing are necessary to arrive at a place of wisdom, including not-knowing. She also is very drawn to the spiral images and birds on the bottom of the page, saying that they speak to her of her ancestors, who made her life possible.

RUMI'S STORY (Figure 16.5)

Rumi talks about what motivates her to stay, and to continue doing what she does is the transpersonal, and her ability to be true to herself. A student who missed an examination early in nursing school sent her this message with a plant during final week of her last semester:

"You are why I am graduating on Friday. I just wanted to say, Thanks." I thought, *Those are the things that keep us going, that we go.* You know what? I let a student take an exam late. She did not call me in advance. She was in the ICU. That was not the important thing. She is going to be, I hope, a wonderful nurse. Sometimes we have to listen to our heart and see that person, that unique individual and respond to that, but it can be hard. It is a difficult balance. I see this as a need to balance it, because I do believe that as educators those are struggles we have. I love the work of Parker Palmer where he talks about a life undivided. He says, "I cannot be one person at home and another person in my work. If I cannot combine those two people and be the same person all of the time, I am going to be in conflict." My collage is Indra's net, and I say on it that I see my students as unique and beautiful and a source of light in

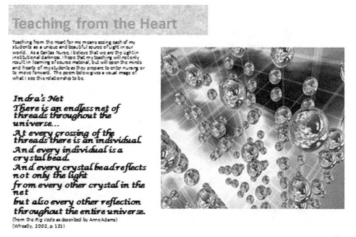

FIGURE 16.5 Rumi's collage.

our world. I believe that as a Caritas nurse we are the light in darkness and I hope that my students in my teaching will open their minds and their hearts as they begin to enter a profession that I see as sacred because it allows us to teach and touch other people at such a deep, spiritual, sacred level as we care for their health needs.

BLAINE'S STORY (Figure 16.6)

The central figure (Figure 16.6) of Blaine's collage is that of a white-haired, elderly female with possibly an indigenous embroidered white cotton dress, hands on her hips, and confident smile: a picture of wisdom and rich life experience. He has lots of delicious food from around the world, and other cultures represented, nature-as-teacher represented by flowers and trees, as well as ducks and eggs to symbolize life and birth. His photo of an adolescent boy depicting "me in my youth" is posted sideways. Regarding the central figure, he explains that considering the concept of gender that he is studying, "This could be me … I mean, she just has had such a life. I look at that. Every wrinkle that you see is a story. As I explore gender fluidity in my own post-doc, why can't this be me?"

Curious about his many depictions of birth and life, this researcher asked him what prompted that focus. Blaine responded that his investment in and enthusiasm for life

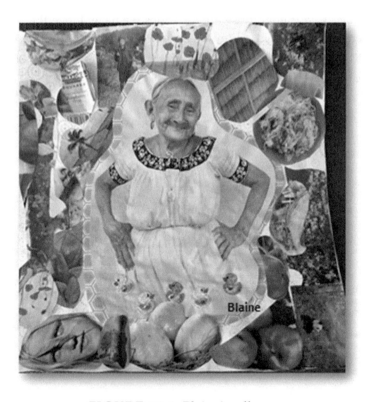

FIGURE 16.6 Blaine's collage.

is a result of having lost so many close friends to the AIDS epidemic in the 1980s and 1990s.

OLD TEACHER'S STORY (Figure 16.7)

Teaching from the heart is the way I convey my passion for wanting other people to be the best that they can be and help other people, particularly nursing students or nurses who are students, to learn to share in that passion and ultimately possess that passion with—it involves more than just teaching about the common physiological types of things that we frequently associate with nursing academics. It involves taking into the thought processes the whole person, his or her place in time when he or she has been, and where he or she is going.

The following six themes were extracted from the stories of the 10 participants as components of the experience of teaching from the heart:

1. Experiencing a hard job

2. Knowing and living caring

3. Embracing vulnerability

4. Learning and growing together

5. Being in right relationship

6. Experiencing spiritual transformation

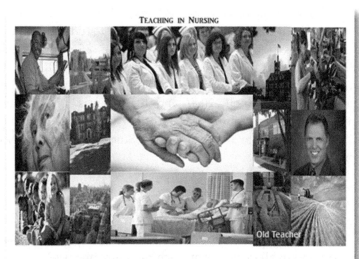

FIGURE 16.7 Old teacher's collage.

CONCLUSION

There are several implications for nursing educators who teach from the heart. Faculty members who participated in this study verbalized a need to connect with other faculty who participated in caring-focused curricula because of a sense of isolation and vulnerability. Participants felt that there was a unifying energy that pervaded the conference calls that boosted their spirits and gave hope. The inspiration this coresearcher felt to hear and read their experiences over and over and to grasp what an extraordinary and intuitive group of teachers they are has not left me. Heart-based teaching and living occur in the community.

Sensing the challenge that teaching from the heart is, Grace asserted, "We need to find ways to sustain ourselves." Shamus (another participant, whose story is not included in this chapter) said that despite working in a caring-focused nursing program, she often felt that other colleagues were uncivil because of her beliefs in the primacy of caring–healing relationships, energy and energetic fields, and spirit-based approaches to teaching and learning. Sandy seemed to feel a sense of isolation when she said that we were on the phone talking at that moment, but when we hung up, she would be by herself, as no one in the city where she lives shares the experience of teaching from the heart within a framework of human caring. The need for connection and community is apparent in this group.

Programs from the Center for Courage and Renewal (www.couragerenewal.org) offer hope to educators through a variety of retreats and other activities. At the Courage to Teach®, retreat participants reflect and re-charge; focus on their own pressing work and life questions; support each other's personal and professional development; and practice deep listening. One of the themes of these workshops is creating "circles of trust."

Creating and participating in an existing online narrative community is one approach to the need for community among caring-focused faculty. Because the numbers of faculty are relatively small and geographically separated, meeting face-to-face is a challenge. Solutions must come at the speed of the Internet. One such arts-based online narrative community of nurses is based in Ontario, Canada (www.theartofexperience.ca). Facebook may also be a location for starting narrative communities. Several recent studies have involved nursing faculty sharing experiences narratively (Cangelosi, Crocker, & Sorrell, 2009; Dattilo, Brewer, & Streit, 2009; Smith, Zahourek, Hines, Engebretson, & Wardell, 2013). A story is the end product of a narrative; however, the telling and retelling of a story is a healing process that is life changing (Clandinin & Connelly, 2000), and this idea was borne out in the interviews when the participants expressed gratitude for the opportunity of being part of the research, of having been "made" to stop, reflect, and create. "Stories are like prayers that heal us" (Chinn & Watson, 1994, p. 50).

NEXT ERA POSSIBILITIES

Education

- How can I demonstrate and share the value of teaching from the heart with other nurse educators and in all instances of teaching in my practice?
- In what ways can nursing curricula at the master's- and doctoral-level programs incorporate heart-based learning and the use of arts and aesthetics to reach a soul and spirit level of knowledge?

Research

- What further Caring Science research is needed that addresses relationship-based, heart-centered nursing education?
- How can nursing use the work of other non-nursing disciplines and general educational theory to advance heart and relationship-based practices?
- How can Caring Science researchers help to translate the more qualitative nature of relationship-focused, heart-based education into a language that quantitatively minded policy makers and decision makers understand, appreciate, and financially support?
- How can I attract young researchers to qualitative research in which the researcher "leans in" to the phenomenon of interest?

Praxis

- How can nursing educators (broadly) and faculty (in degree-seeking programs) draw upon the nursing research into civility/incivility to enhance the "soft skills" of communication, loving-kindness, teamwork, self-care, mentoring, and others to create a kinder, gentler, and more loving discipline for students and for nurses in practice?
- Which dimensions of practice can I improve right now with a greater understanding of the importance of heart-based learning approaches?
- Which of my current work-related outcomes can be reframed to create a kinder, gentler environment for teaching-learning?

Theory and Knowledge Development

- What additional relationship-heart-spirit-centered processes need further study to make education an emancipatory process for nurses?
- What role do self-care and self-reflection play in the development of compassionate, loving, wise, and caring faculty?
- How would I expand the idea of teaching from the heart to include my specialty? Does it fit with patient education? With orientation to a nursing position? What changes would I make?
- How does my own educational philosophy mesh with the phenomenon of teaching from the heart? What ideas would I add to those described in this chapter?

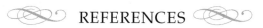

REFERENCES

Affordable Care Act, HR3590 U.S.C. § 1 *et seq.* (Government Printing Office 2010).

Apps, J. W. (1996). *Teaching from the heart.* Malabar, FL: Krieger.

Benner, P., Sutphen, M., Leonard, V., & Day, L. (2010). *Educating nurses: A call for radical transformation.* San Francisco, CA: Jossey-Bass.

Bevis, E. O., & Watson, J. (2000). *Toward a caring curriculum: A new pedagogy for nursing.* Sudbury, MA: Jones & Bartlett.

Boykin, A. (1994). *Living a caring-based program.* New York, NY: National League for Nursing Press.

Butler-Kisber, L. (2010). *Qualitative inquiry: Thematic, narrative, and arts-informed perspectives.* Thousand Oaks, CA: Sage.

Caine, V., & Steeves, P. (2009, September 29). Imagining and playfulness in narrative inquiry. *International Journal of Education & the Arts, 10*(25), 1–14. Retrieved from http://www.ijea.org/v10n25

Cangelosi, P. R., Crocker, S., & Sorrell, J. M. (2009, November/December). Expert to novice: Clinicians learning new roles as clinical nurse educators. *Nursing Education Perspectives, 30,* 367–371.

Carper, B. A. (1978). Fundamental patterns of knowing in nursing. *Advances in Nursing Science, 1,* 13–23. Retrieved from https://journals.lww.com/advancesinnursingscience/Citation/1978/10000/Fundamental_Patterns_of_Knowing_in_Nursing.4.aspx

Casey, B. (2009). Arts-based inquiry in nursing education. *Contemporary Nurse, 32*(1–2), 69–82.

Chinn, P. L., & Watson, J. (Eds.). (1994). *Art and aesthetics in nursing* (pp. 19–40). New York, NY: National League of Nursing Press.

Clandinin, D. J., & Connelly, F. M. (2000). *Narrative inquiry: Experience and story in qualitative research.* San Francisco, CA: Jossey-Bass.

Clark, C. M. (2014, October 31). *Brock Lectureship.* Oklahoma City: Oklahoma State University Institute of Technology.

Clark, C. M., & Springer, P. J. (2010). Academic nurse leaders' role in fostering a culture of civility in nursing education. *Journal of Nursing Education, 49,* 319–325. doi:10.3928/01484834-20100224-01

Dalansky, M., & Moore, S. (2013). Quality and safety education for nurses: The key is systems thinking. *The Online Journal of Issues in Nursing: A Scholarly Journal of the American Nurses Association.* Retrieved from http://www.nursingworld.org/Quality-and-Safety-Education-for-Nurses.html

Dattilo, J., Brewer, M. K., & Streit, L. (2009, August). Voices of experience: Reflections of nurse educators. *The Journal of Continuing Education in Nursing, 40,* 367–370. doi:10.3928/00220124-20090723-02

Davidson, A. W., & Topolski, S. (2011). Theoretical issues and methods for increasing understanding of complex health care systems. In A. W. Davidson, M. A. Ray, & M. C. Turkel (Eds.), *Nursing, caring, and complexity science for human-environment well-being* (pp. 61–94). New York, NY: Springer Publishing.

Diekelmann, N., & Diekelmann, J. (2009). *Schooling learning teaching: Toward narrative pedagogy.* Bloomington, IN: iUniverse.

Dossey, B. M. (2009). Theory of integral nursing. *Advances in Nursing Science, 31*(1), E52–E73. doi:10.1097/01.ANS.0000311536.11683.0a

Dystrophic Epidermolysis Bullosa Research Association of America. (2017). Home page. Retrieved from http://www.debra.org

Freire, P. (1972). *Pedagogy of the oppressed.* London, UK: Penguin Books.

Hills, M., & Watson, J. (2011). *Creating a caring science curriculum: An emancipatory pedagogy for nursing.* New York, NY: Springer Publishing.

hooks, b. (1999). Embracing freedom: Spirituality and liberation. In Glazer (Ed.), *The heart of learning: Spirituality in education* (113–129). New York, NY: Tarcher/Putnam.

Institute of Medicine. (2001). *Crossing the quality chasm: A new health system for the 21st century.* Washington, DC: National Academies Press.

Institute of Medicine. (2003). *Health professions education: A bridge to quality.* Washington, DC: National Academies Press.

Ironside, P. M. (2001, March). Creating a research base for nursing education: An interpretive review of conventional, critical, feminist, postmodern, and phenomenologic pedagogies. *Advances in Nursing Science, 23*(3), 72–87. Retrieved from https://journals.lww.com/advancesinnursingscience/Abstract/2001/03000/Creating_a_Research_Base_for_Nursing_Education__An.7.aspx

Lakoff, G., & Johnson, M. (Eds.). (1980). *Metaphors we live by* (pp. 224–235). Chicago, IL: University of Chicago Press.

Lindsay, G. (2006). Experiencing nursing education research: Narrative inquiry and interpretive phenomenology. *Nurse Researcher, 13,* 30–47. doi:10.7748/nr2006.07.13.4.30.c5988

Lindsay, G. (2008). Thinking narratively: Artificial persons in nursing and healthcare. *Nurse Education Today, 28,* 348–353. doi:10.1016/j.nedt.2007.06.009

Lindsay, G. (2011). Patterns of inquiry: Curriculum as life experience. *Nursing Science Quarterly, 24,* 237–244. doi:10.1177/0894318411409422

Luparell, S. (2011). Incivility in nursing: The connection between academia and clinical settings. *Critical Care Nurse, 31*(2), 92–95. doi:10.4037/ccn2011171

McCraty, R. (2001). Introduction to HeartMath. Retrieved from http://www.heartmath.org/research/science-of-the-heart/introduction.html

McCraty, R. (2015). *Science of the heart: Exploring the role of the heart in human performance.* Boulder Creek, CA: HeartMath Institute.

McCraty, R., Bradley, R., & Tomasino, D. (2005). The resonant heart. *Shift: At the Frontiers of Consciousness,* (5), 15–19. Retrieved from https://www.heartmath.org/assets/uploads/2015/01/the-resonant-heart.pdf

McCraty, R., & Childre, D. (2010, July/August). Coherence: Bridging personal, social, and global health. *Alternative Therapies in Health and Medicine, 16*(4), 10–24. Retrieved from https://www.heartmath.org/assets/uploads/2015/01/coherence-bridging-personal-social-global-health.pdf

Noddings, N. (1984). *Awakening the inner eye: Intuition in education.* New York, NY: Teachers College Press.

Noddings, N. (1992). *The challenge to care in schools: An alternative approach to education.* New York, NY: Teachers College Press.

Palmer, P. (1987). *The courage to teach: Exploring the inner landscape of a teacher's life.* San Francisco, CA: Jossey-Bass.

Palmer, P. (1999). The grace of great things: Reclaiming the sacred in knowing, teaching, and learning. In S. Glazer (Ed.), *The heart of learning: Spirituality in education* (pp. 15–32). New York, NY: Penguin Putnam.

Pearsall, P. (1998). *The heart's code: Tapping into the wisdom and power of our heart energy.* New York, NY: Broadway Books.

Reverby, S. (1987). *Ordered to care: The dilemma of American nursing, 1850-1945.* New York, NY: Cambridge University Press.

Sherwood, G. D., & Horton-Deutsch, S. (2012). Attention to self as nurse: Making sense of practice. In G. D. Sherwood & S. Horton-Deutsch (Eds.), *Reflective practice: Transforming education and improving outcomes* (pp. 189–210). Indianapolis, IN: Sigma Theta Tau International.

Simmons, N., & Daley, S. (2013, July 6). The art of thinking: Using collage to stimulate scholarly work. *Canadian Journal for the Scholarship of Teaching and Learning, 4*(1), 1–11. doi:10.5206/cjsotl-rcacea.2013.1.4

Smith, M. C., Zahourek, R., Hines, M. E., Engebretson, J., & Wardell, D. W. (2013, September). Holistic nurses' stories of personal healing. *Journal of Holistic Nursing, 31,* 173–187. doi:10.1177/0898010113477254

Tenzin Gyatso (The 14th Dalai Lama). (1999). Education and the human heart. In S. Glazer (Ed.), *The heart of learning: Spirituality in education* (pp. 85–95). New York, NY: Tarcher/Putnam.

Vitali, N. (2017). *Nursing faculty experience of teaching from the heart.* (Unpublished doctoral dissertation). Watson Caring Science Institute, Boulder, CO.

Watson, J. (2008). *Nursing: The philosophy and science of caring* (Rev. ed.). Boulder: The University Press of Colorado.

Watson, J., & Smith, M. C. (2002). Caring science and the science of unitary human beings: A Transtheoretical discourse for nursing knowledge development. *Journal of Advanced Nursing, 37*(5), 452–461. doi:10.1046/j.1365-2648.2002.02112.x

17

Developing Values and Philosophies of Being

Lisa Lally Flack and Donnean Thrall

CARITAS LITERACIES

By the end of this chapter, the caring-healing nurse will be able to

1. Examine the evolution of caring in nursing and nursing curricula.

2. Explore philosophies and theories of being and becoming that anchor a Caring Science curriculum.

3. Understand how alternative educational pedagogies support the values of a Caring Science curriculum.

4. Summarize the ways in which a Caring Science curriculum can help nurses develop Caring Literacies through various classroom pedagogies, development of a community of caring/learning, and self-care.

5. Identify ways to embody (through being/becoming) Caritas Literacies in nursing education to promote the development of caring-healing nurses.

❧

Drop a Pebble in the Water

Drop a pebble in the water: just a splash, and it is gone;
But there's half-a-hundred ripples circling on and on and on,
Spreading, spreading from the center, flowing on out to the sea.
And there is no way of telling where the end is going to be.

Drop a pebble in the water: in a minute you forget,
But there's little waves a-flowing, and there's ripples circling yet,

And those little waves a-flowing to a great big wave have grown;
You've disturbed a mighty river just by dropping in a stone.

Drop an unkind word, or careless: in a minute it is gone;
But there's half-a-hundred ripples circling on and on and on.
They keep spreading, spreading, spreading from the center as they go,
And there is no way to stop them, once you've started them to flow.

Drop an unkind word, or careless: in a minute you forget;
But there's little waves a-flowing, and there's ripples circling yet,
And perhaps in some sad heart a mighty wave of tears you've stirred,
And disturbed a life was happy ere you dropped that unkind word.

Drop a word of cheer and kindness: just a flash and it is gone;
But there's half-a-hundred ripples circling on and on and on,
Bearing hope and joy and comfort on each splashing, dashing wave
Till you wouldn't believe the volume of the one kind word you gave.

Drop a word of cheer and kindness: in a minute you forget;
But there's gladness still a-swelling, and there's joy circling yet,
And you've rolled a wave of comfort whose sweet music can be heard
Over miles and miles of water just by dropping one kind word. (Foley, 1911/2009, pp. 17–18)

Developing values and philosophies of "being" is a critical component of a caring-healing nurse. Dr. Lisa Lally Flack and Dr. Donnean Thrall started a new RN-to-BS program at Siena College in upstate New York, providing a unique opportunity to create a curriculum based fully on the philosophy of Caring Science. As postdoctoral scholars working with Dr. Jean Watson at the Watson Caring Science Institute, the authors' goal as nurse educators is to expand the reach of Caring Science and to advance research on Caring Science in nursing education. The authors, being fully immersed in the work of Caring Science, are focused on creating a nursing program focused on developing nurses who embody a culture of caring. Dr. Watson beautifully articulates this philosophy when she states, "It is ironic that nursing education and practice require so much knowledge and skill to *do* the job, but very little effort is directed toward developing how to *Be* while doing the real work of the job" (Watson, 2008, p. 47). In infusing Caring Science throughout the curriculum, the authors are developing Caritas Literacy and Caritas Consciousness among graduates. What often seems as if dropping a pebble into the water to make a wave in the nursing profession, the authors felt what better place to start the tide of change than from within a nursing curriculum that models and brings caring to the front and center of its mission.

Siena College is a Franciscan institution, and the mission of the college and the nursing program align and complement each other. The college's commitment to service, compassion, diversity, breadth of experience, and dignity of the human experience prepares a registered nurse in his or her profession. The Franciscan mission of the college fully mirrors the nursing profession through service and care of others. As St. Francis of Assisi was known for providing loving care to lepers and breaking down barriers caring for a vulnerable population, the inclusion of nursing at a Franciscan College is a clear extension of the mission, "This is our vocation; to heal wounds, to bind what is broken, to bring home those who are lost" (St. Francis of Assisi, from Legend of the Three Companions.) As the Franciscan Friars further explain:

> Franciscan education has as much to do with opening the *heart* to love, as it does with opening the mind to truth. It values interpersonal skills as much as intellectual abilities. It defines human flourishing, not in terms of how much one gains for oneself, but how much one gives of oneself to others. (Friars of Siena College, 2012, p. 5)

Furthermore, in the Franciscan tradition, leadership has been described as an encounter with those other than our own "tribe" in a manner that awakens our empathy and compassion and enlarges our sense of belonging, power, and hope. This leads to a shift from "us versus them" to "we." In nursing, we are in a unique position to be servant leaders who bring caring and compassion to those we serve. Watson (2012) describes nurses as having a social and ethical responsibility to be guardians of human caring, stating, "If nursing does not fulfill its societal mandate for sustaining human caring, preserving human dignity and humanness in self, systems, and society, it will not be carrying out its covenant to humankind and its reason for existence as a profession" (p. 42).

The Department of Nursing created a mission statement to this end that integrates both Franciscan ideals and Caring Science philosophies:

> It is the mission of the Department of Nursing to co-create a community of learning that fosters an engaged heart in the process of transpersonal human caring. This is realized through our commitment to living a caring science curriculum.
>
> We embrace Siena College's core Franciscan values to create lifelong learners, compassionate leaders, and innovative professionals.
>
> We honor the unique lived experience of all people, including the student and faculty. Caring for self is integral to this process, and we believe this supports the development of effective, compassionate, and authentic practitioners.
>
> We are dedicated to graduating students who embrace servant leadership by partnering with our community to promote health through advocacy and service.
>
> The experience of a caring science curriculum results in graduates who are full partners on the healthcare team and who uphold the ethical, moral, and professional responsibilities within the discipline of nursing to be guardians of human caring. (Siena College, 2017)

General information about the Baldwin Nursing Program is given as follows and is also available on the college's website: www.siena.edu/programs/nursing

---

Baldwin Nursing Program at Siena College, Loudonville, NY

The nursing program at Siena College began in 2016 with the development and approval of a bachelor of science degree in nursing. The first program approved was the RN to BS Nursing program. This program is a hybrid program where nurses come to campus one-day per week to take both nursing and liberal arts coursework. Currently, we have over 20 students in the program. This past year, we developed and received approval for our Dual Degree Nursing Program established in 2017. This is a unique collaboration between an associate degree nursing program and Siena College to create a seamless pathway for students to earn their bachelor of science degree in nursing. In our inaugural year, we will have 25 students attending as freshmen.

Both our tracks to a bachelor of science degree in nursing have been created with a Caring Science philosophy. During our first year with the RN to BS nursing students, this has shown to be not only effective but life-changing for them.

For more information about our Nursing Department, please visit www.siena.edu/nursing

---

This chapter reviews the evolution of caring in nursing and nursing curricula over the years. The philosophical framework of Caring Science is discussed and the authors share their own pedagogical methods used to create an environment that embodies caring in nursing education. The meaning and values of being and becoming a nurse grounded in Caring Science are also discussed. Finally, the authors propose the many benefits of framing a nursing curriculum in Caring Science, including student affirmations of this process.

EVOLUTION OF CARING IN NURSING AND NURSING CURRICULA

Almost 30 years ago, as part of the Curriculum Revolution, nursing educators engaged in a shared dialogue about the future of nursing education. These pioneering educators argued for a shift away from the dominant behaviorist paradigm in nursing education to one that advances research-based, alternative pedagogies (Diekelmann, Ironside, & Gunn, 2005). This call for innovation and reform lives on today, specifically with a continued need for a paradigm shift from a content-laden curriculum to one more focused on the in-depth study of key concepts of nursing framed within a nursing rather than a biomedical model (Benner, Sutphen, Leonard, & Day, 2009; National League for Nursing, 2003). The scholars of the curriculum revolution called for a *caring* curriculum using new pedagogies suited for a practice discipline, one capable of developing nurses who could be leaders in healthcare reform (Tanner, 2007).

The work of early nursing theorists such as Madeleine Leininger and Jean Watson laid the groundwork for the development of today's focus on caring in nursing curricula and praxis. Leininger (1978) identified caring as the essence of nursing and a dominant component of the profession, and Watson (1979/1985) proposed that nursing is the art and science of human caring. She goes on to describe nursing is a discipline, which incorporates not only empirical knowledge but also aesthetic, personal, spiritual, moral, and ethical knowing. As Watson (2012) states:

> This sense of a caring moment, caring is a moral ideal rather than an interpersonal technique … it entails a commitment to a particular end. The end is the protection, enhancement, and preservation of the person's humanity and human dignity, which helps to restore inner harmony, wholeness, and potential healing. (p. 71)

This unitary worldview of nursing integrates all ways of knowing and caring-healing practices within healthcare. It is essential that the discipline of nursing identifies our science as the phenomena of human caring and human health-illness experience for all (Hills & Watson, 2011). This encompasses an ethical and moral responsibility to sustain nursing's global covenant with humanity to ensure human caring-healing-health for all (Watson, 2017).

Inspired by Caring Science scholars and the curriculum revolutionaries, the authors are striving to make a paradigm shift by ensuring that students engage in a spirit of inquiry and are able to identify what nursing knowledge is and how this knowledge can be integrated into a healthcare system heavily dominated by the medical model. We seek to advance disciplinary clarity in nursing through the development of a Caring Science curriculum. As Nightingale (1860) first asserted, we hope to contribute to sustaining the future of nursing by graduating nurses who can speak to what nursing knowledge *is* and *what it is not* in a new era where caring is first and foremost the central focus of the discipline of nursing. Barrett (2017) contends "it is time to claim that what nurses do is based on what nurses know, and the essence of this broad knowledge is education in discipline-specific nursing knowledge" (p. 129). The authors hope that this integration of a caring-based curriculum at Siena will support a foundation to guide the nursing profession and the professional from the inside out rather than the outside in, grounded in the discipline of nursing.

DEVELOPMENT OF CARING SCIENCE NURSES THROUGH THE EXPERIENCE OF A CARING SCIENCE CURRICULUM

Developing caring-healing nurses within the framework of a Caring Science curriculum, the following principles of a caring adult learning environment are critical. A Caring Science teaching-learning philosophy creates a sense of being cared for and in turn nurtures both the students' and the faculty's ability to care for others. It is important to respect, foster, and celebrate each person's unique lived experience and contributions to the learning community. In doing so, the authors believe this will enhance each student's ability to find his or her own voice within the discipline of nursing. Caring Science nursing education is more emancipatory by a relationship built on shared learning and equalism where dialogue and discourse on assumptions are the norm so that the process of learning is valued over the outcome of learning (Hills & Watson, 2011). This education values the voice of students and guides them to develop confidence so they can have a strong voice to advocate for their patients and themselves to further the profession of nursing. This section addresses the facets of the Siena College Nursing Department's Caring Science curriculum and its theoretical underpinnings. The topics of civility, hierarchical structure, cocreation of a community of caring in the classroom, teaching-learning methods, and self-care are addressed.

CIVILITY

Creating a caring environment for nursing students begins with a discussion of civility in the classroom, among and between all parties in the educational setting including student to student, student to faculty, faculty to student, and faculty to faculty. Drawing on Clark's (2013a) work on civility in nursing, students and faculty at Siena explore ways in which a change from a predominately negative paradigm can be shifted to one of mutual respect and shared learning, not only in the classroom but also extending into the clinical settings. Clark (2013b) describes the five "RITES" of civility acronymically: "**R**aise awareness and expose effects of incivility; **I**nspire action and catalyze change; **T**ake responsibility for creating civility; **E**ngage and commit to personal and organizational change and **S**ustain results and generate more change" (p. 1). During the first class of the RN-to-BS program, students read Clark's article and complete a self-reflection on their own civility toward others. This leads to a discussion board where students share the process of their self-reflection, and the impact incivility has had on them, their patients, and their workplace. The common theme that resonates from the stories the nurses tell is how they have witnessed and been part of incivility, but realize that they can stop this cycle by their own awareness and actions. Introducing this critical concept and modeling civility in the classroom establishes a framework grounded in a caring philosophy in nursing that hopefully will find a translation into the workplace.

HIERARCHICAL STRUCTURE

Breaking down the hierarchical structure within the classroom is one of the main tenets of a Caring Science pedagogy (Hills & Watson, 2011). This pedagogy is essential to extend beyond the conventional behaviorist pedagogies of nursing education that have traditionally been used. Reducing oppression in the classroom and nursing as a profession can begin a process of liberation and emancipation. A caring, humanistic curriculum whereby the students are active learners and partners with their teachers allows for a liberating experience. De Lissovoy (2010) argues that making the human connection between the student and the teacher leads to liberation. He goes on to say, "teaching, then, is a work on being and the invention of possibility of an authentic encounter between beings outside of domination" (p. 208). In this environment, education is shared, and the dominance of the teacher relationship turns to negotiation. Freire (1970) spoke of the movement of education in the classroom away from the "banking concept" where the teacher directs learning and the student is a depository of information, toward a reciprocal relationship of bidirectionality between the teacher and the student. Freire proposed that this type of education would fulfill a love of life through the cultivation of personal being as one becomes with the work and not of it. Education such as this will liberate the student by practicing freedom and emancipation as opposed to domination (Freire, 1970).

Feminist pedagogy supports these ideals from Freire and De Lissovoy where the relationship within the classroom is participatory and liberating with power being shared. Chinn (1989) articulates this in nursing as feminist praxis that rejects the notion of "power over" and seeks to empower the nurse in the educational process. Chinn further explains that both faculty and students share responsibility for learning in the classroom. A faculty member has a responsibility to decrease the fear of the unknown (grading, assignments, etc.) and demystify the processes involved in all planned activities (Chinn, 1989). The notion of power as creative energy and potential rather than domination is one that is central to this concept. This leads to empowerment in the classroom and allows for the students to claim their education for themselves, generating opportunities for growth and, ultimately, leading to the students' ability to find their own voices (Shrewsbury, 1993).

The authors agree with Hills and Watson (2011) when they declare that, although the authority of the faculty members is acknowledged by virtue of their role/position, they should be in no way authoritarian in their approach to teaching-learning. Their authority is used to increase the power and voice of all. Authentic power is shared power; it is power with, not power over (Hills & Watson, 2011). The teacher becomes a role model to help the class become a community of learners with a shared vision and understanding of the purpose of the classroom, one that will ultimately lead to a similar philosophical shift outside the classroom (Shrewsbury, 1993).

To create a Caring Science classroom that embodies these philosophies and values of being, one must be explicit in defining what this classroom experience is. Nurses have often felt exposed and vulnerable in their education and practice settings, faced with an environment on the basis of a hierarchical, oppressive, and authoritarian culture. Freire (1970) describes this environment as being one in which oppression occurs on the basis of power, and, in this case, the power of an educator to an educatee. In nursing, this notion has been used to explain horizontal violence and bullying that occur when "nurses eat their young." Bevis (1989) has explained historically how nurses have been an oppressed group with more division than union both academically and in practice. She goes on to say that "we are almost more ready to fight each other than to unite against a common threat" (Bevis, 1989, p. 115). As Hills and Watson (2011) eloquently state, "One way to overcome this negativity and to live a culture of caring is to choose to be *in power with relationships*" (p. 130). Traditional nursing education has lived a power-over relationship with students, leading to a more oppressive learning environment for far too long. When this shifts to a notion of shared power and a relational perspective, a caring culture begins within an emancipatory relational pedagogy (Hills & Watson, 2011).

A Caring Science philosophy exposes this traditional nursing education paradigm and seeks to begin the process of changing the culture. When students enter into the RN-to-BS program, they are not expecting an emancipatory learning experience. Instead, students enter the program from within the context of their prior experiences, portraying fearfulness, and are guarded about the educational process. The environment created at Siena allays their concerns and students find that the traditional culture they are familiar with is not part of a Caring Science classroom.

COCREATING A COMMUNITY OF CARING IN THE CLASSROOM

Physical Environment. Beginning with the desk formation in a circle, students enter the classroom noticing immediately that there is no beginning or end, no front or back, and no one person is the center of focus. Although this may be a simplistic way to describe the equalization of power, a Socratic seminar-style classroom creates a constructivist approach to the process of teaching-learning where all participants are equal, sharing experiences and voice. The Socratic seminar motivates students to build a dialogue that encourages them to question their thinking and remain open to the viewpoints of others. This in turn enhances critical thinking and problem solving and enhances students' own values (Cojocariu & Butnaru, 2014).

The tenets of a Caring Science philosophy are shared during orientation at Siena, and a community of caring is cocreated. There is an opportunity for students and faculty to reflect on previous academic and workplace experiences and how these experiences might have been different from or similar to the Siena caring philosophy. Students and faculty dialogue about the importance of a cocreated learning approach and students begin to express feelings of welcome and acceptance. Metaphorically speaking, students embrace this with open arms and are no longer guarded and ready to fight. We have created a "blessing of the hands," used during orientation to further welcome students into the Siena community. Lavender oil is placed on each student's hand, and together we say: "May your hands and heart bring comfort and promote healing to the mind, body, and spirit. May you radiate love, compassion and a spirit of inquiry. You are welcomed into Siena's community of caring."

To further enhance the caring environment, each class starts with sharing a centering meditation. Caring for self is integral to a Caring Science philosophy and in the nursing program at Siena, we recognize the busyness of all of our lives and take 3 to 5 minutes to practice a mindful meditation. As Kabat-Zinn (2012) explains, "Mindfulness is awareness, cultivated by paying attention in a sustained and particular way: on purpose, in the present moment, and nonjudgmentally" (p. 1). Introduction of mindfulness and centering in the classroom creates a calming environment where the students and faculty can take a moment to become fully present in the classroom. Watson (2008) posits that in the midst of our busy pace, the simple act of connecting with that "still point" we all have deep inside can change our consciousness and allow us to be more present to whatever is in front of us to do/be. Students in the nursing program are working nurses, going to school as well as caring for their families. For some of them, this is the first time experiencing a centering activity, and they appreciate the opportunity to decompress and refocus on their classes. Calming essential oil aromatherapy is also present in the classroom. Although this is subtle, it is also another way to decrease stress and anxiety to promote wellness and ease in the classroom. In the nursing classroom/community room, tea and coffee are readily available, and students often bring in healthy snacks to share. This setting creates a comfortable environment for the students to feel respected while also enhancing an overall sense of community.

The Flexibility of Assignments. Part of the community of caring includes the cocreation of the class by both the students and the faculty. One aspect of this Caring Science philosophy from which students have expressed great benefit is the program's flexibility in due dates for assignments. It is a tremendous juggling act for a nurse to return to school while working and, for many, taking care of a family. A weekly check-in at the beginning and end of each class is done to see how everyone is handling the workload and if any adjustments are needed. The faculty member holds ultimate responsibility for curriculum design and creates the course syllabus and schedule of assignments at the beginning of the semester as he or she would for any college course. The students and faculty then discuss any changes that might be necessary for the students to complete the coursework without causing them or the faculty member great distress along the way. A simple change of moving an assignment, paper, or test ahead a day or even a week can be the difference between rushed performance and glossing over the material and greater depth in learning. The overall experience with this approach has been positive, and students have not taken advantage of this method or become complacent with due dates. Students recognize that the due date that is decided upon is the date by which they need to complete the work to be considered on time. Providing this level of flexibility and cocreation of the learning environment in the educational process supports the Caring Science philosophy including the importance of self-care and having life balance.

Caritas Community Discussion Board. One example of fostering open communication between faculty and students is through the use of a discussion board within the learning management system. The Caritas Community discussion board is designed for students to have a safe place to discuss curricular questions, concerns, updates, and so on. This discussion board is located in every course shell and is monitored by both the faculty and the students. When a student has a question about an assignment or other class activity, he or she is encouraged to use this forum to post his or her question so that all course members can benefit from hearing the answers and updates from the instructor and other students. The program is rich with individuals who bring diverse nursing experience to the class, and within this Caritas Community discussion board, they support and encourage each other. This forum provides much-needed clarity to course concerns and builds community, and important information can be referred back to easily by everyone.

TEACHING-LEARNING METHODS

Because *how* we teach is as critical as *what* we teach (Sherwood & Horton-Deutsch, 2012), nursing classes are structured around conventional pedagogies as well as case-based learning, video vignettes, activities, dialogue/storytelling, and a reflective approach to inquiry. This mix of instructional design and delivery methods allows for the structure necessary to meet accreditation standards while advancing the Nursing Department's Caring Science philosophy. For example, the use of narrative pedagogy within the Caring Science framework helps students develop their interpretive skills and seek new ways to understand experiences from multiple perspectives (Ironside & Hayden-Miles, 2012). Narrative pedagogy focuses on exploring multiple ways of knowing, thinking, and interpreting as central to understanding the nature of experiences (Diekelmann, 2001).

All classes in the RN-to-BS program meet 1 day a week face-to-face and have an online component for 30% to 50% of class time. The program is delivered in a hybrid format, so there is an even greater opportunity to hear the voices of each student through online discussion forums and other activities. This method helps develop the student's ability to analyze a topic, explore its meaning, and hear the experiences and opinions of others as a way of developing a spirit of inquiry that is so critical to nursing praxis. According to Chinn

(2007), there are many advantages to online teaching and learning that support the use of feminist pedagogies. In the online environment, every individual has equal access to speaking without interruption; students who may be silenced in the face-to-face classroom can find their voice and are more able to speak their own truth online in ways they might be less comfortable to speak face-to-face (Chinn, 2007).

SELF-CARE

After experiencing some of the many aspects of self-care that the nursing program offers throughout the semester, students have begun to recognize the importance of caring for self and have shown personal growth and development in this area. Many students have never experienced or even considered it important to their lived experience as a nurse. Caring for self is an integral component of Caring Science philosophy and a core concept of Watson's Theory of Human Caring/Caring Science, "We need to love, respect, care for ourselves, and treat ourselves with dignity, before we can respect, love, and care for others and treat them with dignity" (Watson, 1988, p. 51). Nurses must both provide physical care and truly *care for* each person/client they encounter. It is critically important to care for oneself to become effective, compassionate, and caring practitioners. Therefore, it is imperative that nurses take care of themselves to effectively care for others. In Caritas Process® 1: *Cultivating the practice of loving-kindness, compassion, and equanimity toward self and other as foundational to Caritas consciousness*, Watson (2008) invites nurses to recognize the importance of caring for self; she states, "Nurses often become pained and worn down by trying to always care, give and be there for others without attending to the loving care needed for self" (p. 47). She further invites nurses "to attend to self-caring and practices that assist in their own evolution of consciousness for more fulfillment in their life and work" (p. 47).

The Siena nursing program embeds this concept of self-care into the nursing curriculum providing opportunities for both the students and the faculty to engage in self-care activities such as meditation, yoga, mindfulness, and integrative healing practices. To promote more opportunities for self-care, for example, a low-impact, 30-minute yoga class taught by a college yoga instructor is offered each day during a free period. This opportunity allows the students time to take care of themselves during a busy day. Now students who have never participated in a yoga class are taking this short class to relax, stretch, and decompress.

Students learn about self-care during their first nursing course at the college. As part of their curriculum, students read *The Art of Extreme Self-Care* (Richardson, 2009). This book is used for students to begin the journey of their own self-care. On the basis of their personal interest, they choose one chapter to read and practice each month. Using journaling and reflection, students write about their experiences that culminate in a self-reflection paper and a self-care plan that is submitted at the end of the semester. This experience has been shown to raise awareness of the simple ways we can care for ourselves and the importance of doing so. As one student reflected:

One way I have taken time for myself personally is by utilizing the small moments while washing my hands forcing myself to have a calm moment in the midst of chaos. This gives me a moment to collect myself and move forward with the tasks at hand. (Student 1, self-caring reflection, December 2016)

Another student shares:

> The emphasis put on self-care in this class has made me rethink how I let myself fall second or third or last in line to all the other demands in life. It has helped me realize how important caring for oneself is in shaping how we are then able to care for others. (Student 2, self-caring reflection, December 2016)

Changes in students' perceptions of caring and self-care throughout the semester are notable, and the faculty at Siena have witnessed an increase in self-care practices and students often encourage their classmates and faculty to do the same.

THE MEANING AND VALUE OF BEING/BECOMING A CARING SCIENCE NURSE

Through a Caring Science philosophy of nursing education, students experience how caring is central to nursing and themselves. Watson's theory recognizes that in the "transpersonal caring moment," both the person cared for and the caregiver are affected by every interaction. During the process, both the nurse and the patient experience "being and becoming" through a caring–healing relationship (Watson, 2008). During the first year of the Siena program, the level of both personal and professional student growth in caring has been significant and can be seen in student caring reflections. As part of their self-reflection activity at the end of the semester, the students wrote about ways in which caring was reframed in their lives. Some examples of student caring reflections are as follows:

> One of the meditations we listened to by Jean Watson was especially eye-opening for me. She spoke about how we need to be in that moment with that patient. How it is our privilege to be there and that it can affect us as much as it affects the patient. This has been a challenge to me to take a few extra seconds or minutes with each patient and try to focus on them in that moment. It has also helped me see that sometimes we are helped by a patient just as much as we are helping them. (Student 3, caring reflection, December 2016)

> I took to heart the caring in nursing practice. I feel my nursing practice has developed for the better because of this course. Working in a very busy department it's easy to lose sight of the actual patient and just focus on the problem or health concern. I have been making an attempt to slow down and actually listen to the patient and converse. Even when they call out for a blanket with three traumas rolling through the door, I provide the blanket with a smile because the patient experience should not suffer because of how busy we are. I feel reframing my culture of caring made me more tolerant and patient. It is still a work in progress, but I plan on continuing to evolve in my role of caring. I have noticed an effect in patient's attitudes. I was thanked by a few patients for just being nice when the nurses before me were hurried and short with the patient. The patients are definitely noticing our attitudes and behaviors. (Student 4, caring reflection, December 2016)

I had the unique experience this semester of studying nursing as a Caring Science at the same time as I assumed supervision of a hospice program. Whatever greater power there is gave me the gift of having this education when I needed it the most. The focus on care of the nurse along with the transpersonal caring philosophy of Jean Watson has given me language, nursing theory, and awareness of the importance of authentic presence in so many situations over the last 2 months. I have found that care of the staff and reminding them to care for themselves needs constant work within a group of nurses at high risk for both burnout and internalization of end of life stresses daily. I have tried to provide support to the nurses focusing on the quality of life they help build for the patient instead of the technical/physical aspects of the dying process … I am so grateful for being able to go to my notes from class and open the references materials to find ways to help [staff] using tools and wording such as "loving-kindness to yourself and others" … I see this class as a starting point with so much more to learn and I am very appreciative of the guiding presence that [faculty] have given us. (Student 5, caring reflection, May 2017)

These moments showcase the subtle and not so subtle changes that a Caring Science philosophy in education is creating. Part of this education is giving language to describe the caring moment/caring occasion, that simple human-to-human interaction that becomes a part of both individuals who experience it (Watson, 1988). Transpersonal caring moments that affect both the patient and the nurse give the motivation to continue the caring cycle. When a nurse is able to be authentic and give himself or herself in a fully present way, both the patient and the nurse benefit. It is through our interconnections with others that we grow and evolve (Watson, 2008). The Siena College Nursing Department seeks to teach the importance of these caring moments as the foundation of the discipline of nursing. Ideally, the integration of a Caring Science philosophy will generate a nursing workforce grounded in caring to sustain the future of nursing.

CONCLUSION

The Siena College nursing curriculum embraces the philosophical framework of Caring Science and emancipatory relational pedagogical methods that create an environment that embodies caring in nursing education. These teaching–learning processes begin with relationships that are built between the students and the faculty and are a key component to the success of this education. Collaborative, caring relationships in the academic setting must be made up of trust, caring, respect, and an equalization of power. Whether the students have been nurses for 2 months or 20 years, each of them brings his or her lived experiences and is integral to the cocreation of learning. The results of nurses being part of this environment can be life changing both personally and professionally. As Siena's nursing program continues on this journey, we are reminded that our efforts are supporting a tide of change in nursing education.

Drop a pebble in the water: in a minute you forget,
But there's little waves a-flowing, and there's ripples circling yet,
And those little waves a-flowing to a great big wave have grown;
You've disturbed a mighty river just by dropping in a stone. (Foley, 1911/2009, p. 17)

NEXT ERA POSSIBILITIES

Acknowledging that we have more work to do to advance our pedagogy with Caring Science, we are looking forward to continuing to broaden our view of teaching-learning and evaluation methods to more fully embrace this philosophy.

Education

- What are innovative ways of evaluating students that are congruent with this Caring Science paradigm?
- What are alternative pedagogies that can be integrated into our curriculum?

Research

- How does a Caring Science curriculum impact the caring behaviors of nursing students?
- What additional ways can the Theory of Human Caring and the Caritas Processes be applied to nursing education to retain a theoretical foundation grounded in the discipline of nursing?

Praxis

- How does a Caring Science education foster an expanded worldview of caring in the workplace?
- How does a Caring Science education foster transformation of self?

Theory and Knowledge Development

- What additional theoretical models will complement and inform existing Caring Science pedagogy to deepen our values and philosophies of being in nursing education?

 REFERENCES

Barrett, E. A. M. (2017). Again, what is nursing science? *Nursing Science Quarterly*, 30(2), 129–133. doi:10.1177/0894318417693313

Benner, P., Sutphen, M., Leonard, V., & Day, L. (2009). *Educating nurses: A call for radical transformation.* San Francisco, CA: Jossey-Bass.

Bevis, E. O. (1989). The curriculum consequences: Aftermath of revolution. *Curriculum revolution: Reconceptualizing nursing education* (3rd ed.). St. Louis, MO: Mosby.

Chinn, P. L. (1989). Feminist pedagogy and nursing education. In National League for Nursing (Ed.), *Curriculum revolution: Reconceptualizing nursing education* (pp. 9–24). New York, NY: Editor.

Chinn, P. (2007). Reflections on feminist pedagogy in nursing education. In P. M. Ironside (Ed.), *On revolutions and revolutionaries: 25 years of reform and innovation in nursing education* (pp. 155–161). New York, NY: National League for Nursing.

Clark, C. M. (2013a). *Creating and sustaining civility in nursing education.* Indianapolis, IN: Sigma Theta Tau International.

Clark, C. M. (2013b). Five-part series: Fostering civility in nursing education and practice. *Reflections on Nursing Leadership, 39*(1), Sigma Theta Tau International Part II — Cindy's "Five RITES" for fostering student-driven civility. Retrieved from http://www.reflectionsonnursingleadership.org/Pages/Vol39_1_Clark_5RITES.aspx

Cojocariu, V.-M., & Butnaru, C.-E. (2014). Asking questions: Critical thinking tools. *Procedia—Social and Behavioral Sciences, 128,* 22–28. doi:10.1016/j.sbspro.2014.03.112

De Lissovoy, N. (2010). Rethinking education and emancipation: Being, teaching, and power. *Harvard Educational Review*, 80(2), 203–221. doi:10.17763/haer.80.2.h6r65285tu252448

Diekelmann, N. L. (2001). Narrative pedagogy: Heideggerian hermeneutical analyses of lived experiences of students, teachers, and clinicians. *ANS. Advances in Nursing Science*, 23(3), 53–71. doi:10.1097/00012272-200103000-00006

Diekelmann, N. L., Ironside, P. M., & Gunn, J. (2005). Recalling the curriculum revolution: Innovation with research. *Nursing Education Perspectives*, 26(2), 70–77.

Foley, J. W. (2009). *The verses of James W. Foley: Book of life and laughter* (pp. 17–18). Charleston, SC: BiblioLife. (Original work published 1911)

Freire, P. (1970). *Pedagogy of the oppressed*. London, UK: Penguin Books.

Friars of Siena College. (2012). The seven tenets of Franciscan education at Siena College. Retrieved from https://community.siena.edu/assets/file_manager/insecure_file/Seven%20Tenets%20of%20Franciscan%20Education.pdf

Hills, M., & Watson, J. (2011). *Creating a caring science curriculum: An emancipatory pedagogy for nursing*. New York, NY: Springer Publishing.

Ironside, P. M., & Hayden-Miles, M. (2012). Narrative pedagogy: Co-creating engaging learning experiences with students. In G. D. Sherwood & S. Horton-Deutsch (Eds.), *Reflective practice: Transforming education and improving outcomes* (pp. 135–148). Indianapolis, IN: Sigma Theta Tau International.

Kabat-Zinn, J. (2012). *Mindfulness for beginners: Reclaiming the present moment—and your life*. Boulder, CO: Sounds True.

Leininger, M. (1978). *Transcultural nursing: Concepts, theories and practices*. New York, NY: John Wiley & Sons.

National League for Nursing. (2003). Innovation in nursing education: A call to reform. Retrieved from http://www.nln.org/docs/default-source/about/archived-position-statements/innovation-in-nursing-education-a-call-to-reform-pdf.pdf?sfvrsn=4

Nightingale, F. (1860). *Notes on nursing: What it is, and what it is not*. London, UK: Harrison.

Richardson, C. (2009). *The art of extreme self-care: Transform your life one month at a time*. New York, NY: Hay House.

Sherwood, G. D., & Horton-Deutsch, S. (2012). *Reflective practice: Transforming education and improving outcomes*. Indianapolis, IN: Sigma Theta Tau International.

Shrewsbury, C. M. (1993). What is feminist pedagogy? *Women's Studies Quarterly*, 15(3/4), 6–14. Retrieved from https://www.jstor.org/stable/40003432

Siena College. (2017). Baldwin nursing program: Mission statement. Retrieved from https://www.siena.edu/programs/nursing/mission/

Tanner, C. A. (2007). The curriculum revolution revisited. *Journal of Nursing Education*, 46(2), 51–52.

Watson, J. (1985). *Nursing: The philosophy and science of caring*. Plainsboro, NJ: Associated University Press. (Original work published 1979)

Watson, J. (1988). *Nursing: Human science and human care: A theory of nursing*. New York, NY: National League for Nursing.

Watson, J. (2008). *Nursing: The philosophy and science of caring*. Boulder: University Press of Colorado.

Watson, J. (2012). *Human Caring Science: A theory of nursing*. Sudbury, MA: Jones & Bartlett.

Watson, J. (2017, July 7). re: Discipline vs. Profession of Nursing. Unpublished Working Manuscript as Watson portion of AAN Expert Panel Draft Paper; shared with Watson Caring Science Postdoctoral Scholars Seminar. Boulder, Colorado.

18

Fostering Metamorphosis Through Caring Literacy in an RN-to-BSN Program

Mark D. Beck

CARITAS LITERACIES

By the end of this chapter, the caring-healing nurse will be able to

1. Describe the how the language of caring, compassion, and connection is foundational in creating a Caring Science pedagogy.

2. Describe strategies of connection in fostering Caritas Literacy within this RN-to-BSN population.

3. Describe the use of the affective domain as the entry point for engaging an emancipatory approach to the ways of being/knowing/becoming.

4. Explore the value of an emancipatory approach to Caring Science education in developing Caritas Literacy through the dialect.

❦

Do you have the patience to wait
Till your mud settles and the water is clear?
Can you remain unmoving
Till the right action arises by itself?
Lao Tzu Tao Te Ching (Mitchell, 1988, Chapter 15)

This chapter describes how a personal journey of embracing Caritas Literacy fostered metamorphosis in an RN-to-BSN curriculum with Caring Science as its theoretical foundation (Hills & Watson, 2011; Horton-Deutsch, 2017). This personal journey of transformation serves as a road map for others wishing to acquire the necessary attitudes, skills, and knowledge (ASK) necessary to embark on their own journey of transformation for the future of nursing. The journey invites sojourners who seek personal transformation as a vehicle for the most human of qualities, sensemaking, belonging, and remembering purpose (Biley, 2017; Madsbjerg, 2017; Watson, 2005a). In the current structure of nursing education, formation is done to them as in the assembly-line formation of a product (Bevis & Watson, 1989). This product is measured for quality, for example, by the passing of the National Council Licensure Examination (NCLEX)® or certification exams to ensure safety, and a baseline knowledge of a particular facet of nursing. This process is about the doing of nursing and not the becoming. Formation as a process of becoming requires the central actor and protagonist be the nurse and not the teacher (Day et al., 2017). This process requires the nurses to embark on their own hero's journey of self-discovery. The invitation in this program is for nurses to embark on their own hero's journey of metamorphosis (Campbell, 1949/2008).

INSPIRATION BY EINSTEIN, BROWN, AND CAMERON

The inspiration for change can come in many guises at differing times in life. This author's guidance in cocreating a Caring Science curriculum was found in the thinking of Albert Einstein. Four memorable sayings of Einstein's guided the thinking of this creation of a Caring Science curriculum. Einstein is mis-credited with defining insanity as "doing the same thing over and over again and expecting a different result." This was actually said by Rita Mae Brown in her book *Sudden Death* (1983). The saying has such allure and simplicity that it is no wonder of its mis-attribution (Calaprice, 2011). Nursing education as currently structured resembles the factory assembly-line output of nurses as product. Nursing education is not about formation but about production as product (nurses; Bevis & Watson, 1989). The industrial model of nursing education is represented in this axiom. Second, "Imagination is more important than knowledge; knowledge is finite, and imagination encircles the world" (www.brainyquote.com/authors/albert_einstein). Imagination is key to a vision of the future discipline and profession of nursing. The third saying is "You cannot solve a problem with the same consciousness that created it" (www.brainyquote.com/authors/albert_einstein). This begs the following question: What new consciousness is needed in nursing and how can it be cultivated? The consciousness that is informed by moral values, beliefs, and attitudes of the discipline becomes nursing praxis, and informs the profession that is ever changing (Watson, 2017). Finally, perhaps the most important mis-attributed quote to Einstein: "Not everything that is counted counts; not everything that counts can be counted." This was actually stated by the sociologist William Bruce Cameron in a paper delivered to the National Education Association (Cameron, 1958). Does the discipline of nursing measure the right things? What are they? How do these measurements help with encountering the human in nursing praxis? This constellation of these sayings informs the gestalt in cocreating a curriculum with other faculty, students, and the program director.

CONTEXT

The author, who is a Caritas Coach™ (someone who has completed a 6-month deep reflective dive into the transformative power of Caring Science), was recruited as a faculty member to assist in designing a newly minted RN-to-BSN program at a Bay Area school of nursing (SoN) in California. The existing program was initially patterned after the prelicensure program that was already part of the SoN. The university recruited this faculty member specifically for his knowledge, skills, and attitude (KSA) grounded in Caring Science. This RN-to-BSN program was the first designed at this university with a formal theoretical framework as its core.

A hero's journey of self-discovery served as the platform for reimagining the existing prelicensure courses and curriculum. Caring Science at its core is all about self-discovery (Downing, 2017; Godkin, 2001; Rosa, 2016; Sandvik, Eriksson, & Hilli, 2015; Touhy & Boykin, 2008). The author's journey of self-discovery in caring for self and the insights gleaned from this journey provided the road map for the reimagining of the leadership and nursing science series.

The RN-to-BSN nursing program consists of five 15-week semesters and 30 Carnegie units, and is approximately 20 months in duration. This program differed from the previous prelicensure program in three significant ways. The first term included a mindfulness-based stress reduction (MBSR) course on the basis of the University of Massachusetts, Amherst, course (Kang, Choi, & Ryu, 2009; Song & Lindquist, 2015; Wang et al., 2017). The course initiated a different tone to the nursing program by placing value on the self-care and well-being of the nursing student. The leadership course, an existing prelicensure course, was redesigned to extend over four of the five terms rather than one and focused on quality, safety informatics, and leadership. Thematically, the leadership series courses tackled transforming the relationship with self, transforming the relationship with other, transforming the relationship with the healthcare team, and, finally, transforming the relationship with organization or system. Foundational for this series was the work of Duffy (2013) noting the relationship of quality care to the quality of relationships (Duffy, 2013; Duffy & Hoskins, 2003). Third, additional redesign of **Patho-P**harmacology and **P**hysical assessment (3Ps) courses was reimagined as a nursing science series over three of the five terms. Thematically, the series was about creating a self-directed, self-identified learning plan for two areas of need in the student's working environments.

A WHOLE NEW NURSE

The industrialization or the factory assembly-line process of nursing education is outdated and is badly in need of an upgrade (Lee & Fawcett, 2013). This upgrade comes in the form of a Whole New Nurse, on the basis of Daniel Pink's 2005 work *A Whole New Mind*. Pink adeptly illuminates the trends that the profession of nursing is facing, that being of left-brained, algorithmic, and data-driven functions augmented by automation, and the availability of cheap outsourcing of labor in the developing world (Pink, 2005). Technology also plays a role in this outsourcing by the use of algorithms and software. The nursing profession has seen the exponential rise in the use of technology and the advent of nursing informatics as a specialty informed with its scope and standards of practice (American Nurses Association, 2015). Although nursing informatics lends a great deal of knowledge to the profession, nurses feel they spend more time with technology than with patients (Kolb, 2017).

Design, story, symphony, empathy, plan, and meaning are all attributes Pink (2005) assigns to the Whole New Nurse. These aspects became the threads used to develop the curriculum for the reimagined leadership and nursing science series for the

RN-to-BSN program at a Bay Area SoN. The following aspects were defined within this RN-to-BSN program:

- **Design**: Gap analysis individualized to the learner on his or her learning needs (nursing science series) designed by the learner (Reilly, Gallagher-Lepak, & Killion, 2012)

- **Story**: Learning to tell their stories so that they can bear witness to the story of another (nursing science-reflective journaling and leadership with reflective discussions; Ray & Turkel, 2014; Spadoni, Doane, Sevean, & Poole, 2015; Wheatley, 2017; Zender & Olshansky, 2012)

- **Symphony**: Understanding complexity theory and complex adaptive systems (CAS) within the context of biopsychosocial processes of both leadership and nursing science (Sandvik et al., 2015; Sheldrake, 2012; Weberg, 2012)

- **Empathy**: Using reflective discussions with responses to classmates in both leadership and nursing science (Neumann & Forsyth, 2008; Ondrejka, 2014; Parse, 2016; Prochaska & Velicer, 1997; Sandvik et al., 2015)

- **Play**: Emphasis on self-care practices and work-life balance (McCraty, 2001; McCraty & Childre, 2002)

- **Meaning**: Deep dive into the meaning of Caritas Processes® in their academic and work practices (Madsbjerg, 2017)

VALUE-ADDED PROPOSITION

The intention in using Caring Science as the framework for the RN-to-BSN curriculum was to create the value-added proposition (VAP). A VAP is that element of a service or product that distinguishes it from the rest of the pack (Sinek, 2009). The design team for the curriculum asked themselves the following: What distinguishes a graduate of this program from other RN-to-BSN programs? Why would an associate degree nurse (ADN) want to choose this program over the plethora of other available programs? Why would an employer want to employ a graduate of this program? After much deliberation, dialogue, and reflection, the answers came in four simple outcomes: (a) discover their vision in the future of nursing; (b) find their voice so that (c) they can tell their stories, which enables them (d) to own their practice.

DISCOVER THEIR VISION

The ADNs defined their job or work by the tasks they were doing or performed (Conner & Thielemann, 2013; Kolb, 2017). Their education has been focused on the requisite knowledge and skills (KS) to pass the NCLEX exam. Their employers value the tasks that are completed in a timely and efficient manner. When asked to articulate how they view themselves in the future of nursing, most answer in terms of specific jobs and employers. Defining their vision engages imagining what their futures look like and helps to define their goals and aspirations (Mead & Docker, 2017; Sinek, 2009). This is a key element in building the resilience to embark on the hero's journey of transformation (Campbell, 1949/2008).

FINDING THEIR VOICE

The voice of nurses at this level reflects the behavior of those in oppressed groups, which is to say "muted" (Freire, 1970/1993, 1997; Roberts, 2000). Finding that voice takes courage, self-awareness, and knowing personal boundaries (B. Brown, 2010, 2012, 2015, 2017; Wheatley, 2009). Boundaries is an essential function of all living organisms, *Homo sapiens sapiens* included (Wheatley, 2017). Developing that voice comes from the sense of self filling the boundaries of identity and the confidence that comes from knowing self (B. Brown, 2010). Lack of identity and voice shows up in the communication issues that plague the healthcare settings in conflict avoidance and accommodating prevalent styles by nurses (Gallison, 2012).

TELLING THEIR STORIES

Narrative pedagogy has become integral to much of medical education and in some nursing curricula (Charon, 2001; Ironside, 2014). Before nurses can attend to the story of another, they must first know and be able to articulate their own stories. This skill comes into awareness when nurses explore what it means to be authentically present (Godkin, 2001; Hickman, 2013). This skill requires the nurse to "be fully present" with the patients and their families. Being authentically present requires the nurses to know their boundaries, know and articulate their own stories to "be fully present," and honor or "bear witness" to the story of "other" (Brown, 2010, 2017; Duffy, 2013). Bearing witness to the story of other is sometimes the hardest part of the patient encounter, as it is "being with" and not "doing" in the fix-it modality in which most nurses live. If the nurse does not have a fully developed identity and understand his or her own story, the practice of authentic presence and bearing witness can be a very uncomfortable situation (Parse, 2016).

OWNING THEIR PRACTICE

Nurses who have imagined themselves in the future of nursing found their voice by accessing their power through the values, beliefs, and attitudes of their identity, are able to articulate their stories and can attend the story of other, and naturally and quite surreptitiously own their practice (Chinn & Kramer, 2015; Cowling & Chinn, 2001; Iacono & Altman, 2015). This process emerges as they gain emancipation from accessing their own power of identity that is aligned with the values, beliefs, and attitudes of the discipline of nursing (Jacobs, Fontana, Kehoe, Matarese, & Chinn, 2005; Ray & Turkel, 2014). This is the ultimate goal of nursing education (Donohue-Porter, Forbes, White, & Baumann, 2017; Hills & Watson, 2011).

DOING VERSUS BEING

The profession of nursing has been focused on the "doing" of procedures, protocols, policies, and now bundles (groupings of interventions focused around a set of objectives). This aspect of the profession has been emboldened by the pursuit of evidence-based practice (Melnyk & Fineout-Overholt, 2011). Doing has "value" in this culture of consumerism with its focus on return-on-investment (ROI). Doing can be measured, tracked, and placed in a dashboard for review by an administrator and have revenue attached to it. The current economics of nursing influence how "change" is measured and justified. The emphasis on empirical ways of knowing with its reliance on data-driven decision making validates the economics of change and ROI. This view is further validated by the magisterium of science's view of reductionism as the orthodox view of science and scientific knowing (Sheldrake, 2012). The epistemic view of the body as a machine is still the dominating metaphor in the nursing profession (Huether & McCance, 2017).

Ontological views from the discipline of nursing emphasizing ways of being have not had the face time in the classroom that the empirical data-driven "doing" approaches have had (L. P. Brown, 2011). Much of the data-driven approach has been, in this author's experience, from the emphasis on the epistemology of empiricism and lack of comfort in teaching in the other ways of knowing (Carper, 1978). The level of self-awareness and identity reflecting the nurses' values, beliefs, and attitudes directly correlate to the comfort level of understanding the ways of knowing in the affective domain (Neumann & Forsyth, 2008; Ondrejka, 2014). It was only when this author went through 6 months of training to become a Caritas Coach did full appreciation and comfort with the other ways of knowing become manifest (Carper, 1978; Horton-Deutsch, 2017). Language informs the metaphors that inform phenomena of interest (Lakoff & Johnson, 1980/2003). Does nursing curriculum draw upon the language of caring, compassion, and connection held within the discipline of nursing (Koithan, Kreitzer, & Watson, 2017; Touhy & Boykin, 2008)? Or does it reinforce the dominating metaphor of science in the profession of doing (Porter, 2010)? Where is the balance between doing and being (Ray & Turkel, 2014; Touhy & Boykin, 2008; Whelan, 2017)? Does the language in the curriculum even address what constitutes being caring, compassionate, and establishing connection (Parse, 1999)? Have we become nurse alchemists, combining differing amounts and types of cognitive and psychomotor aspects of learning expecting to create the gold of caring, compassion, and connection in the affective domain?

Nursing education has long focused on the cognitive and psychomotor domains of learning in moving the profession forward toward a more evidence-based practice approach. This model of education has its origins in the industrial model of production from which education was originally designed to meet the needs of the factories of the Industrial Revolution (Robinson, 2011). Nursing education has changed little since its inception, that is, the production of skilled labor for the delivery of nursing care in hospitals. Nurses trained at the associate degree level of nursing (ADN) are focused on the KS to pass the NCLEX so they can enter the workforce and make their contributions felt (Conner & Thielemann, 2013). Time is the most precious factor in this industrial model of nursing education, as it is in all assembly-line production. As time is precious within the allotted time frame for the curriculum, the delving into the values, beliefs, and attitudes of the discipline of nursing is attenuated. It is no surprise that nurses who graduate and practice from this industrial model of nursing education define their practice in the language of "doing." The most common refrain from this population is "just tell me what I need to know and how to do it and I'll do that." The product is uniform nurse widgets. The meme "a nurse is a nurse is a nurse" still thrives today in the service leadership arena. This approach is further validated when concerns arise in the delivery of care, and the nurses need to be "reeducated" or "retooled" to address the area of deficiency. "Reeducating" with a cognitive approach because it can be measured and implemented quickly is the preferred method of "quality control" within the profession, yet rarely achieves the long-term desired goal. As Bevis & Watson (Bevis & Watson, 1989) noted so eloquently:

> … without emancipation, education is an oppressive tool. It is an assembly line industry producing nurse-workers who on average follow the status quo. They may make waves, but they stay within the rules while living lives. (p. 162)

Which according to Bevis and Watson (1989):

> are circumscribed by the inflexibility of large medical empire-bureaucracies and bear the inevitable stamp of banality and mediocrity. Emancipatory education encourages learners to ask the unaskable, confront injustices and oppression and be active agents in their lives and in their work. (p. 162)

TAXONOMIES REVISITED

Bloom's taxonomies have long been used by educators to create curricula commensurate with their discipline's body of knowledge. The cognitive, affective, and psychomotor domains have been the bulwark of curriculum designers, accreditation bodies, and state boards of nursing practice (Ondrejka, 2014). The well-rounded nurse has KSAs that the profession has ascribed to the various levels of nursing practice (Amer, 2013; Sherwood & Barnsteiner, 2012).

COGNITIVE AND PSYCHOMOTOR DOMAINS

The traditional workhorses of nursing education are the cognitive and psychomotor domains of learning. These domains are the easiest to industrialize in the production environment through real-time and online testing and presentation strategies. They are the most amenable to objective data-driven outcomes. Although delivery of the evidence-based protocols, procedures, and bundles creates the environment of doing that is most conducive to metric-based measurement, the delivery of "caring" (which is what most patients and families come for) is relationship-based. Quality care comes as a result of the quality of relationships within the organization (Duffy, 2013; Duffy & Hoskins, 2003). Focusing on establishing a connection, authentic presence, and attunement with self, other, teams, and organization are the foundation of quality care and well-being (Biley, 2017; Charon, 2001; Cowling, Smith, & Watson, 2008; Duffy, 2013; Duffy & Hoskins, 2003; Hickman, 2013). For most nursing curricula, the operationalization of "caring for and about" is taught via cognitive methodologies. Caring has been translated into doing the right intervention, at the right time, in the right venue, for the right condition. Although this is certainly an aspect of caring, it is not all encompassing. Caring at its most profound is about sensemaking about the human experience and true belonging for the nurse as well as the patient and family (B. Brown, 2017; Madsbjerg, 2017; Watson, 2005a).

Does the cognitive approach to caring align with the latest neuroscience or cognitive research? Is caring, compassion, and connection a skill (Drummond & Oaks, 2016; Jinpa, 2015; Jones, 2005; Kagan, Smith, Cowling, & Chinn, 2010; McGonigal, 2017b)? If it is a skill, where in the curricula is this skill being taught? Are we teaching in our pathophysiology courses the biology of caring and its implication for health of the nurse as well as the delivery of healthcare (Zender & Olshansky, 2012)? If caring is at the heart and essence of the discipline of nursing, where is the language of caring, compassion, and connection in the curricula (Drummond & Oaks, 2016; Langley, Fonseca, & Iphonfen, 2006; McCraty & Childre, 2002; McGonigal, 2017a)? Where is the ontological content for the formation of the nurse in the curricula?

Nursing education curriculum development is focused on the meeting of elements of the Essentials of Baccalaureate Education for Professional Nursing Practice (American Association of Colleges of Nursing [AACN], 2008) in the case of BSN preparation, and State Boards of Nursing requirements for those in ADN preparation. These elements serve as drivers for the accreditation process with the Commission on Collegiate Nursing Education (CCNE; www.aacnnursing.org/CCNE). Curriculum designers and school administrators are focused on meeting the criteria for accreditation.

AFFECTIVE DOMAIN

The affective domain, home of values, beliefs, and attitudes, those areas that motivate and guide behaviors, has the least face time in the classroom or online setting (Valiga, 2014). These areas are the least amenable to the industrialization of content and standardization. Nursing faculty has varying degrees of comfort with teaching within this realm. This author had no formal training in the affective domain until his Caritas Coach course. Standardizing this content has been attempted in the scripting of discourse for patient satisfaction with mixed results (Hogan, 2013). The affective domain is most often associated with the "soft skills" of the profession, that of caring, compassion, and connection.

The essence of nursing has been described as embodying caring, compassion, and connection (American Nurses Association, 2015; Fowler, 2015). Yet there is no standardized language for these so-called "soft skills." These "soft skills" have become of extreme importance in the era following the implementation of the Affordable Care Act (ACA) and the reimbursement reformulation to include patient satisfaction scores.

REIMAGINING QUALITY, SAFETY, INFORMATICS, AND LEADERSHIP SERIES

The leadership course that was one semester in length on the basis of the prelicensure curricula was reimagined to incorporate the following content: nursing informatics, quality, and patient safety as well as leadership. This required the content to be covered over four semesters from the one in the prelicensure curricula. Caring Science being the framework alongside Duffy's quality caring model naturally created the following thematic semesters: transforming relationship with self, transforming relationship with other, transforming relationship with healthcare team, and finally transforming relationship with organization or system (Duffy, 2013; Hills & Watson, 2011; O'Nan, Jenkins, Morgan, Adams, & Davis, 2014; Watson, 2003, 2005b). The premise that quality care was correlated with the quality of relationship within the profession and with the patients and families was a natural fit with this reimagining. Integration of the Institute for Healthcare Improvement (IHI) courses on basic patient safety certification was incorporated into the four semesters. This provided the basis for understanding quality care from the perspective of an external organization predicated on process and quality improvement. Completion of the 13 online modules is required for the completion of the leadership series.

Technology as a caring competency was also incorporated into the nursing informatics content spread over three of the four semesters (Locsin & Purnell, 2015). Technology is a large part of the delivery of healthcare and has had experiential rollouts focused on the technological aspect of accuracy and efficiency of clinical documentation to the detriment of the caring connection (Kolb, 2017).

TRANSFORMING RELATIONSHIP WITH SELF

This introductory semester is thematically focused on the introduction of Caring Science, leadership and management theories, and the understanding of who the nurse is as a person. In this term, the following concepts are given emphasis: communication through authentic presence, authentic communication, who the nurse is as a personality type (Myers-Briggs Type Indicator (MBTI), what the preferred learning styles are (Learning Type Measure [LTM]), team-work (MBTI types), and creation of their vision board for themselves in the future of nursing.

Reflective discussion with responses to classmates is a foundational aspect of this cur-riculum. The nexus of transformation occurs where the cognitive concepts encounter the self in the act of reflection (Horton-Deutsch, 2017; Sherwood & Horton-Deutsch, 2015, 2017). Here the nurses encounter understanding and becoming in a visceral way (Sandvik et al., 2015). The digital vision board is another modality used to help the nurse see aesthetically the art of nursing through images. This modality evokes many varied visceral responses as they present themselves through the art they share. The IHI modules serve as the student's introduction to patient-centered care and introduction to leadership.

TRANSFORMING RELATIONSHIP WITH OTHER

This semester the focus is on the connection with other, whether that of the patient or families. Carper's Ways of Knowing are introduced to the nurses with reflective exercises. Introduction of the quality improvement process is presented during this term along with the IHI modules for quality improvement (Carper, 1978). Students work in groups to establish a quality improvement problem refining an AIM statement, researching the background, per-forming a literature search, identifying stakeholders, and determining how Caritas Processes #5 and #7 can be used in the project. Integration of the Caritas Processes into each of the stu-dent's projects is required so that Caring Science is not seen as merely concepts or words in a document or on a wall, but rather a part of the very lens used by nurses in their approach to problem solving (Foss-Durant, McDermont, Kinney, & Triner, 2015).

TRANSFORMING RELATIONSHIP WITH HEALTHCARE TEAM

The focus this semester is on transforming relationships within the healthcare team. The nurses take the Thomas-Kilmann Conflict Mode Instrument (TKI) learning about their preferred conflict mode styles and how they show up when conflict arises (Sportsman & Hamilton, 2007). Communication has a large focus this semester with introduction to the TeamSTEPPS™ training. Reflections on communication as a moral construct are required to help bring the ways of knowing into practical relevance. Students continue with their quality improvement projects, this term focusing on innovative processes such as discovery interviews, Caritas Processes #6 and #8, and interprofessional analysis of the team process. The IHI patient safety modules are the content of this semester. Once these modules are completed, students will have earned their Basic Certificate in Patient Safety.

Transforming Relationship With Organization or System

This final term is focused on how the nurses show up within the organization and the power a single voice can have. The final project is the students' e-portfolio and digital vision board outlining their journey within the program. The final presentation is a group discussion of the VAPs of the program, discovering their vision, finding their voice, telling their stories, and owning their practice. They have a final essay on their Caritas journey through the program and the transformation that has or has not happened. One such reflection about a student hero's journey is as follows:

> I have come to understand and accept the mantle of the "moral call" to my chosen profession. It is not only, I have learned, about doing good things. The current runs much deeper than that and involves recognition of ethical dilemmas, applying personal integrity to situations, and leading by example. I now aspire to come into a greater understanding of these principles. When this program began, I entered into it with the idea of completing a life goal in obtaining a bachelor's degree. In that, I am successful as graduation is nearly upon me. What I could not have known from the beginning is that I would rediscover a love for academic learning and decide to continue my education in pursuit of a nurse practitioner's license. In truth, this was an epiphany of just a few short weeks before writing this essay. Watson poses the question of "How do you envision your life?" as a way to know the other and one's self. Caritas #8 Creating healing environment at all levels, whereby wholeness, beauty, comfort, dignity, and peace are potentiated. This is how I envision my life being informed as a practicing nurse both at my current level of education and practice and at the level I will achieve (L. Snyder, personal communication, 2017).

REIMAGINING PATHOPHYSIOLOGY-PHARMACOLOGY AND PHYSICAL ASSESSMENT AS NURSING SCIENCE

The template from the prelicensure program included courses in physical assessment and patho-pharm. These students were licensed and practicing nurses, so these subjects offered the opportunity to reimagine these courses into learning how to learn. This population, as noted earlier, is very task oriented and seeking guidance from the faculty. The students are familiar with having the outline of content and testing for courses to be done by someone other than themselves. Lifelong learning and how to create learning plans have always been created by someone else. Here was the opportunity to teach students how to create these for themselves.

NURSING SCIENCE 1

This course is about introducing the science of learning (P. C. Brown, Roedinger III, & McDaniel, 2014), attitudes of a growth mindset (Dweck, 2006), and the creation of a gap analysis. Establishing a baseline knowledge was a challenge for these seasoned nurses. The decision was made to use the National League for Nursing (NLN) achievement exams for the anatomy and physiology, pharmacology, and physical assessment courses. The nurses were introduced to each of the segments with examples of excellent work from previous cohorts to guide them. The sections of the gap analysis were as follows: baseline assessment, populations served, gap analysis, Specific, Measurable, Attainable, Realistic, and Time-Bound (SMART) goals, and mind mapping of the plan. The intention behind this gap analysis was to help students understand the steps in assessing a learning gap, how to formulate a plan, engage the right brain in the visualization of the plan (mind mapping), and the creation of SMART goals for the populations that students specifically serve (Novack & Cañas, 2008; Rustler, 2012; Schuster, 2016).

The concept of Unitary Caring Science (previously known as unitary-transformative model) is introduced to these students. The faculty guide the students in their grappling with these complex ideas of being, becoming, and belonging with some amazing results (Cowling et al., 2008; Koithan et al., 2017; Lee, Palmieri, & Watson, 2017; Watson, 2017). Here is a reflective journal entry detailing one of these unexpected results:

> One of the most impactful significant lessons in nursing science was the unitary transformative model: being able to care for self and others' entire being; allowing myself to be vulnerable in each moment and interaction with others. Prior to this program, my thought process was very one directional. Looking back at my career and personal life, I was narrow minded; however I did not realize it at the time. The tools given to me with the nursing science course will stay with me my entire life. This course gave me the confidence to face my fears. I have shared the information I have learned with my coworkers, management, and my family. The transformation within myself has changed the environment around me. The new ways of learning, (e.g., the mind map analysis) allowed me to learn important clinical information that my practice was lacking in a creative way. Once I faced my fears of learning in a new fashion and embraced the process, I really enjoyed the process.

NURSING SCIENCE 2

The focus of the nursing science course is to implement the plan designed by the student over the next two semesters. The outcomes are a dashboard with a variance report on the progress of the task of the plan. This acquaints the nurse with how to monitor a plan, and create the variance report if the goals are not met, or need to be modified and why. The thematic focus for this semester is outpatient and continuum of care. The operative concepts for this semester are geriatrics and pain management. Simulations using an acute geriatric pain assessment and encounter are completed with standardized patients (SPs) in a simulation exercise. The goals of the encounter are as follows: (a) geriatric pain assessment and plan, (b) team communication and cohesion, and (c) establishing caring, compassion, and connection with the patient and significant other. The SPs have been specifically coached on what to look for in the three objectives of the encounter. They give specific feedback with regards to these objectives at the conclusion of the scenario. Group debriefing is completed following the SP feedback session.

Reflection of the SP feedback, the group debriefing, and the viewing of the simulation via videotaping are then required. The encounter is repeated as a follow-up clinic visit after the TeamSTEPPS training (Agency for Healthcare Research and Quality, 2013; Gaston, Short, Ralyea, & Casterline, 2016). This allows the adult learner to successfully complete the recommendations that were identified in the reflection, thus allowing the learner to be successful (Clarke, 2014; Husebø, O'Regan, & Nestel, 2015).

A reflective journal is required in this series with the goal of outlining how student learning concepts impact the practice environment of the students. The concepts of nursing science and leadership bleed over into the practice domain as was predicted. The reframing of what nursing practice is begins to show up in their journaling and continues into the next semester (Fairhurst & Saar, 1996).

Nursing Science 3

The focus of this semester is CAS and acute complex issues. Complexity theory and CAS are explored in the following conditions including the inflammatory processes of all conditions using sepsis as the prototype, and the role of the human microbiome in health and disease (Chaffee & McNeill, 2007; Hunt, Walsh, Voegeli, & Roberts, 2010; Lithgow & Covington, 2005; Mira et al., 2017; O'Doherty, Virani, & Wilcox, 2016; Shern, Blanch, & Steverman, 2016).

Outcomes for this semester are the same as for the previous semester in the advancing of the implementation plan for student's gap analysis and variance report, as well as the reflective journaling detailing the application of how learning concepts are being reflected in his or her practice environment.

Tying the Bow

This final term with no real new learning objectives allows for the tying up of the threads for the series, both the nursing science and the leadership series. This coming together has a profound impact on how students have changed the lens from which they view their practice as a nurse and the discipline and profession of nursing.

A subset of one cohort during their final term submitted and presented their work at the International Caritas Consortium in San Mateo, California, in 2017. The students presented their work and talked of their profound transformation in their practice and personal lives. Students have learned the language of caring, compassion, and connection. Students see "theoria" so differently now in how they approach their roles as nurse in the patient encounter, their relationships with their colleagues, and how they have grounded themselves in the principles and framework of Caring Literacy (Watson, 2017). They truly have embraced the South African concept of Ubuntu (Downing, 2017) and joy (Lama, Tutu, & Abrams, 2016).

A student summarized the tying of the bow with the following reflection from her Caritas essay for her e-portfolio as her final deliverable for the leadership series:

The Caritas principles woven into the RN-to-BSN program have given me a fuller, deeper understanding of nursing and caring. Through applying individual principles to scientific, leadership, quality and community I have become a better nurse and coworker. I can meet my patients and fellow caregivers where they are and nurture their spirit and mine as we together build healing environments. I have a platform to guide my practice and interactions. My Caritas journey has only begun and I look forward to where it will take me.

Further confirmation of the impact of this program to transform is illuminated in the observation of a spouse of a participant in this program. He observes:

Aside from "simply" getting her BSN, Karen has gone through a remarkable transition. The program itself along with the people she has met have given her a confidence and self-awareness I never imagined she would have. She is much more self-assured in dealing with her patients, her management, and in dealing with me (thanks for that). She is no longer a "victim" at work. Her way of dealing with a horrible management situation at work has changed from being one that comes home and "complains" about treatment to one that now says we can do this ... maybe we can do that. She looks for and finds solutions; she solicits input from others where before she would not want to get others involved. She has become the leader of her group of nurses, not just in her own department (the neonatal intensive care unit [NICU]), but also for Mother-Baby Unit, Labor & Delivery, and other departments that she has nothing to do with. She is now solicited for her input and advice (W. Green, personal communication, 2017).

The industrialization of nursing education needs to be reimagined as the formation of nurses as a lifelong process of becoming and not just doing. This will require that we (as a discipline and profession) establish a mentorship process throughout the life span of the career of a nurse. Mentorships at different stages will perhaps need different mentors. Understanding of these milestones from a career standpoint needs to be illuminated and researched. Being and becoming require different skill sets than cognitive and psychomotor skills. These skill sets require the faculty to be authentically present and cocreate the curriculum with the students. They require the awareness of within (interoception) and between (interception) in the creation of the teaching-learning environment (Siegel, 2010, 2012a, 2012b, 2017).

CONCLUSION

Theoria in the postclassical Latin and Greek means to contemplate or viewing or seeing. How is theory helping the discipline and profession of nursing to "see" differently? Is the epistemic of the theory translatable into praxis for the bedside nurse? Or does it remain in the realm of the priestly class of doctoral-prepared nurses? The language of the theory of caring must become the lingua franca of the discipline to reshape the profession. If the essence of nursing is in the human-to-human relational context, then language must describe that phenomenon (Graham, 2013). The language of the theory must be taught to all nurses in formation so that it becomes their lingua franca in describing their work and duty. Without the language, the discipline and profession will cease to be "nursing." Adoption of the language of other disciplines, medicine, business, and finance is the adoption of the language of the oppressor in the act of assimilation (Freire, 1970/1993, 1997). The act of assimilation is how a dominate culture diminishes the subsumed culture of another. The loss of language means the loss of identity. The moral imperatives of the discipline and profession of nursing are on the basis of its values, beliefs, and attitudes (Watson, 2017). As noted earlier, the language of the theory must roll off the tongue of every nurse as he or she imagines his or her daily work. The work of nursing is the work of healing. The etymology of the English word for "health" comes from the Anglo-Saxon for "wholeness." Yet it is defined as the absence of illness or disease. Nursing is at the nexus of the healthcare reform. It is time that its voice and value are heard and known. This is an axial point in the survivorship of the discipline.

NEXT ERA POSSIBILITIES

Education

- How can nursing education reimagine nursing from one of "doing" to a lifelong process of becoming?
- How can nurse faculty grow and learn in the affective domain of education?
- How does nursing education prepare each graduating nurse to be an artful reflective practitioner and conversant in the ways of knowing?
- Are we teaching nurses to create their own learning plans to truly own the responsibility for their own learning?
- Is the discipline and profession of nursing making full engagement in its research of all ways of knowing?

Research

- Research foci should include what lifelong mentorship would look like. Are there differing characteristics and needs at different stages in the life span of a career? Does this follow a pattern or is this process dependent on the progress of the individual along the hero's journey? Or have we created dependencies for learning on the basis of relicensure or certification credits?
- Where is the research that demonstrates the use of self and the knowledge that comes from that understanding (interception = within person) and the becoming in between persons (interoception = between persons) as a relational matrix that creates the healing environment?

Praxis

- How is the discipline and profession of nursing teaching the art and science of healing versus curing?
- The profession draws upon the metaparadigmatic elements of the discipline for its moral imperatives. Do these elements need to be updated to redefine the moral imperative in praxis?

- Or does the profession need to speak the language of nursing as its ethical and identity foundation, while being conversant in the languages of medicine, business, and finance?

Theory and Knowledge Development
- How is theory helping the discipline and profession of nursing to "see" differently?
- Is the epistemic of the theory translatable into praxis for the bedside nurse? Or does it remain in the realm of the priestly class of doctoral-prepared nurses?

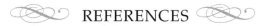 REFERENCES

Agency for Healthcare Research and Quality. (2013). TeamSTEPPS pocket guide, 2.0. Retrived from https://www.ahrq.gov/sites/default/files/publications/files/pocketguide.pdf

Amer, K. (2013). *Quality and safety for transformational nursing.* Boston, MA: Pearson.

American Association of Colleges of Nursing. (2008). *The essentials of baccalaureate education for professional nursing practice.* Retrieved from https://www.bc.edu/content/dam/files/schools/son/pdf2/BaccEssentials08.pdf

American Nurses Association. (2015). *Nursing informatics: Scope and standards of practice (2nd ed.).* Silver Spring, MD: Nursebooks.org.

Bevis, E. O., & Watson, J. (1989). *Toward a caring curriculum: A new pedagogy for nursing.* New York, NY: National League for Nursing.

Biley, A. (2017). *Remembering purpose* (Unpublished doctoral dissertation). Watson Caring Science Institute, Boulder, CO.

Brown, B. (2010). *The gifts of imperfection.* Center City, MN: Hazelton.

Brown, B. (2012). *Daring Greatly: How the courage to be vulnerable transforms the way we live, love, parent and lead.* New York, NY: Penguin/Random House.

Brown, B. (2015). *Rising Strong: How the ability to reset transforms the way we live, love, parent and lead.* New York, NY: Random House.

Brown, B. (2017). *Braving the wilderness: The quest for true belonging and the courage to stand alone.* New York, NY: Penguin/Random House.

Brown, L. P. (2011). Revisiting our roots: Caring in nursing curriculum design. *Nurse Education in Practice, 11*(6), 360–364. doi:10.1016/j.nepr.2011.03.007

Brown, P. C., Roedinger III, H. L., & McDaniel, M. A. (2014). *Make it stick: The science of successful learning.* Cambridge, MA: Belknap Press of Harvard University Press.

Calaprice, A. (2011). *The ultimate quotable Einstein.* Princeton, NJ: Princeton University Press.

Cameron, W. B. (1958). Tell me not in mournful numbers. *National Education Association Journal, 47*(3), 173.

Campbell, J. (2008). *The hero with a thousand faces.* Novato, CA: New World Library. (Original work published 1949)

Carper, B. (1978). Carper's Ways of Knowing. *Advances in Nursing Science, 1*(1), 13–23. doi:10.1097/00012272-197810000-00004

Chaffee, M. W., & McNeill, M. M. (2007). A model of nursing as a complex adaptive system. *Nursing Outlook, 55*(5), 232–241. doi:10.1016/j.outlook.2007.04.003

Charon, R. (2001). Narrative medicine: A model of empathy, reflection, profession and trust. *Journal of the American Medical Association, 286*(15), 1897–1902. doi:10.1001/jama.286.15.1897

Chinn, P. L., & Kramer, M. (2015). *Knowledge development in nursing: Theory and process.* St. Louis, MO: Elsevier.

Clarke, N. M. (2014). A person-centred enquiry into the teaching and learning experiences of reflection and reflective practice–part one. *Nurse Education Today, 34*(9), 1219–1224. doi:10.1016/j.nedt.2014.05.017

Conner, N. E., & Thielemann, P. A. (2013). RN-BSN completion programs: Equipping nurses for the future. *Nursing Outlook, 61*(6), 458–465. doi:10.1016/j.outlook.2013.03.003

Cowling, W. R., & Chinn, P. L. (2001). Conversations across paradigms: Unitary-transformative and critical feminist perspectives. *Scholarly Inquiry for Nursing Practice, 15*(4), 347–365.

Cowling, W. R., Smith, M. C., & Watson, J. (2008). The power of wholeness, consciousness, and caring: A dialogue on nursing science, art, and healing. *Advances in Nursing Science, 31*(1), E41–E51. doi:10.1097/01.ANS.0000311535.11683.d1

Day, L., Ziehm, S. R., Jessup, M. A., Amedro, P., Dawson-Rose, C., Derouin, A., … Remen, R. N. (2017). The power of nursing: An innovative course in values clarification and self-discovery. *Journal of Professional Nursing, 33*(4), 267–270. doi:10.1016/j.profnurs.2017.01.005

Donohue-Porter, P., Forbes, M. O., White, J. H., & Baumann, S. L. (2017). Transforming nursing education and the formation of students. *Nursing Science Quarterly, 30*(2), 134–142. doi:10.1177/0894318417693287

Downing, C. (2017). Practices of caring: A South African perspective. In S. Lee, P. Palmieri, & J. Watson (Eds.), *Global advances in human caring literacy.* New York, NY: Springer Publishing.

Drummond, S., & Oaks, G. (2016). A curriculum founded on human becoming: Educational endeavoring. *Nursing Science Quarterly, 29*(1), 25–29. doi:10.1177/0894318415614628

Duffy, J. R. (2013). *Quality caring in nursing and health systems.* New York, NY: Springer Publishing.

Duffy, J. R., & Hoskins, L. M. (2003). The quality-caring model: Blending dual paradigms. *Advances in Nursing Science, 26*(1), 77–88. doi:10.1097/00012272-200301000-00010

Dweck, C. (2006). *Mindset: The psychology of success.* New York, NY: Ballantine Books.

Fairhurst, G., & Saar, R. (1996). *The art of framing: Managing the language of leadership.* San Francisco, CA: Jossey-Bass.

Foss-Durant, A., McDermott, S., Kinney, G., & Triner, T. (2015). Caring science: Transforming the ethic of caring-healing practice, environment, and culture within an integrated care delivery system. *Permanente Journal, 19*(4), e136–e142. doi:10.7812/tpp/15-042

Fowler, M. D. M. (2015). *Guide to Nursing's Social Policy Statement: Understanding the profession from social contract to social covenant.* Silver Spring, MD: American Nurses Association.

Freire, P. (1993). *Pedagogy of the oppressed.* New York, NY: Bloomsbury Academic. (Original work published 1970)

Freire, P. (1997). *Pedagogy of the heart.* London, UK: Bloomsbury Academic.

Gallison, B. (2012). Conflict resolution and caring science theory. *Beginnings,* 10–13.

Gaston, T., Short, N., Ralyea, C., & Casterline, G. (2016). Promoting patient safety: Results of a TeamSTEPPS(R) initiative. *Journal of Nursing Administration, 46*(4), 201–207. doi:10.1097/NNA.0000000000000333

Godkin, J. (2001). Healing presence. *Journal of Holistic Nursing, 19*(1), 5–21. doi:10.1177/089801010101900102

Graham, L. (2013). The power of names in culture & mathematics. *Proceedings of the American Philosophical Society, 157*(2), 229–234.

Hickman, C. (2013). Authentic presence in nursing: Is it necessary? *International Journal for Human Caring, 17*(4), 74–78.

Hills, M., & Watson, J. (2011). *Creating a caring science curriculum: An emacipatroy pedagogy for nursing.* New York, NY: Springer Publishing.

Hogan, B. K. (2013). Caring as a scripted discourse versus caring as an expression of an authentic relationship between self and other. *Issues in Mental Health Nursing, 34*(5), 375–379. doi:10.3109/01612840.2013.768734

Horton-Deutsch, S. (2017). Thinking, acting, and leading through caring science literacy. In S. Lee, P. Palmieri, & J. Watson (Eds.), *Global advances in human caring literacy.* New York, NY: Springer Publishing.

Horton-Deutsch, S., & Sherwood, G. (2017). *Reflective practice: Transforming education and improving outcomes* (2nd ed.). Indianapolis, IN: Sigma Theta Tau International.

Huether, S., & McCance, K. (2017). *Understanding pathophsyiology.* St Louis, MO: Elsevier.

Hunt, K. J., Walsh, B. M., Voegeli, D., & Roberts, H. C. (2010). Inflammation in aging part 1: Physiology and immunological mechanisms. *Biological Research for Nursing, 11*(3), 245–252. doi:10.1177/1099800409352237

Husebø, S. E., O'Regan, S., & Nestel, D. (2015). Reflective practice and its role in simulation. *Clinical Simulation in Nursing, 11*(8), 368–375. doi:10.1016/j.ecns.2015.04.005

Iacono, L., & Altman, M. (2015). AACN CSI academy, part 2: Nurses emerge as change leaders. *Nursing Management, 46,* 40–43. doi:10.1097/01.NUMA.0000469354.49071.32

Ironside, P. M. (2014). Enabling narrative pedagogy: Inviting, waiting, and letting be. *Nursing Education Perspectives, 35*(4), 212–218. doi:10.5480/13-1125.1

Jacobs, B. B., Fontana, J. S., Kehoe, M. H., Matarese, C., & Chinn, P. L. (2005). An emancipatory study of contemporary nursing practice. *Nursing Outlook, 53*(1), 6–14. doi:10.1016/j.outlook.2004.04.015

Jinpa, T. (2015). *A fearless heart: How the courage to be compassionate can transform out lives.* New York, NY: Hudson Street Press.

Jones, D. A. (2005). Are we abandoning nursing as a discipline? *Clinical Nurse Specialist, 19*(6), 275–277. doi:10.1097/00002800-200511000-00001

Kagan, P. N., Smith, M. C., Cowling, W. R., & Chinn, P. L. (2010). A nursing manifesto: An emancipatory call for knowledge development, conscience, and praxis. *Nursing Philosophy, 11,* 67–84. doi:10.1111/j.1466-769X.2009.00422.x

Kang, Y. S., Choi, S. Y., & Ryu, E. (2009). The effectiveness of a stress coping program based on mindfulness meditation on the stress, anxiety, and depression experienced by nursing students in Korea. *Nurse Education Today, 29*(5), 538–543. doi:10.1016/j.nedt.2008.12.003

Koithan, M. S., Kreitzer, M. J., & Watson, J. (2017). Linking the unitary paradigm to policy through a synthesis of caring science and integrative nursing. *Nursing Science Quarterly, 30*(3), 262–268. doi:10.1177/0894318417708415

Lakoff, G., & Johnson, M. (2003). *Metaphors we live by.* Chicago, IL: University of Chicago Press. (Original work published 1980)

Lama, D., Tutu, D., & Abrams, D. (2016). *The book of joy.* New York, NY: Penguin/Random House.

Langley, P., Fonseca, J., & Iphofen, R. (2006). Psychoneuroimmunology and health from a nursing perspective. *British Journal of Nursing, 15*(20), 1126–1129. doi:10.12968/bjon.2006.15.20.22298

Lee, R. C., & Fawcett, J. (2013). The influence of the metaparadigm of nursing on professional identity development among RN-BSN students. *Nursing Sceince Quarterly, 26*(1), 96–98. doi:10.1177/0894318412466734

Lee, S., Palmieri, P., & Watson, J. (2017). *Global advances in human caring literacy.* New York, NY: Springer Publishing.

Lithgow, D., & Covington, C. (2005). Chronic inflammation and breast pathology: A theoretical model. *Biological Research for Nursing, 7*(2), 118–129. doi:10.1177/1099800405280823

Locsin, R. C., & Purnell, M. (2015). Advancing the theory of technological competency as caring in nursing: The universal technological domain. *International Journal for Human Caring, 19*(2), 50–54. doi:10.20467/1091-5710-19.2.50

Madsbjerg, C. (2017). *Sensemaking: The power of the humanities in the age of the algorithm.* New York, NY: Hachette.

McCraty, R. (2001). *Science of the heart: The role of the heart in human perfomrance.* Boulder Creek, CA: Insititute of HeartMath.

McCraty, R., & Childre, D. (2002). *The appreciative heart.* Boulder Creek, CA. Institute of HeartMath.

McGonigal, K. (2017a). *The neuroscience of change: A compassion-based program for personal transformation.* Boulder, CO: Sounds True.

McGonigal, K. (2017b). *The science of compassion.* Boulder, CO: Sounds True.

Mead, D., & Docker, P. (2017). *Find your why: A practical guide for discovering purpose for you and your team.* New York, NY: Profolio/Penguin.

Melnyk, B., & Fineout-Overholt, E. (2011). *Evidence-based practice in nursing and healthcare.* Philadelphia, PA: Wolters Kluwer/Lippincott Williams & Wilkins.

Mira, J. C., Gentile, L. F., Mathias, B. J., Efron, P. A., Brakenridge, S. C., Mohr, A. M., … Moldawer, L. L. (2017). Sepsis pathophysiology, chronic critical illness, and persistent inflammation-immunosuppression and catabolism syndrome. *Critical Care Medicine, 45*(2), 253–262. doi:10.1097/CCM.0000000000002074

Mitchell, S. (Trans.). (1988). *Tao te ching: A new English translation.* New York, NY: Harper & Row.

Neumann, J. A., & Forsyth, D. (2008). Teaching in the affective domain for institutional values. *Journal of Continuing Education in Nursing, 39*(6), 248–252. doi:10.3928/00220124-20080601-07

Novack, J. D., & Cañas, A. J. (2008). The theory underlying concept maps and how to construct and use them. Technical Report IHMC CmapTools 2006-01 Rev 01-2008, Florida Institute for Human and Machine Cognition. Retrieved from http://cmap.ihmc.us/Publications/ResearchPapers/Theory UnderlyingConceptMaps.pdf

O'Doherty, K. C., Virani, A., & Wilcox, E. S. (2016). The human microbiome and public health: Social and ethical considerations. *American Journal of Public Health, 106*(3), 414–420. doi:10.2105/AJPH.2015.302989

O'Nan, C. L., Jenkins, K., Morgan, L. A., Adams, T., & Davis, B. A. (2014). Evaluation of Duffy's quality caring model on patients' perceptions of nurse caring in a community hospital. *International Journal for Human Caring, 18*(1), 27–34. doi:10.20467/1091-5710-18.1.27

Ondrejka, D. (2014). *Affective teaching in nursing.* New York, NY: Springer Publishing.

Parse, R. (1999). Nursing: The discipline and the profession. *Nursing Science Quarterly, 12*(4), 275–276. doi:10.1177/089431849901200401

Parse, R. R. (2016). Human becoming hermeneutic sciencing: Reverence, awe, betrayal, and shame in the lives of others. *Nursing Science Quarterly, 29*(2), 128–135. doi:10.1177/0894318416630109

Pink, D. (2005). *A whole new mind: Why right-brainers will rule the future.* New York, NY: Riverhead Books.

Porter, S. (2010). Fundamental patterns of knowing in nursing: The challenge of evidence-based practice. *Advances in Nursing Science, 33*(1), 3–14. doi:10.1097/ANS.0b013e3181c9d5eb

Prochaska, J. O., & Velicer, W. F. (1997). The transtheoretical model of health behavior change. *American Journal of Health Promotion, 12*(1), 38–48. doi:10.4278/0890-1171-12.1.38

Ray, M. A., & Turkel, M. C. (2014). Caring as emancipatory nursing praxis: The theory of relational caring complexity. *Advances in Nursing Science, 37*(2), 132–146. doi:10.1097/ANS.0000000000000024

Reilly, J., Gallagher-Lepak, S., & Killion, C. (2012). Affective domain and online learning. *Nursing Education Perspectives, 33*(2), 101–105.

Roberts, S. (2000). Positive professional image. *Advances in Nursing Science, 22*(4), 71–82. doi:10.1097/00012272-200006000-00007

Robinson, K. (2011). *Out of our minds: Learning to be creative.* Chichester, UK: A Wiley & Sons.

Rosa, W. (2016). *Nurses as leaders: Evolutionary visions of leadership.* New York, NY: Springer Publishing.

Rustler, F. (2012). *Mind mapping for dummies.* West Sussex, UK: John Wiley & Sons.

Sandvik, A. H., Eriksson, K., & Hilli, Y. (2015). Understanding and becoming: The heart of the matter in nurse education. *Scandinavian Journal of Caring Sciences, 29*(1), 62–72. doi:10.1111/scs.12128

Schuster, P. M. (2016). *Concept mapping: A critical-thinking approach to care planning* (4th ed.). Philadelphia, PA: F. A. Davis.

Sheldrake, R. (2012). *Set science free.* New York, NY: Random House.

Shern, D. L., Blanch, A. K., & Steverman, S. M. (2016). Toxic stress, behavioral health, and the next major era in public health. *American Journal of Orthopsychiatry, 86*(2), 109–123. doi:10.1037/ort0000120

Sherwood, G., & Barnsteiner, J. (2012). *Quality and safety in nursing.* West Sussex, UK: John Wiley & Sons.

Sherwood, G., & Horton-Deutsch, S. (2015). *Reflective organization: On the front lines of QSEN & reflective practice implementation.* Indianapolis, IN: Sigma Theta Tau International.

Siegel, D. (2010). *Mindsight: The new science of personal transformation.* New York, NY: Bantam Books.

Siegel, D. (2012a). *The developing mind: How relationships and the brain interact to shape who we are.* New York, NY: Guilford Press.

Siegel, D. (2012b). *Pocket guide to interpersonal neurobiology.* New York, NY: W. W. Norton.

Siegel, D. (2017). *Mind: A journey to the heart of being human.* New York, NY: W. W. Norton.

Sinek, S. (2009). *Start with why.* New York, NY: Protfolio/Penquin.

Song, Y., & Lindquist, R. (2015). Effects of mindfulness-based stress reduction on depression, anxiety, stress and mindfulness in Korean nursing students. *Nurse Education Today, 35*(1), 86–90. doi:10.1016/j.nedt.2014.06.010

Spadoni, M., Doane, G. H., Sevean, P., & Poole, K. (2015). First-year nursing students: Developing relational caring practice through inquiry. *Journal of Nursing Education, 54*(5), 270–275. doi:10.3928/01484834-20150417-04

Sportsman, S., & Hamilton, P. (2007). Conflict management styles in the health professions. *Journal of Professional Nursing, 23*(3), 157–166. doi:10.1016/j.profnurs.2007.01.010

Touhy, T., & Boykin, A. (2008). Caring as the central domain in nursing education. *International Journal for Human Caring, 12*(2), 8–15.

Valiga, T. M. (2014). Attending to affective domain learning: Essential to prepare the kind of graduates the public needs. *Journal of Nursing Education, 53*(5), 247. doi:10.3928/01484834-20140422-10

Wang, S. C., Wang, L. Y., Shih, S. M., Chang, S. C., Fan, S. Y., & Hu, W. Y. (2017). The effects of mindfulness-based stress reduction on hospital nursing staff. *Applied Nursing Research, 38*, 124–128. doi:10.1016/j.apnr.2017.09.014

Watson, J. (2003). Love and caring: Ethics of face and hand--an invitation to return to the heart and soul of nursing and our deep humanity. *Nursing Administration Quarterly, 27*(3), 197–202. doi:10.1097/00006216-200307000-00005

Watson, J. (2005a). Caring Science: Belonging before being as ethical cosmology. *Nursing Sceince Quarterly, 18*(4), 304–305. doi:10.1177/0894318405280395

Watson, J. (2005b). *Caring science as sacred science.* Philadelphia, PA: F. A. Davis.

Watson, J. (2017). Global advances in human caring literacy. In S. Lee, P. Palmieri, & J. Watson (Eds.), *Global advances in human caring literacy.* New York, NY: Springer Publishing.

Weberg, D. (2012). Complexity leadership: A healthcare imperative. *Nursing Forum, 47*(4), 268–277. doi:10.1111/j.1744-6198.2012.00276.x

Wheatley, M. (2009). *Turning to one another: Simple conversations to restore hope to the future.* Oakland, CA: Berrett-Koehler.

Wheatley, M. (2017). *Who do we choose to be?* Oakland, CA: Berret-Koehler.

Whelan, J. (2017). The caring science imperative: A hallmark in nursing education. In S. Lee, P. Palmieri, & J. Watson (Eds.), *Global advances in human caring literacy.* New York, NY: Springer Publishing.

Zender, R., & Olshansky, E. (2012). The biology of caring: Researching the healing effects of stress response regulation through relational engagement. *Biological Research for Nursing, 14*(4), 419–430. doi:10.1177/1099800412450505

19

Nursing Doctorally Prepared Caring Scientists

Sara Horton-Deutsch, Kathy Oman, and Karen Sousa

CARITAS LITERACIES

By the end of this chapter, the caring-healing nurse will be able to

1. Describe the philosophy behind the modern understanding and structure of science and how it relates to a Caring Science (CS) orientation.

2. Identify the role of the CS researcher in advancing caring knowledge and practices.

3. Recognize the unique meaning of being/knowing/becoming a CS researcher and how it influences Caritas Literacy.

4. Explore the value of an emancipatory approach to CS education and its complementary nature to understanding of healing, health, wholeness, and humanity.

This chapter addresses the development of an interprofessional doctorate of philosophy program with a focus on CS. As explored in Chapter 13, "Ways of Being/Knowing/Becoming," the evolution of the human caring concept of Caring Literacy, Caritas (Universal Love) brings forth new dimensions of our Ways of Being/Doing/Becoming. Having fluency in caring introduces new meaning to deepen ways of knowing and cultivating how to *be* deeply human/humane, and how to be caring and have a healing presence. Nurse faculty scholars are called to build the science of caring through theory-guided research methodologies and through mentorship of the next generation of caring scientists.

In response to the need for human caring literacy and to advance the science of caring, Dr. Jean Watson developed a doctoral program through her Watson Caring Science Institute (WCSI) in 2012. This transformative and unique program was guided by the British model of graduate study that was based on self-directed and self-paced research rather than formally structured graduate study. The program was interdisciplinary, nontraditional, introspective, and nonaccredited. In 2014, Dr. Watson expressed an interest in relocating the WCSI program to the University of Colorado (CU) College of Nursing (CON) and adapting it in a way that met university criteria for an accredited degree. In July 2014, to prepare for this transition, Drs. Karen Sousa and Sara Horton-Deutsch audited a week-long intensive with Dr. Watson's current doctoral students. This provided a sense of how the program was organized and how to modify and build on the best of what was. In September 2014, Dr. Watson and Dr. Hills (director WCSI PhD program) met with a team of CU faculty and staff to review both the WCSI PhD program and the current CU PhD program. Members then explored how the two converged and crafted a CS focus program plan that would be offered along with the other two focus areas within the existing PhD program.

EVOLUTION OF SCIENCE AND THEORY DEVELOPMENT

Before exploring the approach, meaning, and value of being and becoming a CS researcher, it is helpful to revisit the philosophy behind our modern understanding and structure of science. Over 50 years ago, Thomas Kuhn (1962), a physicist and philosopher, as a student, read Aristotle and realized he did not understand him. Kuhn concluded that neither he nor Aristotle was unwise, but the nature of the realities they dwelled in had changed so drastically they no longer spoke the same scientific language. Eventually, Kuhn wrote the landmark text on the philosophy of science, *The Structure of Scientific Revolution*, where he challenged the long-standing linear notions of science and how it progresses. He argued that transformative ideas do not rise from a gradual process of experimentation and data accumulation but from breakthrough ideas that occur outside of normal science. He also contended that scientific revolutions bring order to the incongruities that amass over time.

Kuhn's (2012) version of how science advanced challenged the notion of steady cumulative progress, as he saw discontinuities and revolutionary phases in which communities of researchers in particular fields entered periods of uncertainty and angst. He termed this a revolutionary phase—for example, from Newton physics to quantum physics—resulting in great conceptual breakthroughs. Kuhn made it clear that to understand scientific development, one must understand the intellectual frameworks within which scientists work. Moreover, over long periods of time, unresolved anomalies accumulate and it gets to the point where some scientists question the current paradigm. When a field enters this period of crisis, it is resolved by a revolutionary change in worldview. This phenomenon, called a "paradigm shift," occurs in human history where social/experiential/intellectual change is so profound that people on either side of the shift can no longer communicate with each other. When competing paradigms are incommensurable, it eventually leads to a shift and a new normal is created, on the basis of a new framework. Sheila Kennedy (2007), a professor of Law and Policy in the School of Public and Environmental Affairs at Indiana University–Purdue University Indianapolis, contends when competing paradigms are irreconcilable such as urban and rural Americans, educated and uneducated Americans, or, from a global perspective, countries with and without basic resources, people begin to live in irreconcilable realities—two competing paradigms.

Another competing paradigm is what counts as science. Kuhn (2012) argued that science be mainly about theory. However, the majority of scientific research over the past 25 years has been data-driven rather than theory-driven. In many ways, this dominant perspective has led to the dehumanization of much of healthcare. We see patients as parts and machines over Spirit-filled human beings. And, despite the inherent differences between science and the humanities, fields of study are changing, expanding, and growing into new dynamic intersections between and among each other. The convergence is seen in mind-body-spirit medicine and new understandings of physics of science, energy medicine, spirituality, and healing (Watson, 2008). The CS theoretical orientation that serves as a more philosophical-theoretical-foundational starting point for research contends there is a need for science that answers questions about humanity, caring, and what it means to be human. To deepen our understanding of common humanity and the human experience, researchers must embrace self-knowledge, self-discovery, and shared human experiences, combined with the study of human emotions and relations (Watson, 2008).

THE VALUE OF BEING/BECOMING A CARING SCIENCE RESEARCHER

Caring moments illuminate what is often hidden from nursing's consciousness and its science; thus, doctoral study in CS yields the most insightful, sensitive, and informed nurse scientist of all (Watson & Smith, 2002). However, before establishing the value of the *CS-informed* nurse researcher, it is necessary to develop what a nurse researcher is and does.

The Significance of the PhD Credential. Doctoral degrees in nursing have been offered since 1933 by Teachers Colleges at Columbia and New York Universities. The initial degree was a doctor of education (EdD). But by the mid-1960s, various doctorates were available for nurses (i.e., EdD, DNS, DNSc, and PhD). Still, however, the PhD uniquely stamped its recipient as a researcher—and this remains the case today. The PhD-trained nurse can (a) ask trenchant/provocative questions, (b) formulate appropriate/innovative strategies for exploring those questions, (c) conduct investigations with high-level precision/competence, and (d) disseminate compelling study results to advance her or his field. At once, the PhD credential conveys to its bearer both a great responsibility and a skillset potent enough to fulfill that responsibility. In short, the PhD-trained nurse is a scholar.

Qualities of a Scholar. Walker, Golde, Jones, Bueschel, and Hutchings (2008), in contributing to the Carnegie Initiative on the Doctorate (2001), identified essential qualities of a scholar:

> *Scholarly integration.* Scholarly integration entails well-roundedness. Bench science proficiency alone is insufficient, as are familiarity with primary/secondary data analysis, pedagogic talent, interventional skill, and writing ability. A scholar must be able to integrate a number of these. A scholar must display versatility in the scholarly craft.
>
> *Intellectual community.* A scholar must be a solid citizen of an intellectual community. Solid citizenry connotes participation, contribution, purposeful interaction with fellow citizens, and respect. The intellectual community also connotes preparation and initiation of the next generation of community members.
>
> *Stewardship.* While the intellectual community is interpersonal, stewardship pertains to the discipline itself. In the capacity of steward, a scholar considers the purposes of the

field and favors responsible application. A steward is mindful of the continuing health of the discipline, separating the best discipline elements from the rest and preserving the best as the inheritance of those who follow in the discipline. (pp. 9–11)

A scholar should be capable of generating and critically evaluating new knowledge; of conserving the most important ideas and findings that are a legacy of the past; of understanding how knowledge—right now—is in the process of transforming the world; and of engaging and communicating knowledge responsibly to others (Atkinson & Tuzin, 1992). The scholar lays herself or himself down as a here-and-now bridge between what has been and what is yet to be. The coordinates of that bridge—the location at which it begins and the point where it touches down—determine in large part the future direction, magnitude, and trajectory of the discipline.

The Development of Caring Science-Informed Scholars. The PhD focus in CS prepares healthcare professionals to strengthen and expand the intellectual, reflective, philosophical, and theoretical underpinnings of CS. PhD-trained, CS-informed nurse scholars will then generate robust research that reintegrates caring-healing into the healthcare profession and infuses healthcare systems with purpose, dignity, and wholeness. The question of what constitutes high-quality healthcare remains a pressing one—any answer not incorporating CS principles advanced by CS scholars is incomplete. CS-informed research hones raw care into purposeful, intentional care.

Carrying Caring Science Into the Future. Leaders in any setting emit a tone that resonates through the setting and vibrates throughout the setting and its citizenry. In this way, CS-informed scholars can broadcast their scholarly perspective, helping guide those around them, in academic environments, in nonacademic environments, or in any environment. The generational knock-on effect—that is, wherein present-day students become teachers for subsequent students—is the process through which PhD-trained, CS-informed nurse scholars will carry their scholarship into a CS-shaped healthcare future.

Developing Caring Science Researchers Through the Study of Human Caring

Thus, we developed a doctorate of philosophy that is both interdisciplinary and introspective, grounded in the intellectual, reflective, philosophical, and theoretical underpinnings of CS as sacred science. It emphasizes unitary consciousness, the artistry of personal growth, creativity, and mindfulness practices. The students' chosen areas of study are explored and developed through theories of transpersonal caring-healing, ancient indigenous wisdom traditions, paradigms of consciousness and sacred healing energy models, the science of the heart, and the unitary Oneness of all (Watson, 1979/1985, 2005, 2008, 2012).

The objectives of the CS focus area correspond to the global objectives of the WCSI:

- Transform the dominant model of Western medical science to a model of unitary CS

- Reintroduce the ethic, energy, and science of caring and Love (Caritas) necessary for healing

- Deepen authentic caring-healing relationships with self, and between self and other

- Restore caring, love, and compassion as the ethical framework for healthcare and all our relations

- Translate model of CS as sacred science into transdisciplinary service in the world

- Transform self/system/society through evolving human consciousness of Oneness of ALL

Doctoral students in the CS focus area complete core courses with doctoral students from the other two focus areas in metatheory, roles of the scientist, and qualitative and quantitative methods. In addition, within the CS focus area, students complete two seminars and three courses. The seminars focus on an introduction to CS and developing CS questions. Courses expand on the seminars with an emphasis on philosophies and theories related to human caring, diverse theories of care, and CS as a transdisciplinary domain for health science education, practice, and research.

THE MEANING OF BEING/KNOWING/BECOMING A CARING SCIENCE RESEARCHER

The seven doctoral students currently enrolled in the PhD program are diverse in their application of CS in practice and their individual research interests. However, what they have in common is an appreciation for the deeper meaning of their work in the world and a desire for deeper ways of attending to and cultivating how to Be, Know, and Become as reflective scholars engaged in caring-healing, health. To cultivate their Being, they complete the Caritas Coach Education Program (CCEP) as the foundation for their scholarship/research. CCEP can be taken for course credit and serves as an elective toward their degree. Their knowing is then expanded through the study of and nature of knowledge that informs their consciousness about what counts as knowledge. Through this process, students begin to transcend conventional ways of knowing and explore whole person ways of knowing—including personal, aesthetic, intuitive, and ethical. From a place of appreciation of these expanded forms of knowledge, they have developed innovative ways to study areas of inquiry including caring leadership, the safety voice of nurses, caring in an online educational environment, palliative care, nurse and provider resiliency, LGBTQ persons and vulnerability, and chronic illness diagnosis and narrative meaning (through the lens of a social worker). Caritas ways of being and knowing flow into ways of becoming through awakening to higher levels of consciousness and connection to infinite source, higher self, infinite love. Although the students' journeys through this course work at the same pace, their personal journeys of being, knowing, and becoming CS researchers are very individual.

DOCTORAL EDUCATION AND ONLINE TEACHING

Doctoral education is personal and reflective and requires deep engagement and interaction with colleagues and faculty. The competencies we expect our CS students to achieve are in addition to the PhD graduate program qualities. Through deep engagement, the faculty and students cocreate a Caritas Literacy throughout the program. Watson (2017) defines Caritas Literacy "as an ontology of being/becoming that emerges from the subjective inner world of the person, morally aroused for reflective and contemplative self-growth, self-caring experiences that contribute to humanity" (p. 7). Caritas Literacy, or as it has evolved to critical Caritas Literacy, goes beyond the task-conscious conventional meaning of book learning and involves being literate in ways that relate to critical reflection and understanding of what it means to be human (Lee, Palmieri, & Watson, 2017). Critical Caritas Literacy is foundational to PhD education and the development of CS researchers.

Our PhD program is a blend of in-person classroom time, called "intensives," for a week at the beginning of the semester, and online discussion postings and synchronous face-to-face meetings in a virtual space. Although the flexibility and self-paced nature of online courses are desirable, the lack of personal interaction and physical connection can be problematic. Students and faculty can feel isolated and disconnected, and learning activities may feel fixed and rigid with discussion board postings being the main form of communication and interaction. In addition, discussion board postings usually rely on written communication and can limit the multiple and aesthetic ways students learn and know. Course design and faculty interaction should encourage student engagement and creativity to foster personal and professional development in the form of critical Caritas Literacy.

HELICOPTER VIEW OF PEDAGOGY

Courses developed from a CS unitary view instill deep caring and engagement between and among the students and faculty. Concepts and activities that reflect the values of CS and some of the 10 Caritas Processes® include the following: starting in-person or synchronous online sessions with a centering activity, using check-in and check-out activities at the beginning and end of either in-person or synchronous sessions (Chinn, 2013), and framing discussions or postings as a SOPHIA (Chinn, 2013). "SOPHIA" is a Greek word for female wisdom and stands for **S**peak **O**ut, **P**lay **H**avoc, **I**magine **A**lternatives. The SOPHIA is used to frame interactions with the readings and peers (Chinn, 2013); incorporating multiple and aesthetic ways of knowing into course assignments is another teaching/learning strategy that fosters critical Caritas Literacy in students (Carper, 1978; Zander, 2007).

Course interaction between the faculty and students follows Sitzman's six exemplars for online pedagogy: (a) offer full presence, (b) acknowledge awareness of shared humanity, (c) attend to the individual, (d) ask for and provide frequent clarification, (e) demonstrate flexibility, and (f) point out favorable opportunities yet acknowledge challenges (Sitzman & Watson, 2017).

CS PhD curriculum requires a transformation of the traditional way graduate nursing programs function. Theory U is a leadership model based on the concept of "presencing," which calls for the student and faculty to look inward, to be open, and to allow future possibilities to emerge (Kreitzer & Koithan, 2014). This five-stage process is used to "discover the future by doing" (Kreitzer & Koithan, 2014, p. 423) and we have created and revised the curriculum by involving the students in coinitiating, cosensing, presencing, cocreating, and coevolving the courses and course content (Kreitzer & Koithan, 2014). The faculty views the CS focus of the PhD program as an evolving, organic, and living process where students are engaged in both the epistemology and the pedagogy as they move into being/knowing/becoming CS research scholars.

CONCLUSION

This chapter has explored the evolution of the first accredited PhD focus area in CS and how it developed from the original created through the WCSI under the leadership of Drs. Watson and Hills. Integrating CS at the doctoral level into formal educational arenas is the next logical step for the advancement of this work in the world. The value of being/becoming a CS scholar shines a much-needed light on the consciousness of caring through research that expands Caritas Literacy. Faculty who create educational environments to support the development of unitary consciousness through mindful practices, authentic dialogue, and deep reflection model the value of caring as the basis for research. As a result, CS-informed scholars serve as an exemplar for others who seek to transform the discipline by developing insightful, sensitive, and informed nursing scientists.

NEXT ERA POSSIBILITIES

To continue to grow the next generation of interprofessional scholars in advancing the art and science of caring requires ongoing evolution of education, theory, research, and praxis. Questions for reflection on next era possibilities include the following.

Education
- How does a CS pedagogy in doctoral education influence the nature of relationships with students and create opportunities for advancing ways of being/knowing/becoming/doing in leadership in academic and healthcare settings?

Research
- How does a PhD-prepared scholar support new knowledge creation for the evolution of CS?
- What are the opportunities for discovering new ways of knowing when we expand our ideas of what counts as data?
- What new models of knowing can be studied to understand the human capacity for evolution toward global consciousness for the care of all living things?

Praxis
- How does CS education ground the learning community in the conscious and intentional discipline of critical reflection and informed moral action?
- How does CS praxis advance a moral ethical worldview and how can a PhD further facilitate this intention and action?

Theory and Knowledge Development
- What paradigms complement CS and through synthesis of their shared worldviews expand ways of knowing?
- What complementary paradigms seek to more deeply explicate the ground of our Being and its expressive characteristics shown through caring and loving actions?

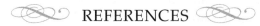 REFERENCES

Atkinson, R. C., & Tuzin, D. (1992). Equilibrium in the research university. *Change, 24*(3), 20–31. doi:10.1080/00091383.1992.10544023

Carnegie Initiative on the Doctorate. (2001). *Overview of doctoral education studies and reports: 1990–present*. Stanford, CA: Carnegie Foundation for the Advancement of Teaching.

Carper, B. A. (1978). Fundamental patterns of knowing in nursing. *Advances in Nursing Science, 1*(1), 13–23. doi:10.1097/00012272-197810000-00004

Chinn, P. (2013). *Peace and power: New directions for building community* (8th ed.). Burlington, MA: Jones & Bartlett.

Kennedy, S. (2007). *God and country: American in red and blue*. Waco, Texas: Baylor University Press.

Kreitzer, M. J., & Koithan, M. (2014). *Integrative nursing*. New York, NY: Oxford University Press.

Kuhn, T. (1962). *The structure of scientific revolutions*. Chicago, IL: University of Chicago Press.

Kuhn, T. (2012). *The structure of scientific revolutions* (4th ed.). Chicago, IL: University of Chicago Press.

Lee, S. M., Palmieri, P. A., & Watson, J. (Eds.). (2017). *Global advances in human caring literacy*. New York, NY: Springer Publishing.

Sitzman, K., & Watson, J. (2017). *Watson's caring in the digital world*. New York, NY: Springer Publishing.

Walker, G. E., Golde, C. M., Jones, L., Bueschel, A. C., & Hutchings, P. (2008). *The formation of scholars: Rethinking doctoral education for the twenty-first century*. San Francisco, CA: Jossey-Bass.

Watson, J. (1985). *Nursing: The philosophy and science of caring*. Boulder: University Press of Colorado. (Original work Published 1979).

Watson, J. (2005). *Caring science as sacred science*. Philadelphia, PA: F. A. Davis.

Watson, J. (2008). *Nursing: The philosophy and science of caring, Revised* (2nd ed.). Boulder: University Press of Colorado.

Watson, J. (2012). *Human caring science: A theory of nursing* (2nd ed.). Sudbury, MA: Jones & Bartlett.

Watson, J. (2017). Global advances in human caring literacy. In S. M. Lee, P. A. Palmieri, & J. Watson (Eds.), *Global advances in human caring literacy* (pp. 3–12). New York, NY: Springer Publishing.

Watson, J., & Smith, M. (2002). Caring science and the science of unitary human beings: A transtheoretical discourse for nursing knowledge development. *Journal of Advanced Nursing, 37*(5), 452–461. doi:10.1046/j.1365-2648.2002.02112.x

Zander, P. E. (2007). Ways of knowing in nursing: The historical evolution of a concept. *Journal of Theory Construction & Testing, 11*(1), 7–11.

20

Advancing Caring Science Through the Missions of Teaching, Research/Scholarship, Practice, and Service

Marlaine C. Smith

CARITAS LITERACIES

By the end of this chapter, the caring-healing nurse will be able to

1. Describe an example of how Caring Science can guide the missions of a college of nursing.

2. Develop a mission, vision, philosophy, and curricular framework consistent with Caring Science knowledge and values.

3. Create curricula and teaching–learning processes consistent with Caring Science pedagogy.

4. Identify strategies to advance the research agenda for Caring Science.

5. Apply Caring Science–based models to guide innovative nurse-led centers and practices.

6. Advance college service projects aligned with a mission centered on Caring Science.

❦

We all search for the ideal place to work and learn. Perhaps such a place is one that supports and nurtures the process of living one's values. In this environment, we feel we are at home, in a place where we can be who we are truly meant to be, where we can express and manifest what matters most to us. In 2006, I moved to a College of Nursing where this was possible for me, and this chapter is about what I have learned about creating environments in an academic setting where our cherished nursing values can be made visible, guide our actions, and nurture the growth of faculty, students, and staff.

Academic settings have the common tripartite mission of teaching, research, and service. Many colleges of nursing have added practice to the mission to differentiate it from university and community service, and to emphasize the development of innovative models that can transform practice. In this chapter, I describe how the knowledge and values of Caring Science have shaped the Christine E. Lynn College of Nursing (CELCON) at Florida Atlantic University and how Caring Science has been advanced through the missions of the College.

BACKGROUND

Florida Atlantic University's Department of Nursing was founded in 1979 with four faculty, a director, and 10 RN-BSN students. The faculty struggled to create a curriculum that responded to the RN students' challenge: "What more can we learn about nursing?"; and the faculty's question: "What is the content of the discipline to be learned in nursing?" (Boykin, 1994). The core concept of Caring emerged as the essence of nursing (Boykin, Touhy, & Smith, 2011, p. 157). This focus has endured for nearly 40 years. The College is known for its singular dedication to Caring. Although the philosophy has evolved, this particular dedication has shaped the identity of the College, attracted students and faculty who resonate with this concept, and distinguished it as a center to advance the study of Caring as a science. There is a reciprocal relationship between the values and the work of the college: The core value shapes the work of the College and the work of the College advances the core value. Many things have changed over this time: Now the College has over 50 faculty and about 1,200 students in programs of study at the baccalaureate, master's, and doctoral levels (both DNP and PhD). But what has not changed is the passion for the substantive knowledge of nursing and the belief that nursing offers a unique and invaluable service to the health of humankind—Caring.

VISION, MISSION, AND PHILOSOPHY

It all begins with articulating core values. The mission, philosophy, and vision statements of any school of nursing are the beacons that guide it in its being and becoming. These statements provide a cogent purpose for its existence, differentiate it from other institutions, and provide the necessary foundations for fleshing out each facet of the mission. In too many situations, the vision, mission, and philosophy of a college of nursing are developed as a required exercise but are not used as a blueprint to guide priority setting, decision making, and day-to-day actions. If we really believe in the significance of these documents, then we would approach them with the reverence they deserve. Developing the mission, philosophy, and vision statements is an organizational spiritual exercise. Each organizational community might approach the process of developing these documents with the understanding that through articulating what matters most to them, they are structuring the heart and soul of their academic community. Within these documents, values about the discipline and profession of nursing, teaching, and learning are made visible.

The mission, vision, and excerpts of the CELCON philosophy appear in Table 20.1. The CELCON defines nursing as "nurturing the wholeness of persons and environment

TABLE 20.1 Mission, Vision, and Excerpts From Philosophy
Mission
The Christine E. Lynn College of Nursing, as an integral part of Florida Atlantic University, is committed to the pursuit of higher education grounded in the arts, sciences and humanities. Faculty of the College support the University mission of teaching, research/scholarship and service within an environment that fosters inclusiveness. The Christine E. Lynn College of Nursing is dedicated to Caring: advancing the science, practicing the art, studying its meaning and living Caring day-to-day.
Vision
Florida Atlantic University's Christine E. Lynn College of Nursing will be the international preeminent leader in advancing caring science through its dynamic, innovative caring based education, research, scholarship and practices.
Philosophy Excerpts
• Nursing is a discipline and a profession. • Scholarship and practice require multiple ways of knowing. • Caring is a mutual process of artistically responding to calls from clients. • Nursing occurs within nursing situations: lived experiences in which caring between the nurse and client fosters well-being. • Person is unique and dynamically interconnected with others and the environment in caring relationships. • Persons choose values, culturally-derived, that give meaning to living and enhance well-being. • Well-being is creating and living the meaning of life. • Well-being is nurtured through caring relationships. • Learning is creating understanding through integration of knowledge in the context of values and meaning. • A caring environment supports learning. • In a caring environment the person is nurtured, supported and celebrated. • The learning environment emphasizes collegial relationships between faculty and students.

Source: Retrieved from Christine E. Lynn College of Nursing. (n.d.-f). Philosophy. Retrieved from http://nursing.fau.edu/about/college-at-a-glance/philosophy.php; Christine E. Lynn College of Nursing. (n.d.-g). Vision and mission statement. Retrieved from http://nursing.fau.edu/about/college-at-a-glance/vision-and-mission.php

in caring" (n.d.-d). It is clear from the mission, vision, and philosophy statements that Caring is the guiding beacon for the CELCON. The prominence of Caring in these documents is essential for any college seeking to create a Caring Science–based program.

THE IMPORTANCE OF LEADERSHIP

Before describing how these Caring values have grounded the missions of the College of Nursing (CON), it is important to acknowledge the importance of leadership. Leaders keep the vision in the foreground, always calling the faculty, staff, and students to its importance. They cocreate an environment where the faculty, staff, and students can live the values important to their academic community and actualize the mission, vision, and philosophy. In addition, leaders articulate and translate the vision, mission, and philosophy to external constituents and mobilize the resources of the organization toward the realization of this vision. I think of leadership as the process of helping others find their way home (Smith, 2004). By "home," I mean being in the right place, being who we truly are, where we can rest in authentic being, and where knowing, being, and doing are integrated. This is a place of feeling at ease, living out what is most important to us, being who we are meant to be, and acting in harmony with our deepest connection to our True Self. Leaders inspire organizations and its members to find their way home—discover and enact their authentic mission in society. Models consistent with caring-based leadership or "leading from the heart" (Turkel, 2014) are servant leadership, mindful leadership (Marturano, 2014), *Peace and Power* principles and processes (Chinn, 2013), strength-based leadership (Rath & Conchie, 2008), and leadership models developed from caring theories (Watson, 2006).

CREATING A CULTURE OF CARING

Beliefs and values of the faculty create the culture of an organization. In a Caring Science–based program, Caring informs the ways of relating to self and others within the academic community. The Dance of Caring Persons (Boykin & Schoenhofer, 2001; Figure 20.1)

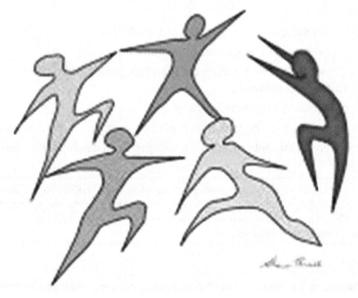

FIGURE 20.1 The dance of caring persons.

Source: Reprinted with permission from Boykin, A., & Schoenhofer, S. O. (2001). *Nursing as caring: A model for transforming practice.* Sudbury, MA: Jones & Bartlett.

is the model used in this College to capture the meaning of organizational caring relationships.

> This model serves as a constant visual re-presentation of right relationship grounded in respect for and valuing of each person. The flat, non-hierarchical, circle conveys that each person in this dance brings unique gifts to the work of the college. No one person's gifts are more important than another's—just different due to roles and responsibilities. For this reason, the College's structure is not usually represented in a traditional organization chart, but instead, a circular, flat structure depicting interrelationships rather than hierarchy. Each person/dancer is viewed as special and caring. Each role is essential to accomplishing the mission and vision of the College. The circle is open as there is always need for others to join the dance to accomplish the mission. The intent of all dancers is to know other as caring person and support each other in living caring uniquely. (Boykin & Schoenhofer, 2001; Boykin et al., 2011, pp. 161–162)

These beliefs are intended to directly guide our way of being in the CELCON, "The declaration that all persons are caring and engaged in caring relationships calls for an understanding of what it means to live caring both in the ordinariness of life and uniquely in the practice of nursing" (Boykin et al., 2011, p. 162). The faculty refers to Mayeroff's (1971) caring ingredients as a template for what it means to live caring in relationships with self, others, and students. These ingredients include knowing, honesty, courage, hope, trust, humility, and alternating rhythms:

> Faculty and students reflect on how each of these ingredients is lived uniquely in their lives. This reflection fosters an understanding of self living caring moment to moment and brings forth the realization that expressions of caring are lived uniquely by each person and the challenge is to grow in an understanding of what it means to live caring. (Boykin et al., 2011, p. 162)

Faculty and students are engaged in a reflective process of growing in Caring. They are invited to intentionally engage in the process of caring for self so critical to the ontological development of a nurse. Examples of activities that promote this reflective process are as follows:

- Beginning each Faculty Assembly meeting with the "Gathering," a time for shared reflections and inspiration

- Walking the labyrinth in the College garden as a tool for self-reflection, self-discovery, and manifesting intentions

- Inviting students to write weekly nursing practice logs to reflect on their Caring within nursing situations

- Structuring times for dialogue about the joys and challenges of teaching in a caring-based program

- Learning ways of caring for self, for example, through HeartMath®, mindfulness practices, Reiki classes or yoga in classes, and less formal presentations and practices

- Inviting students to center before each examination

- Integrating experiential strategies within courses, for example: creating aesthetic representations of caring moments, exploring the artistry of their work using Cameron's (1992) book, *The Artist's Way*, using dance or movement to capture processes of practice

DESIGNING A HOME ON THE BASIS OF CARING VALUES

In 2006, a 75,000-square foot new home for the College of Nursing was completed. This home was the fruition of a dream by Dean Anne Boykin and the faculty and funded by Christine E. Lynn, the College's generous benefactor and namesake, a nurse herself, who recognizes the importance of nursing to the health of the community. The College of Nursing "home" was designed to create a healing environment on the basis of three guiding ideas: (a) the College philosophy of Caring and definition of Nursing; (b) reverence for the environment and its centrality to health; and (c) harmonious flow of energy through attention to structure and design. The latter concept is known as *feng shui* in Chinese philosophy, "The purpose of the building was to create a living, breathing place that invites, teaches, houses, protects and nurtures" (Boykin & Raines, 2006, p. 45). The reminder of the core values and philosophy of the College, the dance of caring persons, is cast in the terrazzo floor of the atrium.

This unique building features a circular design to reflect wholeness and connectedness; three floors of windows overlooking a healing garden with a labyrinth; and unique spaces for living the CELCON caring-healing philosophy such as a meditation room, yoga room, and treatment room. A Center for Caring is available to welcome visitors to the building, and a Museum and Archives of Caring houses important artifacts marking the caring movement in nursing and the original writings of international caring scholars. Representation of the five elements of earth, wood, fire, water, and metal is integrated throughout the offices, learning spaces, and service areas of the building to enhance the flow of ch'i or the life force. These elements are represented with wall colors and symbols in the carpet tiles. The walls and staircases curve to create an unobstructed flow of energy. Any sharp corners are remedied by the placement of crystals (Boykin & Raines, 2006). The building is a gold-certified Leadership in Energy and Environmental Design (LEED) building, built in accordance with principles of sustainability and environmental sensitivity (Boykin & Raines, 2006).

When people enter the building, there is a palpable sense of peace and calm. Through the intentional design features of the building, the concepts of reflection/mindfulness, aesthetic appreciation, healing environments, human-environment integrality, holistic health, and the significance of self-care to the being-becoming of the nurse are prominent. These design features are related to the philosophy of caring that underpins the College (Boykin & Raines, 2006).

CARING AND THE TEACHING MISSION

Curricular Structure

The philosophy of caring guides the teaching mission of the College of Nursing through the curricular model, program outcomes, teaching–learning processes, and student support services. The curricular model is represented in Figure 20.2. The visual model

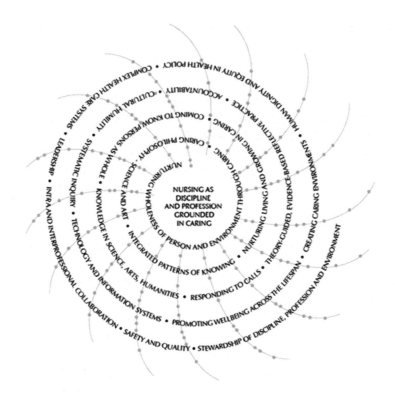

FIGURE 20.2 Curriculum model.

Source: Christine E. Lynn College of Nursing. (n.d.-b). Curriculum Model. Retrieved from http://nursing.fau.edu/academics/curriculum-model.php

emerged as a synthesis of concepts from Martha Rogers, Albert Einstein, the myth of *Indra's Net*, and complexity science. The model is represented as a net composed of bands, strands, and pearls. The circular bands represent the College of Nursing's philosophy and program outcomes. The net is open, without boundary, representing the openness and evolving knowledge that continues to in-form and re-form the curriculum. The strands of the net that emanate outward from the center cross the circular bands and represent the units of instruction within the curriculum. The pearls in the net are nursing situations, the approach to studying nursing in our curriculum. The image of a net represents the interconnectedness of these concepts throughout the curriculum with the pearls as a reflection of the interconnectedness in the nursing situation (CELCON Curriculum Model; CELCON, n.d.-b).

The bands emanate from the Center of the model: *Nursing as a discipline and profession grounded in caring.* The next band is the College's definition of Caring: *Nurturing the wholeness of person-environment through caring.* The following band is *Caring philosophy, science, and art,* encompassing the values within the philosophy of the College, the theories, and research that constitute Caring Science and the art of caring arrived at through aesthetic knowing and performed in practice. Remaining circular bands reflect the major concepts reflected in the program outcomes such as *integrated patterns of knowing; nurturing self, living and growing in caring; foundational knowledge from the sciences, arts, and humanities; theory-guided, evidence-based reflective practice; accountability;* and *cultural humility.* The threads emanating from the center are the levels of instruction: four degree programs, courses, or units that include the content bands.

The curricula are structured with 12 outcomes common to all four-degree programs (CELCON, n.d.-b). The outcomes are leveled and individualized for the focus of each of the four academic programs. Table 20.2 shows an example of two of the program outcomes and how they are leveled for all four-degree programs.

Course titles in the degree programs reflect the focus on Caring and nursing situations as the locus of studying Caring Science. A few of the examples of course titles across programs are as follows: *NUR 3465L The Developing Family: Nursing Situations in Practice, NUR 3115 Foundations of Caring in Nursing Situations, NUR 3171 Creating Healing Environments, NUR 4638 Population Health: Nursing Situations, NUR 6110 Advanced Practice Nursing Grounded in Caring, NGR 7115 Caring: An Essential Domain of Nursing Knowledge,* and *NGR 7661 Population-Based Caring for Aging Populations.*

The faculty decided that it was important to reflect the Caring Science–based curricular model in each course. To do so, "subjectives" were developed to structure course outcomes. The meaning of the term "subjectives" is the formative becoming of the student as caring nurse. "Subjectives" are based on Roach's six Cs: Compassion, Confidence, Commitment, Comportment, Conscience, and Competence. Course objectives are content- or competency-based and are clustered under relevant "subjectives" (Table 20.3). With this structure, the importance and centrality of Caring Science to the curricula are clearly visible to faculty and students in each course in every degree program.

Students at all levels (BSN, MSN, DNP, and PhD.) begin their programs of study with courses that provide knowledge of Caring that is consonant with their levels. The baccalaureate level course is *Foundations of Caring in Nursing Situations*; the master's-level course is *Advanced Nursing Practice Grounded in Caring*; and the doctoral-level course is *Caring: An Essential Domain of Nursing Knowledge*. All four programs have been endorsed by the American Holistic Nursing Credentialing Corporation, and because of the integration of holistic nursing standards and values, certification in holistic nursing is available to students through examination following graduation.

The "nursing situation" guides the study of nursing; this is the ground from which students grow in their knowledge of Caring Science (Barry, Gordon, & King, 2015). Nursing situations are lived experiences in which the caring between the nurse and the client fosters well-being within a cocreative experience (CELCON, n.d.-f). The nursing situation is a story about the nurse–person encounter. All the knowledge needed for nursing is embedded in the story. In this way, the knowledge related to signs and symptoms, medications, treatments, and technologies is contextualized within the experiences of the persons nursed and their significant others in their environment. Students are asked to identify calls for nursing and the responses from the nurse (Boykin & Schoenhofer, 2001; Paterson & Zderad, 1976), "Through authentic presence, as caring person, the nurse is able to enter the world of the other, hear the calls for nursing, and respond appropriately to nurture wholeness" (Touhy & Boykin, 2008, p. 8). Boykin and Schoenhofer (2001) reflected that the conventional nursing process that guides nurses to assess and identify a problem—the nursing diagnosis—does not fit with the intention of our praxis. Rather, the "challenge for nursing is coming to know the other as caring person and to nurture the person in situation specific, creative ways" (p. 30). For them, nursing is "unfolding and guided by intention," and by engaging in the linear process specified by nursing diagnosis we "rob the situation of all the beauty that is nursing" (p. 30).

TABLE 20.2 Two Sample Program Outcomes for Four Programs

OUTCOME #2:

Practice nursing reflectively guided by a caring philosophy and integrating a broad base of knowledge that includes theory and best evidence

BSN Program

1. Synthesize knowledge from the sciences, arts, and humanities as a foundation for generalist practice in nursing
2. Use nursing theories and research to guide caring-based reflective nursing practice

MSN Program	DNP Program	PhD Program
Integrate a broad base of knowledge grounded in caring that includes theory and best evidence for advanced nursing practice	Create innovative models for advanced practice or nursing administration that are grounded in caring, best evidence, and integrate relevant knowledge from nursing and other disciplines	Develop and evaluate theory-guided and evidence-based approaches that inform Caring Science for practice

OUTCOME #3:

Integrate multiple complex patterns of knowing in coming to know persons and responding critically and reflectively to calls within nursing situations

BSN Program

Integrate multiple complex patterns of knowing in coming to know persons and responding critically and reflectively to calls within nursing situations in generalist practice

MSN Program	DNP Program	PhD Program
Integrate multiple complex patterns of knowing in coming to know persons and creatively responding to calls within nursing situations in advanced nursing practice	Integrate multiple complex patterns of knowing in coming to know populations of persons and creatively responding to calls for leadership within nursing situations in advanced nursing practice	Integrate multiple complex patterns of knowing in creation of innovative research designs and methods

Source: Christine E. Lynn College of Nursing. (n.d.-b). Curriculum Model. Retrieved from http://nursing.fau.edu/academics/curriculum-model.php

---

TABLE 20.3 Examples of Course Subjectives With Objectives

1. Becoming competent (subjective)
   - Use SBAR communication to provide a complete, organized report to collaborating nurses and other health professionals that reflects knowing of the whole person
   - Demonstrate assessment and skill in safe dosage calculation and medication administration
2. Becoming compassionate (subjective)
   - Listen to the story of the older adult's health experience to understand and respond to calls for nursing
   - Use touch appropriately to convey presence and understanding

---

SBAR, situation, background, assessment, recommendation.

Source: Information retrieved from Christine E. Lynn College of Nursing. (n.d.-b). Curriculum Model. Retrieved from http://nursing.fau.edu/academics/curriculum-model.php

Caring is both science and art. Caring Science encompasses the substantive knowledge of Caring in the philosophies, theories, and research on Caring. The art of nursing is the creative application of that knowledge in practice choreographed through the unique nurse–person relationship. Each nurse manifests his or her own unique expressions of caring. Each response to a particular nursing situation portrays the singular beauty of that nurse's caring. In this way, the art of nursing is created by each nurse in each situation. Sharing this art deepens our understanding of the richness of our practice and provides an opportunity to reflect on the range of knowledge essential for expert nursing care, "Studying nursing in this way assists students in developing and celebrating nursing knowledge. They grow in their substantive understanding of Caring Science and their appreciation of nursing's unique contribution to the health and wholeness of persons" (Boykin et al., 2011, p. 169).

Empirical patterns of knowing from the prerequisite and supporting courses in the program of study, such as pathophysiology, pharmacology, health assessment, technologies, and psychology, are drawn upon as students engage with the nursing situation. This is only one pattern of knowing; the faculty member calls students to center on the Caring between the nurse and the person. In this way, the Caring becomes the "figure" and any disease processes, treatments, signs, and so on, become the "ground." "Emphasis in nursing courses is on critical reflection and integration of knowledge in specific nursing situations, and creation of nursing responses. The study of Caring is integral to knowing nursing and is a focus in each nursing course at all levels of the program" (Boykin et al., 2011, pp. 169–170).

Learning to teach from nursing situations is an evolving process and our faculty is continuously growing in this area. A book by Barry et al. (2015) featuring nursing situations in a variety of settings has been a valuable teaching resource for mentoring faculty in this approach. Creating videos and digital stories of nursing situations is another useful teaching approach used by the College; for example, YouTube videos presenting series on "Living Caring: Transculturally"; "Caring Colloquium"; and "Theory of Nursing as Caring" appear on the Anne Boykin Institute (ABI) site (nursing.fau.edu/outreach/anne-boykin-institute/youtube_videos.php).

TEACHING–LEARNING PROCESSES

The teaching–learning processes reflect the CELCON philosophy that "a supportive environment for learning is a caring environment. A caring environment is one in which all aspects of the human person are respected, nurtured and celebrated. The learning environment emphasizes collegial relationships with faculty and students" (CELCON, n.d.-f). This type of environment is facilitated through dialogue, debate, and engagement rather than lecture or the "banking" method of education (Friere, 2007) where experts deposit their knowledge into students' empty minds. Instead, faculty and students enter the learning experience as colearners, each with distinctive roles and responsibilities, but both open to the possibilities that emerge in the experience. Critical reflection, self-knowledge, and aesthetic awareness are fostered. Some of these aesthetic representations are found in *Nightingale Songs* or the *Journal of Art and Aesthetics in Nursing and Health Sciences*, CELCON journals containing poems and prose that express Caring. Faculty has published on the importance of aesthetics to the pedagogy of Caring Science (Barry & Purnell, 2008).

The use of technology in nursing education is growing and is integrated thoughtfully and intentionally as teaching–learning processes. For example, simulations featuring the use of mannequins have become standard in most nursing programs. The traditional approach is to use these mannequins to teach skills and critical thinking in response to pathophysiological changes that are programmed into the mannequin. Simulations reflecting a nursing grounded in Caring Science are designed differently (Eggenberger & Keller, 2008). Students are introduced to a situated patient–family drama in which the nursing situation evolves. They become actors in the drama as they not only practice skills and think critically about their responses and priorities but also comfort patients in pain, explain procedures to family members, and support the patient and family in the dying process. The hospice simulation features a host of actors playing the roles of a patient's (mannequin) daughter and healthcare team members. Those witnessing the simulation are often moved to tears.

Online courses provide access to education for students who could not enroll in classes otherwise. The teaching-learning strategies used in these courses foster virtual Caring communities (Watson, 2002). For example, in a hybrid course, Chinn's (2013) *Peace and Power* process is used to engage all participants as collaborators in teaching-learning. Faculty engage in a variety of strategies to create virtual caring communities in online classes. A doctoral student studied the process of virtual presence mediated by technology to inform strategies of communicating caring through email and social media (Grumme, Barry, Gordon, & Ray, 2016).

The caring philosophy and values of the College guide the development of academic policies. It is important to understand that Caring does not mean lowering standards. Quite the opposite. Competence is one of the qualities of Caring described by Roach (1984), and students must demonstrate competent practice to ensure our covenant of Caring for those we serve. Students and faculty approach evaluation with Mayeroff's (1971) definition of Caring as "helping the other to grow" (p. 1), and with the ingredients of knowing, honesty, patience, humility, courage, hope, trust, and alternating rhythms (Mayeroff, 1971). Students are nurtured in their growth in Caring, and policies and services are designed to promote this growth.

CARING AND THE RESEARCH MISSION

The research mission of the CELCON is advancing Caring Science within the discipline of nursing:

> Caring Science, in the discipline of nursing, is the body of knowledge, arrived at through intentional research and theory development, focused on the relationship of caring to health, healing and well-being of the whole person within the context of the family, community, society and within the global environment. (CELCON, n.d.-c, "Our Unique Focus on Caring")

The research mission is advanced through the CELCON's organizational structure, faculty recruitment, and a mentoring program for new faculty. The organizational structure to support the research mission includes an Office of Research and Scholarship and PhD Studies. This Office has an associate dean for Research and Scholarship, two research coordinators who support faculty in preparing and managing grants, an editor to assist faculty with manuscript development, and a statistician.

The associate dean leads a Research Advisory Committee whose work involved the development of goals for the CELCON Strategic Plan that include the following: Specifying the meaning of Caring Science and its importance to the discipline of nursing; delineating caring frameworks and/or models that capture, define, and/or operationalize caring constructs to advance Caring Science; initiating strategies to increase funding for work in advancing Caring Science; evaluating the connection of the College's research focus areas to University priorities; and creating a culture that supports a research-intensive environment (CELCON Strategic Plan 2016–2021). A well-funded intramural grants program exists to support pilot work with the expectation that this work will lead to proposals for external funding. The criteria for awarding this intramural funding include the development of an explicit connection to Caring Science. The guidelines for applicants state: "How does the proposed work emerge from a Caring philosophy and fit into your ongoing research program?" In this way, the College encourages faculty to shape their research trajectories within a Caring Science–based framework (Boykin et al., 2011).

Faculty recruitment is perhaps the most important activity for the future of any college. The faculty is recruited to the CELCON who have a passion for nursing as a discipline and value Caring Science. The prospective faculty is invited to frame their research, scholarship, and/or practice within Caring Science. Interview questions include queries about their understanding and appreciation of the philosophy and how they view their work within the context of advancing Caring Science. Prospective faculty has the opportunity to be reflective and intentional in their choice to join our community.

The faculty has clustered their research in Caring Science under four main areas: Healthy Aging, Health Equity, Holistic Health, and Transforming Practice Environments. Examples of faculty research projects include the following: caring communication patterns between spouses when one of them has memory loss; using HeartMath techniques for persons with depression; moral distress in chief nurse executives, addressing incivility (horizontal violence) in the workplace; what matters most to caregivers of people with mild to moderate dementia; and addressing disparities in genetic screening in underserved minority populations. In each of these diverse research projects, the faculty has made some explicit relationship to advancing Caring Science through their theoretical grounding.

Mentoring is essential to developing the research mission. Every new faculty is assigned to a mentoring team. The team consists of senior faculty who support the faculty in teaching and research. Research mentors assist new faculty in connecting their ideas to Caring Science, identifying research collaborators and resources for funding, and writing grants and manuscripts. The associate dean for Research meets with the faculty and mentors. Teaching mentors assist faculty in learning the curriculum, Caring Science resource literature, and teaching from nursing situations (Boykin et al., 2011).

CARING AND THE PRACTICE MISSION

The practice mission of the CELCON encompasses the development of innovative Caring Science–based practice models. The practices become vibrant learning laboratories where faculty practice and students learn. In addition, the practices are the site for research. The College has two nurse-led centers and other school-based faculty practices. One is the Louis and Anne Green Memory and Wellness Center, with a unique mission grounded in Caring Science, The mission of the Center "is to meet the complex needs of persons with memory disorders … and their families through a comprehensive array of services, compassionate and innovative programs of care, research and education" (CELCON, n.d.-e, para. 1). The Center has an interprofessional team of gerontological nurse practitioners, nurses, neuropsychologists, social workers, art therapists, yoga teachers, physical therapists, and activity coordinators. The explicit intention of the Center is to treat the whole person "with dignity and respect, enabling each client to function at his or her personal best while maximizing their quality of life" (CELCON, n.d.-e, para. 1) The Center's two buildings house a diagnostic clinic, a dementia-specific adult day center, counseling, and educational and research activities. One of the two buildings features a healing room, an art room, and flexible space for yoga, dance, and other activities. Baccalaureate, master's, and doctoral students in the College have practicum experiences at the Center. In this way, students can witness and engage in nursing practice guided by Caring Science. The Center becomes a vibrant learning laboratory where Caring is lived, learned, and studied (Boykin et al., 2011).

The College of Nursing's Community Health Center (CHC) is located in an underserved area and serves a diverse community of people. The CHC provides an array of services through Caring Science–based interprofessional team-based care including integrated, culturally safe, primary and mental healthcare, diabetes specialty care, women's healthcare, and outreach for primary and secondary prevention. The staff includes advanced practice nurses, a physician, nurse diabetes educators, case managers, social workers, community outreach workers, medical assistants, nutritionists, and pharmacists. The Center is directed by an advanced practice nurse who knows the needs of the community. Students in the Colleges of Nursing, Medicine, and the School of Social Work have practicum experiences at both nurse-led centers. The CON philosophy guides the practice in the Center described by the patients as a family or home-like environment where they feel welcomed and respected.

The Nursing Leadership Institute (NLI) fosters the leadership development of nurses at all levels. The Institute offers evidence-based programs and resources to local and regional nursing administrators using a relationship-based approach to leadership, consistent with Caring Science. The goal is to help nurses to develop their leadership skills through continuing education programs and sharing of best practices. Dialogues with nursing leaders in the community inform the programs offered by the NLI.

The Initiative for Intentional Well-Being, a part of the Christine E. Lynn Center for Caring, offers programs related to holistic health and humanizing healthcare. For example, yoga classes are offered several days a week, and nutrition, therapeutic touch, integrative nurse coaching, and Reiki classes have been offered to nurses in the community. A room for providing massage, therapeutic touch, or Reiki is available. The purpose of the initiative is to integrate holistic caring practices into nursing education and practice.

Academic-practice partnerships have been created to transform practice environments through implementing caring-based practice models. For example, the Port St. Lucie Medical Center partnered with the College of Nursing to adopt Boykin and Schoenhofer's (2001) Theory of Nursing as Caring as a model for the entire organization. The Caring-based Academic Practice Partnerships (CAPP), the Recruitment, Education and Employment of Primary Care Providers (REEP), and the Caring-based Academic Partnership in Excellence (CAPE) grants, funded by the Health Resources and Services Agency, have provided resources to develop practicum sites for nurse practitioner students that serve diverse, underserved populations.

CARING AND THE SERVICE MISSION

Faculty and students fulfill the service mission of the College and University through volunteer work with the local, regional, national, and global communities. This service is consistent with the mission, vision, and philosophy of the College of Nursing. Service learning is a component of several courses where students engage with communities in projects identified as important by the community. For example, students have developed recreational programs in assisted-living facilities or offered health screenings in communities. Faculty combines a study abroad trip to Guatemala with our service mission by collecting donations for vented wood stoves and installing them for families who suffer effects of smoke inhalation from cooking within their nonventilated homes. The Student Nurses Association and the CELCON Sigma Theta Tau chapter adopt needy families for the holidays, participate in fundraising for healthcare organizations, and volunteer for peer tutoring. Faculty, students, and alumni have partnered with organizations in Haiti, Guatemala, and Uganda to provide nursing education and critically needed nursing care.

CONCLUSION

CONTINUING THE WORK

Sustaining and growing a Caring Science–based program in a university setting requires commitment, vigilance, and nurturance. Transitioning leadership, faculty turnover, funding pressures, and the next bandwagon in nursing can threaten its existence. There are several initiatives in place to promote the sustainability of the program. First is the ABI for the Study of Caring in Nursing. The Institute, created in 2011, offers Summer Academies with focused topics. The agendas of previous Academies were Caring-Based Education, Research in Caring Science, and Interprofessional Practice Grounded in Caring. The Institute is funded by an endowment with a mission to provide "the global leadership for nursing education, practice, and research grounded in caring; [promote] the valuing of caring across disciplines; and [support] the caring mission of the Christine E. Lynn College of Nursing" (CELCON, n.d.-a, "Mission").

Next, the CELCON established the Archives of Caring in Nursing with the mission of preserving the history of Caring in Nursing, inviting the study of Caring, advancing Caring as a science and an essential domain of nursing knowledge, and creating meaning for the practice of nursing (nursing.fau.edu/outreach/archives-of-caring/index.php). The presence of the Archives is a commitment to the legacy of the College. By securing the papers of Caring scholars, the Archives is a rich access for Caring scholars. This preserves the caring knowledge of the past as a springboard for knowledge development for the future.

Nurturing the growth of the next generation of Caring Science scholars is essential. Doctoral students are the intellectual lifeblood of any college. The PhD students advance Caring Science through their theory development and research, whereas the DNP students lead the transformation of healthcare through implementing Caring Science–based practice models. Those prepared at the doctoral levels will seed and grow Caring Science in other educational and practice environments.

With an increasing number of national and international nursing scholars studying Caring Science, alternative educational models that can be offered to those who want to study Caring Science are essential. This could be in the form of certificate programs, webinars, and YouTube videos. Some of these are already available. The Caritas Coach Program and the Watson Caring Science hospital affiliates offered through the Watson Caring Science Institute (www.watsoncaringscience.org) and the Watson Caring Science Center provide educational opportunities and resources outside of degree programs. The ABI for the Advancement of Caring in Nursing has offered a colloquium, summer academies, webinars, and videos that can engage nurses in exploring aspects of Caring Science (nursing.fau .edu/abi). The College is launching an international postdoctoral fellowship program in Caring Science.

Finally, the Carnegie Report on the future of nursing education (Benner, Sutphen, Leonard, & Day, 2010) calls for reforms that align with a Caring Science–based approach to education: "This report recommends a situated, contextual approach to learning through the use of narratives, patient interviews and case studies that engage students in clinical reasoning and clinical imagination" (Boykin et al., 2011, p. 183). This approach is consistent with using nursing situations for studying Caring in Nursing. The use of a simulation for practicing expressions of Caring "transforms it from an exercise in technical know-how and critical thinking to a rehearsal of ethical comportment and growing ontological competencies," so important to living caring in practice situations (Boykin et al., 2011, p. 183).

The CELCON has fully integrated Caring Science within its teaching, research, practice, and service missions. Caring Science is visible in the mission, vision, values, and philosophy of the CELCON and explicit in its curricular model, program outcomes, and courses. The culture of living caring within the community is strong, and as in any culture, it will endure with mentoring and orientation programs. Growing and sustaining this program will require commitment, vigilance, and continuing passion for the importance of this work in the transformation of the discipline and enhancing health and healing of those we serve.

NEXT ERA POSSIBILITIES

Education

- What are the advantages of having a curriculum model grounded in Caring Science?
- Describe examples of pedagogies that are caring-based. What makes them so?

Research

- How can a college of nursing evaluate the difference that a Caring-based approach to teaching-learning makes in student outcomes?
- What research focus areas can constitute Caring Science?

Praxis

- How can teachers help students grow in Caring?
- How can faculty evaluate the Caring behaviors of students?

Theory and Knowledge Development

- Provide an example of how a concept from a Caring theory can be taught, modeled, and evaluated in a teaching-learning situation.
- Create a curriculum model on the basis of a selected Caring theory.

 REFERENCES

Barry, C. D., Gordon, S. C., & King, B. M. (2015). *Nursing case studies in caring across the practice spectrum.* New York, NY: Springer Publishing.

Barry, C. D., & Purnell, M. (2008). Uncovering meaning through the aesthetic turn: A pedagogy of caring. *International Journal for Human Caring, 12*(2), 19–23.

Benner, P., Sutphen, M., Leonard, V., & Day, L. (2010). *Educating nurses: A call for radical transformation.* San Francisco, CA: Jossey-Bass.

Boykin, A. (1994). *Living a caring-based program.* New York, NY: National League for Nursing.

Boykin, A., & Raines, D. A. (2006). Design and structure as an expression of caring. *International Journal for Human Caring, 10*(4), 45–49.

Boykin, A., & Schoenhofer, S. O. (2001). *Nursing as caring: A model for transforming practice.* Sudbury, MA: Jones & Bartlett.

Boykin, A., Touhy, T. A., & Smith, M. C. (2011). Evolution of a caring-based college of nursing. In M. Hills & J. Watson (Eds.), *Creating a caring science curriculum: An emancipatory pedagogy for nursing* (pp. 157–184). New York, NY: Springer Publishing.

Cameron, J. (1992). *The artist's way: A spiritual path to higher creativity.* New York, NY: J. P. Tarcher.

Chinn, P. L. (2013). *Peace and power: New directions for building community* (8th ed.). Burlington, MA: Jones & Bartlett.

Christine E. Lynn College of Nursing. (n.d.-a). Anne Boykin Institute for the Advancement of Caring in Nursing: Mission vision history. Retrieved from http://nursing.fau.edu/outreach/anne-boykin -institute/mission-vision-history.php

Christine E. Lynn College of Nursing. (n.d.-b). Curriculum Model. Retrieved from http://nursing.fau.edu/academics/curriculum-model.php

Christine E. Lynn College of Nursing. (n.d.-c). History & introduction. Retrieved from http://nursing.fau.edu/about/college-at-a-glance/index.php

Christine E. Lynn College of Nursing. (n.d.-d). Introduction. Retrieved from http://nursing.fau.edu/academics/student-resources/graduate/introduction.php

Christine E. Lynn College of Nursing. (n.d.-e). Louis and Anne Green Memory & Wellness Center. Retrieved from http://nursing.fau.edu/outreach/memory-and-wellness-center/index.php

Christine E. Lynn College of Nursing. (n.d.-f). Philosophy. Retrieved from http://nursing.fau.edu/about/college-at-a-glance/philosophy.php

Christine E. Lynn College of Nursing. (n.d.-g). Vision and mission statement. Retrieved from http://nursing.fau.edu/about/college-at-a-glance/vision-and-mission.php

Eggenberger, T., & Keller, K. (2008). Grounding nursing simulations in caring: An innovative approach. *International Journal for Human Caring, 12*(2), 42–46.

Friere, P. (2007). *Pedagogy of the oppressed (30th anniversary edition)*. New York, NY: Continuum.

Grumme, V. S., Barry, C. D., Gordon, S. C., & Ray, M. A. (2016). On virtual presence. *Advances in Nursing Science, 39*(1), 48–59. doi:10.1097/ANS.0000000000000103

Marturano, J. (2014). *Finding the space to lead: A practical guide to mindful leadership*. New York, NY: Bloombury Press.

Mayeroff, M. (1971). *On caring*. New York, NY: Harper Perennial.

Paterson, J., & Zderad, L. (1976). *Humanistic nursing*. New York, NY: Wiley.

Rath, T., & Conchie, B. (2008). *Strengths-based leadership: Great leaders, teams and why people follow*. New York, NY: Gallup Press.

Roach, S. (1984). *Caring: The human mode of being: Implications for nursing*. Ottawa, ON: Canadian Hospital Association Press.

Smith, M. (2004). *Leadership lessons learned along the yellow brick road*. Presentation at Sigma Theta Tau Alpha Kappa Chapter-at-Large Research Day, Denver, CO.

Touhy, T., & Boykin, A. (2008). Caring as the central domain in nursing education. *International Journal for Human Caring, 12*(2), 8–15.

Turkel, M. C. (2014). Leading from the heart: Caring, love, peace, and values guiding leadership. *Nursing Science Quarterly, 27*(2), 172–177. doi:10.1177/0894318414522663

Watson, J. (2002). Metaphysics of virtual caring communities. *International Journal for Human Caring, 6*(1), 41–45.

Watson, J. (2006). Caring theory as an ethical guide to administrative and clinical practices. *Nursing Administration Quarterly, 30*(1), 48–55. doi:10.1097/00006216-200601000-00008

V

Authenticating Caring Science Through Scholarly Inquiry

V

21

Leading From the Heart: Caring, Love, Peace, and Values Guiding Leadership*

Marian C. Turkel

CARITAS LITERACIES

By the end of this chapter, the caring-healing nurse will be able to

1. Reframe the traditional language of nursing leadership into one grounded in Caring Science and the unitary-transformative paradigm.

2. Provide additional Caring Science exemplars to Tables 21.1 and 21.2.

3. Reflect on the meaning of love in the role of nursing leadership.

With the emergence of the American Nurses Credentialing Center (ANCC) Magnet Recognition program®, recognizing excellence in professional nursing practice, nursing theory is being used to guide practice in a variety of healthcare settings and systems around the world. Contemporary nursing practice positioned within the worldview of the unitary-transformative paradigm focuses on Caring Science, caring values, and creating caring-healing environments for nurses, patients, and families. Within the context of this paradigm, the concepts of relationships, patterns, values, healing, authentic presence, cocreating, being, engaging, caring, complexity, humanity, and intentionality are used to describe nursing practice grounded in theory-guided professional practice models. Theories framed in Caring Science are being used to inform and transform nursing practice at both the national and the international levels. As direct care (staff) registered nurses are integrating caring theory into practice, they are leading the profession and, in reality, using Parse's

*Reprinted with permission from Turkel, M. (2014). Leading from the heart: Caring, love, peace, and values guiding leadership. *Nursing Science Quarterly*, 27(2), 172–177. doi:10.1177/0894318414522663

humanbecoming leading-following model (Bournes, 2013; Parse, 2008) as they are providing nursing care with respect and dignity, reaffirming their own values, and finding their voice as they integrate caring practices with authenticity and intentionality. As informed theory-guided practice or praxis emerges, it is simultaneously freeing or emancipatory for registered nurses. One nurse shared the following: "We open up our hearts to do what we need, it is out of love as our patients are so vulnerable, we just do it, we don't ask permission, it reaffirms why we are in nursing" (Ray & Turkel, 2014).

The ANCC Magnet program recognizes transformational leadership. In the past, transformational leadership focused on concepts such as skilled communication, collaboration, effective decision making, outcome measurement, and financial management in terms of productivity, and strategic planning. Contemporary transformational leadership focuses on authentic leadership styles, relational caring, meaningful recognition, creativity, building trust, relationships, participative decision making, dialogue with time for reflection, and innovation (Boykin & Schoenhofer, 2010; Boykin, Schoenhofer, & Valentine, 2014; Ray & Turkel, 2012; Watson, 2006). Sullivan-Marx (2013) added to this expanding body of knowledge by using Carper's Ways of Knowing as a framework for nursing leadership. This paradigm shift is occurring at the same time the U.S. healthcare system is making the shift from volume-based payments to value-based payments. The purpose of this chapter is to illuminate how concepts from the unitary-transformative paradigm and Caring Science can be integrated within nursing leadership practice, to invite nursing leaders to make these concepts explicit in their own transformational leadership journey, and to offer ways of reframing traditional organizational language. As you read this chapter, I extend an invitation to you to reflect on the future and what transformational leadership will look like when nursing leaders make decisions on the basis of love, caring, and values instead of fear related to regulatory practices, business, and economics.

Through the Lens of the Unitary-Transformative Paradigm: Relevance of Theoretical and Philosophical Tenets to Leadership

The original focus of scholarly discourse and critique of extant literature within the discipline of nursing centered on the relationship of the nurse to the patient (human being), health, and/or the environment. Nurse scholars provided meaningful contributions to advance the disciplinary perspective of what constitutes nursing knowledge and the practice of nursing (Smith, 1999). Nursing's disciplinary focus continues to be advanced by theorists and scholars. Knowledge development informed by central tenets from the unitary-transformative paradigm recognizes the commonalities of philosophical, theoretical, and conceptual frameworks related to Caring Science and complexity science, and the congruence among the concepts of relationships, patterns, energy, mutuality, wholeness, belonging, and connectedness.

The original thesis of nursing knowledge and theory development did not make explicit the role of the nurse leader in relationship to the health and well-being of those they are leading. However, this is changing as theory transcends practice and theory-guided practice is being actualized by registered nurses. Nurse leaders are recognizing their role in creating practice environments that are congruent with the values of caring theory, sustaining positive, supportive work environments, and integrating theoretical concepts into their practice of leadership (Boykin et al., 2014; Ray & Turkel, 2012; Watson, 2006). Extant nursing theories situated within the unitary-transformative paradigm can serve as the philosophical framework that honors and gives meaning to the art and science of nursing leadership and provides a new way of conceptualizing the practice of nursing leadership.

Building on Rogers's Science of Unitary Human Beings and its concepts of pattern recognition, human as energy fields, open systems, and continuous and innovative change in human-environment energy fields (Smith, 2011), a new approach in practice is emerging that is situated within complex systems. Rogers viewed caring as important within nursing practice but not as a substantive area within the discipline (Smith, 1999). Today, changes related to healthcare reimbursement, healthcare economics, efficiency standards, productivity measures, intense focus on quality scores, regulatory policies and procedures, and technological advances are accelerating faster than in the previous two decades. Leaders can recognize their own energy pattern and how their energy influences relationships with colleagues and the system. Personal or system imbalance creates negative energy patterns within the system as a whole, whereas creativity, innovation, and openness allow for transformation to occur.

Parse's *humanbecoming school of thought* advanced from her original works includes the theoretical concepts of lived experiences, presence, human science, meaning, transcendence, rhythmical patterns of relating, and uncertainty (Parse, 2010). *Humanbecoming theory* serves as the theoretical framework for the humanbecoming leading-following model (Parse, 2008). Bournes (2013) illuminated how the model guided the practice of nursing where formal leaders mentored and developed staff nurses to lead research projects related to patient-centered care and quality of work-life. Bournes (2013) referred to the three essences of Parse's humanbecoming leading-following model as deliberately innovating, potent engaging, and persistently pursuing excellence. This humanbecoming leading-following model thus can serve as a framework for creating professional models of care, identifying future visions for practice, reframing organizational values, and reenergizing the spirit of colleagues to reconnect with their true passions.

Watson's (2008) *theory of human caring,* grounded in the ontology and epistemology of Caring Science, allows for the creation of authentic Caring Science transformational leadership practices and for caring and healing to occur within self and system. Watson's (2008) 10 *Caritas Processes*® give a voice and language to the practice of nursing and inform nursing leadership. Theoretical concepts include authentic presence, patterns, energy, relational ontology, open emergence, love, altruistic values, being, intentionality, and evolving consciousness. Watson's (2003) philosophical reflection on love and caring within the practice of nursing makes explicit the connection among caring, love, and humanity that is needed for transformation of self and system. Watson's most recent innovation involves inviting healthcare systems to be designated as an *International/National Caring Science Affiliate* of the *Watson Caring Science Institute* (WCSI). Caring Science Affiliates are invited on the basis of the chief nurse executive's (CNE) visionary leadership, commitment, and continued dedication to Caring Science theory informing scholarship, and professional practices within his or her hospital or system. WCSI Caring Science Affiliates have demonstrated tangible authentic human caring value-guided foundational changes and outcomes. The affiliate CNEs work in collaboration with Watson to identify and establish defining criteria for authenticating Caring Science at a system-wide level in the areas of practice, research, education, and leadership.

Early in the evolution of Caring Science, at the first National Conference on Caring in 1978, Ray (1981) presented a philosophical inquiry on the study of caring. Her claim that caring was the essence of nursing involved a philosophical analysis using the works of Marcel, Buber, and Mayeroff, the nursing source, Nightingale, and a qualitative inquiry with children and women to illuminate the essence of caring as *copresence and love*, oblative love or *other-directedness* characterized by the unfolding of mystery, authentic presence, interest, empathy, touch (touching the heart), and dialogue (communication).

Ray and Turkel (2012) have been studying caring within complex systems from the perspective of nursing leaders, staff nurses, patients, and administrators for over 20 years. Ray and Turkel's *theory of relational caring complexity* was generated from research on caring and economics within complex systems and is viewed as a metatheory (Ray & Turkel, 2012) originating from the sentinel *theory of bureaucratic caring*, and informed by the theories of *struggling to find a balance, relational complexity*, and *relational self-organization*. (Please refer to the 2012 source for a detailed reference list of the scholarly works of Ray; Ray and Turkel; Turkel; and Turkel and Ray.) Research (Ray & Turkel, 2012) related to the *relational caring questionnaires* demonstrated a link between caring and economics. Findings from a multi-site study showed that the hospital with the highest mean scores related to organizational caring had a slightly lower number of registered nurses per shift, the lowest number of patient falls, and the lowest cost per adjusted patient day. These findings validated what registered nurses verbalized in the quantitative research, "Living the caring values in everyday practice makes a difference in nursing practice and patient outcomes" (Ray & Turkel, 2012, p. 34).

The *theory of relational caring complexity* and associated research findings serve as a guide for nursing leadership in practice by advancing the notion of caring economics, valuing caring resources, and highlighting the ethical choice making related to resource allocation. Concepts within the theory and concepts derived from research include patterns of relationship, interconnectedness, self-organizing, cocreative process, ethical caring, openness, and values.

The *Theory of Nursing as Caring: A Model for Transforming Practice* advanced by Boykin and Schoenhofer serves as a framework for nurses in practice, the practice of nursing leadership, nursing education, and research. Within the theory (Boykin & Schoenhofer, 2010), caring is recognized as an "altruistic, active expression of love and is the intentional and embodied recognition of value and connectedness" (p. 372). Boykin and Schoenhofer (2010) believe that the focus of the practice of nursing is nurturing persons living caring and growing in caring, always unfolding, guided by intentionality, occurs with the nursing situation, and the commitment to know self and other as caring persons. Boykin and Schoenhofer (2001) were among the first scholars to make explicit the role of nurse leaders in creating caring environments within healthcare systems. Their most recent work (Boykin et al., 2014) illustrates how the theory and the model *dance of caring persons* can be used to transform healthcare systems by creating an authentic culture of caring grounded in Caring Science, caring values, and respect for the gifts that all employees bring to the organization and nursing situation. This theoretical and philosophical approach to praxis recognizes the value of authentic caring and is very different than customer service approaches to transformation where scripted language that is used consistently and repeatedly, and hourly rounding are "tactics" to increase patient satisfaction scores.

PEACE

Peavey (cited in Chinn, 2013) describes "heart politics as the merging of power with openness, connectedness, and love, and part of the important work of evolving a way of creating and working with power" (p. xi). Chinn's (2013) work on *Peace and Power* offers suggestions, guides, and practices to create meaningful communities where all are valued and respected, and differences are resolved in a manner that creates peace. The intention of peace is the commitment to shared values and actions that foster harmony and trust. According to Chinn (2013), "at the heart of all approaches to being at peace with one's self and with others is the ability to love, and to feel and to act from a place of genuine respect for another as people" (p. 9). PEACE (Chinn, 2013) is the acronym for **P**raxis, **E**mpowerment, **A**wareness, **C**ooperation, and **E**volvement and reflects a commitment that guides the ways leaders choose to relate with colleagues within the context of meetings or dialogue. Chinn (2013) identified Peace and Power processes that are driven from values. The following PEACE Powers are not inclusive of all the PEACE Powers noted by Chinn (2013), but were selected for their relevance to *leading from the heart* and concepts from the unitary-transformative paradigm. The *Power of the Whole* values the flow of new thinking and energy from all; the *Power of Collectivity* values the power of each person as being integral to the well-being of the group; the *Power of Nurturing* honors life and experiences as resources to be cherished and respected; the *Power of Intuition* makes one sense which action to take on the basis of perceptions of human experience; the *Power of Consciousness* recognizes ethical behaviors and long-term outcomes; the *Power of Creativity* values actions taken on the basis of imagination and ingenuity; and the *Power of Trust* focuses on building genuine human relationships. Take a moment to think about your leadership practices and your way of being when collaborating with colleagues. Which power best reflects your leadership practice? Which power do you need to enhance? And which power makes you uncomfortable?

FOCUSING ON SELF-CARE AND MANIFESTING INTENTIONS

I have written about the value of self-care in the past (Turkel & Ray, 2004), and have committed to a personal plan for self-care, integrated caring for self into college curricula, created caring healing rooms and retreats within the practice setting, and incorporated self-care into evaluations for registered nurses; however, it has only been with the past 3 years that I can honestly say that I have fully come to realize that the *practice of loving-kindness to self* (Watson, 2008) is truly foundational to *leading from the heart*. Understanding the science behind the relationship among heart energy, consciousness, and communication allowed me to truly value that what we carry in our hearts matters most (Watson & Browning, 2012). With advances in science, measurement of the electromagnetic waves of the heart as far as 6 to 8 feet away from the human body has been recorded (Watson, 2011). According to Watson (2011) "the heart, the most powerful of all electromagnetic generators in the body serves as a mini-radio tower, radiating out whatever vibration we hold within our hearts" (Figure 21.1).

When we carry caring, compassion, love, and peace, we radiate, vibrate, and give out caring, compassion, love, and peace. When we are carrying fear or anger in our hearts, we radiate, vibrate, and give out fear or anger.

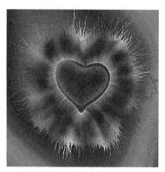

- What energy are you vibrating to others?
- Caritas leaders are *creating caring environments for self-renewal.*
- Caring for self is important to have the energy to lead others.

FIGURE 21.1 What we carry in our hearts matters most.

Cocreated by faculty Watson Caring Science Institute; Turkel, M. (2014). Leading from the heart: Caring, love, peace, and values guiding leadership. *Nursing Science Quarterly*, 27(2), 172–177. doi:10.1177/0894318414522663. Figure 1, p. 175.

Figure 21.1 illustrates the energy field of the heart and serves as a point of reflection for nurse leaders: What energy do you vibrate to others? A leader who is holistic and self-caring vibrates harmony and peace, actively listens, and practices authentic presence in the caring moment with colleagues or staff. If the leader does not care for self, it is impossible for him or her to compassionately care for others.

Manifesting intentions (Smith, 1999) is also foundational to *leading from the heart*. Smith identified manifesting intentions as the first constitutive meaning of caring from the unitary perceptive. In her writing, Smith (1999) defines manifesting intentions as "creating, holding, and expressing, thoughts, images, feelings, beliefs, desires, will (purpose) and actions that affirm possibilities for human betterment or well-being" (p. 21).

Figure 21.2 illustrates the interrelationship among the energy field of the heart, practice of loving kindness to self, and manifesting intentions to allow for the emergence of caring and healing. Within the WCSI, faculty associates teach about the caring moment. Nurses are taught about the power of subtle energy, and creating a healing

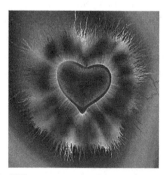

Intentionality or manifesting intention

- Practice of loving kindness to self allows one to enter the caring relationship with others with intention to become the energetic environment that potentiates caring and healing.

FIGURE 21.2 What we carry in our hearts matters most.

Cocreated by faculty Watson Caring Science Institute.

environment, so they become conscious of centering, releasing stress, and establishing positive intentionality in their hearts as they enter into any patient care experience (Watson, 2008).

When teaching Transformational Leadership classes or doing scholarly presentations on Caring Science leadership, I close with the ritual of moving forward by letting go. Those in attendance are invited to participate in a centering meditation and to let go of any feelings or thoughts that are blocking their hearts and not allowing them to be open to new possibilities, creative emergence, and making decisions on the basis of caring, love, peace, or values. Participants leave with a candle and lavender oil as a reminder to make time for reflection and self-care, a Peace stone to consider PEACE Power, and a heart touchstone to remember that what we carry in our hearts matters most. Following are two examples of leaders' stories.

HONORING PRACTICE EXEMPLARS

As part of my personal leadership journey of exploring what leading from the heart looks and feels like, I invited leaders to share personal stories of caring, love, peace, or values guiding their practice or decision making, and to reflect on what that experience was like for them.

Love

I love my nurses and I am comfortable telling them that I love them; when I come back from vacation I hug them and let them know I miss them. I am always letting them know that I appreciate and honor them for the work they do every day with our patients. We celebrate everything; I bake and bring in food. When a nurse passes a national certification exam we have banners in the unit. Coming to know and love myself as a caring person began when I was studying caring theory at a deeper level and has made it easier for me to be more comfortable with the word LOVE. It is love of humanity; we are all humans, myself, my nurses, the patients, the families and the physicians. Nurses work of caring is LOVE in action, practice comes from the heart. I LOVE the concept of LOVE so much that I began a doctoral program and will be studying LOVE for my doctoral dissertation. Some may think that LOVE and caring are just the soft part of nursing but I have made a difference and transformed my unit. When I started as the manager of the Neurological Intensive Care Unit over 7 years ago, I had a high vacancy rate, high turnover rate, low morale, and the unit was always over budget.

I integrated caring theory into the care nurses provide to patients and families and also into my own leadership style. We have an engaged Shared Governance Committee and the registered nurses make patient-centered decisions that improve unit quality outcomes and processes. Over the past 3 years, the unit's scores for nursing quality based on data from the National Database Nursing Quality Indicators (NDNQI) and patient satisfaction scores compiled by Press Ganey have been in the 95 percentile and the highest for any unit within the six hospital system.

The vacancy rate for the last 3 years has been zero, I have a waiting list of nurses who want to transfer into the unit, and my unit is always within budget. The nurses don't just have great skills and competence; they LOVE their patients and work from the heart center.

Making Decisions Based on Love, Not Fear

An opportunity in a collective bargaining negotiation served as a way to live our shared values. I recently had the opportunity to lead from the place of caring and love in this very challenging situation. Knowing that we would all need to work together after the agreement, making decisions from love and not fear or personal ego was important. After a year of fruitless talks and negotiation, both sides of the negotiation were tired, angry, and frustrated. The imposition of "a worker versus management paradigm" does little to bring peace and much to encourage discord. The key to avoiding talks breaking down and things going from bad to worse centered on one simple thought: After the agreement is reached, what will be important? For us that future was the entire team working in collaboration and unity to care for our community. That vision became the framework for leadership behavior during the negotiations. Winning was irrelevant, especially if winning resulted in hurt feelings or worse, and meant we could not work in collaboration and unity to care for our community. Then what was truly won? As leaders, we no longer thought in terms of winners and losers. The only winner had to be our community, our patients. I hosted meetings with department leaders and discussed what it meant to be a caring leader. The department leader's role was to focus on caring for our community. Accepting that staff were advocating for what they valued was respected by the leaders and they realized that outsiders involved in the process were stirring up strong emotions and that "retaliating" would not allow for collaboration and unity. At 2 o'clock in the morning, all were exhausted, frustration high, many were ready to give up, and to move forward with a strike and pick up the pieces. One leader focused on keeping the group talking, and more importantly, listening. The negotiators agreed to move on to another day. The sun rose, the negotiations continued and a unanimous agreement was reached, all through love, not fear.

REFRAMING THE LANGUAGE

Words and language convey meaning and intent from those speaking to those listening. Zukav (1990) reminds us that a thought is energy or light informed by our consciousness. According to Zukav (1990), negative emotions of anger, blame, or fear have a lower energy frequency than positive emotions of love, compassion, appreciation, or recognition. When emotions are expressed through words, the negative energy drains our own system and negativity radiates to others, whereas positive energy expressed through words is uplifting to our systems and radiates peaceful, calm, or soothing energy to others.

In my own leadership practice, I intentionally reframe language to convey authentic presence, caring, appreciation, and support when situations occur that traditionally focus on blame: What went wrong? And what regulations or policies were not followed? The following is my personal story:

Approximately 2 years ago, we had two patient deaths in a short time period in one of the hospitals within the network where deaths do not usually occur. Leaders were involved in the "root cause analysis" and nursing staff were overwhelmed with questions related to policies, procedures, and regulatory requirements. As we all know, given the complexity of the human body, death occurs even when all procedures are followed. I spent 3 days at the hospital with a caring healing cart, gave hand massages to any employee who wanted to experience human touch, and invited them to share what the experience was like for them. I asked them, "How are you feeling?", "What was the experience like for you?", and "How can I help you?" My most memorable experience was crying with a novice nurse as he shared what it was like to be part of his first emergency code blue, witness a patient dying, and feeling helpless. He thanked me for hearing his story instead of focusing on documentation and policies. As leaders, we have an ethical responsibility to assure competent care, patient safety, and evidence–based practice; however, we also have an ethical responsibility to integrate caring and humanity into our dialogue when situations occur that require followup.

Within Einstein Healthcare Network Caring Science, language is integrated into policies and procedures, the plan of care, and performance evaluations. Examples include changing the word "body" to "deceased person" in the postmortem policy; asking patients, "What is most important to you today?"; infusing the care plans with the words of caring-healing modalities: collaboration, connection, reflection; and having all nursing employees write a caring moment and plan for self-care on their evaluations. Tables 21.1 and 21.2 reflect the

TABLE 21.1 Reframing the Language of Leadership

Traditional	Caring Science
• Full-time equivalents (FTEs)	• Registered nurses
• Discipline	• Performance accountability
• Management by walking around/rounding on staff	• Honoring caring moments through authentic presence
• The budget data	• A caring story
• Making decisions out of fear	• Making decisions out of LOVE
• LOVE MONEY and use people	• LOVE PEOPLE and use money
• Compliance	• Participation

Source: Created with authenticity and intentionality by WCSI Faculty Associates. Reprinted with permission from Turkel, M. (2014). Leading from the heart: Caring, love, peace and values guiding leadership. *Nursing Science Quarterly, 27*(2), 172–177. doi:10.1177/0894318414522663. Table 1; p. 177.

TABLE 21.2 Reframing the Language of Leadership

Traditional	Caring Science
• Hourly rounds	• Authentic visitation
• Tactics	• Innovations, caring practices
• Strategic plan	• Future visions
• Targets	• Visions of excellence
• Scripts	• Authentic voice
• Bottom line	• Caring economics
• Throughput	• Safe transition/patient journey
• Low performers	• Recognize individual gifts

Source: Created with authenticity and intentionality by WCSI Faculty Associates. From Turkel, M. C. (2014). Leading from the heart: Caring, love, peace and values guiding leadership. *Nursing Science Quarterly*, 27(2), 172–177. doi:10.1177/0894318414522663. Table 2; p. 177.

ongoing work of my colleagues at the WCSI and caring leaders as we are always looking to reframe the traditional industrial paradigm of leadership. I invite you to use these words and to add to this body of knowledge.

CONCLUSION

BEING WITH OTHERS AS A CARING LEADER

In closing, I leave you with the following quotes that reflect the relationship among caring, love, and peace, for self and system:

Never believe that a few caring people can't change the world. For, indeed, that's all who ever have.
Margaret Mead

Always the most important hour is the present.
Always the most important person is the one you are facing.
Always the most important act is Love.

Meister Eckhart

If there is light in the soul,
There is beauty in the person;
If there is beauty in the person,
There is harmony in the house;
If there is harmony in the house,
There is order in the nation (system);
If there is order in the nation; (system),
There will be peace in the world.
Ancient Chinese proverb: anonymous (word system added by Dr. Jean Watson)

NEXT ERA POSSIBILITIES

Education

- How can nursing faculty integrate the concepts of relationships, patterns, values, healing, authentic presence, cocreating, being, engaging, caring, complexity, humanity, and intentionality into baccalaureate-, graduate-, and doctoral- (PhD/DNP) level nursing leadership courses?
- How can nursing faculty integrate caring for self into the nursing curricula for baccalaureate-, graduate-, and doctoral- (PhD/DNP) level nursing students?
- What teaching-learning experience could faculty create to allow students at the baccalaureate, graduate, and doctoral (PhD/DNP) levels to share personal stories of leading from the heart?

Research

- What is the meaning of love from the perspective of chief executive officers, chief financial officers, and chief nursing officers?
- What is the meaning of the "power of intuition" and "power of trust" from the perspective of nurse managers and direct care registered nurses?
- What organizational changes (human and economic) occur when leaders at all levels lead from the heart?

Praxis

- How can nurse leaders create caring-healing practice environments?
- How can leaders at all levels of the organization reframe their language into one grounded in Caring Science?
- What practices can leaders at all levels of the organization integrate to allow for the *Power of Consciousness* and *Power of Creativity* to become part of the heart and soul of the organization?

Theory and Knowledge Development

- How can the concepts of leading from the heart (relationships, patterns, values, healing, authentic presence, cocreating, being, engaging, caring, complexity, humanity, and intentionality) be framed into a middle-range theory?
- How would this middle-range theory inform nursing knowledge in the year 2020?
- How do the PEACE Powers presented in this chapter inform nursing knowledge?

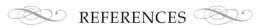 REFERENCES

Bournes, D. A. (2013). Cultivating a spirit of inquiry using a nursing leading-following model. *Nursing Science Quarterly, 26*(2), 182–188. doi:10.1177/0894318413477154

Boykin, A., & Schoenhofer, S. (2001). The role of nursing leadership in creating caring environments in health care delivery systems. *Nursing Administration Quarterly, 25*(3), 1–7. doi:10.1097/00006216-200104000-00003

Boykin, A., & Schoenhofer, S. (2010). Anne Boykin and Savina Schoenhofer's nursing as caring theory. In M. Parker & M. Smith (Eds.), *Nursing theories and nursing practice* (3rd ed., pp. 370–385). Philadelphia, PA: F. A. Davis.

Boykin, A., Schoenhofer, S., & Valentine, K. (2014). *Healthcare system transformation for nursing and healthcare leaders: Implementing a culture of caring*. New York, NY: Springer Publishing.

Chinn, P. (2013). *Peace and power: New directions for building community* (8th ed.). Burlington, MA: Jones & Bartlett.

Ray, M. A. (1981). A philosophical analysis of caring within nursing. In M. Leininger (Ed.), *Caring: An essential human need* (pp. 25–36). Thorofare, NJ: Charles B. Slack.

Ray, M. A., & Turkel, M. C. (2012). A transtheoretical evolution of caring science within complex systems. *International Journal for Human Caring, 16*(2), 28–49.

Ray, M. A., & Turkel, M. C. (2014). Social justice and human rights and caring as emancipation in nursing: The theory of relational caring complexity. *Advances in Nursing Science, 37*(2), 132–146. doi: 10.1097/ANS/0000000000000024

Rizzo Parse, R. (2008). The humanbecoming leading-following model. *Nursing Science Quarterly, 21*, 369–375. doi:10.1177/0894318408323492

Rizzo Parse, R. (2010). Rosemarie Rizzo Parse's humanbecoming school of thought. In M. Parker & M. Smith (Eds.), *Nursing theories and nursing practice* (3rd ed., pp. 277–289). Philadelphia, PA: F. A. Davis.

Smith, M. (1999). Caring and the science of unitary human beings. *Advances in Nursing Science, 21*(4), 14–28. doi:10.1097/00012272-199906000-00006

Smith, M. (2011). Philosophical and theoretical perspective related to complexity science in nursing. In A. Davidson, M. Ray, & M. Turkel (Eds.), *Nursing, caring, and complexity science: For human-environment well-being* (pp. 1–20). New York, NY: Springer Publishing.

Sullivan-Marx, E. M. (2013). The bear and the canyon: Toward an understanding of personal leadership. *Nursing Science Quarterly, 26*(4), 373–375. doi:10.1177/0894318413501961

Turkel, M. C. (2014). Leading from the heart: Caring, love, peace and values guiding leadership. *Nursing Science Quarterly, 27*(2), 172–177. doi:10.1177/0894318414522663

Turkel, M. C., & Ray, M. A. (2004). Creating a caring practice environment through self-renewal. *Nursing Administration Quarterly, 28*(4), 249–254. doi:10.1097/00006216-200410000-00004

Watson, J. (2003). Love and caring: Ethics of face and hand—an invitation to return to the heart and soul of nursing and our deep humanity. *Nursing Administration Quarterly, 27*(3), 197–202. doi:10.1097/00006216-200307000-00005

Watson, J. (2006). Caring theory as an ethical guide to administrative and clinical practices. *Nursing Administration Quarterly, 30*(1), 48–55. doi:10.1097/00006216-200601000-00008

Watson, J. (2008). *Nursing: The philosophy and science of caring* (2nd Rev. ed.). Boulder: University Press of Colorado.

Watson, J. (2011, September). *CARITAS: Caring Science*. Keynote presentation Atlanta Research Measurement Conference, Atlanta, Georgia.

Watson, J., & Browning, R. (2012, August). Caring science meets heart science. *American Nurse Today, 7*(8). Retrieved from https://www.americannursetoday.com/viewpoint-caring-science-meets-heart-science-a-guide-to-authentic-caring-practice

Zukav, G. (1990). *The seat of the soul*. New York, NY: Fireside, Simon & Schuster.

22

Evaluation of Authentic Human Caring Professional Practices*

Barbara B. Brewer and Jean Watson

CARITAS LITERACIES

By the end of this chapter, the caring-healing nurse will be able to

1. Describe authentic professional human-caring practices.

2. Identify five Caritas Processes® inherent in human caring.

3. Describe a research study designed to measure human-caring behaviors of caregivers from the perspective of their patients.

⟨≈⟩

The purpose of this chapter is to report on a Caring Science research project, which measures patient's experience of authentic professional human caring practices. This Caring Science practice approach applies to caregivers toward each other as well as patients/families and communities.

BACKGROUND

SCRIPTING AS AN INTERVENTION TO DEMONSTRATE CARING

As hospitals seek approaches to improve patient satisfaction and address finances, many administrators resort to "scripting" as one way to solve nurse–patient communication and improve outcomes. Perhaps there is some benefit to scripting as a means to guide communication and interactions; however, inauthentic communication is detected immediately by patients (Hogan, 2013). Leadership wisdom dictates that administrators can have the greatest strategy to improve patient care, but "it is culture, which will eat strategy for lunch" (Coffman & Sorensen, 2013). To be successful, communication and nurse–patient relations require "authentic presence" and ways-of-being that are reflective, sensitive, and present to the patient/family situation in the moment—connecting human-to-human (Watson, 2008). Personal self-reports from nurses in hospitals where "scripting" is used find the requirement intrusive, artificial, demoralizing, and insulting (Sweeney, 2014). This is especially true for nurses committed to theory-guided, professional Caring Science practice. Caring Science hospitals and staff hold a sacred covenant with their patients. When nurses are most in touch with that covenant, they appreciate the need to form trusting relationships with patients/families and to be "authentically present" during interactions, and even brief moments of communication (Clarke, Watson, & Brewer, 2009).

Attempts at *scripting* a "caring moment" (Sitzman & Watson, 2014) and any authentic interaction is an oxymoron. Such a structured approach, based on administrative attempts to improve outcomes, undermines the possibility for an authentic human-to-human connection (Hogan, 2013). Moreover, scripting goes against long-standing, educational teachings of "therapeutic use of self," common to all nurses, embedded in the timeless, classic teachings of Peplau (1952), and more recently, practices informed and guided by Caring Science theoretical values, philosophy, and ethic as a mature professional model (Watson, 1979, 2008). Indeed, recent Institute of HeartMath research affirms that inauthentic communication is detected immediately, energetically, and intuitively, and affects the larger field of communication. So, both philosophically and empirically, scripting is not a solution to improved patient care and hospital outcomes (Institute of HeartMath, 2015).

The maturing of nursing professional practice models, in spite of the dominant medical disease hospital system and conventional administrative attempts to "scripting" as a way forward, is revolutionary. Magnet® hospital's success in instituting a professional nursing model has had major impact on hospital staff, patients, and society alike (Stimpfel, Rosen, & McHugh, 2014; Tonges, McCann, & Strickler, 2014). However, even with these best-practice hospital successes, and with the maturing of nursing as a distinct discipline and profession, the professional practices for improving patient care are still surrounded by an outdated scientific Western worldview. This worldview is confined to physical body care, medical—disease, acute sick—care hospital practices, compounded by external technical interventions. This approach to patient care and models of care delivery is based on latent and overt norms established by the institutional, industrial product-line, hospital culture of this so-called modern era (Sitzman & Watson, 2014).

Evolution to Health

Global shifts are upon us in healthcare. These shifts are awakening toward philosophical value-guided health approaches toward whole-person/whole-system caring-healing-health. The human consciousness shifts toward wellness are awakening to energetic models and possibilities of inner healing and emotional mental health; they are oriented toward subjective, experiential indicators such as individual self-love, self-caring, self-knowledge, self-control and self-healing health approaches, addressing individual and collective human suffering. This evolving view for humankind and population health returns us to the heart of our humanity and heart of nursing; it invites and requires practices for sustaining a healthy environment and human environment caring for our well-being (Watson, 2008).

What is happening today in this era in human history, demands an expanded, dramatically different worldview, quantum shift. The quantum move is away from episodic sick care and from material medicine and external interventions and cure of body, at all costs—physically, mentally, economically, and spiritually. New research models are needed to generate data that explore authentic human caring-healing and health, in contrast to the physical cure and biomedical views of sick care (Watson, 2010, 2014a, 2014b).

METHODS

To shift the focus from objective, problem-oriented criteria and measures that address the status quo, this study, grounded in Caring Science, represents an expanded framework for healthcare and subjective outcomes, guided by authentic human-to-human caring and assessing core variables of patient experiences of caring. The study uses a descriptive design and is part of an ongoing national comparative database project. Participants submit quarterly responses from a random sample of patients who are hospitalized on adult acute care and rehabilitation units. Further description of the data collection procedure is in the following text. The results reported here are from the second quarter of 2014.

SAMPLE AND SETTING

The sample consists of 1,010 patient responses from 48 units in eight hospitals located throughout the United States. All hospitals are either affiliates or research partners of Watson Caring Science Institute (2018). Quarterly hospital coordinators from each of the eight hospitals collect a random sample of patient surveys from each of the 48 units and submit them to the database. Because the unit of comparison is patient care units, all individual patient responses are aggregated to the patient care unit. Patient care units in the sample represent 10 different unit types, which are illustrated in Figure 22.1. The most frequent unit type is medical-surgical (MS; $n = 15$) and the least frequent is moderate acuity in an adult ($n = 1$).

Patients reported a mean age of 58.7 years (16.9), had been on the hospital unit for 5.8 (7.3) days, had 3.1 (2.3) health problems, and had a pain score of 3.1 on a scale of 1 to 10, 1 indicating no pain and 10 the worst possible pain (values in parentheses represent standard deviations). In addition, the sample was 54% female ($n = 537$), with an equal proportion (40% each) reporting bad and very bad health. Forty-five percent ($n = 437$) came to the hospital with an emergency condition, 55% ($n = 554$) were White, and 43% ($n = 437$) were on bed rest, whereas 37% ($n = 370$) were able to sit in a chair at the bedside.

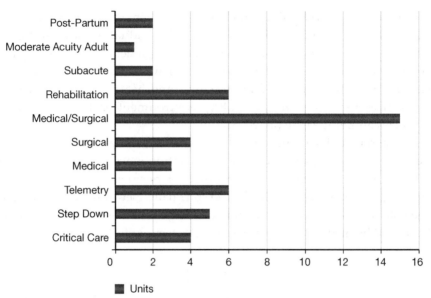

FIGURE 22.1 Frequency of participating units by type of unit.

MEASURES

The measurement assessment is *Watson Caritas Patient Score*® (WCPS) (Figure 22.2; Brewer & Watson, 2013), capturing the patient's experiencing of caring. The five items of the WCPS emerged from the Watson Theory of 10 Caritas Processes (Figure 22.3) as universals of caring phenomena and foundational indicators of human caring (Watson, 2008; Watson & Brewer, 2015). Response options for each item range from 1 (never) to 7 (always). The items empirically assess the patient's subjective experience of receiving caring; the items refer to such indicators as loving-kindness, trust, dignity, healing environment, and honoring of beliefs and values (Table 22.1). The scale demonstrates satisfactory internal consistency reliability, Cronbach alpha = 0.90 (Watson, Brewer, & D'Alfonso, 2010). Construct validity has been evaluated using exploratory factor analysis with principal components using varimax rotation, which resulted in a single factor explaining 76% of variance. Table 22.1 presents factor loadings by item, which ranged from 0.766 to 0.906. The second measure used in the study is a 10-question demographic survey, which asks standard questions such as age, number of health issues, reason for hospitalization, ethnicity, mobility level, educational level, and current pain level.

PROCEDURE

The project received approval from the University of Arizona human subjects review board as well as at each hospital. Following human subjects approval, a hospital coordinator from each site received training regarding all project procedures. Each site selected and trained data collectors. Project requirements specified that data collectors not be employed on the unit where they collected data to reduce possibilities of biasing patient responses.

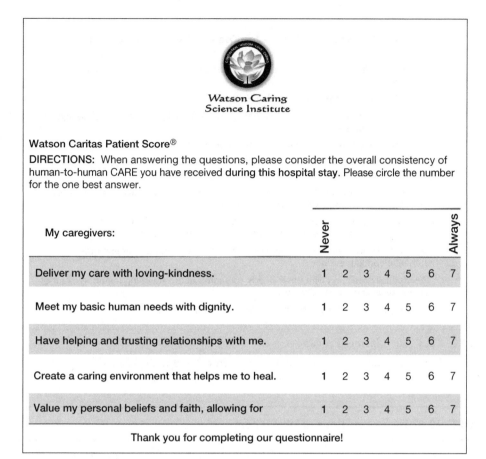

FIGURE 22.2 Watson Caritas Patient Score® (WCPS).

Source: Reprinted with permission from Watson, J., Brewer, B. B., & D'Alfonso, J. (2014). *Watson Caritas Patient Score (WCPS)®.* Boulder, CO: Watson Caring Science Institute. Retrieved from https://www.watsoncaringscience.org

Patient surveys were distributed to a random sample of patients who had been hospitalized on the current unit for a minimum of 24 hours, were 18 years or older, and were cognitively able to complete a survey in English. Surveys were distributed throughout the quarter and all but one site, which collected data using a tablet, used paper surveys.

All site coordinators, with the exception of the one using the tablet, entered data through a secure online portal. Individual hospital and comparison reports are accessed through a different page on the same online portal.

DATA ANALYSIS

All data analyses were done using Statistical Package for Social Sciences (Armonk, NY). Individual-level data were aggregated to the unit level and evaluated for group-level validity using the criteria recommended by Shortell and colleagues (1991). Descriptive statistics were used to evaluate differences across unit types and hospitals. Nonparametric

---

TEN CARITAS PROCESSES® – Jean Watson Theory of Human Caring

1. Humanistic-Altruistic Values – Practice of Loving Kindness and Equanimity with self/other;
2. Being Authentically Present -Enabling Faith-Hope;
3. Being Sensitive to self/others by cultivating own spiritual practices – beyond ego- to transpersonal presence;
4. Developing and Sustaining loving, trusting-caring relationships;
5. Allowing for expression of positive and negative feelings – authentically listening to another person's story;
6. Creatively problem-solving – 'solution-seeking' through caring process; full use of self – use of all ways of knowing;
7. Engaging in transpersonal teaching-learning within context of caring relationship; staying within other's frame of reference – shift toward coaching;
8. Creating a healing environment at all levels; subtle environment for energetic authentic caring presence;
9. Reverentially assisting with basic needs as sacred acts – touching mindbodyspirit of other; sustaining human dignity;
10. Opening to spiritual, mystery, unknowns – allowing for miracles.

FIGURE 22.3 Ten Caritas Processes.

Ten Caritas Processes, Watson's Theory of Human Caring. Used with permission.

TABLE 22.1 Factor Loadings of WCPS Items

Item	Loading
Create a caring environment that helps me to heal	0.906
Deliver my care with loving-kindness	0.904
Have helping and trusting relationships with me	0.899
Meet my basic human needs with dignity	0.868
Value my personal beliefs and faith, allowing for hope	0.766

WCPS, Watson Caritas Patient Score.

Source: Reprinted with permission from Brewer, B. B., & Watson, J. (2015). Evaluation of authentic human caring professional practices. *Journal of Nursing Administration, 45*(12), 622–627. doi:10.1097/ NNA.0000000000000275. (Table. 1); p. 625.

correlations (Spearman's rho) were performed to examine relationships among caring items and unit-level quality indicators.

RESULTS

All individual items and the scale score met the criteria of Shortell et al. (1991) ($F > 1.4$, $p < .05$) for aggregation of individual items to reflect a group (patient care unit) score. Mean scores for each of the five items and the total scale ranged from 5.7 to 7. There were

TABLE 22.2 Watson Caritas Patient Score by Hospital

Hospital	Mean	SD	F	p
A	6.69	0.13	3.042	.012
B	6.37[a]	0.24		
C	6.70[a]	0.03		
D	6.54	0.17		
E	6.49	0.25		
F	6.48	0		
G	6.65	0.19		
H	6.41	0.21		

[a]$p < .05$.

SD, standard deviation.

Source: Reprinted with permission from Brewer, B. B., & Watson, J. (2015). Evaluation of authentic human caring professional practices. *Journal of Nursing Administration*, 45(12), 622–627. doi:10.1097/NNA.0000000000000275. (Table. 2); p. 626.

statistically significant differences in three of the five items and the total scale score among the eight hospitals in the sample. Table 22.2 provides the breakdown of hospital scale means and standard deviations. As can be seen from the table, two of the eight hospitals exhibited statistically significant differences in the WCPS.

Each of the five items and the WCPS were correlated with Hospital Consumer Assessment of Healthcare Providers and Systems (HCAHPS) scores (HCAHPS, 2015) for the participating patient care units. The HCAHPS items selected for the analysis were communication with nursing, responsiveness of hospital staff, pain control, communication about medicines, quiet of hospital environment, cleanliness of physical environment, discharge information, overall hospital rating, and recommendation of hospital to family and friends. The items were selected because they were believed to be most sensitive to nursing care and the practice environment (American Nurses Association, 1995). Two of the HCAHPS items, communication with nursing and responsiveness of hospital staff, correlated with three of the WCPS items. Communication with nursing correlated with three items: meet my basic needs with dignity (Spearman's rho = 0.33, $p < .05$); helping and trusting relationships (Spearman's rho = 0.36, $p < .05$); and create a caring environment that helps me to heal (Spearman's rho = 0.43, $p < .01$). Responsiveness of hospital staff correlated with one item, helping and trusting relationships with me (Spearman's rho = 0.33, $p < .05$).

DISCUSSION

The WCPS items and scale were able to discriminate across unit types and hospitals. The scale demonstrates satisfactory internal consistency, reliability, and validity. Its use, whether for research as in this case or in practice for understanding caring from the patient's perspective, invites a very different conversation from other patient experience measures.

Anecdotally, hospital site coordinators have told the authors they have used the instrument on units other than those in the study as a means for engaging patients in conversations, because both staff and patients appreciate the meaningful discourse the questions engender.

Three of the WCPS items correlated with two HCAHPS items, communication with nursing and responsiveness of hospital staff. This finding is consistent with the findings of a systematic review examining the effects of caring and patient satisfaction of hospitalized adult patients (Wolf, 2012) and the findings of Esmaeili, Cheraghi, and Salsali (2014) who found that cardiac critical care patients described behaviors associated with patient-centered care as careful listening to them by the nursing staff.

In addition, relationships between caring behaviors of the staff and satisfaction with nursing support the findings of Tonges et al. (2014) who found that nurse satisfaction scores increased with the implementation of a professional practice model on the basis of caring.

LIMITATIONS

This study is part of a larger ongoing comparative research project the participants of which are all Watson Caring Science Affiliate hospitals or research partners. As a result, the caring scores are higher than what might be expected across all hospitals, which may have blunted the magnitude of correlations between the caring items and the nurse-sensitive quality indicators. When correlation coefficients are calculated using scores from a restricted range (as in this case, higher caring scores than might be seen across all hospitals), the strength of the correlation may appear that there is no, or a weak, relationship between two variables (Kiess & Green, 2010). In addition, although the sample was random, it may not fully represent all patients on the participating patient care units because of the small number of patients sampled within the quarter of analysis.

IMPLICATIONS FOR MANAGEMENT

In the past few years, there has been a shift toward measurement of patient subjective experiences versus objective criteria alone. The WCPS provides some insight into a patient's subjective experience of caring staff behaviors. Despite the move to measurement of more subjective experiences, reality still remains that unless systems have indicators of caring and patient experiences, it is not reliable or possible to have data relating caring process of nursing to outcomes. The WCPS gives nurse leaders some evidence of the effectiveness of their professional practice model through the patient's eyes. This direction for assessing and validating caring provides new forms of evidence consistent with transformation within systems for whole person/whole system shifts related to healthcare reform and evolved consciousness of the public beyond medical technical care alone.

CONCLUSION

The WCPS is a valid and reliable tool that may be used by nurse leaders who have built professional practice environments on the basis of human-caring theory to evaluate their effectiveness. The tool has successfully been used to compare caring staff behaviors across hospitals and unit types and has shown relationships to patient assessment of nursing communication and staff responsiveness. It may provide an alternative measure of patient subjective feelings of the care they have received.

NEXT ERA POSSIBILITIES

Education
- How can I integrate Caritas Processes into nursing curricula?
- How can I ensure that new graduate nurses link theory to their practice?

Research
- What future research studies can be developed using the WCPS?
- What research methods can be used to link Caritas Processes to patient and staff outcomes?

Praxis
- How can I build practice environments where clinical care is guided by human Caring Science principles?
- How can I ensure that all patients receive care that they perceive was delivered with human kindness?

Theory and Knowledge Development
- How can I make explicit relationships between human-caring theory concepts and patient outcomes?
- Do human-caring theoretical concepts mediate or moderate relationships between clinical practices and patient outcomes?

 REFERENCES

American Nurses Association. (1995). *Nursing care report card for acute care*. Washington, DC: American Nurses Publishing.

Brewer, B. B., & Watson, J. (2013, November). *Dare to care: National comparative database of caring professional practice indicators through the patient's eyes*. Poster presented at International Nursing Administration Research Conference, Baltimore, MD.

Brewer, B. B., & Watson, J. (2015). Evaluation of authentic human caring professional practices. *Journal of Nursing Administration, 45*(12), 622–627. doi:10.1097/NNA.0000000000000275

Clarke, P. N., Watson, J., & Brewer, B. B. (2009). From theory to practice: Caring science according to Watson and Brewer. *Nursing Science Quarterly, 22*, 339–345. doi:10.1177/0894318409344769

Coffman, C. W., & Sorensen, K. (2013). *Culture eats strategy for lunch: The secret of extraordinary results. Igniting the passion from within*. Denver, CO: The Liang Addison Press.

Esmaeili, M., Cheraghi, M. A., & Salsali, M. (2014). Cardiac patients' perception of patient-centred care: A qualitative study. *Nursing in Critical Care, 21*(2), 97–104. doi:10.1111/nicc.12148

Hogan, B. K. (2013). Caring as a scripted discourse versus caring as an expression of an authentic relationship between self and other. *Issues in Mental Health Nursing, 34*(5), 375–379. doi:10.3109/01612840.2013.768734

Hospital Consumer Assessment of Healthcare Providers and Systems. (2015). Retrieved from http://www.hcahpsonline.org

Institute of HeartMath. (2015). Welcome to HeartMath Research. Retrieved from http://www.heartmath.org/research/research-home/research-center-home.html

Kiess, H. O., & Green, B. A. (2010). *Statistical concepts for the behavioral sciences* (4th ed.). Boston, MA: Allyn & Bacon.

Peplau, H. E. (1952). *Interpersonal relations in nursing: A conceptual frame of reference for psychodynamic nursing. Modern nursing series.* New York, NY: Putnam.

Shortell, S. M., Rousseau, D. M., Gillies, R. R., Devers, K. J., & Simons, T. L. (1991). Organizational assessment in intensive care units (ICUs): Construct development, reliability, and validity of the ICU nurse-physician questionnaire. *Medical Care, 29*(8), 709–726. doi:10.1097/00005650-199108000-00004

Sitzman, K., & Watson, J. (2014). *Caring science, mindful practice: Implementing Watson's human caring theory.* New York, NY: Springer Publishing.

Stimpfel, A. W., Rosen, J. E., & McHugh, M. D. (2014). Understanding the role of the professional practice environment on quality of care in Magnet® and non-Magnet hospitals. *Journal of Nursing Administration, 44*(1), 10–16. doi:10.1097/NNA.0000000000000015

Sweeney, C. (2014). "We love scripting"...Said no nurse ever. *Arizona Nurse, 67*(4), 3.

Tonges, M., McCann, M., & Strickler, J. (2014). Translating caring theory across the continuum from inpatient to ambulatory care. *Journal of Nursing Administration, 44,* 326–332. doi:10.1097/NNA.0000000000000077

Watson Caring Science Institute. (2018). National Caring Science affiliates of WCSI. Retrieved from https://www.watsoncaringscience.org/national-wcsi-affiliates/

Watson, J. (1979). *Nursing. The philosophy and science of caring.* Boulder: University Press of Colorado.

Watson, J. (2008). *Nursing: The philosophy and science of caring* (Rev. ed.). Boulder: University Press of Colorado.

Watson, J. (2010). *Postmodern nursing and beyond* (2nd ed.). Boulder, CO: Watson Caring Science Institute.

Watson, J. (2014a). Integrative nursing caring science, human caring, and peace. In M. J. Kreitzer & M. Koithan (Eds.), *Integrative nursing* (pp. 101–108). New York, NY: Oxford University Press.

Watson, J. (2014b). Social/moral justice from a caring science cosmology. In P. N. Kagan, M. C. Smith, & P. L. Chinn (Eds.), *Philosophies and practices of emancipatory nursing: Social justice as praxis* (pp. 64–70). New York, NY: Routledge.

Watson, J., & Brewer, B. B. (2015). Caring science research: Criteria, evidence and measurement. *Journal of Nursing Administration, 45,* 235–236. doi:10.1097/NNA.0000000000000190

Watson, J., Brewer, B. B., & D'Alfonso, J. (2010, September). *Caritas: A theory guided scale to measure human caring.* Poster presented at The 2010 State of the Science Congress on Nursing Research, Washington, DC.

Watson, J., Brewer, B. B., & D'Alfonso, J. (2014). *Watson Caritas Patient Score (WCPS)*©. Boulder, CO: Watson Caring Science Institute. Retrieved from https://www.watsoncaringscience.org

Wolf, Z. R. (2012). Systematic review of effect of a caring protocol provided by nursing staff on patient satisfaction of adult hospitalized patients. *International Journal for Human Caring, 16*(4), 58–70.

23

The Evolution of Knowledge Development Related to Caring in Online Classrooms and Beyond

Kathleen Sitzman

CARITAS LITERACIES

By the end of this chapter, the caring-healing nurse will be able to

1. Recognize the increasingly central role that distance technology plays in effective student, professional, and client education.

2. Discuss key research findings related to caring in online teaching and learning settings.

3. Describe teaching learning practices that will support caring in online teaching and learning settings.

WATSON'S CARING SCIENCE IN EDUCATION AND PRACTICE

"Caring is considered by many as one central feature within the metaparadigm of nursing knowledge and practices" (Watson & Smith, 2002, p. 456). As the nursing profession evolves over time, day-to-day practice of professional caring also evolves. Ongoing exploration of what it means to care in all areas of nursing practice is key to preserving caring as nursing's core. Definitions of nurse caring through time have focused on nurses attending to the physical and emotional needs of others during face-to-face encounters (Judd & Sitzman, 2014; Nightingale, 1859). Extensive knowledge development has clarified how caring in the nursing profession can be perpetuated through face-to-face interactions that model caring in educational activities, peer interactions, and nurse–client encounters among teachers, students, and professional colleagues (Bevis & Watson, 2000; Touhy & Boykin, 2008). Watson's Human Caring Theory, introduced in nursing literature in 1979 (Watson, 1979), has provided an enduring theoretical foundation for exploring, understanding, and enacting key caring dimensions in nursing and beyond. Fundamental elements of this theory include the following:

- Transpersonal Caring Moments/Caring Occasions, wherein "the one caring connects with and embraces the spirit of the other through authentic, full attention in the here and now, and conveys a concern for the inner life and personal meaning of another" (Sitzman & Watson, 2014, p. 19)

- Ten Caritas Processes® to support caring comportment (Sitzman & Watson, 2014):
  1. Demonstrate loving-kindness, compassion, and equanimity with self and others.
  2. Be fully and authentically present.
  3. Nurture personal sensitivity through spiritual awareness and practice.
  4. Cultivate trusting-loving-caring relationships.
  5. Engage in authentic, nonjudgmental listening/interacting in both positive and negative situations.
  6. Promote creative problem solving through full use of self and resources.
  7. Use transpersonal teaching and learning methods that honor the learner's frame of reference.
  8. Create holistically healing environments at all levels.
  9. Assist with basic needs as sacred acts.
  10. Open oneself to mystery and unknowns, and allow for miracles.

The emergence of the digital age has expanded the role of the nurse to include interactions in cyberspace where face-to-face contact is largely absent and digital interactions such as email, texting, and online learning are integral (Sitzman, 2016a; Sitzman & Watson, 2017). Because digital interactions are now elemental to the nursing role in most professional settings, understanding how to model, teach, convey, and sustain digital caring is critical to maintaining caring as a core value in nursing. Watson (2002) anticipated this trend before digital interactions in nursing practice became widespread and commonplace:

The interface of technology and human technology changes the basic ontological position of separation and embraces—or is required to be open to—an ontological position of unity, connectedness, and transpersonal consciousness and technology that transcend time, space, and physicality … The implications invite new horizons of human technology evolution, which can embrace virtual and real, nonphysical and physical caring in a new order for new meanings [to emerge]. (p. 43)

Watson (2002) describes electronic/digital/virtual human interactions as nonlinear and disembodied experiences where caring and connection can be nurtured in new ways that are not limited by proximity, time, or space. Watson's Human Caring Theory has provided a lens through which digital interactions can be conceived as opportunities for reaching across distance and time to convey, teach, and share caring and love with any and all who have access to digital resources.

EIGHT STUDIES THAT EXPLORED DIGITAL CARING

Knowledge development related to caring in online nursing education has illuminated the nature of caring practice in everyday digital teaching/learning/interacting situations where physical proximity is absent, and a myriad of nonproximal interactive opportunities are routinely used to maintain ongoing human-to-human caring connections. Results from eight studies that used Watson's Caring Science as a guiding framework have validated the applicability of Watson's work in this environment (Leners, & Sitzman, 2006; Mann, 2014; Mastel-Smith, Post, & Lake, 2015; Sitzman, 2010; Sitzman, 2015; Sitzman, 2016a; Sitzman, 2016b; Sitzman & Leners, 2006). Table 23.1 provides a brief overview of findings from each of the eight studies.

Four of the studies focused on nursing student perceptions of caring in online classrooms. Sitzman and Leners (2006) published results of a pilot study that focused on 11 undergraduate nursing students' perceptions of caring and uncaring in online classrooms. Themes emerged that clarified student preferences and concerns in the online classroom setting. Leners and Sitzman (2006) replicated the study by Sitzman and Leners (2006), this time focusing on 39 graduate nursing students' perceptions of caring and uncaring in online classrooms. Themes emerged that provided insight into the caring needs of graduate nursing students in online classroom settings. Sitzman (2010) then completed a larger national study, on the basis of results of the two pilot studies (Leners & Sitzman, 2006; Sitzman & Leners, 2006) discussed earlier, with 122 undergraduate nursing students that clarified specific student-preferred caring behaviors for instructors who teach online. Mann (2014) replicated the study by Sitzman (2010) with 48 online RN-BSN students. Study participants identified three important activities an instructor could do to create a caring online learning environment.

Three subsequent studies explored nursing faculty perceptions of caring in online classrooms. Sitzman (2016b) asked nursing instructors to indicate what student cues prompted caring interventions in online classrooms. The first study (Sitzman, 2016b) had 56 respondents who provided brief answers to questions in three areas of inquiry that included identification of student cues that prompted caring interventions, the nature of the caring interventions, and student response to caring interventions. Results yielded information about specific caring cues and responses in online nursing classrooms. Twenty-six of the 56 respondents in this study also provided unsolicited rich narrative detailing their day-to-day experiences of caring in online nursing classrooms, which resulted in an additional nested study (Sitzman, 2015).

Three themes emerged (Figure 23.1) that described an iterative process for interacting with students in a caring manner in online nursing classrooms:

- **Sense** circumstances through full attention to cues provided in the online setting:
  - Tone of messages
  - Frequency of communications
  - Timing of communications
  - Changes in usual pattern of written communication or use of technology
  - Absence of communication when it is needed
  - Decreased quality of work

TABLE 23.1 Eight Studies Related to Digital World Caring

Study	Findings
Sitzman and Leners (2006) explored 11 under-graduate nursing students' perceptions of instructor caring in online nursing classrooms	Eight themes emerged that highlighted the importance of providing the following: • *Frequent feedback:* Reaching out to communicate at least once a week • *Timeliness:* Responding within 24 hours or less • *Reciprocity of caring online:* Recognizing that caring goes both ways • *Personal connection and empathy:* Being fully human and fully present • *Clarity:* Taking the time to create clear and accurate content and communications • *Multiple contact opportunities:* Being available by phone, email, text, and other means • *Second-fiddle worries:* Assuring the other of his or her importance despite lack of physical proximity • *Teacher's commitment to learning:* Expressing purpose and joy in digital settings
Leners and Sitzman (2006) explored 39 gradu-ate nursing students' perceptions of instructor caring in online nursing classrooms	Six themes emerged: • *Empathic perspective:* Cultivating inclusion and full presence • *Timeliness of communication:* Responding in 24 hours or less • *Tone of appreciation:* Acknowledgment of effort, involvement, and work • *Being the best I can be:* Encouraging the best in self and others • *Finding a chord of harmony:* Establishing a collaborative and collegial environment • *Feeling the passion of caring online:* Valuing, appreciating, and demonstrating excellence in digital environments
Sitzman (2010) completed a national study in which 122 undergraduate nursing students clarified what they perceived to be caring online instructor behaviors in online classrooms	Four general caring online behavioral attributes were identified: Clarity/Expertise, Timeliness, Empathic Presence, and Full Engagement/ Accessibility (Sitzman, 2010, p. 176). Preferred behaviors included the following: • Providing clear and detailed written instructions for course activities and assignments • Engaging in timely communication • Demonstrating excellence, passion, and enthusiasm in relation to teaching/ learning

(continued)

TABLE 23.1 Eight Studies Related to Digital World Caring *(continued)*

Study	Findings
	• Providing individual, private guidance when needed • Referring to specifics in students' work so they know it has been read • Ensuring accessibility so students are able to get help when needed • Sharing ongoing online challenges and remedies so students know they are not alone
Mann (2014) replicated the study by Sitzman (2010) with 48 RN-BSN students at historically Black colleges and universities	The three most important activities an instructor could do to create a caring online learning environment included the following: • Paying attention to detail in organization and clarity • Providing prompt and detailed assignment feedback • Promptly responding to students' questions
Sitzman (2016b) completed a national study involving 56 nursing instructors who were asked to identify student cues that prompted caring interventions in online classrooms, the nature of the caring interventions they initiated, and student response to caring interventions	Cues that prompted caring fell into six categories: • *Academic struggle:* Declining or failing grades • *Appeals for help:* Asking for help directly or commenting frequently about stress • *Concerning behaviors:* Negative or despairing comments • *Withdrawal:* Decreased level of communication or participation • *Personal problems:* Illness, divorce, financial struggles, deployment, other challenges for self, family, or significant others • *Positive events:* Wedding, pregnancy, awards, promotions, other accomplishments for self or significant others Instructor responses fell into three categories: • *Reaching out:* Calling, emailing, texting, other • *Concrete academic support:* Offering help from existing resources • *Intentional caring comportment:* Creating unique, meaningful, and personalized ways to express caring Student responses fell into three categories: • *Gratitude:* Wanting to say "Thank you" • *Finding their voice:* Feeling confident about expressing needs in a positive and productive way • *Academic improvement:* Improving grades, increasing confidence and participation

(continued)

TABLE 23.1 Eight Studies Related to Digital World Caring *(continued)*

Study	Findings
Twenty-six of the 56 respondents in the national study by Sitzman (2016b) provided unsolicited rich narrative detailing their experiences of caring in online nursing classrooms, which resulted in an additional nested study **(Sitzman, 2015)** that further explored instructor perceptions of caring in online settings	Three themes emerged that described an iterative process for interacting with students in a caring manner online: • *Sensing* circumstances • *Connecting* through reaching out • *Facilitating* growth and learning based on individual needs
Sitzman (2016a) then analyzed information in previous caring online studies (Sitzman, & Leners, 2006; Leners, & Sitzman, 2006; Sitzman, 2010; Mann, 2014; Sitzman, 2016b; Sitzman, 2015) to assess whether consistent caring communication patterns were evident	Six consistent communicative elements emerged (see Table 23.2 for suggested caring language): • Offering full presence • Acknowledging shared humanity • Attending to the individual • Asking for and providing frequent clarification • Demonstrating flexibility • Acknowledging challenges and pointing out favorable opportunities
Mastel-Smith et al. (2015) explored faculty perceptions and expressions of caring presence in online classrooms and integrated findings with Watson's Caritas Processes	Four themes emerged from the data: • *Online teaching experiences* that encompassed feelings about online teaching, teaching philosophy, technology, communication, teaching methods, and student engagement • *Similarities and differences between online and face-to-face teaching* including absence of physical proximity, online interaction as a great equalizer, time management, availability to students, disclosure/anonymity, and knowing students • *Online presence* defined by course preparation, communication patterns with students, and being part of the students' learning experiences • *Online caring presence* including valuing student success, conveying positive/helpful affirmations, offering caring feedback, and engaging in active cultivation of a caring community/environment

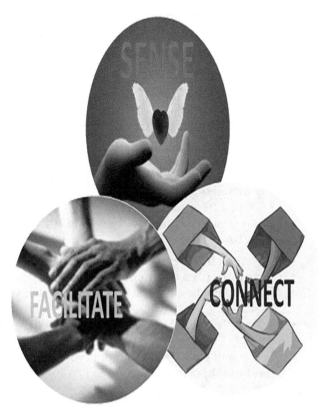

FIGURE 23.1 Digital caring cycle.

- **Connect** when cues warrant further attention to promote productivity or success:
  - Call, email, or text to invite caring communication related to observed concerns.
  - Engage in Caritas Process nursing practice to create a safe, caring, and productive sharing space where productivity and positivity are cultivated.
  - Work together to create productive ways to move forward.

- **Facilitate**:
  - Offer appropriate individual, departmental, organizational, community, and other resources to support productive outcomes and further growth/learning.
  - Create structure, as needed, to support accountability and positive/productive outcomes.
  - Allow for failure while providing a clear path forward toward hope and dignity.

When these three iterative phases are practiced continually, they support digital caring.

Sitzman (2016a) then analyzed information in the six studies discussed earlier (Leners, & Sitzman, 2006; Mann, 2014; Sitzman, & Leners, 2006; Sitzman, 2010; Sitzman, 2015; Sitzman, 2016b;) to determine whether there were consistencies in caring communication patterns that could be discerned from the study data. Six consistent communicative elements emerged that outline parameters of a caring lexicon that could be used in digital environments. Table 23.2 provides examples of specific caring language that may be used in online settings as is or modified to reflect personal style and preferences.

TABLE 23.2 Suggested Caring Language for Online Teaching and Learning Settings

Caring Communication Exemplar	Suggested Terminology
Offer full presence	• I am here for you • I am working online all day today—call/email/text if you need me • My thoughts are with you • I see you have sent a message that I cannot fully address at this time. I will respond fully by (day/time)
Acknowledge shared humanity	• We are in this together • Let's learn from one another • I will do my best for you and hope that you will do your best also • I struggled with this topic when I was in nursing school • If you will work hard to support your success, I will work hard to support your success too
Attend to the individual	• I want you to be successful • You are important to me • I see you missed an assignment, which is not your typical behavior … • You showed a lot of insight when you said … • I missed seeing your contributions in the last discussion board • I really appreciate your attention to detail (or promptness, or sense of humor, or sensitivity, or experience, etc.)
Ask for clarification	• Do you understand? • Is everything okay? • Are you prepared for the upcoming (test, assignment, presentation, etc.)? • Do you need clarification or assistance? • How is your day today? • Is there anything I can do to help you right now? • How are you feeling about …?
Propose flexible solutions	• I do not understand what you meant … How about if we discuss things further in a phone call or video chat rather than by email? • Because you turned your assignment in early with good effort, I will give you an additional 3 days to redo the sections where content was missed

(continued)

Caring Communication Exemplar	Suggested Terminology
TABLE 23.2 Suggested Caring Language for Online Teaching and Learning Settings *(continued)*	
	• I would like to work with you to create a learning contract so that we have clear instructions related to what you and I will need to do to move productively forward • I am inviting input from everyone regarding how to make the assignment/rubric/test question(s)/course instructions, and so on, clearer
Acknowledge challenges and point out favorable opportunities	• I know you are struggling, but I would like to help and mentor wherever possible • Although they can be challenging, group assignments cultivate collaborative skills that are critical to productivity in every working environment • I can sense your frustration/disappointment/sadness, and I am offering to work with you to better understand and help • We (or your group) productively worked together in this difficult situation and found good ways to move forward

Source: Adapted from Sitzman, K. (2016a). Mindful communication for caring online. *Advances in Nursing Science, 39*(1), 38–47. doi:10.1097/ANS.0000000000000102

Mastel-Smith et al. (2015) explored faculty perceptions and expressions of caring presence in online classrooms and integrated findings with Watson's Caritas Processes #1 to #9. Four themes emerged from the data that characterized similarities and differences between face-to-face and online instruction and presented dimensions of online caring presence.

Examples of Caring Science and the Digital Realm

Examples of Transpersonal Caring Moments and Caritas Practices in digital settings were evident in the words of researchers and study participants in all eight studies and are represented in Table 23.3.

Examples of digital Transpersonal Caring Moments include the following:

- (Researcher Comment) "… elements of intuitive interaction were also identified … and referred to as inherent in an empathic approach to online education. Students stated that online caring involved 'being in tune with the thoughts and feelings of others' and faculty ability to 'sense overload from a distance'" (Leners & Sitzman, 2006, p. 317).

- (Faculty Comment) "Each student needs to know that you are there, there for them, and care about them and their success" (Sitzman, 2016b, p. 67).

TABLE 23.3 Digital Caritas Process

Caritas Processes	Corresponding Digital Examples
1. Demonstrate loving-kindness, compassion, and equanimity with self and others	(Faculty comment) "I encourage you to be kind to yourself as you embark on this … you do not have to be perfect" (Mastel-Smith, Post, & Lake, 2015, p. 148). (Faculty comment) "I value the sacrifices you are making to be in school and believe that you want to do your best. Here is an area that needs your reflection on how to improve" (Sitzman, 2016b, p. 67).
2. Be fully and authentically present	(Student comment) "Letting us know they were there—by actually reading what was posted and responding—let the students know there was someone there that really cares" (Sitzman & Leners, 2006, p. 256). (Faculty comment) "[Sometimes I say to the student] I notice that you seem overwhelmed. Tell me what is concerning you. How can I help?" (Sitzman, 2015, p. 27).
3. Nurture personal sensitivity through spiritual awareness and practice	(Faculty comment) "… you must check your ego at the door and put on your caring attitude once you sit down at the computer …" (Sitzman, 2015, p. 27). (Faculty comment) "I have given many students spiritual gift tests, and then I meet with them over the phone or online [to discuss results]" (Sitzman, 2015, p. 27).
4. Cultivate trusting-loving-caring relationships	(Researcher comment) "… [student] respondents discussed the belief that caring online is a reciprocal process that requires commitment" (Sitzman & Leners, 2006, p. 256). (Student comment) "Caring is taking the time to assure that both parties understand what is expected and needed from the other" (Sitzman & Leners, 2006, p. 257).
5. Engage in authentic, nonjudgmental listening/interacting in both positive and negative situations	(Student comment) "… caring instructors actively sought feedback regarding graded evaluations, for example, confusing exam questions, written homework [sic] and may change grading if appropriate" (Sitzman, 2010, p. 176). (Faculty comment) "[I] encourage expression of thought and feeling … expression is a form of self-reflection and learning. I also share with them during difficult situations; reflection and expression can be therapeutic and helpful …" (Sitzman, 2015, p. 27).
6. Promote creative problem solving through full use of self and resources	(Faculty comment) "Students were encouraged to be creative and 'think outside the box. You will be the innovator, the creator, the trailblazer'" (Mastel-Smith, Post, & Lake, 2015, p. 148).

(continued)

TABLE 23.3 Digital Caritas Process *(continued)*

Caritas Processes	Corresponding Digital Examples
7.	(Faculty comment) "I will usually take time to respond with examples or step-by-step instructions so that the students are able to figure out whatever it is they are frustrated with. I provide many details and explanations to help them along. I've also asked questions or inquired if they have tried a different approach toward solving the problem" (Sitzman, 2016b, p. 66).
8. Use transpersonal teaching and learning methods that honor the learner's frame of reference	(Student comment) "Try to understand and respect the learning that is taking place on the students [sic] part even if it is not in a way that the instructor might have intended" (Sitzman, 2010, p. 176). (Faculty comment) "I always start any response/email … by saying something like 'Thank-you for inquiring into …' I also tell students that if they are asking this question, then other students are also thinking the same …" (Sitzman, 2016b, p. 66).
9. Create holistically healing environments at all levels	(Student comment) "… it is important to have class schedules, requirements, postings, and so on easily accessible and understandable so it isn't a nightmare trying to figure out what you need to do and how to turn in your work" (Sitzman, 2010, p. 175). (Student comment) "Online faculty caring helps me be the best I can be …" (Leners & Sitzman, 2006, p. 317).
10. Assist with basic needs as sacred acts	(Faculty comment) "I cannot stress [enough] the importance of treating each student as a valuable member of your course. Each student email ends with a thank you for their questions, or a thanks for sending information … if they make a suggestion I thank them for their time and interest. It is important the student know that they are a valuable member of the course and that [the nursing program] cares about each one" (Sitzman, 2016b, p. 67). (Faculty comment) "Our priority is communicating with you, so if there are any problems, we will work to solve them" (Mastel-Smith, Post, & Lake, 2015, p. 148).
11. Open oneself to mystery and unknowns, and allow for miracles	(Faculty comment) "They [the students] really are beautiful people, you just need to figure out where they are coming from and then deal appropriately" (Sitzman, 2015, p. 28). (Faculty Comment) "I contact students when I notice … a difference … I inquire if something is happening that is impacting their ability to fully participate at the expected level and ask that they reply to me so that I can understand what is happening and offer suggestions to help them improve performance" (Sitzman, 2015, p. 26).

Source: Adapted from Sitzman, K., & Watson, J. (2014). *Caring science, mindful practice: Implementing Watson's human caring theory.* New York, NY: Springer Publishing.

CONCLUSION

When considered as an integrated whole, knowledge development stemming from the eight studies discussed in this chapter represents confirmation that Watson's Human Caring Theory is relevant and applicable in digital settings. Comments from researchers and study participants illuminate an ongoing dynamic process of interpretation and application related to constructing ways to care in digital environments.

Effective integration of a theoretical framework into two vastly different settings such as digital and face to face is a hallmark of universality and elemental resonance. Human Caring Theory is fluidly applicable in both of these contexts because the basic tenets of Watson's work resonate with the primal core of love from which caring intentionality originates before emerging into face-to-face, digital, or other domains of being. Watson's work transcends time, space, and proximity, allowing it to serve as an effective framework for exploration and discovery now and into the future as new ways of interacting, connecting, loving, and caring unfold.

NEXT ERA POSSIBILITIES

Education

- How can I consciously build caring practices into every online course and interaction I engage in for my clients, colleagues, and both near and extended community?
- In what ways do current online educational offerings in both professional and academic realms need to be reimagined so that they reflect caring in structure, language, and content?

Research

- What further research is needed to fully describe caring online pedagogy?
- How can caring online research be extended into quantitative inquiry?

Praxis

- What educational practices can we all improve right now to convey better caring on digital and online settings?
- What policies and practices related to online and digital interactions could be enhanced with caring guidelines?

Theory and Knowledge Development

- What are additional actions needed to fully develop and implement a distinct digital caring pedagogy in professional and academic settings?
- Given my specialty, where can I contribute to the expansion of digital caring?
- How does my own understanding of nursing blend with the practices discussed in this chapter? How can I expand my vision of caring possibilities within the digital realm?

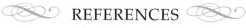 REFERENCES

Bevis, E. O., & Watson, J. (2000). *Toward a caring curriculum: A new pedagogy for nursing.* Sudbury, MA: Jones & Bartlett.

Judd, D., & Sitzman, K. (2014). *A history of American nursing: Trends and eras.* Burlington, MA: Jones & Bartlett.

Leners, D. W., & Sitzman, K. (2006). Graduate student perceptions: Feeling the passion of caring online. *Nursing Education Perspectives, 27*(6), 315–319. doi:10.2202/1548-923X.1267

Mann, J. C. (2014). A pilot study of RN-BSN completion students' preferred instructor online classroom caring behaviors. *Association of Black Nursing Faculty Journal, 25*(2), 33–39.

Mastel-Smith, B., Post, J., & Lake, P. (2015). Online teaching: "Are your there, and do you care?" *Journal of Nursing Education, 54*(3), 145–151. doi:10.3928/01484834-20150218-18

Nightingale, F. (1859). *Notes on nursing: What it is and what it is not.* London, UK: Harrison and Sons.

Sitzman, K. (2010). Student-preferred caring behaviors for online nursing education. *Nursing Education Perspectives, 31*(3), 171–178. Retrieved from https://journals.lww.com/neponline/Abstract/2010/05000/Student_Preferred_Caring_Behaviors_for_Online.9.aspx

Sitzman, K. (2015). Sense, connect, facilitate: Nurse educator experiences of caring online through Watson's lens. *International Journal for Human Caring, 19*(3), 25–29. doi:10.20467/1091-5710-19.3.25

Sitzman, K. (2016a). Mindful communication for caring online. *Advances in Nursing Science, 39*(1), 38–47. doi:10.1097/ANS.0000000000000102

Sitzman, K. L. (2016b). What student cues prompt online instructors to offer caring Interventions? *Nursing Education Perspectives, 37*(2), 61–71. doi:10.5480/14-1542

Sitzman, K., & Leners, D. (2006). Student perceptions of caring in online baccalaureate education. *Nursing Education Perspectives, 27*(5), 254–259. Retrieved from https://journals.lww.com/neponline/Abstract/2006/09000/Student_Perceptions_of_CARING_in_Online.10.aspx

Sitzman, K., & Watson, J. (2014). *Caring science, mindful practice: Implementing Watson's human caring theory.* New York, NY: Springer Publishing.

Sitzman, K., & Watson, J. (2017). *Watson's caring in the digital world: A guide for caring when interacting, teaching, and learning in cyberspace.* New York, NY: Springer Publishing.

Touhy, T., & Boykin, A. (2008). Caring as the central domain in nursing education. *International Journal for Human Caring, 12*(2), 8–15.

Watson, J. (1979). *Nursing: The philosophy and science of caring.* Boston, MA: Little, Brown.

Watson, J. (2002). Metaphysics of virtual caring communities. *International Journal for Human Caring, 6*(1), 41–45.

Watson, J., & Smith, M. C. (2002). Caring science and the science of unitary human beings: A transtheoretical discourse for nursing knowledge development. *Journal of Advanced Nursing, 37*(5), 452–461. doi:10.1046/j.1365-2648.2002.02112.x

VI

Touching the Space of Praxis

24

Caring Inquiry Methodology: The Aesthetic Process in the Way of Compassion[1]

Marilyn A. Ray

CARITAS LITERACIES

By the end of this chapter, the caring-healing nurse will be able to

1. Describe Caring Inquiry Methodology for purposes of seeking to understand Caring Science as the journey of compassion and love and researching Caring Processes.

2. Appreciate the art of caring in nursing as the "compassionate we," the "speaking together" of the one caring and the one cared for to reveal the human, spiritual, and environmental contexts.

3. Distinguish Caring Inquiry as aesthetic knowing that illuminates creativity, the quality of presences, spirituality and reflective intuition of the meaning of the life world experiences, and the meaning of meaning (pre-flective experience or experiences as we live through them) related to caring and compassion.

4. Identify the steps of the human caring-healing science approaches of phenomenology (description) and phenomenological hermeneutics (interpretation) to study persons who are sharing experiences of their life world.

5. Understand the constitutive meanings in the textual data as themes and metathemes to understand the meaning of being and becoming through caring.

⁂

[1]From Ray, M. A. (1991). Caring inquiry: The esthetic process in the way of compassion. In D. A. Gaut & M. M. Leininger (Eds.), *Caring: The compassionate healer* (pp. 181–189). New York, NY: National League for Nursing, Permission to reprint granted by the National League for Nursing, New York, NY.

Comprehend phenomenological reduction and the process of intuiting to grasp the unity of meaning as a direct, unmediated apprehension of the whole of the meaning of meaning of the experience, a transcendence, a theory of the whole of the experience.

Years ago, an elderly woman bedridden with a stroke looked at me with her stark, piercing blue eyes. Though I usually didn't like loud music, I turned up the radio to drown the sorrows of the sick room I was in—to drown out the sounds and, in some strange way, the sight of the suffering one before me. Unspeaking, I looked at her. She spoke with her heart. Uncomfortable in her presence, but responding to the life of compassion deep within my heart and soul, I turned off the radio. The journey of sharing the pain—that is, nursing—began.

I wrote this chapter to share ideas and an approach to the method that may capture the complexity of researching—caring. I have spent much time researching and reflecting on the nature of caring and feel intensely that it is the way of compassion, a journey of love. Caring and love are synonymous (Ray, 1981, 1997*). Inquiring about caring touches the heart and translates through the soul: the "speaking together" between the one caring and the one cared for. It is an immersion into the human encounter that also reveals the human, environmental, and spiritual contexts that are nursing.

The metaphorical heart and soul are the symbols and synonyms for life, living, sensitivity, reason, and integrity. These symbols represent a creative process: the gradual or, more often, abrupt shifting of consciousness from focus on the "they" or "I" to a compassionate "we" (Kidd, 1990), which is also spiritual (and divine*; which deepens and moves one forward and upward; Kandinsky, 1977). Compassion is a wounding of the heart by the other, where the "other" enters into us and makes us other. In the minutes of presence and dialogue with the other, we have the transformative powers of the aesthetic (and spiritual)—the understanding of forms of meaning within the sheer presence of the other and of dialogue or language that exercises the most penetrative authority over consciousness (Steiner, 1989).

In the compassionate way of being, the forms of "other" in consciousness communicate a depth of felt-realness or authenticity, which is intuitive (Steiner, 1989) and depends on the granting to the other to whom one communicates a share in one's being (Buber, 1965). The aesthetic act in a compassionate way of being thus communicates in the understanding of forms of meaning a simultaneous immanence and transcendence—human choice to share in the life of the other, and an intuitive knowing, which, as we become "other," can be translated into a call to a deeper life, a more integrated wholeness, and a coming to understand more fully what we have understood.

What does this mean for nursing and nursing inquiry? Real presence and dialogue as choice and intuition in compassionate forms of meaning in understanding are an act of creation for nursing. This aesthetic act, this conceiving and bringing into being, is a birthing and growth of the divine or spiritual life within. Steiner (1989) intimated that in an aesthetic act, there can be no experience that does not wager on a presence of sense that is, finally, theological (God-centered or love*). He states, "So far as it [the esthetic act] wagers

_____

Asterisk (*) indicates additional references or clarification in the chapter.

on meaning, an account of the act of reading in fullest sense, of the act of the reception and internalization of significant forms within us, is a metaphysical and, in the last analysis, a theological one; [t]he meaning of meaning is a transcendent postulate" (1989, pp. 215–216). Transcendence in the felt-realness of the compassionate encounter is the unwritten theology. The meaning of meaning or transcendence as unwritten theology is an apprehension of the "radically inexplicable presence, facticity and perceptible substantiality of the created, it is; we are" (p. 201) because there is creation.

For nursing inquiry as the way of compassion, the aesthetic (creative) act of *knowing about* the meaning of the meaning of nursing as caring presumes creation—the conceiving of and bringing into being a knowledge of the substantiality of the created. There is transcendence that is also theological (love or of God*). There is a presence that, as the researcher dwells with the data to read "being anew" or to apprehend the nature of caring, "is the source of powers, of significations in the text, in the work [that is] neither consciously willed nor consciously understood … [t]he unmastered 'thereness' of a secret-sharer [God-centeredness or love*], of a prior creation with and against which the art [esthetic] act has been effected" (Steiner, 1989, pp. 211–212). In essence, the felt-realness of compassion (caring) in nursing and nursing research, because of the focus on the compassionate "we," is a theological (loving) enterprise. As Emily Dickinson notes in one of her poems (Stone, 1990), "The soul selects her own society—Then, shuts the door" (p. 9).

CARING INQUIRY: THE PHENOMENOLOGY OF AESTHETIC RESEARCH

Caring Inquiry as an aesthetic process in research is a unique method of presence and dialogue. It attends to both immanence—communion with and transcendence—and reflective intuition. When a researcher engages in Caring Inquiry, the compassionate "we" is enacted. Encountering the "other" to learn anew the world of caring, not the world as encoded earlier by scientific analysis, is where the word and compassion (love) interact (Steiner, 1989). Both description (phenomenology) and interpretation (phenomenological hermeneutics) and aesthetic knowing of the experience of caring are the means by which questions about the meaning of caring are illuminated. Phenomenology and phenomenological hermeneutics (van Manen, 1990, 2014*) are human sciences that study persons who are experiencing the life world. Aesthetic knowing in caring research attends to creativity, sensitivity, and the quality of presences. It is an approach of describing and understanding the meaning of being and becoming through caring. In bringing to reflective awareness the nature of caring in the events experienced in the world of nursing, the researcher (as well as possibly the research participant) is transformed, contributing to the fullness of being and the call to a deeper life—a life of integrated wholeness and openness to creative forces within and without.

Thus, what makes phenomenological hermeneutics an aesthetic enterprise is an investment of one's own being in the process of the events of the research. The response to the descriptions and interpretations of the events of caring in aesthetic inquiry is one of pure receptivity and responding responsibly, or being answerable to the text in the specific sense, which is at once moral, spiritual, and psychological (Steiner, 1989). The translation of data communicated as text from "shared remembrances" of participants of the meaning of caring into the general perspective of human recognition is teaching the way of the compassionate heart and soul. It illuminates a valuation of the theological or spiritual. The phenomenology of aesthetic research of caring presupposes and validates an enmeshment in the metaphysical and theological. What the method is seeking is integrity—a coming to understand more fully what we have understood—where the word and love are a synthesis.

The following is a methodological process I developed on the basis of the ideas of Husserl (Natanson, 1973), van Manen (1990; 1997/2016; 2014), Reeder (1984, 1988), and other philosophers of human science, art, and theology. The process is outlined as follows (Ray, work in progress-Not published, 1991, 2013):

1. The Intentionality of Inner Being of the Researcher

2. The Process of Dialogic Experiencing

3. The Process of Phenomenological-Hermeneutical Reflecting and Transforming

4. The Movement of Phenomenological-Hermeneutical Theorizing to a Theory of Meaning

5. Dialoguing With Written Texts: Examining Similarities and Differences

6. Credibility and Significance of the Process of the Phenomenology of the Aesthetic Act

The general research question relates to the meaning of the experience of caring or compassion in nursing research. A specific question could be: What is the meaning of caring in your experience? This methodology also could be used for any other phenomenological-hermeneutical question in nursing.

THE AESTHETIC PROCESS IN CARING INQUIRY

A dynamic, disciplined, dialectical, reflective, and creative approach among the following activities forms the process of the aesthetic phenomenological-hermeneutical inquiry and is outlined as follows (Ray, work in progress-Not Published):

A. The Intentionality of Inner Being of the Researcher
   1. Imagining the vision of the caring in nursing—past, and future within the present
   2. Listening to the "voices" within embodied consciousness, as a feeling and a form of discourse about the meaning of caring in nursing
   3. Focusing on and identifying one's presuppositions of caring in nursing
   4. Practicing bracketing to hold in abeyance one's prehistory and presuppositions about the caring in nursing

B. The Process of Dialogic Experiencing
   1. Developing the proposal* and [s]electing the participants for the study grounded within the imagined vision
   2. Engaging with the participants to discuss the roles of interviewer and interviewee, and securing informed consent signatures

3. Copresencing/sensing the other by recognizing the immediate impact of each other's being on each other—the "compassionate we"

4. Conversing with participants in tape-recorded, intensive dialogical interviews lasting approximately 1 hour, about the meaning of caring in nursing by asking the phenomenological question: What is the meaning of caring in your experience?

5. Engaging in a cue-taking, talk-turning, researcher-bracketed, dialogical-dialectical interactive process on the basis of the participants' experience to penetrate the meaning and experience of how caring nursing is constructed for or understood by the other. The researcher at this time of dialogic interviewing holds in abeyance, or temporarily sets aside, his or her knowledge of caring that is a part of his or her embodied consciousness. There is continued controversy over the issue of bracketing in phenomenological philosophy (Stapleton, 1983). For the purpose of this research approach, bracketing of presuppositions about caring is used during the interviews by moving from the lead question of the meaning experience of caring followed by the cue-taking, talk-turning interaction of the actual dialogue itself.

C. The Process of Phenomenological-Hermeneutical Reflecting and Transforming: The Flow of Analysis occurs through:

1. Reflecting and feeling the presencing of the participants' beings in one's consciousness

2. Transcribing the phenomenological data of the meaning of the art of nursing as texts through a computer-assisted data text and analytic system (Seidel, 1988) or any qualitative data analysis software (QDAS) such as multiplex quantitative DNA array (MQDA), NVivo, Atlas.ti, and so forth (Goransson, Ehrenberg, Ehnfors, & Fonteyn, 2006)*. Although many phenomenologists argue against computer-assisted data analysis, Goransson et al. (2006) remarked that phenomenologists could reconcile this disagreement with careful selection of the best technology that explores their phenomenon, such as, in this situation, caring*.

3. Bracketed reflecting for a pure descriptive phenomenology or receptive knowing in consciousness while engaging in the first encounter with the transcribed data (bracketing one's interpretive tendency in relation to one's history and presuppositions about the phenomenon)

4. Attending to the speaking of language in the texts. If a transcriber, other than the researcher, transcribes the data, the researcher should listen to the tapes at the time of encountering the texts for the first time.

5. Highlighting the descriptive experiences of the art of nursing, caring-healing in the texts by using a highlighter pen or technological* device to illuminate the participants' language of experience

6. Interpretive reflecting (hermeneutic-thinking or unbracketed reflecting) to reveal the immanent themes (linguistic dimensions) emerging in the data. Unbracketed reflecting is the foundation for phenomenological-hermeneutical interpretation. Rather than bracketing one's preassumptions of caring, the history or horizon of meaning of the researcher is brought into being in the dialectic of consciousness and the text.

7. Moving back and forth in understanding the meaning of the textual data to and in consciousness (copresencing and dialoguing with the data in consciousness)

8. Writing and transforming the themes in the transcribed text to cocreate the metathemes that are linguistic abstractions of the themes

9. Phenomenological reducing or intuiting—turning to the nature of the transcendental meaning of the phenomenon by intuiting or grasping the unity of meaning as a direct, unmediated apprehension of the whole of the experience. This process is an intersubjective universal—a transcendent experience of knowing wherein the researcher as knower makes a connecting leap of insight and the separateness of the phenomenon melds into a whole. The universal is reached by a "coming together" of the variations. Thus, variations or similarities of the experience are intuitively and authentically grasped and constituted in consciousness—the primordial material of sensation out of which arises the knowing of the meaning of experience (the possibility of the phenomenological genesis or beginning, i.e., what has been experienced as apart comes together as insight/new awareness, but is not put together from the different dimensions). References to the data, or themes, of experiences-as-meant of the meaning of caring in nursing from participants' experiences undergo transformation into the researcher's intentional life, and stand out as a component of the researcher's concrete essence. A new way of experiencing, thinking, and theorizing thus is opened up for the researcher. (This experience may occur at any time in the process of reflection.) A metaphor(s) too may be grasped as the unity of meaning at this time.

10. Composing linguistic transformation of data to themes, metathemes, or metaphor (metatheme and metaphor may be the transcendent experience)

D. The Movement of Phenomenological-Hermeneutical Theorizing to a Theory of Meaning

1. "Putting together" a theory of meaning, which when constituted by the descriptions, themes, metathemes, and/or metaphor(s), and transcendent unity of meaning, becomes the *form* or *structure* of the phenomenological meaning of caring. The theory as form may be represented as a visual model showing all the dimensions of the experience. A theory in phenomenological philosophy and method may seem contradictory given the fundamental notion of the continuous, experiencing process of the living world. However, the idea of theory in a sense is a way of giving form to the intentional acts of the research itself—where the knower and the known are one, are integral (Reeder, 1984), and where the researcher communicates to the world the integrality of understanding the aesthetic act itself. Theory in this sense aims at making explicit the universal meaning of the whole of the experience. Note the etymology of theory—Theo and eros—God and love.

E. Dialoguing With Written Texts: Examining Similarities and Differences

1. Relating the theory of meaning to literary writings in art or nursing to enhance the epistemic development of nursing theory is expressed by illustrating and

illuminating similarities and differences from the phenomenological analytic data and theory or theories advanced earlier. The form or structure of the meanings, that is, the phenomenological theory, gives rise to its value in relation to the existing theories or literary works and subsequently to the implications or recommendations of nursing education, practice, administration, and research.

F. Credibility and Significance of the Process of the Phenomenology of the Aesthetic Act
    1. *Recognizing*, *believing*, and *acknowledging* are the dynamics of credibility of the research. The phenomenological evidence of the reality-as-meant of caring is what has been lived and communicated by the participants. Reality, as expressed in experience, is not inauthentic. Meanings convince, and the meanings of the experience alter the sensibilities of those dwelling in the phenomenological written text—the researcher and other readers. Phenomenology enlarges human awareness directly or expands the range of human perception with new ways of experiencing, rather than with new, objective, mechanistic interpretations as in traditional science. Deepening and expanding the possibilities of being—the quality of making humans more human, humane, and spiritual (the ontologic)—rather than more mechanistic is the valid experience of phenomenological aesthetic inquiry.
    2. *Affirming* and *confirming* the meaning of the lived experience are the dynamics of the significance of the research and are expressed and understood not as an agreement, conformity, or generalization, but moving toward the universal that is paradoxical. The capacity to grasp and communicate the meaning of the whole of the experience is articulated and "tested" through the reflective intuition and individuality of the researcher. The universal is deep. It is a sympathetic relationship through which the researcher is transposed into the interior lives of others. The universal is undifferentiated wholeness or caring wisdom that is ultimately both within and without—a reflective symmetry, which brings together into a unity the reflective interiority of the researcher with the possibilities and contradictions of historical-cultural horizons. The quest for meaning is a social signifier and therefore exists in the relationship between the personal-mutual, the individual-community, and the specificity-commonality of culture. The movement of phenomenological theorizing to a theory of meaning captures, through the solitude of the researcher's reflection on the meaning, the researcher's capacity to bridge participants' meaning of experience of caring and the universality of human action as aesthetic. Thus, the transformations or possibilities in experiencing (the epistemologic) are open or available to all readers in the reflective symmetry or synthesis encapsulated in the theory.

CONCLUSION

This chapter focused on the sharing of ideas and an approach to the method that reflects the complexity and creative power of Caring Inquiry as a way of compassion and an aesthetic act. What I have affirmed by expressing the interiority of compassion as presence and dialogue through metaphysical and epistemological means is that caring and Caring Inquiry, in the final analysis, are spiritual and theological. The density of theological presence in nursing research has been effectively communicated by its absence in the past few decades, possibly because of the logical positivist teachings of science, or the newer dimensions of deconstructionist philosophy. It may well be that forgetting the question of the theological, in a sense forgetting to address the mystery of the hidden, yet revealed an interiority of the heart and soul that will continue to drain from nursing its creative, authentic caring potential, and the entire sphere of the aesthetic—the meaning of meaning. The crisis in nursing science and practice today demonstrates an emptiness that echoes of the loss of the theological. I have communicated the loss. It could be, however, more from silence than emptiness. This chapter has given voice to this silence.

QUESTIONS FOR REFLECTION
[ADDED IN THE 2013 PUBLICATION]

BACCALAUREATE

1. What did you observe about Ray's (1991, 2013*) views on caring, love, and compassion?

2. Why is a phenomenological approach effective in investigating the aesthetic process of conducting a Caring Inquiry?

3. How does an investigator who used phenomenological hermeneutics become enmeshed in the research process, according to Ray (1991, 2013)? Describe.

MASTER'S

1. How is the text or material of phenomenological studies obtained by investigators?

2. What did you learn about how Ray (1991, 2013*) created the methodological process to study the experience of caring or compassion in nursing research and the meaning of caring in the researcher's experience? What are the sources used in this new method?

3. What affects you about the way Ray (1991, 2013*) looked at Caring Inquiry?

DOCTORAL

1. What are the steps of the methodological process outlined by Ray (1991, 2013*)? Briefly summarize three steps.

2. What follow-up information do you need to expand your understanding of phenomenological reducing or intuiting?

3. What did you learn about the study of caring from a phenomenological method after reading Ray's chapter?* Please also see the research of Czerenda (2006)* and Shields (2007).*

NEXT ERA POSSIBILITIES

Education

- In what way can caring scientists help faculty more prepared in quantitative or mixed methods understand the authentic *meaning* of holistic nursing and caring-healing—the "compassionate we"?
- How can caring scientists help faculty to appreciate the beliefs and principles of intentional consciousness and reflective intuition in understanding the journey of Caring Inquiry Methodology?
- In what ways can faculty engaged in nursing curricula development integrate the philosophy of Caring Inquiry Methodology into Qualitative Nursing/Caring Research at all program levels?
- How can Caring Science educators, through ideas presented in this Caring Inquiry Methodology, integrate and teach aesthetic action, the holistic foundations (body, mind, spirit) of caring, including the expansiveness of life world/universal experiences, the philosophies of phenomenology and hermeneutics, and the quest for ever-deepening interpretive reflective knowledge to intuit meaning and advance understanding of the unfolding of phenomenological theory in their qualitative/caring research courses?
- What is the phenomenology of technological caring in the student–teacher learner experience or the nurse–patient teaching-learning process?

Research

*Graduates who have used the method in their research, specifically, Dr. A. Judith Czerenda and Dr. Deborah Shields, have contributed to this section.

- Given the claim that "caring is the essence of nursing" and caring–healing is a process of caring literacy, how can Caring Scientists address the value of and implement Caring Inquiry Methodology at a time when advanced quantitative methods or mixed methods using description are taking over in nursing research?
- How does one share a method that values caring and healing and spirituality to funding agencies and policy makers who value primarily quantitative statistics or big data?
- How does the nature of the "compassionate we" and the aesthetic act of the "way of compassion—as a way of life" and as method fit into traditional phenomenological and hermeneutical philosophy research approaches?
- What is reflective intuition and immanent and transcendent meaning, the spirituality named "compassion"?
- How can Caring Inquiry Methodology be used in Mixed Methods research approaches?
- How can an interpreter be used in conjunction with Caring Inquiry Methodology?
- What is the value of the use of QDAS in Caring Inquiry data analysis?
- How does Caring Inquiry Methodology relate to the Sciences of Complexity—the sciences of interconnectedness, holism, and quality?

Praxis

- What does "compassion" and the "compassionate we" mean to me?
- How can clinical and administrative practices be improved by knowledge and use of Caring Inquiry as a journey of compassion? How can the "compassionate we" be appreciated?

- Can the processes of the aesthetic caring-healing action of the Caring Inquiry Methodology be used in everyday interaction with patients, families, clinicians, administrators, and communities?
- How can praxis with a focus on critical caring ethical inquiry for individual and collective human and cultural rights and social justice in practice for nurses, patients, and families be designed and developed or improved by the knowledge and use of Caring Inquiry Methodology?
- How can Caring Inquiry be implemented in practice with, in many countries, the adoption of medically assisted death? How are conflicts reconciled?

Theory and Knowledge Development

- How is the new cosmology/vision of the universe transforming science and spiritual life?
- How is or is the new cosmology transforming nursing science?
- Is there any such thing as objective science?
- Does caring theory phenomenologically relate to theory as truth, as correspondence— what is right and just, and also pragmatic, technical, and bureaucratic (the Western view); or as disclosure, unconcealment, withdrawal, and openness—the study of meaning (the ancient Greek view), as stated by Heidegger (in van Manen, 2014, pp. 342–343)?
- Can science or even the sciences of complexity be redefined using caring, love, and healing as foundations?
- What nursing action can be taken in nursing or healthcare organizations and in research generally to recognize the value of qualitative Caring Inquiry as a legitimate and joint scientific and aesthetic method to study nursing, caring, healing, transcultural interaction, global/planetary nursing and health, dying, and death?
- Reflect upon and outline the aesthetic action and inquiry processes for the development of reflective intuitive theory (immanence and transcendence) using the Caring Inquiry Methodology as a foundation.
- What new Caring Inquiry methods can evolve after contemplating the nature of "caring as the essence of nursing" and caring and love as the essence of nursing and health?
- Could Caring Inquiry as a revealer of truth or meaning be designed as forms of quantitative methods and associated with big data?
- Is it possible to use Caring Inquiry or other caring methods to study humanoid robots from the perspective of the technological "being"?

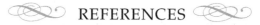 REFERENCES

Buber, M. (1965). *The knowledge of man*. New York, NY: Harper & Row.

Czerenda, A. J. (2006). *"The show must go on": A caring inquiry into the meaning of widowhood and health for older Indian widows* (Doctoral dissertation). Boca Raton: Florida Atlantic University.

Goransson, K., Ehrenberg, A., Ehnfors, M., & Fonteyn, M. (2006). The use of qualitative data analysis software (QDAS) to manage and support the analysis of think aloud (TA) data. *Studies in Health Technolgies & Informatics, 122*, 143–146.

Kandinsky, W. (1977). *Concerning the spiritual in art* (M. T. Sadler, Trans.). New York, NY: Dover.

Kidd, S. (1990). Birthing compassion. *Weavings: A journal of the Christian spiritual life, 5*(6), 18–30.

Natanson, M. (1973). *Edmund Husserl: Philosopher of infinite tasks.* Evanston, IL: Northwestern University Press.

Ray, M. A. (1981). A philosophical analysis of caring within nursing. In M. M. Leininger (Ed.), *Caring: An essential human need* (pp. 25–36). Thorofare, NJ: Charles B. Slack.

Ray, M. A. (1991). Caring inquiry: The esthetic process in the way of compassion. In D. A. Gaut & M. M. Leininger (Eds.), *Caring: The compassionate healer* (pp. 181–189). New York, NY: National League for Nursing.

Ray, M. (1997). Illuminating the meaning of caring: Unfolding the sacred art of divine love. In M. Roach (Ed.), *Caring from the heart: The convergence of caring and spirituality* (pp. 163–178). New York, NY: Paulist Press.

Ray, M. (2011). Complex caring dynamics: A unifying model of nursing inquiry. In A. Davidson, M. Ray, & M. Turkel (Eds.), *Nursing, caring and complexity science: For human-environment well-being* (pp. 31–52). New York, NY: Springer Publishing.

Ray, M. (2013). Caring inquiry: The esthetic process in the way of compassion. In M. C. Smith, M. C. Turkel, & Z. R. Wolf (Eds.), *Caring in nursing classics: An essential resource* (pp. 339–345). New York, NY: Springer Publishing.

Reeder, F. (1984). Philosophical issues in the Rogerian science of unitary human beings. *Advances in Nursing Science, 6*(2), 14–23. doi:10.1097/00012272-198401000-00005

Reeder, F. (1988). Hermeneutics. In B. Sarter (Ed.), *Paths to knowledge* (pp. 193–238). New York, NY: National League for Nursing.

Seidel, J. (1988). *The ethnograph.* Littleton, CO: Qualis Research Associates.

Shields, D. (2007). *The meaning of the lived experience of receiving therapeutic touch in people with heart failure* (Doctoral dissertation). Cincinnati, OH: The Union Institute & University.

Stapleton, I. J. (1983). *Husserl and Heidegger: The question of a phenomenological beginning.* Albany: State University of New York Press.

Steiner, G. (1989). *Real presence.* London, UK: Faber and Faber.

Stone, J. (1990). *In the country of hearts.* New York, NY: Delacorte Press.

van Manen, M. (1990). *Researching lived experience: Human science for an action sensitive pedagogy.* London, ON, Canada: Althouse Press.

van Manen, M. (2014). *Phenomenology of practice: Meaning-giving methods in phenomenological research and writing.* Walnut Creek, CA: Left Coast Press.

van Manen, M. (2016). *Researching lived experience: Human science for an action sensitive pedagogy* (2nd ed.). New York, NY: Routledge. (Original work published 1997.).

25

Holding Sacred Space for Loving-Kindness and Equanimity for Self/Others

Joseph Giovannoni

CARITAS LITERACIES

By the end of this chapter, the caring-healing nurse will be able to

1. Define the meaning of "holding sacred space" as it relates to the practice of nursing.

2. Apply the ontology of a unified mind into praxis of human caring.

3. Explain how we can transcend from ego consciousness to unitary consciousness.

4. Explain the process of dissolving the ego-divided consciousness toward experiencing a unified consciousness.

5. Explain how embodying the 10 Caritas Processes® promotes human caring and a healing environment.

❧

Holding sacred space is being in the moment, still, silent, and connected with Source, our deepest sense of knowing. All of humanity is connected to Source, a consciousness that is holographic, pandimensional and nonlocal, and universal, and expresses infinite Love (Watson, 2008). Space, time, matter, and consciousness are created by a universe that is alive and predisposed toward love and compassion.

Watson reminds us that our work as nurses has a sacred dimension because "We dwell in mystery and the infinity of cosmic Love as the source and depth of all life" (Watson, 2008, p. 9). Nurses hold sacred space when they look deeply into another without judgment to dissolve all barriers.

Holding space for blissful silence is the first step in rising above the ego, a separate sense of self, and connecting with Source, the light of unitary Consciousness. Centering in silence with heart-centered breathing (HeartMath.com) unites us with our deepest sense of know-ing that we are interconnected with everything and dissolves all barriers between the self and others. In silence, we can observe and discern our own internal processes and actions in relation to others with compassion and without judgment. This self-care practice con-nects us to the wisdom of universal consciousness and understanding that all of humanity belongs to infinite Source that unites us for healing to emerge. The nurse who holds sacred space to be and become an extension of unitary Consciousness sustains compassion for all of humanity. Intentionally holding space for loving-kindness, peace, and understanding brings us closer to experiencing caring moments with others.

BACKGROUND

I was born and raised in the historical walled city of Lucca, Italy, near Florence, where I felt enriched by my exposure to the aesthetic works of the masters of the Renaissance period. The human body has evolved into a magnificent work of art as depicted in masterpieces such as Michelangelo's *David*, da Vinci's beautiful *Mona Lisa*, and Botticelli's *The Birth of Venus*. Humans have been enamored with the physical body as witnessed in the advertise-ments of a multibillion-dollar cosmetic industry, cosmetic surgeries, diet remedies, and bodybuilding with sacred stories such as the creation of Adam and Eve. This reflects our collective ego's attempt to understand and maintain a sense of control and purpose in life. For the most part, people define their identity through their physical body, the ego person-ality, and, therefore, experience consciousness as a separate self. Humankind has tried to understand the source of consciousness through philosophy, religion, and science; overall many people remain perplexed as to what to believe is the source of their being. We must have faith that we are connected to a higher Source of consciousness and hold sacred space to listen and trust that guidance will unfold for us all in perfect time and order.

Over the past 5 years, my focus has been to understand the ego's mode of operation. I am not attacking this aspect of my own humanity. My intention is to understand the ego, dissolve its irrational fears, distorted perception of separation, and its judgment of self and others. This requires the courage to revisit my own wounds and grievances toward those who have hurt me. I had to be willing to cross the dark bridge of separateness by placing my faith and trust in the wisdom of other scholars, philosophers, mystics, quantum physicists, human caring theorists, and seekers of unity of mind. On this path, I have become more aware of my own verbiage of separateness, thoughts of fear, judgment, and anger. Forgiveness became a daily ritual to dissolve the bombardment of these thoughts as they surface. To dissolve the ego, I knew I had to practice compassion toward this aspect of the split mind by holding sacred space to forgive the thoughts and core beliefs that divide me from others seeing the futility of the core beliefs that kept me in the dark. I placed faith in the unknown, Source, and trusted that compassion and forgiveness for myself and others acquiesced the ego moment by moment.

HOLDING SACRED SPACE FOR UNITARY CONSCIOUSNESS

Consciousness does not reside in the brain or the body (Dossey, 1991; van Lommel, 2010; Watson, 2008). Science has *not* been able to prove that consciousness and memory are ware-housed in the brain. Scholars of phenomenology have questioned whether consciousness is endless, preexisting before the body, and will continue after death. The ego self relies on the input from a five-sensory system that perceives consciousness as a separate individual entity operated by the brain, and is terminal with death (Zukav, 2014). Science has attempted to localize consciousness in the brain; however, no scientific proof has been able to verify the source of consciousness. What is known is that the ascending reticular activating system, the brainstem, the thalamus, and the hippocampus connect with copious groups of neurons in the frontal lobes of the brain to enable the experience of consciousness (Edelman & Tononi, 2000; van Lommel, 2010). Pure consciousness is whole and extends beyond the physical body and can distinguish between objective and subjective experiences.

One's darkest thoughts and emotions originate in the belief of separation. This is exemplified in thoughts such as "I am right, you are wrong"; "I am better, you are worse"; or "I am worse, you are better." This form of consciousness depicts the ego at war with itself. It is self-destructive and contributes to stress and human suffering. We need to hold space for Source, to illuminate our consciousness, to uncover our deepest illusions of separation so that we can forgive these illusions that contribute to conflict and poor relations with others. Forgiveness to dissolve the ego illuminates the mysteries of life and eases our journey to being more peaceful, rather than feeling despair and fighting for external control. Metaphorically, sitting and having tea, and a dialogue with our ego, while forgiving the futility of its tenacious belief in separateness, organically brings unitary consciousness to fruition and grants us the opportunity to experience the authentic internal power of healing.

HOLDING SACRED SPACE FOR COMPASSION TO DISSOLVE THE EGO

The ego self provides a limited consciousness that is dependent on the input of our five senses and constructs our five-sensory personality (Zukav, 2014). The ego creates the illusion of self as separate, and it often sees the self as a victim of others. Relying solely on the input of five senses—taste, touch, smell, sight, and hearing—to define the world restricts us from experiencing a pandimensional, holographic consciousness that connects with the wisdom of the universe. We are a projection of divine consciousness that is shadowed in darkness by the ego's identity with the body and its survival. Being grounded in our body and relying solely on our five senses to inform our consciousness limits our view of the world. We are vulnerable to experiencing a divided worldview that focuses on fear, greed, conflict, and the multiplicity of human struggles. Living and relying on the ego perception is a barrier to rediscovering our divine consciousness that is holographic, pandimensional, and interconnected with universal Source. The repeated practice of holding sacred space to connect with universal Source opens our hearts to extend loving-kindness for self and others and dissolves the ego. It elevates us to a multisensory consciousness of unity, compassion, wisdom, understanding, and boundless love. We are universal beings interconnected with the universal inspiration of Love.

Human beings are a projection of divine consciousness that is shadowed in darkness by the ego's identity with the physical body and its survival. Being grounded in body and relying solely on the five senses to inform consciousness limits our view of the world/universe. Believing that consciousness is encased in the skull makes us vulnerable to experiencing a divided self, a worldview that focuses on fear, greed, conflict, and the multiplicity of human struggles. The ego perception of separateness always creates problems that stem from a perceived lack of love. Living and relying on the ego perception is a barrier to rediscovering divine consciousness that is holographic. It is only our acceptance of the truth that we, as individuals, are the extension of the presence of a unified mind of Love that will facilitate discovering our pandimensional consciousness that interconnects with the universe. This consciousness frees the perception of any need at all, and so it is embracing the unity of mind and love that heals all problems of separation. Living in a pandimensional world does not deprive us of anything that the body needs on this journey on earth. The repeated practices of holding sacred space to connect with this universal Source opens the heart to envision humanity as interconnected; we are one, and as we extend loving-kindness to others, we also extend it to ourselves. Contemplating the unity of mind elevates us to a consciousness filled with compassion, wisdom, and understanding where boundless love flourishes. We are universal beings interconnected through the universal inspiration of Love.

Understanding the Evolution of a Separate Self

Our early ancestors depended on their instincts to inform their ego, the five-sensory personality for strength and survival. They were conditioned to fight with or flee from any perceived threat. Over the millennia, the human body has evolved to reflect our expanded capacity for thought and invention. Simply put, we need less brute strength than we did then. Yet this does not seem to be the case when we turn on the news and witness cruelty, violence, and human despair. Despite our advanced humanity and knowledge, we still desire to know the meaning of our existence. We need to acknowledge that we still carry a vestige of our ancestors' survival skills that are embedded in our ego self. The ego uses the five senses to program the brain to respond to its environment with a primary purpose to preserve the body and maintain external power. To survive, it must be constantly vigilant for threats.

We are projections of divine consciousness and are born innocent, and enter the physical realm from the spirit world. We are influenced by our environment and those who are responsible for nurturing and protecting us. We are informed by social, cultural values and beliefs, and adapt to our environment, often focusing on survival and self-gratification. The ego's physical realm is rooted in the brain's ventral tegmental area (VTA) and the limbic system, which includes the hippocampus, the hypothalamus, and the amygdala or the emotional center. These physical structures and associated neural pathways filter the input delivered by our five senses from outside the body and evoke neural signals of information to our cerebral cortex. Collectively we can think of the limbic system as the center for emotional responsiveness, motivation, memory formation and integration, olfaction, and the mechanisms to keep ourselves safe. The limbic system controls fear, anger, and the survival of the body. This is the root of all personal ego agendas that divide one from another. These brain structures respond to danger or trauma by triggering a fight-or-flight response. The VTA and medial forebrain also serve as our pleasure circuit. We are hardwired to catch a pleasure buzz by the release of dopamine (Linden, 2011). The VTA is triggered by the intake of food and psychoactive drugs such as opiates and nicotine, and can cause habituation or addictions. These structures and their associated neural circuitry store memories in the cortex. Memories of pleasure, pain, and addictions are closely intermingled.

From the spirit world, we carry a divine innate intuition and the desires for connection with others to love and be loved. This can be overshadowed by the ego's personal agendas and love is often extended with conditions. Divine consciousness is authentic, unconditional, forgiving, and compassionate. Rumi, the 13th-century Persian mystic and poet, addresses the struggle of the ego and reminds us of the source of our being, stating, "Although you appear in earthly form your essence is pure Consciousness. You are the fearless guardian of Divine Light. So, come and return to the root of the root of your own soul" (www.brainyquote .com/quotes/authors/r/rumi.html). With compassion toward self, our ego will dissolve and we will return to the seat of our soul (Hawkins, 2012; Zukav, 2014), the divine light of the Universe.

Mindful practices quiet the brain and override the impulsive reactivity of the VTA and medial-lateral forebrain (Siegel, 2011). Holding sacred space for mindful practices brings us in alignment with Source and empowers a deeper aspect of ourselves. Mindfulness opens our consciousness for compassion and facilitates impulse control over our pleasure center in the brain that could evolve in a problem of impulsive immediate gratification. Pleasure is a human experience that should be celebrated as long as it is not at the expense of exploiting, manipulating, and coercing another, and does not harm self/other.

The ego's informed perception of self as separate creates barriers that interfere with authentic selfless interpersonal relationships. It builds core beliefs that divide us from one another rather than uniting us. We need to be gentle with our self and avoid identifying with the collective ego that holds the belief of a separate self that dehumanizes others. The collective ego consciousness of separation is often witnessed in religious ideology and politics. A divided self temporarily escapes discomfort and suffering by seeking immediate relief from pain, and desires immediate gratification, a dopamine fix from the pleasure center and an adrenalin rush. This makes the body, whose consciousness focuses on being a divided self, vulnerable to addictive behaviors. The ego consciousness of duality and separation creates a feeling of powerlessness and the need to seek external control over others. This can be observed in systems where those in authority need to control others rather than creating a forum for collective sharing of wisdom toward creative solutions.

In my 40 years of experience as a forensic practitioner, I believe the desire for external control and power is at the core of domestic violence, sexual assault, and criminal behavior. It is the metaphor of the elephant in the room that creates division and prevents us from understanding a problem that needs cocreative solutions. It is the ego's denial that we are deeply connected with each other and the universe that creates a pandemic of violence. The ego feeling powerless makes us void of empathy toward self and others. A fundamental reason for humanity's struggle with warfare first occurs within our brain and then externally is projected by being at war with others. It leads to the rationalization and excuses to justify devaluing and attacking others. It prevents us from seeing the similarities that unite humanity in love and compassion. All religions' central theme seems Cosmic. However, the division created by the collective ego that tells us that we are separate from one another rather than being united with the consciousness of Love creates dogmatic beliefs that we are separate from one another and perpetuates division. This is often observed with righteous fundamentalist religions. It has divided and created discord between Christians and Muslims as well as political factions. Our ego consciousness is threatened by the ontological belief that we are multidimensional divine beings living multidimensional lives that are interconnected with others and the universal Source of Love. The ego is in love with itself as it related to the body and enjoys the optical illusion that we are separate, different, better than, and perhaps stronger or weaker than others.

Philosophy, religion, metaphysics, epistemology, political ideology, and the sciences grounded in numerical evidence have attempted to provide humanity with knowledge, the meaning of our existence, an understanding of human nature, and how to protect the survival of humanity. Humanity's primary struggles are the worship of the ego-divided self. Numerical data will never prove the existence of Universal Love. There is no yardstick that can measure Love; it is infinite. Love is absence of the belief in sin. The ego has turned to imaginary idols for answers to the calamities that humanity faced in history, distorting the message from powerful authentic icons such as Jesus, Buddha, Muhammad, and Gandhi who understood the multidimensional consciousness of Love.

The choice to hold sacred space to connect with the Source of Love opens our hearts and minds for creative solutions, solutions to inner and outer conflict that we experience in life. Conflict does not start outside the self but rather from within and is then projected outward. The repeated mindful practices that facilitate blissful silence, holding space for self-forgiveness and self-compassion, release the grasp of the fearful ego's need for external power. Through compassion and forgiveness, we hold space for divine Light to help us make a connection with all of humanity. Through our ability to hold sacred space, we will stop fighting over ideologies and work together to cocreate solutions that advance humanity to a higher consciousness that expresses universal Love. We will stop exploiting the Earth. We will nurture each other to return to the light of our Divine nature. Our Divine nature is well expressed by St. Paul in his definition of Love.

> Love is patient, love is kind. It does not envy, it does not boast, it is not proud. It does not dishonor others, it is not self-seeking, it is not easily angered, it keeps no record of wrongs. Love does not delight in evil but rejoices with the truth. It always protects, always trusts, always hopes, always perseveres. (Corinthians 13:4-7)

The desire to know and understand the meaning and purpose of our life is shrouded by the dynamics of our and the collective ego consciousness with which we identify. The ego experiences dissonance to the ontology that as a living human being we are interconnected with everything in the universe. As we continue to see ourselves as separate from one another, we remain vulnerable to experiencing conflict with self and others, and neglect creation as sacred and interconnected.

A New Paradigm of Science

Caring Science Theory predicates the view that humanity resides in a unitary or undivided field of consciousness (Levinas, 1969/2000; Levinas, Poller, & Cohen, 2003; Watson, 2008). The vision that we are interconnected with everything in the universe facilitates our intention to be present, and heart centered to hold loving space to observe our inner and outer world, discerning for wisdom about human nature. Seeing our interconnectedness enables the capacity to extend loving-kindness and compassion to self/others and caring moments. Unitary caring science professionals hold sacred every encounter as they touch the face, hand, and heart of those who are in their care (Watson, 2005).

Caring Science-Sacred Science (Watson, 2005) is a new paradigm of science and ethics that informs compassionate healthcare and praxis of nursing to preserve compassion, caring, and human dignity of self and others in a healthcare system, which is becoming progressively mechanical and impersonal. As a patient who has undergone several medical procedures, I have experienced nurses and other health science specialists performing their tasks with proficiency yet void of loving-kindness. I felt as if I was another body, a number to be tested, to be probed on a medicalized conveyer belt system whose bottom line seemed to be focused on moving patients on an assembly line of/for profit. I was not acknowledged as a person with thoughts and feelings concerning the procedures that I was undergoing. Many competent advanced practice nurses empowered with prescriptive authority and independent practice seem to have become medicalized and focus on external control to fix the body. They have come to neglect the importance of humility, and to stop and be present with those who are suffering. We need to return to the sacred practice of nursing by incorporating and honoring the perceptions and subjective meaning the patients have given to their illness. Nurses need to remember "the body has the power at some intrinsic level to heal itself" (Watson, 2008, p 65). Holding this sacred consciousness can intrinsically empower advanced practice nurses to more effectively use their scientific skills to facilitate health and healing.

The financial stability of an organization can be enhanced when its administration and employees take responsibility to create space: a caring-healing environment for self and the patients they serve in the system they sustain. Holding sacred space begins with loving-kindness toward self and practicing self-care (Watson, 2008). Caring Science informs us that the heart is much more than a pump (Rosch, 2015) and that the powerful practice of heart-centered breathing can lower stress and create positive relationships. The human heart extends an electromagnetic field of energy that radiates outward. Our emotions affect our physiology and the heart's magnetic field. We must hold sacred space to be heart centered and heart focused, take a deep breath, and repattern our presence to be the energetic healing field when we connect with someone who is in pain.

A fast-paced technological, medical system that provides sacred space for its employees to take a break for self-care helps to lower their stress. A stressful healthcare environment creates emotionally indifferent, detached caregivers who radiate negative emotional energy. This can have a negative impact on the patients being cared for. When I conduct forensic evaluation and lead cognitive behavioral groups, I engage in micropractices such as pausing, breathing into my heart, and visualizing that behind the mask of an angry, disgruntled patient there remains an unchanged loving energy that is being denied by his or her ego self. Self-care, being heart-centered with loving-kindness and compassion toward self, is essential before we can extend this compassion and loving-kindness to others (Giovannoni, 2017; Watson, 2008). Being still for a moment and focusing on the breath before entering a patient's room or performing a procedure facilitates a sense of well-being and equanimity, and a caring field for the health science professional to be more focused to deliver a procedure with authentic caring. Aesthetic posters with high-energy statements placed on the walls facilitate a healing environment and remind both patients and caregivers to open sacred space to be heart centered, promoting caring and healing. Mindful microcaring science practices such as conscious, intentional breathing into our heart and saying, "breathe in love" and breathing out, "releasing fear," facilitates sacred space for inner peace and equanimity, and radiates loving-kindness (see Figure 25.1). With this consciousness, the nurse becomes the healing environment.

HOLDING SACRED SPACE FOR THE ESSENCE OF MIND

Connecting with Source, a higher consciousness that is holographic, pandimensional and nonlocal,   universal, and infinite Love, requires practicing loving-kindness for self and others (Watson, 2008). We must hold faith that we can advance to a multisensory consciousness of unity, compassion, wisdom, understanding, and boundless love. We must hold sacred space to be mindful of our connection with one another and everything in creation. Then our life journey will tell a story of dignity, equanimity, joy, compassion,

BREATHE IN LOVE
BREATHE OUT FEAR

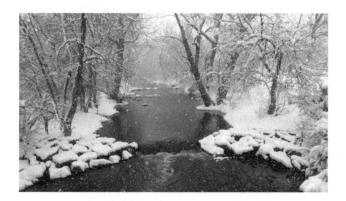

Love Prevails Over Fear
BE HEART CENTERED
BE HEART FOCUSED
BE HEART FEELING
Practice loving kindness to self/others.

Dr. Giovannoni DNP, APRN, Postdoctoral student WCSI

Watson Caring
Science Institute

FIGURE 25.1 Breathe in love.

inner peace, and respect for others and the Earth. Source will reveal the wisdom, the grand design of the universe.

Caring Science theory as conceived by nursing theorist Dr. Jean Watson is founded in the Unitary theory of the French Philosopher Levinas (Levinas, 1969/2000). Watson states, "We dwell in mystery and the infinity of cosmic Love as the source and depth of all life" (Watson, 2008, p. 9). The essence of mind is universal Source, Cosmic Love. Universal Mind views all living things as "connected on vibrational energy levels" (Hawkins, 2012). The brain is not our mind. The neurons in our brain and its sophisticated neural pathways operate the functions of the systems of the body. It imprints diverse core beliefs that are learned from life experiences that most often reflect a perception of separateness. The universal Mind extends cosmic Love that unites humanity. The mind is not separated by biology, ideology, religion, dogma, or cultural beliefs.

Comprehending and merging with the mind of cosmic Love requires enabling, sustaining, and honoring faith, hope, and a deep belief in our inner subjective connection with Source (Watson, 2008). This begins with quieting our brain from the chatter of our thoughts that focus on separateness. Being heart centered with loving-kindness and focusing on our breath clears our consciousness of negative thoughts, negative emotions, and judgments, and is the entrance to a multisensory awareness. As human beings, we are not just a mortal physical body but also universal energy that is interconnected with everything. The desire to become connected with cosmic Love facilitates the inner subjective experience of oneness with Source and embodies the consciousness of compassion. The ego no longer reigns over our existence by focusing on the material world and separation. Our consciousness focal point becomes an "intrinsic wellspring of loving-kindness, caring and friendliness" (Watson, 2008, p. 58).

Oneness can be experienced only when we are still, and quiet the inner chatter of our thoughts. To experience a united consciousness, we must attend to our perceptions, the thoughts and emotions that are filtered by our five senses as our brain wonders without reacting to anything. When our brain chatter is noiseless of fearful, angry thoughts of separation, compassion and forgiveness of self and others emerge and we will embrace our human diversity. Nurses who hold space with the intention to look deeply into the other without judgment begin to dissolve all barriers. They understand that they hold the life energy of their patients in their hands and authentically care for them (Watson, 2008).

In blissful silence with self-compassion, we can begin to observe and understand our own inner experiences and become enlightened by the vision that we are interconnected. We stop focusing on the problem and our differences. Holding scared space for loving-kindness, peace, and understanding creates an energetic field for creative solutions that benefit all of humanity. It is a state of being and becoming the universal mind of Love as we sustain others in maintaining their emotional, physical, mental, and spiritual well-being.

The practice of mindful silence and introspection opens our awareness of our connection with Source; then our body integrates the five senses with a multisensory consciousness (Zukav, 2014). This awareness has helped me age with dignity, and facilitates inner peace, equanimity, and joy as I continue my work with a challenging population. In my career, I have seen many individuals die in fear and despair. Holding sacred space for compassion for the ego and forgiving its illusions of separateness has helped me peacefully contemplate my own finiteness as a physical being.

At 72 years of age and 50 years of nursing practice, my journey has revealed that making peace with my own ego-divided self requires holding space for self-compassion as I recognize those thoughts that descend upon my sense of self into darkness, fear, anger, and judgment. Gracefully dissolving the ego requires a process of observing and discerning these thoughts, associated core beliefs, and their origin, and letting them go (Giovannoni, 2015, 2016, 2017).

We need to set sacred space to recognize the ego's illusions that prevent us from being in good relations with self and others. We need to practice loving-kindness and self-compassion by forgiving and letting go of our grievances toward others. Forgiveness is a healthy practice (Watson, 2008) because authentic love holds no grievances. Self-compassion is a healthier way to treat our self (Giovannoni, 2017) as we move from ego toward unitary Consciousness. To connect with universal Source, we must have faith that "we come from the spirit world and return to the spirit source" (Watson, 2008, p. 9). To connect with Source, the universal infinite field of Love requires holding space to practice loving-kindness to self and others (Watson, 2008) and the silent practices of mindfulness, meditation, and prayer.

HOLDING SACRED SPACE FOR SELF-CARE

As a forensic nurse, I work with a challenging population. My patients are referred by the judicial system and rarely seek help voluntarily. An angry, hostile, life-energy depleting demeanor is not uncommon. A new patient's mood can radiate a disturbing frequency that can set a stage for a "biocidic interaction" (Halldorsdottir, 1991; Watson, 2008). I need to be conscious not to react. Biocidic interactions can trigger relationships that decrease the well-being of the helper and the person being helped. Holding sacred space for loving-kindness toward self to repattern the field is essential to maintain equanimity. I need to be clear about my intention, not to react, and be mindful to ask for guidance from Source to gain the strength to make a connection with the patient so that I can be of service to him or her. Where there is darkness and potential biocidic interactions, it is important that I authentically role-model human caring and compassion while setting limits, while listening to my patient express his or her negative emotionality.

The breath is one of the most important self-care techniques. Consciously breathing helps hold sacred space in the moment. The breath is a life force that increases energy, promotes wellness, and facilitates relaxation (Angelo, 2012). Being mindful of our breath in difficult encounters, and with full awareness or in conjunction with compassionate statements, can be helpful. The mindful practice of consciously centering on the heart, breathing in loving-kindness for self, and breathing out and releasing fear and angry thoughts has positive physiological effects (Homma & Masaoka, 2008; Roozendaal, McEwen, & Chattarji, 2009). Consciously taking rhythmic breaths and focusing on our heart can facilitate our ability to achieve a high state of heart rate variability coherence (HRVC; Edwards, 2015). Intentionally raising our HRVC promotes positive emotions and we can set a sacred space to facilitate unity with others with whom we are communicating (Morris, 2010). Focusing on positive emotions helps manage stress in toxic situations we may encounter with patients and colleagues.

A healthcare agency that holds space, a self-care room for moments of rest and revitalization, reduces employees' stress in the work setting. There are significant benefits in creating and holding such sacred space. Self-care is important for healthcare providers before they begin to take care of others, and for job satisfaction (Hozak, Nelson & Gregory, 2016). The outcome of self-care interventions leads to more compassionate care. I have visited a hospital in Cashel, Ireland that provides such a space. The staff of St. Patrick Hospital has a special room for solitude, and a quiet space for meditation (see Figure 25.2). A self-care room can have a massage chair, aromatherapy, pleasant mindful music for quiet time, and mindfulness meditation for the staff to set sacred space. Encouraging the practice of self-care should be considered as a strategy to enhance outcomes such as improved interpersonal communication, stress reduction, and job satisfaction. In a busy hospital or clinic, holding sacred space can be as simple as the microcosmic practice of taking 3 minutes for handwashing between patients while being mindful of heart-centered breathing, for example, breathing in "I am calm" and breathing out "I am smiling." When I practice this in a group or between individual sessions, I feel my facial muscles relaxing into a gentle smile. The walls of my clinic are absorbed with mindful, caring science posters I created (www.josephgiovannoni.com).

AN EXAMPLE OF HOLDING SCARED SPACE FOR A PATIENT

Some interactions with patients can be toxic, and energy depleting. I work with challenging patients who have sexually assaulted children and adults, and present other mental health comorbidities. Mr. Dark came for a sex offense–specific evaluation. He sexually abused his 12-year-old stepdaughter for 3 years. Mr. Dark was angry and blamed his attorney claiming that his attorney had failed him by suggesting that he plead no contest to avoid a long prison sentence. Mr. Dark blamed the legal system for the unjust treatment he received presentence. He did not take any responsibility for abusing his stepdaughter. He blamed his wife for not supporting him and his stepdaughter for being seductive and making up stories that were not true. Mr. Dark resented seeing me and having to subject himself for an evaluation. He viewed himself as the victim. Mr. Dark's anger could have triggered my ego to respond to his negative, abrasive demeanor by allowing my own limbic system to be triggered. My own ego perception wanted to throw Mr. Dark out of the office and send him back to his probation officer. I reminded myself to hold sacred space, and sit with him to observe and

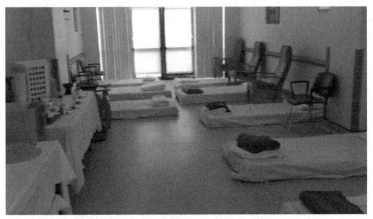

FIGURE 25.2 St. Patrick Hospital self-care room.

discern without judgment the drama that unfolded before me. I reminded myself that at some deeper level our humanity was interconnected. I focused on my breath and being heart centered. Before proceeding with the risk assessment, which requires asking personal questions, I took a deep breath and asked Source for guidance. I consciously reminded myself that every healing/helping relationship serves not only the patient but the therapist as well. This was an opportunity for me to cultivate loving-kindness to self by maintaining equanimity. I did not allow my ego to stray into making judgments. While breathing in love and breathing out the tension in my body, I told Mr. Dark that my philosophy was to help him find his true self. I encouraged him to be open to minister to himself by being honest and we could cocreate a helping relationship that would benefit him to understand his thinking, beliefs, and circumstances that contributed to his predicament. I told Mr. Dark that I would do everything in my power to help him heal himself and his family. I encouraged him to open his heart to see the truth of the darkness of the human ego that feels powerless and needs external power. As the interview progressed, Mr. Dark's ego that engaged in the seeing himself as the victim began to dissolve. Mr. Dark became less defensive and together we explored the thoughts, feelings, and salient events that led him to target his victim for his self-centered need for immediate gratification.

HOLDING A SACRED SPACE IN MY PROFESSIONAL WORK

For the past 35 years as a forensic advanced practice nurse, I have attempted to rehabilitate patients who are adjudicated sex offenders, drug abusers, and domestic violence abusers. My work is guided by the legal system and evidence-based research on sex offender's recidivism (Marshall & Laws, 2003). Concern for others has been identified in sex offender risk assessment as an important need to be attended to in treatment (Hanson & Harris, 2000). The work is largely an interprofessional collaboration that requires joint commitment and mutual trust, because rehabilitation requires patients to waive their confidentiality to ensure community safety. The professionals working jointly with me are Society's Safe-Keepers® (SSKs; Giovannoni, 2015). They believe in justice and human dignity, and promote faith, hope, and peace for our society. They believe that protecting society from tyranny requires a philosophy of caring and respect for all of humanity. They are role models of human caring and compassion. I have experienced colleagues whose intention is not to collaborate or cocreate but rather to enhance personal ego agendas and focus on the problem rather than on the solution. It is important as we work with others to intentionally hold space to create and become the healing environment; to affirm and value the diversity of the team to become aware of and relinquish personal ego agendas, differences that distract the team from collaborating and maintaining a healing environment with professionals who are biogenic, life giving, and life receiving (Watson, 2008). Members of any interprofessional team need to relinquish personal ego agendas. We need to be courageous to acknowledge and address our own personal wounds and long-held beliefs that separate us from others with self-compassion and self-forgiveness. It is important to protect victims from further victimization and empower them and not keep them stuck in biocidic anger at their perpetrators.

Engaging in reflective practices is setting space for self-care by helping us become more consciously aware of how our work affects us personally. In my work, I realized that I was heading for burnout. Caring Science, being mindful, and patiently engaging in the repeated practice of the 10 Caritas Processes (Watson, 2008), helped me "to see" and understand more deeply the nature of violence (see Table 25.1).

For example, Caritas Process #5, Allowing for the expression of positive and negative emotions and authentically listening to another's story, creates a space for my patients to become more transparent and self-disclosing of their struggles. Furthermore, it facilitates an authentic helping and trusting relationship (Caritas Process #4). Shifting my focus from a punitive posture to one of practicing a more conscious loving-kindness generates space for my patients to see the errors of their thinking and develop concern for others. Through role-modeling caring in practice, I can bring the light of caring to others who dwell in darkness, are violent, and lack concern for others.

Unity of the mind, the relationship between compassion, love, and restorative justice, needs to be understood and embraced. Chaos in society cannot be corrected by force but rather by a life-giving philosophy that unites humanity. Compassionate universalism bridges separation and reminds us to shift from a perception of duality, separation, and ego-centeredness to a vision of oneness (Giovannoni, 2016). Before being introduced to Watson's theory and integrating it into my forensic practice, I became exhausted and I was heading for burnout. I did not have a good relationship with myself or my colleagues. Embodying the Watson's caring theory helped me to be present with challenging patients within my practice. I trained as a Caritas Coach at the Watson Caring Science Institute in 2013. A Caritas Coach transforms self and systems by intentionally holding sacred space to integrate and restore caring, healing, and love into one's life, work, and the world. A Caritas Coach promotes a deeper meaning, purpose, dignity, and wholeness in other healthcare

TABLE 25.1 Watson's 10 Caritas Processes

Practice of Loving-Kindness With Self/Others

Enabling Faith and Hope, Being Present Authentically

Sensitivity to Self-Others, Ongoing Spiritual Development

Developing Authentic, Trusting-Caring Relationships

Allowing Expression of Positive-Negative Feelings: Listening to Another's Story

Creative Problem-Solving, Solution Seeking

Relational Teaching and Coaching

Creating Healing Environments/Becoming the Caritas Field

Assist With Basic Needs-Sacred Acts

Open to Existential-Spiritual Unknowns: Allow for Mystery and Miracles

providers, patients, institutions, and society. A Caritas Coach is interested in facilitating caring and healing environments and promoting helping and trusting relationships. It begins by self-discovery through self-reflection, and self-compassion. A Caritas Coach practices self-care and makes a sacred covenant to alleviate the suffering of humanity, understanding that "love is the highest level of consciousness and the greatest source of all healing in the world" (Watson, 2008, p. 22). Love is universal energy that interconnects all of humanity. Being a Caritas Coach requires embodying this mind-set, an expanded consciousness that views all of creation as sacred and interconnected. I am reminded that "in transpersonal caring and healing, we will need to sustain the existence of a community of healers which is committed to the domain of art, beauty, and soul care to accompany and transform the usual ways of doing medicine" (Watson, 2010, p. 199).

HOLDING SACRED SPACE FOR PERSONAL HEALTH

In the healthcare field, it is essential that we work closely with colleagues to identify creative solutions to improve the health and quality of life for self and others. This requires becoming aware and letting go of acrimonious personal ego agendas, holding space to quiet the mind, and with each in-breath forgiving and on the out-breath extending compassion. Forgiveness does not imply that we do not hold accountable those who inflict pain and suffering on others. I am clear that it is an act of caring to contain someone who is eminently capable of hurting others. However, we must align ourselves with creative solutions to the problem of violence. To be effective a penal justice system needs to focus on rehabilitation. Professionals such as correctional officers, in addition to being trained in containing "prisoners," need training in human caring literacy.

I have conceived the term Society's Safe-Keepers (SSKs) for these individuals who make up this interdisciplinary team. The strength of an SSK is to uphold compassionate human dignity while implementing best practices (Giovannoni, McCoy, Mays, & Watson, 2015). SSKs need to be positive role models for those who have behaved recklessly and uncaring. They are professionals who dedicate themselves to protecting society. They are not administrators of punishment. They believe in justice and human dignity, and promote faith, hope, and peace for our society. They are responsible for correcting individuals who have violated the human rights of others. This process of being and becoming an SSK requires holding sacred space to develop a unitary consciousness guided by compassion and love.

COMPASSION, LOVING-KINDNESS, HUMAN CARING SHOULD NOT BE USED AS "BUZZ" WORDS

In the healthcare system, we must be cautious not to use love, compassion, and human caring as "buzz words" to promote personal or corporate ego's agendas. I have seen these concepts being used by healthcare agencies, in universities' schools of nursing advertisements and mission statements, yet their actual implementation and outcome is not being embodied or measured as promoted. Human caring in nursing is not just about doing or practicing advanced skills efficiently and safely. Authentic human caring requires holding sacred space to being and becoming the energetic healing field. Therefore, I am proposing that nurses, health science professionals, and institutions be clear about their intention when they are using the words such as "caring," "compassion," and "love." Health science professionals need to authentically cultivate the practice of loving-kindness and equanimity toward self and extending it to others, patients and colleagues (Watson, 2008). Through self-care and the repeated practice and embodiment of the 10 Caritas Processes, as health science professionals, when conflict arises, we can be authentic, compassionate, and loving. It is unfortunate that often personal ego agendas create biostatic and biocidic environments. We all want to be seen and heard, and our opinion valued by our colleagues and those in leadership positions. We must ask ourselves, "What is it that I am holding onto that I need to let go to be at peace, and be in good relations with self and others?" Having good relations with others is important to cocreate solutions that benefit the whole. To let go, we must be willing to take a grueling and dangerous descend into our personal and collective shadow with which we identify. We need to acknowledge our personal ego agendas, and fears, so that we can bring the light of an understanding of how the human ego separates us from another. We can do this when we pause and set sacred space to be more present, trust our intelligent heart, and practice heart-centered breathing (HeartMath.org) so that we can elevate our consciousness for compassion for self and others to work together to develop creative solutions.

The 10 Caritas Processes give language and are guidance for practicing human caring. Practicing and embodying them assist us in developing, becoming, and being the energetic field that sets sacred space to return to the mind of love.

Love is rarely used in a healthcare setting, especially in my field. Some argue and say, "What has love got to do with scientific best practices in a healthcare system?" Watson (2008) reminds us that love is the highest level of consciousness and healing. Watson intentionally uses the Latin word, Caritas, meaning love and charity to invoke an explicit "connection between caring and love, Love in its fullest universal infinite sense" (Watson, 2008, pp. 39–40). Personal ego agendas must be relinquished before we can hold sacred space to embody caring and love in our work. The medical system focuses primarily on fixing parts of the mechanical body that are broken or become diseased. Holding space for mind, body, and spirit (the capacity of humanity to express universal love) keeps us interconnected and not separate. Embodying *Caritas* heals the mind of our misperception of separateness and connects us with the universal energy of Love. It means being present, to discern, cherish, appreciate, and give special, loving attention to everything that is being presented to us without placing any judgment. We can extend loving-kindness as we hold people accountable for the choices they make and help them identify and correct those core beliefs that manifest in behavior that causes pain and suffering. Health science professionals, advanced practice nurses, and auxiliary personnel who embody loving-kindness and the 10 Caritas Processes enhance the capacity for supporting the medical model to cure the body and support healing the mind toward unity of spirit.

CONCLUSION

Holding sacred space to connect and to evolve a higher consciousness that is unitary and pandimensional, and expresses boundless love requires the willingness to acknowledge our own darkest thoughts and beliefs that separate us from others. It is a continuous practice of being mindful with silence to practice self-forgiveness and self-compassion to dissolve the illusion of the ego-separate self. When we practice the 10 Caritas Processes, we embody Caritas and create a healing environment that facilitates a patient's collaboration with his or her treatment plan. We can let go of personal ego agenda and comingle and cocreate with colleagues in developing and implementing best practices with authentic human caring, dignity, and compassion.

The practice of human caring by embodying Caritas can be applied to any profession or human endeavor to improve relationships and promote collaboration, and for creative solutions to humanity's problems.

NEXT ERA POSSIBILITIES

Education

- How can I integrate the practice of holding sacred space in my clinical practice, and with colleagues?
- In what ways can I provide nursing education related to holding sacred space to colleagues and others to facilitate the practice of loving-kindness to self?
- How can I provide education on holding sacred space to registered nurses in the practice setting to enlighten their practice?

Research

- How can I use Caring Science research to address the mindful practice of holding scared space in relation to positive outcomes for practitioners and patients?
- What qualitative research study can I design to understand the lived experience of holding sacred space?
- How will I use research findings related to holding sacred space to advance Unitary Caring Science?

Praxis

- Which dimension of practice can I improve right now with a greater understanding of the mindful practices of holding sacred space?
- How can I embody *Caritas* to correct my misperception of separateness and connect with the universal energy of Love for equanimity and lower my job-related stress?

Theory and Knowledge Development

- How can the mindful practices of holding sacred space enhance my ability to dissolve personal ego agendas and support my vision of a unified mind?
- How can I advance creating sacred space as a middle-range nursing theory?
- How can the concept of holding sacred space advance nursing disciplinary-specific knowledge?

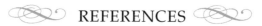 REFERENCES

Angelo, J. (2012). *Self-healing with breathwork*. Rochester, VT: Healing Heart Press.

Dossey, L. (1991). *Meaning and medicine*. New York, NY: Bantam Books.

Edelman, G., & Tononi, G. (2000). *A Universe of consciousness*. New York, NY: Basic Books/Perseus Books.

Edwards, S. D. (2015). Heartmath: A positive psychology paradigm for promoting psychophysiological and global coherence. *Journal of Psychology in Africa*, 25(4), 367–374. doi:10.1080/14330237.2015.1078104

Giovannoni, J. (2015). Probation officers reduce their stress by cultivating the practice of loving-kindness with self and others. *International Journal of Caring Sciences, 8*(2), 325–343.

Giovannoni, J. (2016). Egoless & interconnected: Suspending judgment to embrace heart-centered health care. In W. Rosa (Ed.), *Nurses as leaders: Evolutionary visions of leadership* (pp. 265–278). New York, NY: Springer Publishing.

Giovannoni, J. (2017). Perspectives: Compassion for others begins with loving-kindness toward self. *Journal of Research in Nursing, 22*(1-2), 173–178. doi:10.1177/1744987116685635

Giovannoni, J., McCoy, K., Mays, M., & Watson, J. (2015). Probation officers reduce their stress by cultivating the practice of loving-kindness with self and others. *International Journal of Caring Sciences, 8*(2), 325–343.

Halldorsdottir, S. (1991). Five basic models of being with another. In D. A. Gaut & M. M. Leininger (Eds.), *Caring: The compassionate healer.* New York, NY: National League for Nursing.

Hanson, R. K., & Harris, A. J. (2000). Where should we intervene? Dynamic predictors of sexual offense recidivism. *Criminal Justice and Behavior, 27*(1), 6–35. doi:10.1177/0093854800027001002

Hawkins, D. (2012). *Letting go: The pathway of surrender.* New York, NY: Hay House.

Homma, I., & Masaoka, Y. (2008). Breathing rhythms and emotions. *Experimental Physiology, 93*(9), 1011–1021. doi:10.1113/expphysiol.2008.042424

Hozak, M. A., Nelson, J., & Gregory, D. (2016). Relationship of hospital architecture to nursing staff caring for self, caring for patients, and job satisfaction. *Interdisciplinary Journal of Partnership Studies, 3*(1). doi:10.24926/ijps.v3i1.121

Levinas, E. (2000). *Totality and infinity.* Pittsburg, PA: Duquesne University. (Original work published 1969)

Levinas, E., Poller, N., & Cohen, R. A. (2003). *Humanism of the other.* Chicago: University of Illinois Press.

Linden, D. J. (2011). *The compass of pleasure.* New York, NY: Viking Penguin Group.

Marshall, W. L., & Laws, D. R. (2003). A brief history of behavioral and cognitive behavioral approaches to sexual offender treatment: Part 2. The modern era. *Sex Abuse, 15*(2), 93–120. doi:10.1177/107906320301500202

Morris, S. (2010). Achieving collective coherence: Group effects on heart rate variability coherence and heart rhythm synchronization. *Alternative Therapies in Health and Medicine, 16*(4), 62–72.

Roozendaal, B., McEwen, B. S., & Chattarji, S. (2009). Stress, memory and the amygdala. *Nature Reviews Neuroscience, 10*, 423–433. doi:10.1038/nrn2651

Rosch, P. (2015). Why the heart is much more than a pump. In M. Dahlitz & G. Hall (Eds.), *Issues of the Heart: The Neuropsychotherapist special issue* (pp. 1–13). Brisbane, Queensland: Dahlitz Media.

Siegel, D. (2011). *Mindsight. The new science of personal transformation.* New York, NY: Bantam Books.

van Lommel, P. (2010). *Consciousness beyond life.* New York, NY: Harper Collins.

Watson, J. (2005). *Caring science as sacred science.* New York, NY: F. A. Davis.

Watson, J. (2008). *Nursing: The philosophy and science of caring.* Boulder: University Press of Colorado.

Watson, J. (2010). *Postmodern nursing.* Boulder, CO: Watson Caring Science Institute.

Zukav, G. (2014). *The seat of the soul* (25th anniversary ed.). New York, NY: Simon & Schuster.

26

Mutual Vulnerability: Creating Healing Environments That Nurture Wholeness and Well-Being

Beth M. King and Charlotte D. Barry

CARITAS LITERACIES

By the end of this chapter, the caring-healing nurse will be able to

1. Discuss the concept of mutual vulnerability for the nurse and the one/ones nursed.

2. Discuss the concept of mutual vulnerability as an integral component of a healing environment.

3. Write a nursing situation grounded in Caring Science and informed by the concepts of healing environment, wholeness, and well-being.

The concept of "vulnerability" has many definitions but as we discuss healing environments in this chapter, the authors invite you to reflect on Daniel's (1998) definition of vulnerability. He stated, "Rather than a state to avoid, vulnerability is a trait to enjoy; for through it, humans celebrate the authenticity of what it is to be human" (p. 191).

The purpose of this chapter is to describe vulnerability as a concept in which both nurse and patient/client/community are mutually vulnerable, not at risk for a problem that needs fixing, but with the "... promise of knowing each other as whole filled with potential" (Parker, Barry, & King, 2015, p. 437). Many nursing scholars have written about the mutuality of the nurse and one nursed in relationship. Nightingale (1859/2007) described this relationship as the reparative process, the patient, the nurse, and the environment unfolding together toward the alleviation of suffering. Later, Paterson and Zderad (1988) described nursing as the intersubjective transaction in which the nurse's "thereness" or presence nurtured the well-being or more being of persons in the "between" (p. 7). Within the between, "both the nurse and the one nursed share a moment of authenticity that moves toward both the potential for well-being and more being" (p. 14). Paterson and Zderad's existential writings in nursing have inspired many of the theories grounded in the science of care/caring Leininger (1981), Leininger and McFarland (2010), Wehbe-Alamah (2015), Ray (1989), Ray and Turkel (2015), Watson (1979/1985, 2015), Boykin and Schoenhofer (2001, 2015), Parker et al. (2015), Sumner (2012), Duffy (2013, 2015), and Locsin (2005, 2015). Each of these theories emphasizes caring in relationship between the nurse and the one nursed.

REVIEW OF THE LITERATURE

HEALING ENVIRONMENTS

Jonas, Chez, Smith, and Sakallaris (2014) have defined optimal healing environments as "a system and place comprised of people, behaviors, educational activities and interventions, and their psychological and physical parameters" (p. 83) with salutogenesis as foundational to the environment. Although this definition includes the construct of healing relationships, others have identified the core tenet of a healing environment as the "intentional caring relationship between a caregiver and the patient and his or her family" (Felgen, 2004, p. 29). The basic tenet of Felgen's model of Relationship-Based Care is the therapeutic relationship, with all systems within healthcare supporting the therapeutic relationship between the nurse and the patient. Felgen believed that "while the physical environment promotes healing, it is the spirit and consciousness of the people providing care that are most crucial" (p. 43).

A scoping review and analysis of the caring moment in a relationship identified preconditions for a caring moment to include: "mutually vulnerable as unique humans in the moment … the closeness and intimacy shared between and within nurses and patients … have consequences and implications for both" (Wolf, King, & France, 2015, p. 18). The caring moment was described by Watson as "transpersonal, each feels a connection with the other at the spirit level … opening up possibilities for healing and human connection" (p. 11). In contrast, Sumner (2008) described the bidirectional communication of a caring moment "that enables the nurse to acknowledge that he or she has her own needs that require meeting as well as the patient needs" (p. 12).

A model that has described a way of being in a caring relationship is the "Dance of Caring Person" (Boykin, Schoenhofer, & Valentine, 2014). The core tenets of this model are, "all persons have the capacity to care by virtue of their humanness; commitment to respect for persons …; and recognition that each participant … has a unique and valuable contribution to make to the whole …" (p. 28). This way of "being in relationship" transforms the traditional healthcare hierarchal way of communicating to one of mutual relationship, which supports a healing environment.

Mutual Vulnerability

Being vulnerable is to be human according to Daniel (1998; Sellman, 2005). Vulnerability is not a state one chooses; all of us are vulnerable, both the nurse and the patient. By recognizing this state of mutual vulnerability, the nurse–patient relationship is based on authenticity and mutual understanding.

Sumner's (2004) work provides a grounding framework for understanding the concept of mutual vulnerability between the nurse and the patient. Using critical social theory and Habermas's theory of moral consciousness, Sumner interviewed 10 practicing nurses to aid in understanding, "What is caring in nursing and is it an impossible ideal?" (p. 39). She described the construct of a nurse in terms of personal self and professional self. The findings identified the characteristics of nurse as personal self as: having a sense of altruism, a sense of power, and a need for self-awareness, and to be honest with oneself. In contrast, the professional self was described as a combination of the "theoretical, experiential, and practice knowledge with the personal self, that leads to the sense of the 'responsibility to care' …" (p. 41). One nurse stated, "If my vulnerability is interfering with what's best for the patient then that is probably something that I would need to address" (p. 40). Sumner postulated that the vulnerability of the nurse may lead to "minimal effort and robot like mechanical action… feeling threatened or frightened … which can promote a defensive response when feeling vulnerable" (p. 42). The analysis indicated that the nurse experts have "needs too" (p. 43) and their personal sense of self needs to be replenished to satisfy their need to "feel good in the role of the nurse otherwise he/she is left unfilled" (p. 43).

Angel and Vatne (2016) lends further understanding of the concept of mutual vulnerability and the nurse's hopes and dreams for caring. They related the nurse's vulnerability to sharing the suffering of the person's difficulties and feelings of shame when wanting to do more for the person, feelings of powerlessness by a patient's unpredictability, and mental harm when feeling less confident and anxious. The mutual relationship between the nurse and the person cared for can lead to a sense of vulnerability and the desire to be "the persons they both want to be" (p. 1435).

A qualitative study by Thorup, Rundqvist, Roberts, and Delmar (2012) explored the ethical formation of 23 nurses through the analysis of their own sense of vulnerability. Findings indicated that both vulnerability and suffering, along with courage, influenced the nurses' ethical development over time. Vulnerability was seen as either a blind spot or a sore point; sore points are facilitated by life experiences and self-reflection and can impact ability to provide care when they turn into blind spots. In contrast, having courage was related to the courage needed to confront the person's vulnerability, to witness the other's suffering, and to trust in oneself.

Another qualitative study by Heaslip and Board (2012) provides further understanding of the vulnerability of nursing staff. They conducted focus groups with nursing staff caring for patients on a unit for persons with dementia. The findings indicated that the staff felt vulnerable with the unpredictability of the dementia process and at times felt threatened by the unpredictability of the clients. In addition, the staff grieved when patients would die and experienced a sense of their own vulnerability of mortality. The issue of professional boundaries initiated both a sense of vulnerability and dissonance of whether to become close to patients or to be distant. The authors concluded that authenticity contributes to both personal and work satisfaction and each nurse must be responsible for his or her own actions.

Another study of nurses by Malone (2000) discussed the life and death situations of the emergency room and the sense of vulnerability for both nurse and patient. This phenomenological study analyzed 40 taped interviews with emergency room clinicians and found that nurses coped with their vulnerability by "distancing themselves … walling off …" and attributing death to destiny (p. 7). In addition, the degree of witnessing the suffering of those cared for impacted the nurses' sense of vulnerability. The suffering nurses witnessed brought forth the vulnerability of both the nurse and the person suffering. Malone concluded that the recognition of mutual vulnerability of both the nurse and the one cared for "preserves on a societal level the value of caring for others" (p. 10).

Sarvimäki, Stenbock-Hult, Sundell, and Oesch-Börman (2017) brought to light the view of vulnerability as a resource, an opportunity for one to experience "openness, sensitivity and closeness to ones feelings" (p. 113). Their secondary analyses of focus groups with four family caregivers were compared with vulnerability identified by nurses. The core theme of being human, that caregiving was "part of life" (p. 114) and "having feelings," was identified by nurses as a component of mutual vulnerability. Both the caregivers and the nurses identified courage by admitting one's limitations and speaking up for the other. Protecting oneself was identified in the caregiver group as a way to dissociate from the experience. Two themes were identified by only the family caregivers: the burden of duty and the feeling of shame that was not identified by nurses as part of vulnerability. They concluded that living authentically may expose a person to pain and suffering, yet openness and courage allowed the nurse to be vulnerable and to care for others with a sense of responsibility and freedom of choice. Mutual vulnerability is an integral component of a caring relationship. Understanding the vulnerability of both the nurse and the one nursed offers the possibility to create healing environments grounded in respect and trust and filled with promise and hope.

THEORETICAL PERSPECTIVE

The caring-based, community nursing practice model (CNPM) developed by Parker and Barry (1999, 2010) and extended by Parker, Barry, and King (2015) guides the understanding of caring in nursing, the concept of mutual vulnerability and healing environments. The CNPM, depicted in Figure 26.1, is based on the caring constructs and values of nursing as nurturing the wholeness of others in caring, respect for persons, and community as a safe place in which members experience shared values, inclusion, and a feeling of being honored. In this model, nursing occurs in nursing situations, which are described as the shared lived experience of caring between the nurse and the one nursed that nurtures wholeness and well-being. The amorphous water color of the model (Figure 26.1) depicts the creative interconnections of the nurses and the one nursed in the core and with others in a widening circle of concern and support for well-being of persons and communities. Using caring constructs and values of respect, inclusion, and collaboration, healing environments emerge through mutual respect, collaborative relationships, and relationships built on respect, trust, and love.

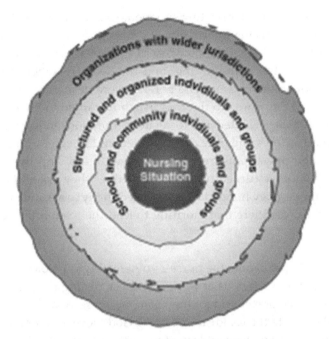

FIGURE 26.1 The community nursing practice model. Concentric circles of empathetic concern.

MUTUAL VULNERABILITY ILLUMINATED IN NURSING SITUATIONS

Nursing situations are stories from practice described as the shared lived experience of caring between the nurse and the one nursed that nurtures wholeness and well-being of both in caring (Barry, Gordon, & King, 2015). The following nursing situations illuminate the existential, mutual, vulnerable relationship between the nurse and one nursed and the healing environments that evolved.

NURSING SITUATIONS AND REFLECTIONS

The Kaddish Prayer of Mourning (Leah Serio)

In the following nursing situation, the nurse's and the family's vulnerability is opened wide to fill with the possibility of hope, solace, and godliness.

> I generally shy away from anything religious at work; however, one night I was called to prayer and I responded. At 5:00 a.m. one morning I was called to work to care for a young man who had been stabbed multiple times in the abdomen, had gone to surgery, and was back in recovery. Intubated and unresponsive, this 17-year-old began to hemorrhage profusely. As fast as I could I pumped blood into him; it flowed out. The surgeon did not leave the room and we worked side by side trying to find the source of the bleeding. We were literally up to our forearms, trying to suction the blood out. But nothing we did helped. We asked the parents to come in to be with their son,

knowing they would enter a devastating situation. As soon as they entered the young man coded and we were trying to save him.

The parents asked us to do all we could until a Rabbi arrived to say the mourner's Kaddish, a prayer for the ailing, dying, and the dead. A Rabbi was called but I knew he would not arrive in time. The parents were desperate for a prayer book; they didn't know all the words to the Kaddish, but wanted to recite it before their son died. I asked if they wanted me to recite it; they looked surprised, relieved, and devastated all at the same time. They agreed and I began to recite it and they joined in. After the prayer was over they allowed us to stop the code. He died within minutes. Once we turned off all the machines they asked the surgeon and me to stay with them. They hugged us both, cried in my arms, and said how grateful they were that I was there that morning to lead their son and them in praying the Kaddish.

Reflection: In this nursing situation, the nurse's vulnerability is palpable; she states that she "shies away from anything religious at work." And yet, feeling the parents' vulnerability, pain, and hope to have the prayer said for their son, she offers to say the prayer and together with the parents they recite the Kaddish imploring God's love and compassion for the boy. This nursing situation illuminates a tableau of mutual vulnerability, the parents, the nurse, and the doctor united in caring for the boy, a son, and the one nursed. Sometimes a response to another's vulnerability begins with reluctance.

Lily and Authentic Presence (Susan Driscoll)

It was 3 o'clock in the afternoon; I entered a clinic exam room. I was exhausted. The patient was distraught. We both quickly assessed and understood the nursing situation at hand, but we kept it locked in the corners, failing to appreciate it within the pattern of the nurse and one nursed relationship that unfolded.

My mind was reeling, bogged down in the stress of the day, work, and family. The clinic had opened at 8:00 a.m. and I had not stopped all day; no lunch and I don't think I even went to the bathroom either. I had just come back to work after maternity leave; I had a 6-month-old and a 2-and-a-half-year-old at day-care; I was working with very little sleep.

The client, I will call Lily, sat fully clothed on the exam table, rocking back and forth holding her abdomen. She looked pale and scared. She described heavy vaginal bleeding over the past week. She said she never had this before and I knew she was not pregnant. She added, "I think the bleeding and pain are less. And I don't have any money, a job, or insurance. I can't afford the ER, is there anything you can do?"

I did a quick observation and thought: She's not that pale; she's having this conversation with me; she can't be in that much pain. Again she said, "What should I do?" I thought that if I examined her, I would have to charge her for a visit, and she said no exam. I told her she should really go to the ER. She said she was scared of the ER and couldn't afford it. I told her that they had to treat her regardless of her ability to pay. She promised me that if the pain and bleeding continued that she would go to the ER.

I made a quick note and did not charge her. And I left the exam room, although I was never really there for her in the first place, and I am not sure Lily was either.

Reflection: Habermas (1995) states that all humans require considerateness of their being, of their vulnerability. Roach's (2001) discussion of commitment can help one understand this nursing situation. Roach defines commitment as "a complex affective response characterized by a convergence between one's desires and one's obligations, and by a deliberate choice with them" (2001, p. 62). This nursing situation causes us to stop and think, and it draws us into understanding that each of us expresses caring uniquely. This nurse expressed caring of Lily by her competent assessment of pallor and togetherness within the context of sociopolitical knowing and also in her courage and humility to share this story.

The following nursing situation, written by an undergraduate nursing student, provides an understanding of the vulnerability of nursing students and the ones they nurse.

The Glasses (Yasmin Heringer, BSN)

My peers and I gathered together for report for the first time on a psychiatric unit. The charge nurse looked at each of us and said, "Be careful with Ms. B, she is very unstable!" As I walked onto the unit, wouldn't you know it—Ms. B yelled out, "YOU!" There she was, Ms. B, pointing her finger at me. I froze in my boots. Scared, I asked, "Me"? She said, "Yes. I just wanted to say I like your glasses."

As I looked at my reflection in the mirror, I felt guilty. How could I be scared of someone I didn't even know; someone I didn't even give a chance to speak to me? She must be afraid; they said she hears voices. If it were me, how would I feel if I heard voices and could not control them? The next time we had clinical, I introduced myself to her and we talked for a long time. I listened to her and how much she was suffering. As I turned my back and walked towards the nurses' station, tears rolled down my face. I could not imagine going through my day while voices were saying evil things, confusing myself about who I really was!

Reflection: The vulnerability of both the student nurse and the one nursed is illuminated in this story. At first, the student withdrew and distanced herself from the situation; however, on reflection, the student began to understand the idea of mutual vulnerability. The caring attribute of courage was evident in the one nursed, to live with voices that only she heard, and the courage of the student to recognize her fears. Mayeroff (1971) states that courage is "informed by insight from past experiences" (p. 34); thus, in this nursing situation, the nurse's courage was guided by her insight on her actions and thoughts. Boykin and Schoenhofer (2001) refer to courage as essential ingredients to live and grow in caring. The student nurse was transformed as she codeveloped a healing environment for her patient and for herself.

The following nursing situation offers a different format. The nursing situation created by a new graduate nurse is described within the context of multiple patterns of knowing and concludes with a Haiku, as an aesthetic representation of the caring between the nurse and the one nursed.

The Caring Moment (Jonathan George)

In my nursing situation, I was able to answer a call for nursing to care for my patient Jack when I saw the look on his face. I used Carper's (1978) ways of knowing to guide my nursing situation. I personally knew the facial expression Jack was wearing in that moment was a facial expression that I would wear if I had something on my mind. In my life, when I have something on my mind, I usually am in one of two positions: I either do not want to discuss the matter with anyone, or I am yearning for someone to simply listen to me. Seeing that facial expression on Jack helped guide my response in that moment to listen to his concerns for growing old.

I used Carper's (1978) ethical way of knowing in understanding my duty to nurture the wholeness of my patient and enhance his well-being to the best of my ability. I empirically understood that a patient who feels cared for has better health outcomes. This was a moment where I could develop trust with Jack. My intention was to care for him by listening. I used Munhall's (1993) unknowing to guide my caring moment with Jack by being open to hear things he had to say, and reflect with him as he reviewed portions of his life with me. I used White's (1995) sociopolitical way of knowing to guide my knowing the context of Jack's life. I had the opportunity to cocreate a healing situation with Jack that would be significant to him and his healing process. This knowing made me value my time with Jack all the more.

I aesthetically knew my nursing situation by understanding the dance of caring needed between Jack and me in that specific moment. As Jack spoke, I knew I had to "dance" with him; I did not want to overpower him, but work with him, bob-and-weave with him to keep the momentum going. The end result of "our dance of caring" was a precious moment that nurtured both Jack and me.

The intensity and simplicity conveyed by haiku poetry also echoed my feelings of caring simply and meaningfully by being authentically present to listen to Jack. And in return I took part in an intense, impactful moment. Since haiku poetry is based on a syllable count, they are short poems, light on words, and heavy in meaning. This reflected my experience in that I was part of a caring moment that did not involve many words, but still had so much meaning for both Jack and me.

Moments
Unmistakable,
Shining, hiding, inviting,
Are caring moments.

Reflection: This nursing situation offers a unique understanding of vulnerability. The nurse's personal knowing of a certain look inspired his response of being there to listen to Jack in a shared moment of mutual vulnerability. Levinas (1961/1996) describes that facial expressions can convey a moral appeal for care. This is further described for health professionals by Gjengedal et al. (2013) as the development of a "clinical eye" (p. 132) that sees beyond the illness and apprehends the whole person. John goes on to further describe his caring moment with Jack. He stated, "I felt rejuvenated after writing the poem; my reflections helped me understand the significance of my response to the man's call to care, and this inspires me to continue to embrace caring moments as I practice."

CONCLUSION

This chapter presented an examination of the concept of vulnerability in nursing through a specific lens of Caring Science explicated in the CNPM. This value-based model inspires and guides nurses in nurturing the wholeness and well-being of self and others in caring. Within this model, persons are understood as whole in the moment and filled with the promise of possibilities unfolding in the nurse–patient relationship.

The review of the literature offered a broad perspective of the concept of mutual vulnerability as an integral component of a caring relationship, nurse and one nursed, as participants in the creation of healing environments grounded in respect, caring, and trust and filled with promise and hope. The nursing situations illuminated and affirmed four specific lived experiences of mutual vulnerability and transformed the review of the literature into real-life nursing practice.

In the nursing situation *The Kaddish*, we read of the nurse's reservation to participate in spiritual matters of her patients. And then we witness the nurse's grace under pressure and metamorphosis to join the family in prayer, and present an exquisite tableau of shared vulnerability.

Lily, the nursing situation that unfolded in a clinic, offers another real-life exemplar of mutual vulnerability: the nurse exhausted on her first day back to work after maternity leave and the one nursed fearful of her pain and bleeding and yet more fearful of not having health insurance. Sometimes for the nurse, competence in skill is the highest expression of caring; and for the one nursed, expressing that she will seek care at an emergency room if the pain and bleeding do not subside.

The Glasses nursing situation invites us into a student nurse's experience of learning the essence of caring for a patient who hears voices, and her understanding of the mutuality of caring relationships in nursing. The student's reflection on her impulse to leave the woman inspired her courage to go back and stay. In doing so, she learned that they were alike: both were afraid, both had courage, and both shared vulnerability.

The *Moment* nursing situation created by a new graduate inspires hope for the advancement of Caring Science. Jack's facial expression offers a clarion call for nursing and acknowledging personal knowing and mutual vulnerability; the nurse responds by offering to listen. The nurse explains that the caring moment created by listening to Jack's concerns was short in words but long in meaning, like a Haiku.

In summary, this chapter presented the concept of vulnerability as a human relational phenomenon and as the basis of caring nurse–patient relationships. The four nursing situations brought the concept to life in the shared lived experience of caring between the nurse and the one nursed and affirmed Daniel's (1998) definition of vulnerability: "Rather than a state to avoid, vulnerability is a trait to enjoy; for through it, humans celebrate the authenticity of what it is to be human" (p. 191). The understanding of mutual vulnerability inspires anew the commitment to create meaning in the lives of nurses and the ones nursed in environments of caring and healing.

NEXT ERA POSSIBILITIES

Research

- What research methodologies can we use to analyze nursing situations and the mutual vulnerability between the nurse and the one nursed?
- What scholarly journals are appropriate for the dissemination of our findings?

Education

- How can we integrate teaching/learning nursing situations into our courses?
- What other pedagogies can we use to teach Caring Science and the essence of caring nurse–patient relationships as we acknowledge the mutual vulnerability of teacher and student?

Praxis

- How would our nursing practice and healing environments change with an enhanced understanding of mutual vulnerability?
- What nursing situations can we reflect on that express mutual vulnerability of the nurse and the one nursed?

Theory and Knowledge Development

- How useful is the CNPM for our nursing practice?
- In what ways can we advance Caring Science through theory-guided practice?

 REFERENCES

Angel, S., & Vatne, S. (2016). Vulnerability in patients and nurses and the mutual vulnerability in the patient–nurse relationship. *Journal of Clinical Nursing, 26,* 1428–1437. doi:10.1111/jocn.13583

Barry, C. D., Gordon, S. C., & King, B. M. (2015). *Nursing case studies in caring: Across the practice spectrum.* New York, NY: Springer Publishing.

Boykin, A., & Schoenhofer, S. O. (2001). *Theory of nursing as caring: A model for transforming practice.* New York, NY: National League for Nursing Press.

Boykin, A., & Schoenhofer, S. O. (2015). Theory of nursing as caring. In M. C. Smith & M. E. Parker (Eds.), *Nursing theories and nursing practice* (4th ed., pp. 341–356). Philadelphia, PA: F. A. Davis.

Boykin, A., Schoenhofer, S., & Valentine, K. (2014). *Health care system transformation for nursing and health care leaders.* New York, NY: Springer Publishing.

Carper, B. A. (1978). Fundamental patterns of knowing in nursing. *Advances in Nursing Science, 1,* 13–23. doi:10.1097/00012272-197810000-00004

Daniel, L. E. (1998). Vulnerability as a key to authenticity. *Image–the Journal of Nursing Scholarship, 30*(2), 191–192. doi:10.1111/j.1547-5069.1998.tb01279.x

Duffy, J. R. (2013). *Quality caring in nursing: Applying theory to clinical practice, education, and leadership.* New York, NY: Springer Publishing.

Duffy, J. R. (2015). Joanne Duffy's quality caring model. In M. C. Smith & M. E. Parker (Eds.), *Nursing theories and nursing practice* (4th ed., pp. 393–409). Philadelphia, PA: F. A. Davis.

Felgen, J. (2004). A caring and healing environment. *Nursing Administration Quarterly, 28*(4), 288–301. doi:10.1097/00006216-200410000-00012

Gjengedal, E., Ekra, E. M., Hol, H., Kjelsvik, M., Lykkeslet, E., Michaelsen, R., … Wogn-Henriksen, K. (2013). Vulnerability in health care: Reflections on encounters in every day practice. *Nursing Philosophy, 14*(2), 127–138. doi:10.1111/j.1466-769X.2012.00558.x

Habermas J. (1995). Reconciliation through the public use of reason: Remarks on John Rawl's political liberalism. *Journal of Philosophy, 92*(3), 109–131. doi:10.5840/jphil199592335

Heaslip, V., & Board, M. (2012). Does nurses' vulnerability affect their ability to care? *British Journal of Nursing, 21*(5), 912–916. doi:10.12968/bjon.2012.21.15.912

Jonas, W. B., Chez, R. A., Smith, K., & Sakallaris, B. (2014). Salutogenesis: The defining concept for a new health care system. *Global Advances in Health and Medicine, 3*(3), 82–91. doi:10.7453/gahmj.2014.005

Leininger, M. M. (1981). *Caring: An essential human need*. Thorofare, NJ: Slack.

Leininger, M. M., & McFarland, M. R. (2010). Madeleine Leininger's theory of culture care diversity and universality. In M. E. Parker & M. C. Smith (Eds.), *Nursing theories and nursing practice* (3rd. ed., pp. 449–460). Philadelphia, PA: F. A. Davis.

Levinas, E. (1996). *Totalitet og uendelighed: Et essay om exterioriteten* [Totality and infinity. An essay on extoriority] (M. Crone, Trans.). Copenhagen, Denmark: Hans Reitzels Forlag. (Original work published 1961)

Locsin, R. C. (2005). *Technological competency as caring in nursing: A model for practice*. Indianapolis, IN: Sigma Theta Tau International.

Locsin, R. C. (2015). Rozzano Locsin's technological competency as caring in nursing. In M. C. Smith & M. E. Parker (Eds.), *Nursing theories and nursing practice* (4th ed., pp. 449–460). Philadelphia, PA: F. A. Davis.

Malone, R. E. (2000). Dimensions of vulnerability in emergency nurses' narratives. *Advances in Nursing Science, 23*(1), 1–11. doi:10.1097/00012272-200009000-00005

Mayeroff, M. (1971). *On caring*. New York, NY: HarperCollins.

Munhall, P. L. (1993). 'Unknowing': Toward another pattern of knowing in nursing. *Nursing Outlook, 41*(3), 125–128.

Nightingale, F. (2007). *Notes on nursing*. New York, NY: Barnes & Noble. (Original work published 1859)

Parker, M. E., & Barry, C. D. (1999). Community practice guided by a nursing model. *Nursing Science Quarterly, 12*(2), 125–131. doi:10.1177/089431849901200211

Parker, M. E., & Barry, C. D. (2010). The community nursing practice model. In M. E. Parker & M. C. Smith (Eds.), *Nursing theories and nursing practice* (3rd ed., pp. 451–459). Philadelphia, PA: F. A. Davis.

Parker, M. E., Barry, C. D., & King, B. M. (2015). The community nursing practice model. In M. C. Smith & M. E. Parker (Eds.), *Nursing theories and nursing practice* (4th ed., pp. 435–447). Philadelphia, PA: F. A. Davis.

Paterson, J. G., & Zderad, L. T. (1988). *Humanistic nursing*. New York, NY: National League for Nursing Press.

Ray, M. A. (1989). The theory of bureaucratic caring for nursing practice in the organizational culture. *Nursing Administration Quarterly, 13*(2), 31–42. doi:10.1097/00006216-198901320-00007

Ray, M. A., & Turkel, M. C. (2015). Marilyn Anne Ray's theory of bureaucratic caring. In M. C. Smith & M. E. Parker (Eds.), *Nursing theories and nursing practice* (4th ed., pp. 461–482). Philadelphia, PA: F. A. Davis.

Roach, M. S. (2001). *Caring, the human mode of being: A blueprint for the health professions* (2nd ed.). Ottawa, ON, Canada: Canadian Hospital Association Press.

Sarvimäki, A., Stenbock-Hult, B., Sundell, E., & Oesch-Börman, C. (2017). The vulnerability of family caregivers in relation to vulnerability as understood by nurses. *Scandinavian Journal of Caring Sciences, 31*, 112–119. doi:10.1111/scs.12325

Sellman, D. (2005). Towards an understanding of nursing as a response to human vulnerability. *Nursing Philosophy, 6*, 2–10. doi:10.1111/j.1466-769X.2004.00202.x

Sumner, J. (2004). The nurse in the caring in nurse relationship: A critical social theory perspective. *International Journal for Human Caring, 8*(1), 37–45.

Sumner, J. F. (2008). *The moral construct of caring in nursing as communicative action: A theory for nursing practice*. Saarbrücken, Germany: VDM Verlag Dr. Müller Aktiengesellschaft.

Sumner, J. F. (2012). Communication as moral caring in nursing: The moral construct of caring in nursing as communicative action. *International Journal for Human Caring, 16*(2), 20–27.

Thorup, C. B., Rundqvist, E., Roberts, C., & Delmar, C. (2012). Care as a matter of courage: Vulnerability, suffering and ethical formation in nursing care. *Scandinavian Journal of Caring Sciences, 26*(3), 427–435. doi:10.1111/j.1471-6712.2011.00944.x

Watson, J. (1985). *Nursing: The philosophy and science of caring.* Boulder: University Press of Colorado. (Original work published 1979)

Watson, J. (2015). Jean Watson's theory of human caring. In M. C. Smith & M. E. Parker (Eds.), *Nursing theories and nursing practice* (4th ed., pp. 321–339). Philadelphia, PA: F. A. Davis.

Wehbe-Alamah, H. (2015). Madeleine Leininger's theory of culture care diversity and universality. In M. C. Smith & M. E. Parker (Eds.), *Nursing theories and nursing practice* (4th ed., pp. 303–319). Philadelphia, PA: F. A. Davis.

White, J. (1995). Patterns of knowing: Review, critique and update. *Advances in Nursing Science, 17*(4), 73–86. doi:10.1097/00012272-199506000-00007

Wolf, Z. R., King, B. M., & France, N. E. M. (2015). Antecedent context and structure of communication during a caring moment: Scoping review and analysis. *International Journal for Human Caring, 19*(2), 7–20. doi:10.20467/1091-5710-19.2.7

27

Integrating Caring Science and Caritas Into Professional Practice

Linda Ryan

CARITAS LITERACIES

By the end of this chapter, the caring-healing nurse will be able to

1. Describe the ethical, professional calling to create caring-healing environments.

2. Explain the psychological, physiological, and financial benefits of creating caring-healing environments.

3. Apply methods and strategies to enhance the role of the Caring Science/Caritas practitioner within the healthcare system.

4. Develop methods and strategies to enrich the domain of practitioners so as to facilitate Caring Science and Caritas integration.

5. Identify caring-healing modalities as activities of the Caritas practitioner.

6. Discuss benefits of integrating Caring Science/Caritas into professional practice related to patient satisfaction, patient outcomes, and nurse satisfaction.

❧

"… nature heals the wound … And what nursing has to do … is to put the patient in the best condition for nature to act upon him."—Nightingale, *Notes on Nursing*, 1859/2007

From the time that Florence Nightingale founded the profession of nursing, nurses have been called to create environments in which natural healing can occur. Caring has been identified as a foundational component in creating such healing environments

(Watson, 2008; Watson, 2009). The American Nurses Association (2010) purports that it is a vital function of nurses to create healing environments by establishing and maintaining caring relationships with those they serve. The International Council of Nurses (2012) espouses that nurses have an ethical obligation not to participate in any activities that undermine caring and healing; thus, they have a responsibility to not contribute to uncaring environments. Caring is essential to nursing as well as all healthcare professionals, because caring potentiates health and well-being (Watson, 2008; Watson, 2009).

Caring is associated with psychological as well as physiological healing. Psychologically, caring practitioner–patient relationships can enhance a person's perception of self-efficacy and fulfill his or her need for social affiliation (Zender & Olshansky, 2012). Physiologically, caring interactions can calm activated autonomic nervous systems, thus mitigating the negative consequences of stress responses that often accompany healthcare encounters (Zender & Olshansky, 2012).

Positive, caring relationships can also have economic benefits for healthcare providers. As part of its value-based purchasing program, Medicare links financial reimbursement to results of the Hospital Consumer Assessment of Healthcare Providers and Systems (HCAHPS) surveys that evaluate patient perception of care on various topics, including provider communication, respectfulness, and responsiveness (Centers for Medicare & Medicaid Services, 2017; Mason, 2015). Hospitals can gain or lose up to 2% of reimbursement dollars based, in part, on their survey scores; better HCAHPS scores protect reimbursement, whereas lower scores place reimbursement at risk (Goodman, 2015; Letourneau, 2016). Because HCAHPS scores are publicly reported, consumers are able to compare hospital scores on these measures. Informed consumers may use these comparisons to influence their decisions regarding which provider they will select for their healthcare needs. Hospitals with better scores may be selected more frequently for healthcare services than those with lower scores, resulting in higher revenues for the selected hospitals.

Despite the ethical covenant that calls for practitioners to create caring-healing environments with those they serve, despite the fact that caring potentiates psychological and physiological well-being, and despite the financial incentives for establishing caring-healing environments, healthcare worldwide is still challenged to maintain such environments (Beck, 2015; Haslam, 2015; Martinsen, 2011; Meehan, 2012; Naburi et al., 2016; Shan et al., 2016). Because of heightened focus on the ethical responsibility of professional healthcare providers to proactively create caring-healing environments, and because of the increased awareness of the benefits of caring-healing environments, both informal and formal innovative healthcare leaders are advocating for the intentional integration of Caring Science and Caritas into professional practice. These leaders realize that caring cannot be assumed. Caring needs to have dedicated attention and nurturing for it to flourish in the hearts of practitioners and subsequently manifest itself throughout the healthcare environment, for the betterment of both the public and the practitioner.

CARING SCIENCE AND CARITAS

Watson (n.d.) espouses that Caring Science embraces a "humanitarian, human science orientation to human caring processes, phenomena and experiences" (para. 1). Caring Science thus incorporates not only science but also the arts and humanities. "A relational ontology of being-in-relation, and a worldview of unity and connectedness to All" underpin Caring Science (Watson, n.d., para. 1). Transpersonal caring is central to Caring Science. Watson intentionally uses the word "transpersonal" in regards to caring, so as to connote the nature of connectiveness inherent within this form of caring. This form of caring "acknowledges unity of life and connections that move in concentric circles of caring—from individual, to others, to community, to world, to Planet Earth, to the universe" (Watson, n.d., para. 1).

Caritas is a key concept in Caring Science. According to Watson (2008), "Caritas" means "to cherish, to appreciate, to give special, if not loving, attention to" (p. 39). Loving attention is paramount for healthcare practitioners because love is "the greatest source of healing in the world" (Watson, 2008, p. 40). When professional practice is guided by Caring Science, there are profound implications for healing not only individuals but also society as a whole. When healthcare professionals embrace and live out the principles of Caring Science within their practice, those professionals help "sustain human dignity and humanity itself while contributing to the evolution of human consciousness, helping to move toward a more humane and caring moral community and civilization" (Watson, 2008, p. 40).

Watson (2008) developed 10 Caritas Processes® as a foundational guide for practice. The Caritas Processes guide practitioners to "practice loving-kindness and equanimity" with self and others; to be authentically present with self and others; to develop their own spiritual practice that encourages them to elicit higher wisdom rather than rely on their own egos; to not only create caring-healing environments through the use of art, music, light, and caring-healing modalities but also actually *become* the caring-healing environment for themselves and others by their authentic, heart-centered presence; and to allow for and recognize everyday miracles around them (p. 34).

Watson (2008) also espouses that through Caring Science–guided practice, sacred caring moments are cocreated between practitioners and the individuals they serve. Caring moments are characterized by spirit-to-spirit connections when one is able to truly "see" and deeply connect with the spirit-filled person behind the patient, the patient's loved one, the practitioner, and each member of the healthcare team. Caring moments touch the spirits of the persons involved and change them on some level. Caring moments go beyond time, space, and physicality and are carried with the involved persons forever.

This discussion has offered a brief, general overview of key tenets of Caring Science and Caritas. Readers are encouraged to gain a more comprehensive understanding of Caring Science by exploring the theories and related research of Caring Science theorists, such as the works of Jean Watson, Marilyn Ray, and Kristen Swanson.

Caring Science and Caritas are integrally related to one another. One cannot practice Caring Science without practicing Caritas. Thus, for the remainder of this chapter, the terms "Caring Science" and "Caritas" are used interchangeably to explore their integration into professional practice.

PROFESSIONAL PRACTICE

One needs to understand what comprises professional practice to integrate the tenets of Caring Science and Caritas described earlier into professional practice. Professional practice is composed of three main components: (a) the role of the practitioner, (b) the domains in which the practitioner functions, and (c) the activities exercised by the practitioner to carry out the role within his or her domains (Poitras, Chouinard, Fortin, & Gallagher, 2016). To fully integrate Caring Science into professional practice, dedicated attention must be given to incorporate caring into all three components of professional practice. The practitioner guided by Caring Science is cognizant of, committed to, and comfortable with his or her fundamental role of manifesting the tenets of Caring Science within his or her domain. The domain in which the practitioner functions refers to the workplace, specialty field, and/or territory in which the practitioner carries out his or her role. When the workplace, specialty field, and/or territory support the tenets of Caring Science, the capacity of the practitioner to manifest those tenets is exponentially enhanced. In such workplaces/specialty fields/ territories, there is a mutual consensus among administrators, practitioners, and allied transdisciplinary healthcare team members to value and prioritize caring, and thus caring is facilitated and encouraged. The supported Caritas practitioner is comfortable with and confident in his or her role and consciously manifests caring through his or her presence and caring activities.

The question arises as to how healthcare systems can pragmatically provide dedicated attention to and nurturing of these three components of professional practice, so as to fully and intentionally weave Caring Science into the fabric of their systems. Fortunately, there are innovative, caring-healing healthcare systems that can serve as exemplars. The methods and strategies that have proven to be successful for such systems are discussed in this chapter, and so also the outcomes these systems have realized owing to their dedicated efforts to integrate Caring Science and Caritas.

DEDICATED ATTENTION TO THE ROLE OF CARITAS PRACTITIONERS

There is a dearth of literature that explains why persons enter healthcare professions in general; however, there are studies that illuminate why nurses enter their field. Research has shown two common themes describing the reasons behind men and women becoming nurses: (a) they have an innate sense that nursing is more than a job—it is, rather, a vocation or calling; and (b) nursing provides them the opportunity to care for others (Eley, Eley, Bertello, & Rogers-Clark, 2012). Empathy and altruistic ideals are often traits of both nurses and nursing students (Eley et al., 2012). When nurses perceive that they are able to fulfill their vocations through opportunities to care for others with empathy and altruistic ideals, they are likely to experience compassion satisfaction. Compassion satisfaction refers to the feelings of gratification caregivers receive from providing care; these positive feelings of gratification nurture and fulfill the caregivers, preserving and restoring their spirits (Smart et al., 2014). The Caring Science/Caritas practitioner role allows nurses, and perhaps the other allied healthcare professionals, to fulfill their vocational desires, and it nurtures their spirits. Dedicated attention to developing and supporting the Caring Science/Caritas practitioner role in healthcare systems is thus imperative.

For the practitioner role to be guided by the tenets of Caring Science, they have to be familiar with and aligned with those tenets. It cannot be taken for granted that all practitioners are knowledgeable of, value, and seek to manifest these tenets in their roles. Caring must be articulated, discussed, and focused on to raise awareness and support the notion that caring is an integral part of the practitioner role. Otherwise, there is a risk for practitioners, even those who enter their fields with altruistic values, to become task-based rather than person-centered in their care delivery. Haslam (2015), the chair of the National Institute for Health and Care Excellence in London, United Kingdom, describes task-based care as impersonal; he acknowledges that task-based care does exist, but counsels that it does not meet the needs of the public, as it desires compassionate, respectful care that preserves its unique dignity.

Caring Science educational sessions, both formal and informal, are paramount for practitioners to affirm their existing caring practices and/or to enhance caring practices. Healthcare organizations nationally and internationally have budgeted resources to provide formal Caring Science educational programs for all disciplines. In addition to educating existing practitioners, healthcare facilities have also assured that new team members become familiar with Caring Science by including relevant education as part of new-employee orientation. These formal educational sessions have included didactic content on Caring Science and Caritas, covering topics such as:

- Why is Caring Science an important foundation for practice?

- How does Caring Science align with and support the healthcare organization's mission?

- An overview of the tenets of Caring Science and Caritas

- Reflective discussion regarding how the 10 Caritas Processes are manifested currently in practice and identifying where there are opportunities for enhancement

Formal educational sessions also have often included experiential content in which attendees were able to be the recipients of and/or practice caring-healing modalities with one another. Examples of these modality experiences included such exercises as heart-centering, music listening, hand massage, guided imagery, meditation, journaling, a physical assessment with intentional loving presence, and authentic listening. Attendees were encouraged to share how these modalities influenced their own feelings of well-being, and how they might incorporate the modalities into their daily practice. Often attendees initiated implementation of such caring-healing modalities into their personal practice and/or their workplace settings after participating in these experiential educational sessions.

One institution engaged nursing students in a formal Caring Science endeavor for their master's program capstone project. These students not only developed a Caring Science educational session but also conducted research to evaluate whether participation in the educational session influenced the attendee's comfort with caring behaviors, and whether this had an impact on patient perception of care as measured by specified patient satisfaction questions. Their research found that those who attended the educational session did increase their comfort with caring behaviors and this increased comfort was sustained over a 6-month period; there were also improvements in patient perception of care in the clinical areas where these attendees practiced (Desmond et al., 2014).

Practitioners can also be educated informally on their role to intentionally manifest caring in their practice. Discussions on Caring Science can be woven into established nursing committees and councils, such as shared governance councils. Besides discussions of caring during these established group meetings, some organizations developed an additional transdisciplinary council that focused primarily on integrating Caring

Science into professional practice. All of these various venues allowed for brainstorming sessions in which practitioners discussed and developed ways to enhance caring within their individual practices and their organizations as a whole. Some healthcare facilities began their committee and/or council meetings with a tenet or quote from Caring Science literature, followed by a caring story exemplifying the tenet or quote. Departments created bulletin boards highlighting caring practices and/or Caritas processes, and acknowledging caring practitioners.

To provide further attention to the role of the Caritas practitioner, in addition to educational endeavors, healthcare facilities invited practitioners to write stories of their caring moments for publication in organizational newsletters. Several facilities gathered those stories and published them as a collection of Caritas practices. These published collections were sometimes given as gifts to practitioners for special occasions, such as Nurses' Week or Hospital Week celebrations. One organization made their published collection available for sale in their hospital's gift shop.

Another method healthcare organizations used to promote the role of the Caritas practitioner was to include caring reflection as part of the practitioners' annual evaluation process. The practitioners would be invited to write a reflective story of a caring moment, and identify which Caritas processes were exemplified in their story. This process of reflective writing helped to value and validate their personal Caritas practice.

This valuing and validating of personal Caritas practice nurtured the notion that caring is integral to the practitioner role; it enhanced the practitioner perception that caring was not an additional duty to be carried out, but it was foundational to who they were in their role. Research has shown that role perception influences performance. Roch, Dubois, and Clarke (2014) found in their study of 292 direct care Canadian nurses that perception of their role was the strongest predictor of caring practice performance. Thus, when practitioners perceive caring as integral to their role, they are more likely to engage in caring practices.

To fully integrate Caring Science/Caritas practice into healthcare organizations, the organizational domain has to support the endeavor. How healthcare domains provide support for such endeavors is discussed in the following section.

DEDICATED ATTENTION TO THE DOMAINS OF CARITAS PRACTITIONERS

Too often in healthcare systems, there is a focus on efficiency and productivity at the expense of authentic caring practices. Certainly, efficiency and productivity are critical aspects for financial viability, but these aspects should not be prioritized over caring practices, as each of these aspects is an important facet in today's healthcare arena.

Caring practices are linked to patient satisfaction. Palese et al. (2011) conducted a study with 1,565 surgical patients from six European countries and found that positive connectedness between patients and nurses was the main dimension that explained patient satisfaction. Caring practices foster positive connectedness, and that, in turn, enhances patient satisfaction. Because, as stated earlier, patient satisfaction is a key indicator that influences reimbursement and patient preferences for healthcare services, caring practices are to be viewed as equally paramount to financial viability as efficiency and productivity.

Administrative leaders not only are called to value caring practices as significantly as they value efficiency and productivity but have a responsibility to role model caring as well (Goodman, 2015; Haslam, 2015; Watson, 2006). Haslam (2015) states, "Compassionate leaders create compassionate organizations" (p. 3). Watson (2006) encourages administrative leaders to develop caring skills and behaviors, including "caring presence in formal and informal relationships with individuals and groups"; she also states that leaders are to "understand and communicate caring as philosophy and ethic for organizational processes, structures, and relationships" (p. 53). Administrative leaders have an obligation to create and maintain a caring milieu within their organization's domain.

Similar to the needs of practitioners, administrative leaders need Caring Science education. Educational sessions for Caritas leaders can have comparable content as Caritas practitioner educational sessions; however, the content can be expanded to include discussions on how caring can become explicit in the organization's mission and vision if it is not already evident. Time can be allocated for reflection on how the leaders can best role model, support, and promote caring practices for those they lead. Some organizations have allotted time within their educational sessions for leaders to create vision boards to artistically express their vision for their own Caritas leadership. Leaders may also need time to discuss the budgeting of necessary resources to support the development and/or enhancement of caring within their organizational culture.

Another strategy that has proven to be helpful in the development of Caritas leadership is devoting time for leadership reflection and discussion regarding the differences between authentic caring and scripted caring practices. There are many customer service models prevalent in today's healthcare arenas that purport benefits of practitioners using scripted language and behaviors during certain key interactions with patients and their significant others. However, scripted language and behaviors are the antitheses of authentic caring. McGee (2014) contends that "Caring and compassion cannot be faked. These are not actions we perform mechanically, but states of being that flow from within to make healing connections with others in need. To be authentically healing requires that we live authentic lives" (p. 725). McGee also emphasizes that persons can immediately tell the difference between authentic caring and scripted caring; he writes, "Anyone who has received care can easily perceive in an instant who authentically cares for them and who does not. Patients value not so much what we say, but how we are as a manifestation of our character as we conscientiously execute our caring roles" (p. 725). Scripted caring language and behaviors thus have the risk of being perceived as inauthentic and mechanical, and can serve as an impediment to developing caring-healing relationships. Authentic caring, guided by the framework of Caring Science, provides the opportunity for practitioners to develop genuine life-supporting and life-giving caring-healing relationships with those they serve.

Another aspect that must be addressed when giving dedicated attention to the domain of Caritas practitioners involves the phenomena of incivility, lateral violence, and bullying that, unfortunately, may be prevalent within healthcare organizations. Incivility pertains to discourteous, offensive, and/or unsociable language or behavior. Lateral violence consists of disruptive and inappropriate, demeaning behavior on the part of colleagues; bullying is similar behavior that is perpetrated by superiors or persons with perceived organizational power. Research has shown that up to 85% of nurses have been victims of lateral violence and up to 93% have witnessed this type of behavior (Jacobs & Kyzer, 2010; Quine, 2001). The

American Nurses Association (2015) has published a position paper in which they purport that all healthcare organizations have an ethical, legal, and moral obligation to create healthy, safe workplaces for every healthcare team member and the public they serve; they also recommend implementation of zero tolerance policies in regards to incivility, lateral violence, and bullying within the organization. As stated earlier, administrative leaders have the responsibility to create and maintain a caring milieu within their organization's domain. They must, therefore, develop effective mechanisms to address any and all instances of incivility, lateral violence, and/or bullying in efforts to move toward a culture of kindness, dignity, and respect.

An additional strategy to promote a Caritas domain is to intentionally make caring explicit in philosophy statements, policies, procedures, professional practice models, and position descriptions. Language that articulates Caring Science tenets and Caritas could be woven into the organization's nursing philosophy. Policy and procedures may include language to indicate that the practitioner is expected to exemplify caring/Caritas as he or she carries out the policy/procedure. The professional practice model would graphically display that his or her professional practice is founded on and guided by Caring Science. In addition, position descriptions could include language articulating that practitioner practice is founded on and guided by the tenets of Caring Science.

Creating restorative spaces for all healthcare team members is another proven strategy to enhance a caring domain. Organizations have allocated spaces and resources and engaged their practitioners in creating restful, peaceful, aesthetic areas to which staff can retreat to restore their spirits during their time at work. Space is often a limited commodity within healthcare facilities, but creative solutions to identify places have been found. Organizations have redesigned storage areas or obsolete treatment rooms for such restorative spaces. Caritas leaders and practitioners have also transformed dull and dreary outside areas into beautiful healing gardens. It is recommended that practitioners be engaged in the process of designing and decorating the spaces once they have been identified, so that those areas reflect their spirits and meet their needs; they should also work collaboratively with their facilities department to assure any furnishings and decorative treatments meet fire and safety regulations as well as building codes.

Finally, the domain can also support the Caritas practitioner by intentionally integrating caring interventions and Caritas language into the clinical documentation system. Caritas practitioners have worked creatively with information system team members to revise their organization's clinical documentation systems, so that practitioners are able to document their caring interventions and patient responses to those interventions in their electronic health records; nurses have found it valuable and affirming to be able to document their caring practices in this manner (Rosenberg, 2006).

DEDICATED ATTENTION TO CARITAS ACTIVITIES

The third component of professional Caritas practice focuses on the activities exercised by the practitioners to carry out their caring role within their domains. Caritas activities involve both *being* and *doing*. As mentioned earlier, Caritas practitioners are encouraged to *be* the caring–healing environment through internal spirit-focused activities. Caritas practitioners also create aesthetically pleasing and holistically supportive external environments for self and others through purposeful planning and design activities. In addition, Caritas practitioners purposefully integrate caring-healing modalities into their practice.

The *being* activities facilitate the Caritas practitioner to *be* the caring-healing environment; these activities involve intention, authentic presence, spiritual/holistic practices, and attention to self-care. Caring is not taken for granted; rather, the Caritas practitioners intentionally bring caring into their consciousness as they enter their domain. Activities that might help the practitioners bring caring into their consciousness may be engaging in mind-body-spirit practices such as heart-centering, guided imagery, meditation, pausing in the midst of chaos to center oneself, deep breathing exercises, and/or purposeful relaxation of tense muscles within their body. Taking time to visually imagine the release of cares and concerns floating away, like a leaf floating away down a river, may help practitioners let go of worries that might preclude them from being authentically present to another. Traditional transition practices may be transformed into sacred passages that help one be more authentically present. For example, when washing hands between patients, practitioners might take this time to pause and intentionally release their focus from their previous patient to center on the next patient; they may offer the previous patient a blessing as they release him or her. Some organizations have placed prayers or reflections over their sinks to assist with this type of intentional transitional practice.

Attention to self-care is imperative for practitioners to have the capacity to *be* a caring-healing environment; practitioners cannot emanate caring-healing energy if their mind-body-spirits are depleted. Caritas practitioners practice self-care through nutritional diets, adequate physical exercise, sufficient rest, and partaking in activities that restore their spirit, whatever those might be. Caritas practitioners and Caritas leaders realize that self-care is not selfish; it is vital to maintaining one's well-being. It is essential to "fill up one's cup" so that one has the energy and capacity to give loving attention to others. Too often our society places high regards on persons who work extensive hours, stress out, and neglect their own personal needs. Sometimes, it can be seen as a competition as to who works the hardest and the longest, with no concerns for holistic well-being. Caritas domains/leaders/practitioners intentionally move from such self-destroying, life-depleting mindsets to self-protecting and life-restoring perspectives.

The *doing* activities involve creating aesthetically pleasing and holistically supportive external environments for self and others through purposeful planning and design, and the integration of caring-healing modalities. Caritas practitioners are attentive to the external environment and evaluate whether it is contributing to or detracting from health and well-being. They intervene whenever possible to reduce noxious noises; adjust uncomfortable ambient temperatures; facilitate soft, relaxing light; arrange for nature views or artwork; and so on. Caritas practitioners are indispensable members of planning teams for renovations or construction of new facilities so that the building design includes aesthetic caring-healing elements.

Caritas practitioners also have integrated caring-healing modalities into their professional practice activities. They may have made music selections available for patients undergoing invasive procedures; music listening of genres that align with patient preferences helped patients relax and reduced their anxiety. Caritas practitioners have collaborated with art suppliers to make art materials available for patients' use while hospitalized, or visitors' use while waiting in waiting rooms. Art activities have been especially well received in pediatric, oncology, and obstetrical units, and in neonatal intensive care waiting rooms where siblings of hospitalized infants spend much time. Caritas practitioners have promoted and facilitated healing arts programs in their organizations. These programs bring in performers, such as comedians, actors, and musicians, to transform the hospital environment. An example of a healing art performer is a harpist who transforms the environment from a sterile, medicalized state to one filled with restful, restorative musical melodies. Patients and healthcare team members alike have shared their appreciation for such transformed environments. Caritas practitioners also have purposefully reintroduced back massages and/or hand massages into their caring-healing practices; these modalities have helped reduce stress and promote rest for patients and their loved ones. Some organizations have even budgeted for massage therapists to be available routinely for patients, families, and employees.

Another modality that was implemented in a faith-based organization was code prayer. This modality involved playing a particular melody over the hospital public address system, signaling that someone within the hospital requested prayer. Anyone could request the melody to be played simply by dialing the operator and requesting a code prayer. Those who heard the melody could respond by silently saying a prayer for whoever had made the request.

Finally, one other "doing" activity that caring practitioners and caring organizations have participated in is the hosting of the International Caritas Consortium. This consortium is a gathering of interdisciplinary professionals who are actively integrating or seeking to integrate the tenets of Caring Science and the theory of human caring into professional practice (Watson Caring Science Institute, 2014). Participants share practical and innovative Caritas practice insights from personal stories and/or research endeavors. Dr. Jean Watson begins the consortium with a heart-centering practice and then opens the venue for sharing of stories among the Caritas practitioners. Dr. Watson shares her Caritas wisdom with and provides authentic loving kindness for the participants, cocreating a caring-healing and inspirational environment. Dr. Watson also provides updates and explicates the future vision for the global movement to integrate Caring Science into professional practice.

OUTCOMES OF INTENTIONAL INTEGRATION OF CARING SCIENCE AND CARITAS

Organizations that have integrated Caring Science into professional practice have realized positive outcomes for both patients and practitioners. Such organizations have realized improvements in overall patient satisfaction (Foss Durant, McDermott, Kinney, & Triner, 2015; Tyrrell, Ryan, & Desmond, 2013). Patients have reported enhanced listening, communication, courtesy, and respect on the part of nurses after Caring Science and Caritas were integrated into professional practice (Desmond et al., 2014; Foss Durant et al., 2015; Tyrrell et al., 2013). These healthcare facilities also linked integration of Caring Science with improved quality indicators; they found that when Caring Science was more fully implemented, there were related decreases in rates of ventilator-associated pneumonia and catheter-associated urinary tract infections (Goldin, 2015), as well as decreases in hospital-acquired pressure ulcers, hospital-acquired *Clostridium difficile* infections, falls with injuries, and bloodstream infections (Foss Durant et al., 2015).

Organizations also saw increases in nurse satisfaction measures after incorporating Caring Science into professional practice. There were improvements in the perceived ability of nurse managers to provide support and leadership to nurses, the practice environment was enhanced, and nurses reported better job enjoyment (Goldin, 2015; Tyrrell et al., 2013). Nurses indicated that they felt more competent in their caring behaviors and attitudes (Desmond et al., 2014). There were also fewer reported incidents of lateral violence and/or bullying after Caring Science implementation endeavors (Tyrrell et al., 2013).

CONCLUSION

Integrating Caring Science and Caritas into professional practice has been associated with enhanced patient satisfaction, improved patient outcomes, heightened practitioner satisfaction and competence, and better work environments. There is no one precise formula to follow to implement the methods and strategies described earlier to successfully integrate Caring Science into practice. However, if organizations provide dedicated attention to weaving Caring Science and Caritas throughout the three main components of professional practice (the role of the practitioner, the domains in which the practitioner functions, and the activities exercised by the practitioner to carry out his or her role within his or her domains), successful integration is likely to occur.

The methods and strategies to integrate Caring Science and Caritas into professional practice described earlier are recommendations that have proven to be beneficial to numerous organizations nationally and internationally. However, every recommendation might not be a fit for all organizations. It is suggested that each organization consider these recommended methods and strategies and adopt ones that best align with their mission, vision, and culture.

Organizations are encouraged to engage caring practitioners and leaders along the way and to be creative with this process. The recommendations provided earlier are a starting point with this creative process, but new possibilities are always on the horizon. The questions in the section "Next Era Possibilities" are meant to explore new possibilities for each organization's unique journey to integrate Caring Science and Caritas into professional practice.

NEXT ERA POSSIBILITIES

Education
- How can I integrate Caring Science/Caritas into the education I provide for colleagues and transdisciplinary team members?
- In what ways does nursing curriculum need to be expanded to include the tenets of Caring Science/Caritas discussed in this chapter?

Research
- What qualitative research studies need to be undertaken to capture the influence of Caring Science/Caritas on the health and well-being of practitioners and the public they serve?
- What quantitative research studies need to be undertaken to measure the impact of Caring Science/Caritas integration into professional practice?

- What meta-analysis and metasynthesis need to be performed to synthesize already published Caring Science research to develop guidelines for best practice?

Praxis
- Which dimensions of practice can I improve right now with a greater understanding of the tenets of Caring Science/Caritas?
- How can I best provide caring-loving attention to myself, my colleagues, my superiors, and the public I serve?
- How can I incorporate caring-healing modalities into my professional practice activities?

Theory and Knowledge Development
- What additional methods and strategies do I believe could be used to facilitate the integration of Caring Science/Caritas into professional practice?
- Given my specialty, what areas could be enhanced to include the tenets of Caring Science/Caritas? What specific contributions can I make?
- How does my own theory of nursing resonate with the ideas discussed earlier? Are there possibilities for me to open up to new ways of being, doing, and knowing so as to optimize my ability to manifest Caring Science/Caritas in the world?

 REFERENCES

American Nurses Association. (2010). *Nursing's social policy statement: The essence of the profession* (3rd ed.). Silver Spring, MD: Nursingbooks.org

American Nurses Association. (2015). Incivility, bullying and workplace violence. Retrieved from http://www.nursingworld.org/MainMenuCategories/WorkplaceSafety/Healthy-Nurse/bullyingworkplaceviolence/Incivility-Bullying-and-Workplace-Violence.html

Beck, C. (2015). *Hermeneutic phenomenological study to explore the experience of native Hawaiian patients in terms of satisfaction/dissatisfaction with nursing care* (Doctoral dissertation). Retrieved from ProQuest Dissertations & Theses Global. (Order No. 10085568)

Centers for Medicare & Medicaid Services. (2017). Hospital value-based purchasing. Retrieved from https://www.cms.gov/Outreach-and-Education/Medicare-Learning-Network-MLN/MLNProducts/downloads/Hospital_VBPurchasing_Fact_Sheet_ICN907664.pdf

Desmond, M. E., Horn, S., Keith, K., Kelby, S., Ryan, L., & Smith, J. (2014). Incorporating caring theory into personal and professional nursing practice to improve perception of care. *International Journal for Human Caring, 18*(1), 35–44. doi:10.20467/1091-5710-18.1.35

Eley, D., Eley, R., Bertello, M., & Rogers-Clark, C. (2012). Why did I become a nurse? Personality traits and reasons for entering nursing. *Journal of Advanced Nursing, 68*(7), 1546–1555. doi:10.1111/j.1365-2648.2012.05955.x

Foss-Durant, A., McDermott, S., Kinney, G., & Triner, T. (2015). Caring science: Transforming the ethic of caring-healing practice, environment, and culture within an integrated care delivery system. *Permanente Journal, 19*(4), e136–e142. doi:10.7812/TPP/15-042

Goldin, M. (2015, November). *Applying caring theory guided leadership to inspire, empower, and improve quality.* Podium session presented at Sigma Theta Tau 43rd Biennial Convention, Las Vegas, NV.

Goodman, M. E. (2015). *Patients' lived experience of caring during hospitalization: A phenomenologic study* (Doctoral dissertation). Retrieved from ProQuest Dissertations & Theses Global. (Order No. 10029780)

Haslam, D. (2015). More than kindness. *Journal of Compassionate Health Care, 2,* 6. doi:10.1186/s40639-015-0015-2

International Council of Nurses. (2012). *The ICN code of ethics for nurses* (Rev. ed.). Geneva, Switzerland: Author.

Jacobs, D., & Kyzer, S. (2010). Upstate AHEC lateral violence among nurses project. *South Carolina Nurse, 17*(1), 1.

Letourneau, R. (2016). Better HCAHPS scores protect revenue. *HealthLeaders Media*. Retrieved from http://www.healthleadersmedia.com/finance/better-hcahps-scores-protect-revenue

Martinsen, E. (2011). Harm in the absence of care: Towards a medical ethics that cares. *Nursing Ethics, 18*(2), 174–183. doi: 10.1177/0969733010392304

Mason, D. (2015). JAMA forum: Does linking payment to patient satisfaction harm or help? *news@JAMA*. Retrieved from https://newsatjama.jama.com/2015/06/17/jama-forum-does-linking-payment-to-patient-satisfaction-harm-or-help

McGee, M. D. (2014). Authenticity and healing. *Journal of Religion and Health, 53*, 725–730. doi:10.1007/s10943-014-9835-1

Meehan, T. C. (2012). The careful nursing philosophy and professional practice model. *Journal of Clinical Nursing, 21*(19-20), 2905–2916. doi:10.1111/j.1365-2702.2012.04214.x

Naburi, H., Mujinja, P., Kilewo, C., Bärnighausen, T., Orsini, N., Manji, K., ... Ekström, A. M. (2016). Predictors of patient dissatisfaction with services for prevention of mother-to-child transmission of HIV in Dar es Salaam, Tanzania. *PLoS One, 11*(10), e0165121. doi:10.1371/journal.pone.0165121

Nightingale, F. (2007). *Notes on nursing.* New York, NY: Barnes & Noble. (Original work published 1859.)

Palese, A., Tomietto, M., Suhonen, R., Efstathiou, G., Tsangari, H., Merkouris, A., ... Papastavrou, E. (2011). Surgical patient satisfaction as an outcome of nurses' caring behaviors: A descriptive and correlational study in six European countries. *Journal of Nursing Scholarship, 43*(4), 341–350. doi:10.1111/j.1547-5069.2011.01413.x

Poitras, M. E., Chouinard, M. C., Fortin, M., & Gallagher, F. (2016). How to report professional practice in nursing? A scoping review. *BioMed Central Nursing, 15*, 31. doi:10.1186/s12912-016-0154-6

Quine, L. (2001). Workplace bullying in nurses. *Journal of Health Psychology, 6*(1), 73–84. doi:10.1177/135910530100600106

Roch, G., Dubois, C. A., & Clarke, S. P. (2014). Organizational climate and hospital nurses' caring practices: A mixed-methods study. *Research in Nursing & Health, 37*(3), 229–240. doi:10.1002/nur.21596

Rosenberg, S. (2006). Utilizing the language of Jean Watson's caring theory within a computerized clinical documentation system. *Computers, Informatics, Nursing, 24*(1), 53–56. doi:10.1097/00024665-200601000-00013

Shan, L., Li, Y., Ding, D., Wu, Q., Liu, C., Jiao, M., ... Ren, J. (2016). Patient satisfaction with hospital inpatient care: Effects of trust, medical insurance and perceived quality of care. *PLoS One, 11*(10), e0164366. doi:10.1371/journal.pone.0164366

Smart, D., English, A., James, J., Wilson, M., Daratha, K. B., Childers, B., & Magera, C. (2014). Compassion fatigue and satisfaction: A cross-sectional survey among US healthcare workers. *Nursing & Health Sciences, 16*(1), 3–10. doi:10.1111/nhs.12068

Tyrrell, S., Ryan, L., & Desmond, M. E. (2013, October). *Caring science professional practice, professional practice model and research: Adventist Hinsdale Hospital.* Poster session presented at the 19th International Caritas Consortium, Oak Brook, IL.

Watson Caring Science Institute. (2014). International caritas consortium. Retrieved from http://www.watsoncaringscience.org/wp-content/uploads/2014/09/WCSI-ICC-DearbornMI_FLYER_2014.09.pdf

Watson, J. (2006). Caring theory as an ethical guide to administrative and clinical practices. *Nursing Administration Quarterly, 30*(1), 48–55. doi:10.1097/00006216-200601000-00008

Watson, J. (2008). *Nursing: The philosophy and science of caring* (Rev. ed.). Boulder: University Press of Colorado.

Watson, J. (2009). Caring as the essence and science of nursing and health care. *Mundo Da Sao Paulo, 33*(2), 143–149.

Watson, J. (n.d.). Caring science theory: Caring science defined. Retrieved from https://www.watsoncaringscience.org/jean-bio/caring-science-theory

Zender, R., & Olshansky, E. (2012). The biology of caring: Researching the healing effects of stress response regulation through relational engagement. *Biological Research for Nursing, 14*(4), 419–430. doi:10.1177/1099800412450505

VII

*Redefining Healthcare Through
Heart-Centered Wisdom*

28

A Blueprint for Caritas Health "Care"

Jacqueline G. Somerville and Susan M. Lee

CARITAS LITERACIES

By the end of this chapter, the caring-healing nurse will be able to

1. Recognize the importance of the practice of loving-kindness, compassion, and equanimity for self and others in advancing the health of those in service and the health of those whom they serve.

2. Understand the blueprint or approach of one organization to create a community of caring.

3. Identify at least one caring practice that can be introduced in the local practice setting to infuse caring science.

Although improvements in curing disease have been impressive, the dissatisfaction remains with care, especially when hospitalized. Many current healthcare delivery systems are impersonal, fast paced businesses designed to fix problems with little attention to the individual experiencing them. Nursing is a major professional group, able to use its knowledge to address these deficits of healthcare delivery—Jones, 2007, p. 167

A friend recently shared two experiences she had in the healthcare system. First, her mother was diagnosed with a seizure disorder and started on levetiracetam. She also suffers from hypothyroidism and takes levothyroxine—you know where this is going. The levetiracetam prescription was filled for levothryroxine, basically doubling her dose. A follow-up EEG showed no improvement in her seizure activity and so the dose was doubled again. She began feeling extremely ill and her daughter—a nurse—asked to see her medications. She discovered the error, returned to the pharmacy, and got her traumatized mother back on the road to recovery. She took the time to listen to her mother's symptoms and to physically look at the medications that she was taking—low tech, high touch. No MRIs or scans. She knew her patient and listened.

That same week, my friend's sister, who recently had surgery for a recurring brain tumor, learned that she qualified for a clinical trial. Just weeks after her surgery, she was required to spend a grueling, 13-hour day getting all the required testing completed to enter the trial, only to be called a few days later and told that she had been worked up for the wrong trial. She was asked to return to an affiliated facility closer to her home to have the correct testing completed, which she did again spending another full day only to be called a second time and told that the incorrect tests were done. The administrative assistant even said to her, "My gut told me this wasn't right, but because the orders came from our flagship hospital I didn't question them."

Each of us could probably tell countless similar stories, especially if you are a clinician and are called upon regularly to help families, neighbors, and friends navigate our broken "sick care" system. Why do these mishaps and errors happen so regularly? Do clinicians not care anymore?

We do not believe that for a second.

NURSING AND CARING: THE HEART OF THE SOLUTION

What we witness are pressures to "do more with less," to spend decreased time with the patient in the name of productivity, to fragment "nursing" into discreet tasks that can be delegated to lower paid technical workers, all in the name of "affordable care." Dr. Jean Watson is clear that caring is a professional and moral ideal, not an affect or task-oriented behavior (Watson, 2008). Instead of focusing on leveraging the caring knowledge of healthcare workers to take the real sources of fragmentation out of the system, most systems focus on what they describe as the biggest cost in the current system from their point of view—the people—and in many organizations the largest professional workforce—nursing.

This approach is exacerbated by the fact that most nurses practice in an employer-based structure, whose goals may be at odds with society's mandate for nurses as professionals. As Porter-O'Grady (2017) notes, although the understanding that professionals must honor society's mandate of their unique profession, "it has not been considered legitimate when applied to nurses" (p. 69). As we move toward employment versus partner models with other colleagues, including physicians, challenges are being faced outside of nursing to the belief that professionals "are self-managed and have exclusive control over their own practice and work as partners with organizations" (Porter-O'Grady, 2017, p. 70). This dissonance in nursing contributes to one in five new nurses leaving his or her first position within his or her first year of practice (Kovner, Brewer, Fatehi, & Jun, 2014). According to Kovner et al. (2014), millennial nurses have some of the highest rates of compassion fatigue in the profession. Kelly, in an interview with Adams, calls upon us to offset such fatigue and dissonance by "determining how to help nurses practice optimally, mindfully and compassionately" and, we would add, with patients, themselves, and interprofessional colleagues (Adams, 2017, p. 80).

We believe, as do so many clinicians, that a transactional approach will not transform the health of our world. It will only cause greater inefficiencies, costs, and human suffering. Instead, we need a transformative approach. If we build systems that support and celebrate our clinicians and staff, they can be fully present to care for the people and communities whom they are called to serve; then and only then will we transform our "sick care" system into a true healthcare system. Medicalization of health has not served humanity well. It is time to reclaim our fundamental practice premise—the unity of mind, body, and spirit and our connection to each other and our universe. Creating space for caring clinicians to ensure that intention matches impact is the path to health for all.

And what do our patients think? We turned to our patient and family advisors to help us guide our journey. Brigham and Women's Hospital (BWH) established 15 patient–family advisory councils across service lines, practice settings, and affinity groups, being the first hospital in the nation to establish a Lesbian, Gay, Bisexual, Transgender, Queer, or Questioning (LGBTQ) Patient Family Advisory Council. What we heard from these experts is what we have known for centuries: They echoed the sentiments of Osler (1963) that the practice of medicine exercises one's heart and mind and is an art whose basis is in science.

In 2013 and 2014, the Schwartz Center conducted focus groups to understand what patients expect from compassionate care (Schwartz Center, 2017). Their language mirrored the Caritas Processes® and is consistent with findings in nursing and Caring Science research. In the Schwartz focus groups, the themes reflected that they valued a clinician who shared information in a way that the patient and family could understand, one that involved the patient in decision making, actively listened, treated them as a whole person, not a disease, and clinicians who showed respect for the patient and his or her family. Here is the power of this information: Focus group participants said that all of the above alleviate some of the mental and emotional distress caused by the healthcare system that then frees up energy to improve health and quality of life. In addition, when clinician behavior was consistent with the above, patients were more likely to seek care and to be honest about their lives with their clinicians.

These themes are consistent with my (Jacqueline G. Somerville [JGS]) research regarding patients' perceptions of feeling known by their nurses (Somerville, 2009). As a clinical nurse, nurse executive, consultant, patient, and family member, I have witnessed the healing power of the nurse–patient relationship. In the current healthcare environment, the ability for nurses and clinicians to "know their patients" is undervalued and placed at risk. Care is often focused on task-driven activities with little time for the nurse to fully respond to the experiences of their patients, families, and communities. Without caring intention and the ability for clinicians to know each of their patients as a whole person, care is experienced as technical and cold and does not advance human healing. We have all seen patients who were cured but not healed as well as patients who were healed but not cured. Relational care is the key. Over and over again we witness this. As a consultant, I led a disease management initiative focused on asthma. We had outstanding clinical algorithms and technology coupled with the intervention of a nurse case manager. We unfailingly witnessed that it was the human presence of a clinician—who bore witness to that which held meaning to the patients, integrated this knowledge into the plan of care, extended hope to their human potential, and helped them tap into their unique patterns of health and illness—that improved their quality of life and advanced their health.

These many experiences drove me to explore patients' perceptions of feeling known by their nurses, a phenomenon that I would later describe and quantify (Somerville, 2009). When patients felt known by their nurses, they felt recognized as unique human beings; they felt safe; and they felt a meaningful, personal, mutual connection with their nurses and, therefore, felt empowered to participate in their care. Isn't that what we are seeking—patients, families, and communities as active participants in their care? With these themes guiding us, we began our journey, which we are honored to share with you.

OUR JOURNEY TO HEALTH "CARE"

From 2011 to 2016, I (JGS) was honored to be the chief nurse and senior vice president of Patient Care Services of BWH in Boston. When asked by nurses what my vision was for the department, I clarified again and again that we would cocreate a future that would build upon and sustain the strong foundational work of caring-healing that was entrusted to us by our predecessors, while continuing to evolve the practice to meet the dynamic needs of those we serve.

I (JGS) began my 5.5-year journey by spending time with clinical nurses in each area to witness their practice. What I experienced was breathtaking and variable. The acuity of the patients was staggering and the cutting-edge technical care and expertise was the best I had ever witnessed. It was the loving-kindness that nurses gave to themselves, each other, their peers, colleagues, patients, and families that was variable. It was nurse-dependent and occurred despite the many competing demands, that is, throughput, in an organization that consistently ran over 100% occupancy, documentation demands to meet regulatory, reimbursement, and pay-for-performance requirements, and productivity measures that often failed to capture the unique and time-sensitive, holistic needs of fragile patients and families in crisis. As a leadership team, we began to strategize to ensure that we supported nurses and teams in providing care that was not simply technically excellent and evidence informed but theory-infused—informed by Caring Science, holding sacred and as evidence that which holds meaning for the patient, family, and community.

Dr. Jean Watson As Visiting Professor

Our first step was to invite Dr. Jean Watson to BWH as a visiting professor. As she began her presentation in her humble way using her singing bowl to ensure that we were centered and present as a collective community, we watched some eyebrows be raised in this Harvard-affiliated, academic medical center. By the end of the lecture, however, we witnessed a transformation of cynicism to tears. Jean connected nurses back to the core of why they had chosen the profession—to know their patients and to preserve and promote their patients' unique humanity through the experience of health and illness. Her theory was not only accessible to clinical nurses but also energizing to their hearts and spirits. Many nurses had witnessed profound human suffering over the course of their careers and without strategies to ensure care for self, and had shut down their hearts to survive and continue to provide expert, technical care. When we gaze into the face, the eyes, the experience of those we serve, we witness our own humanity and come face to face with our own vulnerability.

To continue this service requires self-care, courage, and compassion for ourselves as well as for others.

Nurses Becoming Caritas Coaches

As we learned more about Caring Science, we recognized the need to invest in local experts through the Watson Caring Science Institute (WCSI) Caritas Coach Education Program (CCEP). I (JGS) decided to enroll in the program and, with the encouragement and financial support of a very wise, philanthropic friend of the department, invited a clinical nurse colleague to join me on the journey. The strategy, to ensure that both formal leadership and clinical nurses were engaged in the learning process together, proved effective and was continued in future courses, creating a critical mass of experts to begin to infuse caring practices across the continuum of care.

Each dyad that was part of the CCEP challenged participants to implement theory-infused practices in their local, clinical setting. We recognized quickly the power of our wonderful nurse leaders and the need for them to care for themselves and each other or they too might risk shutting down their hearts and going through the motions. As Dr. Watson always affirms, it was an invitation for those ready to begin this very personal journey—not a mandate. "The decision to live by design rather than by default is a deeply personal one" (Pipe, 2017, p. xiii). We, including this chief nurse, gathered twice weekly, checking in with one another and offering support to those in need. We used the singing bowl and heart-centered breathing to ensure full presence and took turns offering leadership intentions to coworkers. It was often as simple as, "May we be fully present to every human soul–patient, family, ourselves, colleagues, and staff to ensure that they feel fully seen, heard, and valued." We committed to heart-centered breathing and repeating the intention at noon and at the end of the day. The practice has evolved and continues today.

Advent of Becoming A Caritas Scholar

In December 2014, BWH became an affiliate of WCSI to make public our commitment to infuse loving-kindness into our practice, a commitment to which we now would hold ourselves and expect others to hold us accountable.

That same year, I (Susan M. Lee [SML]) came to BWH as a senior nurse scientist while also studying as a postdoctoral fellow in WCSI with Dr. Watson. I was thrilled to continue my relationship with Dr. Watson at BWH. After the completion of the fellowship in 2015, I then became a Caritas Scholar, a name given to those who have completed advanced training in Caring Science. This dovetailed beautifully with BWH's goals to advance Caritas nursing, first among nurse leaders, and then throughout the institution. I was called upon to provide bimonthly seminars in which we organically developed the essence of Caritas leadership, expanding upon the Caritas Processes, described in the following text.

Building Upon Caring-Healing

The director and program manager of Caring and Healing Modalities began to explore how to bring the idea of self-care to our broader community, beyond the department of nursing. BWH was in need of intentional acts of healing, particularly after the Boston

Marathon bombing in 2013 and when a staff surgeon was shot and killed in the hospital by a distraught family member in 2015. BWH received many victims from the Boston Marathon bombing and cared for their peer in the wake of the shooting; staff across settings from the emergency department to the operating rooms to the intensive care unit not only witnessed the trauma of the victims and families but also experienced the trauma of their world being disrupted. Boston was a safe home to many and the BWH was truly a safe haven. These events shattered both of these assurances. In collaboration with the director of Occupational Health, drop-in sessions were held to provide staff access to mental health counselors, chaplains, Reiki, and other restorative modalities.

The group also began to infuse our science with a Caritas framework. They studied the impact of an auricular acupuncture intervention over the course of several weeks on stress and anxiety reduction in healthcare providers in a burn/trauma unit and sought to understand whether auricular acupuncture impacts provider capacity for developing caring relationships with patients (Reilly, Buchanan, Vafides, Breakey, & Dykes, 2014). Compared with baseline, participants had a significant reduction in state anxiety, trait anxiety, burnout, and secondary trauma scores, and significant increases were noted in courage and patience, two dimensions of the Caring Ability Inventory. They had made the case for why the investment in caring knowledge workers was critical to patients and organizational success.

Our Diversity and Inclusiveness Committee met with Dr. Watson and began to integrate Caring Science into its mission to ensure that every person—patient, family, and staff member—who entered any BWH door felt welcomed and cared for. It established a Lotus award, named by a BWH physician, to recognize and celebrate a formal leader, clinician, and a clinical and nonclinical support staff member who exemplified this ethic. The lotus symbolizes rebirth, the growth of pure beauty from the muddy water in which it is rooted. Its unfolding petals represent expanding consciousness and expansion of the soul.

Many other initiatives came from our growing cohort of Caritas Coaches including enlisting volunteer units to set an intention at the beginning of each shift, integrating nurse-presented personhood into medical rounds, and adopting loving-kindness toward self, peers, and patients by the interprofessional team in a primary care practice. Another strategy introduced by a clinical nurse Caritas Coach was to post one of the Caritas Processes over the entrance of each of the rooms on her 10-room unit.

CARITAS ROOMS

Caritas rooms began to appear across several of the BWH units. These tiny rooms became a tangible and symbolic sign of clinical nurses' commitment to self-care to bring their highest and best self to patients and peers. Each room reflected the unique culture of the unit but held some commonalities. There was a massage recliner, some soft music or nature sounds, dim lights, a reflection journal for staff to enter thoughts, and a book of poetry or positive affirmation cards. Staff would use these rooms intermittently throughout the day to regroup and center. It might be a way to begin their day before entering the sacred space of the care environment or to reflect after the death of a patient. It was inspiring to hear staff members who visited these spaces on a sister unit become champions to establish these sacred spaces within their own clinical unit.

Caritas HeartMath

The director and program manager for Caring and Healing Modalities, which includes the largest volunteer Reiki service in the country, stepped forward and became Certified Caritas HeartMath Trainers. They continue to offer monthly courses to interprofessional staff which are consistently, fully subscribed. Most often used to center self, stories of how this technique impacted patients began to emerge. The nurse director of a neuroscience intermediate care unit described a particularly compelling event of a patient whose escalating behaviors were threatening the safety of staff. One day, as she observed him beginning to escalate, she stood in the doorway of his room and coached him to close his eyes, to focus on the area in and around his heart, to place his hand over that spot, and to breathe in light and to breathe out gratitude. She watched him begin to deescalate and HeartMath, instead of security presence, became the first step in addressing his anxiety. Another patient described HeartMath as "what kept me alive" during the stress of an acute hospitalization.

As a leadership team, we continued to look for every opportunity to infuse Caring Science into the language and practice. As we onboarded graduate and doctoral students, we introduced Caring Science as a foundation for them to consider in guiding their theses, capstones, or dissertations. One compelling study (Hogan, 2016) observed high-risk case managers' interactions with their patients and discerned that the healing presence of the nurse, the nurse who cared about—not just provided care for—the patient, appeared to be the most impactful intervention from both the patient and the nurse perspective. In the sentiments of Annie Warburton Goodrich (1973), all nurses must speak with the language of science as well as that of the people.

RESEARCH

Caritas and HCAHPS Pilot

BWH participated in a nationwide pilot with Press Ganey that added the Watson Caritas Patient Scale (WCPS), a five-item scale designed to measure patients' perceptions of caring practices, to our postdischarge, patient satisfaction or Hospital Consumer Assessment of Healthcare Providers and Systems (HCAHPS) survey.

The WCPS rates patients' experiences with the following statements. My caregivers:

1. Deliver my care with loving-kindness.

2. Met my basic human needs with dignity.

3. Have helping and trusting relationships with me.

4. Create a caring environment that helps me to heal.

5. Value my personal beliefs and faith, allowing for hope.

The results demonstrated a high concordance between the Caritas Processes and the patient's experience of care as measured by HCAHPS.

CARITAS LEADERSHIP DEVELOPMENT AND RESEARCH

The importance of nurse leaders' influence on professional practice/work environments and patient and organizational outcomes has been well described (Adams & Ives Erickson, 2011). I (JGS) aimed to ensure that *caring* remained the central focus of the Department of Nursing (DON) at BWH. My overall aim was to improve the professional practice environment through leadership development. Infusing the Theory of Human Caring is directly aligned with the organization's "highest quality, safe care" commitment that bases a healthy work environment and the patient experience of care on the Caritas Processes.

I (JGS) sponsored the Leadership Seminar, a 2-hour, bimonthly forum funded and sponsored by the DON. It brings together the chief nursing officer (CNO) with the assistant chief nursing officers (ACNOs), nurse executive directors, nurse directors, and nursing program directors for ongoing leadership development and mentoring of members. Described in detail (Somerville, 2017), the incorporation of the Caritas Processes into the fabric of BWH is an ongoing, multipronged approach. In 2016, six intensive leadership development seminars took place. Baseline data were collected in March 2016 and postprocedure data were collected monthly after the conclusion of the intervention in 2016.

I (SML) served as faculty for the seminars, which were interactive forums that consisted of small group activities and didactic sessions. A main theme of the education was promoting respect in our professional practice environment, particularly around Caring leadership. An important component of our professional practice model is "true collaboration," which entails skilled, respectful, and effective communication. Many of the role-plays and other teachings concentrated on respectful communication. During this time, the Caritas Processes were applied as Caritas Leadership Practices.

The perceptions of nursing leaders were tracked over the course of the program to determine how these new concepts were being incorporated into their leadership practices. The Caring Factor Survey—Caring by Managers (Nelson & Watson, 2012), a 10-item, Likert-style self-report instrument, was adapted for use by asking nurse leaders to respond "as their staff would." Responses ranged from 1 (strongly disagree) to 7 (strongly agree). The two highest responses (agree and strongly agree) were tracked from baseline on each of the 10 items. Next, the mean scores were used to determine progress over time. Knowing that words in the Caritas Processes were unfamiliar to many nurses, or that they were not typically used in clinical conversations (e.g., "loving-kindness"), I (SML) developed a second instrument to determine the level of resonance with Caritas Processes over four time periods and found that nurse leaders achieved greater literacy (27% increase) and had indeed enacted these strategies in their practice.

CARING AND CIVILITY STUDY

We were interested to understand, as part of our professional value of caring, the current state of caring among nurses. We administered to 3,000 nurses the Caring Factor Survey: Caring for Co-Workers (Nelson & Watson, 2012) and the Negative Acts Questionnaire-Revised (NAQ-R; Einarsen, Hoel, & Notelaers, 2009) in the fall of 2015 to serve as a baseline prior to any caring interventions among staff. The Caring Factor Survey: Caring for

Co-Workers is a 10-item scale that is based on the 10 Caritas Processes, the language of which would be new to our nurses. Scores on the instrument ranged from 0 to 10 with higher scores indicating greater caring. A 7-point Likert scale, ranging from 0 = Strongly Disagree to 7 = Strongly Agree, was used. The instrument exhibited good reliability (Chronbach's alpha = 0.94). The NAQ-R is a 22-item, 5-point Likert scale that is weighted as follows: 0 = never; 2 = now and then; 6 = monthly; 25 = weekly; and 125 = daily with total scores ranging from 0 to 2,750. Weighted scores separate those actions that happen occasionally from those that happen daily or weekly, per the definition of bullying (Einarsen et al., 2009). Higher scores indicate more negative acts. The scale, used worldwide, exhibited good reliability (alpha Cronbach = 0.93). The study was deemed exempt by our institutional review board because it was an anonymous, online survey.

Item means of the Caring Factor Survey items ranged from 4.33 (SD = 1.6) to 5.34 (SD = 1.3; Table 28.1). Most of the 1,005 nurses who responded (mean age 45 [SD = 12.11]) were female (93%), non-Hispanic (97%), and White (91%), held a BS in Nursing, and had over 10-year (71.2%) tenure.

TABLE 28.1 Caring Factor Survey: Caring for Coworkers

Items	Mean (SD)
1. My coworkers acknowledge and respect my belief system.	5.34 (1.3)
2. My coworkers have established a helping and trusting relationship with me.	5.33 (1.5)
3. As a team, my coworkers are good at creative problem solving to meet each other's individual needs and requests.	5.30 (1.4)
4. When part or all of the team needs to learn something new, my coworkers are good at making sure we use teaching methods that everyone will understand.	5.19 (1.4)
5. My coworkers respond to me as a whole person, helping me respond to all my needs and concerns.	4.96 (1.5)
6. Every day I am here, I see staff members caring for each other with loving-kindness.	4.92 (1.6)
7. I feel that I can talk openly and honestly about what I am thinking, because my coworkers respect my feelings, no matter what my feelings are.	4.63 (1.7)
8. My coworkers encourage me to practice my own spiritual beliefs that are part of my self-caring and healing.	4.61 (1.4)
9. My coworkers acknowledge and are supportive of my beliefs regarding a higher power.	4.57 (1.3)
10. Our healthcare team always seeks to create a healing environment that recognizes the connections between body, mind, and spirit.	4.33 (1.6)

Key: Range: 1 to 7 (1 = strongly disagree to 7 = strongly agree).

The mean score for the NAQ-R was 63.60 that indicated a very low level of nurse-to-nurse lateral violence. We found our scores to be lower than or equal to those of other published findings (Olender, 2013; Simons, 2008). As expected, among both male and female nurses, caring was inversely related to negative acts (r = −.442, p = .000); nurses who perceived caring from coworkers were less likely to perceive nurse-to-nurse lateral violence. The top three reported negative acts were of particular interest to us, which were as follows: (a) being ignored or excluded, (b) having opinions or views ignored, and (c) spreading gossip and rumors about you.

The survey also provided space for the respondents to comment after each item. The qualitative data were analyzed into themes, again, to promote understanding of the culture of the organization. The qualitative themes extended our understanding of the quantitative findings and included descriptions of (a) hurtful behaviors by coworkers, (b) poor teamwork, and (c) cliques that caused nurses to feel excluded and ignored.

We believe that research findings must be shared with nurse-participants as a means to foster dialogue and understanding. We shared the findings in several meetings, including nursing grand rounds. Finally, we compared our findings with our values in the BWH professional practice model. Findings solidified our commitment to caring and inclusivity that will continue to be the North Star for the department of nursing.

CONCLUSION

In this chapter, we have provided a blueprint for Caritas Health "Care," hoping this will be helpful to those who are interested in building caring literacy among frontline professional staff (Lee, 2017; Somerville, 2017). I (JGS) chose to first implement caring at the leadership level to promote fluency and authenticity among middle and senior levels prior to full-scale implementation. Not everyone will choose to follow a caring philosophy (Watson, 2008), but we have been encouraged by the admirable and innovative work that many leaders and clinical nurses have initiated and sustained on our units. I recall a comment from a nurse director who said that she believed the adoption of caring led to care that was "different." The care, she believed, was intentional, and similar to Pipe's (2017) notions—it happens by design and not simply by default to regulatory requirements and tasks delegated to nurses by other disciplines. She described a sense of reclaiming nursing's role and contribution in a collaborative team as well as in their autonomous nursing practice. In this nursing director's words: "It's who we are and how we choose to bring ourselves to our practice. Once your heart and eyes are opened, you can never go back."

We believe, as Jones stated at the start of the chapter, that nursing is uniquely positioned to bring "health" back to the healthcare system. "We are moving from attention to the patient as an object to attention to the we in relationship, from fixing things to attending to the meaning of the whole ... It is time to break with a paradigm [focused] on power, manipulation, and control and move to one of reflective, compassionate consciousness" (Newman & Jones, 2007, p. 122). This is what society is demanding and we have the knowledge to meet their call. We have, as Dr. Watson points out, a responsibility to repattern the healthcare system. If we as nurse professionals and leaders do not seize this opportunity and return to our caring roots, others will be accountable for shaping the system and nursing's role in the future.

NEXT ERA POSSIBILITIES

Education

- How can graduate nursing education be expanded to include Caritas leadership principles?
- What are the best ways to integrate Caritas leadership principles into the service setting?

Research

- What methodologies can be developed to capture caring systems–level changes?
- What measures will help to establish a business model for caring?

Praxis

- What are the essential components of caring that should be captured in electronic medical records to make caring explicit?
- What are the most effective strategies to integrate care for selves and teams in the service setting?

Theory and Knowledge Development

- How can we advance the theory of Caritas leadership so that it is easily translated to the practice environment at both leadership and clinical levels?
- How do we advance unique knowledge of embodied spirit as a valued and unique source of evidence, integrating theory-infused and evidence-informed care?

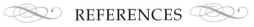 REFERENCES

Adams, J. M. (2017). The influence of emerging nursing administrative and leadership researchers: An interview with Dr. Lesly Kelly. *Journal of Nursing Administration, 47,* 79–81. doi:10.1097/NNA.0000000000000442

Adams, J. M., & Erickson, J. I. (2011). Applying the Adams influence model in nurse executive practice. *Journal of Nursing Administration, 41,* 186–192. doi:10.1097/NNA.0b013e3182118736

Einarsen, S., Hoel, H., & Notelaers, G. (2009). Measuring exposure to bullying and harassment at work: Validity, factor structure and psychometric properties of the Negative Acts Questionnaire-Revised. *Work & Stress, 23*(1), 24–44. doi:10.1080/02678370902815673

Goodrich, A. (1973). *The social and ethical significance of nursing.* New Haven, CT: Yale University School of Nursing.

Hogan, J. (2016). *Examining caring behaviors of RN care coordinators in complex care management* (Unpublished doctoral dissertation). Massachusetts General Hospital Institute for Health Professions, Charlestown.

Jones, D. (2007). A synthesis of philosophical perspectives for knowledge development. In C. Roy & D. A. Jones (Eds.), *Nursing knowledge development and clinical practice* (pp. 163–176). New York, NY: Springer Publishing.

Kovner, C. T., Brewer, C. S., Fatehi, F., & Jun, J. (2014). What does nurse turnover rate mean and what is the rate? *Policy, Politics and Nursing Practice, 15*(3-4), 64–71. doi:10.1177/1527154414547953

Lee, S. M. (2017). Advancing Caritas literacy in practice, education, and health systems. In S. M. Lee, P. A. Palmieri, & J. Watson (Eds.), *Global advances in human caring literacy* (pp. 13–21). New York, NY: Springer Publishing.

Nelson, J. W., & Watson, J. (2012). *Caring: International research on Caritas as healing.* New York, NY: Springer Publishing.

Newman, M. A., & Jones, D. A. (2007). Experiencing the whole: Health as expanding consciousness (State of the Art). In C. Roy & D. A. Jones (Eds.), *Nursing knowledge development and clinical practice* (pp. 119–128). New York, NY: Springer Publishing.

Olender, L. D. (2013). *Nurse manager caring and workplace bullying in nursing: The relationship between staff nurses' perceptions of nurse manager caring behaviors and their perceptions of exposure to workplace bullying within multiple healthcare settings* (Unpublished doctoral dissertation). Seton Hall University, South Orange, NJ.

Osler, W. (1963). *Aequanimitas*. New York, NY: W. W. Norton.

Pipe, T. (2017). Foreword. In S. M. Lee, P. A. Palmieri, & J. Watson (Eds.), *Global advances in human caring literacy* (pp. xiii–xiv). New York, NY: Springer Publishing.

Porter-O'Grady, T. (2017). A response to the question of professional governance versus shared governance. *Journal of Nursing Administration, 47*(2), 69–71. doi:10.1097/NNA.0000000000000439

Reilly, P. M., Buchanan, T. M., Vafides, C., Breakey, S., & Dykes, P. (2014). Auricular acupuncture to relieve health care workers' stress and anxiety: Impact on caring. *Dimensions of Critical Care Nursing, 33*(3), 151–159. doi:10.1097/DCC.0000000000000039

Schwartz Center. (2017). Understanding what patients want. Retrieved from http://www.theschwartzcenter.org/partnering-with-patients/understanding-what-patients-want

Simons, S. (2008). Workplace bullying experienced by Massachusetts registered nurses and the relationship to intention to leave the organization. *Advances in Nursing Science, 31*(2), E48–E59. doi:10.1097/01.ANS.0000319571.37373.d7

Somerville, J. (2009). Development and psychometric evaluation of Patients' Perceptions of Feeling Known by their Nurses (PPFKN) Scale. *International Journal of Human Caring, 13*, 27–43.

Somerville, J. (2017). Creating intentionality and heart-centered leadership in the hospital setting. In S. M. Lee, P. A. Palmieri, & J. Watson (Eds.), *Global advances in human caring literacy* (pp. 89–99). New York, NY: Springer Publishing.

Watson, J. (2008). *Nursing: The philosophy and science of caring* (Rev. ed.). Boulder: University Press of Colorado.

29

Kaiser Permanente Patient Care Services Northern California: The Adaptation of Caring Science

Anne M. Foss-Durant and Shawna M. McDermott

CARITAS LITERACIES

By the end of this chapter, the caring-healing nurse will be able to

1. Identify the characteristics and responsibilities of Caritas leaders at all levels of the organization in creating environments that support and sustain an ethic of human caring in day-to-day operations.

2. Develop an understanding of key strategies, tactics, and methods that can be implemented when transforming systems to caring-healing "total health"–oriented environments.

3. Appreciate the various sources of evidence used to assess and measure transformation and return on investment as the creation of a human-caring organizational culture unfolds.

4. Develop an understanding of how to frame and respond to Human Resource (HR) concerns and business/financial needs of the organization, demonstrating the value of fostering a caring ethic.

This chapter is intended to share the processes used to integrate Caring Science across a hospital system in Northern California. "When we human beings want to understand or describe singular people in particular situations that unfold over time, we reach naturally for narrative, or storytelling, to do so" (Charon, 2006, p. vii). Narrative is a powerful tool for adult and organizational learning, and is often underutilized in favor of empirical science and data. By sharing the narrative of our journey, we hope to allow others to see new possibilities for their organizations.

This is not the work of one individual; it was the work of a small number of individuals whose hearts resonated with Caring Science, who dedicated time to become involved and pursued advanced learning and Caritas teaching. I would be remiss if I did not recognize the contributions of the following individuals:

- Esther Kearn Frolich, who was my colleague in this work at the beginning

- Linda Ackerman, who joined Esther and me on the Caring Science journey from the Maternal Child perspective

- Shawna McDermott, a caring spirit who assisted in guiding the process at the system level. She was my thought partner and codesigner of the work at a regional level

- Gwen Kinney and Trudy Triner, who joined Shawna and me in our multicenter integration

- Anita Zuniga and Sandy Small, for taking the risk on a new idea and whole-heartedly supporting the implementation at a senior leadership level

- Jim N. D'Alfonso, who collaborated with Kaiser to pilot the Level I Human Caring Program (HCP). Jim now oversees the future work of Caring Science in Kaiser Permanente Patient Care Services (PCS), Northern California

- All of the Caritas Coaches, HeartMath Trainers, and Level I graduates in the Kaiser system who keep this work alive at their local medical centers

IN THE BEGINNING

In 2004/2005, California was beginning to implement a nurse-to-patient ratio law applicable to inpatient hospital settings. The staffing requirements for nursing provided an opportunity to reestablish the role of the RN as central to the coordination of patient care and quality of care in the inpatient setting. The law specified minimum RN staffing for defined types of units. For example, in a 24-bed medical surgical unit, there would be no more than five patients assigned to each RN each shift; in addition, there would be a requirement to have an unencumbered nurse available to relieve each nurse for meal periods and breaks. In essence, this law "skilled up the workforce"; where we once had three teams of a nurse paired with a nursing assistant on a 24-bed unit and varied staffing across the shifts, we would now have six nurses on the same-size unit, capable of the full scope of nursing practice across all shifts, five in direct care and one available to relieve for breaks and lunches. This change required that we begin to think differently about how care at the bedside was being delivered.

The nursing leaders at Kaiser Permanente Vallejo used this opportunity to examine how we could improve the care of our patients, and how we could become more "service oriented" or patient focused. In our minds, these were two separate and yet overlapping work streams, transition to a new staffing model and also an opportunity to implement a professional practice nursing model. These two work streams often were muddled as the same nursing leaders worked on the logistics of staffing at the higher nurse-to-patient ratio and cocreated how to design a practice model that was patient centric. The chief nursing officer and the clinical nursing directors led this work. As I reflect back, this confusion across these two work streams, particularly for the non-nursing leaders, may have contributed to the low level of executive support for this work.

We began the professional practice model design by developing an understanding of "what was," the values, behaviors, and practices that shaped nursing culture within Kaiser Permanente Vallejo. Accordingly, the clinical nursing directors sought to gain staff's perspective on the challenges and issues they faced day to day, obtaining data through interviews, simulations, and shadowing exercises. We engaged in dialogue with direct care nurses, nursing assistants, and managers to develop a clear model for what nursing practice looked like at that point in time.

We learned the following:

- There was a lot of activity on the units, yet not a lot of nursing care.
  - Nurses were drawing labs, running to get supplies or medications that were not stocked on the unit.
  - They would leave the unit to obtain dietary trays for patients waiting for nourishment.

- Nurses were anxious and defeated before they even looked at their assignments, feeling overwhelmed and dispirited at the long list of tasks.
  - They were unable to prioritize patient needs. They blindly worked through an endless checklist of tasks, hoping to complete "all of their assigned duties" by the end of their shifts.
  - When they entered a room, they never stopped or acknowledged the person in the bed. They simply focused on what they needed to get completed and then left the patient's room, going on to the next task.

- They were showing signs of compassion fatigue: Some reported feeling ill as they drove to work. Others spoke of being overwhelmed and would delay leaving the report room as they knew they could not possibly get everything completed.
  - The leadership team was equally as overwhelmed, not knowing how to begin to solve the problem and unsure whether anyone even recognized the issues.

The director group began contemplating how the characteristics of a Magnet®-designated Hospital were similar to our desired future state. Nurses who work in Magnet-designated hospitals are engaged and participate in decision making; they take pride in continual learning and pursue higher education and certifications and look for opportunities to research clinical issues or apply research in the practice setting. Although the Magnet journey was not embraced by our organization, the directors explored what it might mean if we were to be more similar to a Magnet facility, realizing there was benefit in the process even if we had no intention of submitting a formal application.

We began our exploration by sending one director to a Magnet conference, Linda Ackerman. The goal was to develop a rudimentary understanding of the Forces of Magnetism, assess if our thinking was on track, and look for examples of how other organizations began this process. When she returned, she shared her observations.

Every Magnet facility had a theory that they adopted to guide nursing professional practice:

- Most organizations adopted or at least referred to the Theory of Human Caring by Dr. Jean Watson.

- Many of the organizations that had chosen the Theory of Human Caring had invited Dr. Watson to their medical center for site visits.

- Organizations with a spiritual affiliation tended to do better engaging the staff in the organizational mission and vision and the associated value of providing patient-centric care.

- The engagement of frontline nursing staff was critical to the success of the organizations in achieving both high performing reliability and a successful Magnet survey process.

Hearing this, the directors began contemplating the question of adopting a theory-guided practice model. It was at that moment that Esther informed the group that we had already selected a theory; it was the Theory of Human Caring by Dr. Jean Watson. We were all surprised: How was it that we had adopted a theory of practice, yet none of the leaders were aware of or able to articulate how our practice was guided by this theory? We were certain our nurses had no knowledge of this either.

Theory provides the framework from which nursing practice is developed. It provides context and common language for the work of nursing and assists in developing a prioritization for the work with some activities more central to care than others. Our next steps became evident: We needed to educate the leadership, our frontline staff, and key stakeholders on the theory, and we needed to consider how to purposefully link the Theory of Human Caring to the strategic and operational priorities of the organization. The question in the room was how to begin: Should we purchase Jean Watson's book *Nursing: The Philosophy and Science of Caring* (2008) for all of our nurses and require they read it; should we hold journal or book club sessions to discuss components of Human Caring Science; or should we forgo the staff reading and provide classes on the Human Caring Theory and how it related to practice? Linda offered that at the Magnet Conference, many organizations had success by inviting Dr. Watson to visit. Organizations reported that Dr. Watson was able to support frontline staff in grasping the concepts and constructs of the Theory of Human Caring from an intellectual, emotional, and spiritual level of understanding.

The director group decided that Esther would reach out to Dr. Watson. Dr. Watson personally responded that she would be happy to travel to our medical center. Esther's passion was reignited; she relished the idea of doing this work and potentially leaving a legacy for the nurses at Kaiser Permanente Vallejo. This work clearly aligned with her core being. After a few planning phone calls, where we shared our current situation and discussed our hopes and vision for nursing in Kaiser Permanente Vallejo, Dr. Watson offered to lead an 8-hour conference where she could introduce the theory, provide exemplars from other organizations using her theory, and conduct an appreciative inquiry exercise to engage the staff in defining our future state. She titled the conference "Taking Time to Make Time." We quickly confirmed dates for the fall of 2006.

The conference was held off-site; we rarely took our staff off-site for events. The registration for the conference was greater than anticipated. As a leader, it was heartwarming and encouraging to see the engagement in the room. Many of the staff had heard of Dr. Watson; some staff had used her work in their nursing school projects and were honored to meet her in person. They were attentive and comfortable enough to speak openly, sharing their reality and pain as well as their hopes for the future. I personally left the conference with renewed hope that it would be possible to change the nursing culture for the betterment of the patients and staff and filled with energy to carry this work forward.

On the basis of some of the exemplars presented at the conference, touchstones and evidence of Human Caring Theory began to appear in each of the units: blessing baskets, centering moment practices, and reminders to assist with centering practices for staff, families, and patients. Only a small fraction of the entire staff had the opportunity to attend the conference, yet those individuals assisted in bringing forward the Theory of Human Caring in daily practice. It was difficult work, having to "reinvent" who we were as a nursing service—there was limited time to do this work as there were a multitude of other organizational priorities. It was slow to see gains and required tenacity for everyone involved.

Our vision and efforts were still largely invisible to the executives of the medical center. As we focused on realizing "Our Destiny," as the staff described it during appreciative inquiry exercises, the patient satisfaction scores slowly began to rise. Just 6 months from the conference with Dr. Watson, Vallejo Medical Center achieved a significant improvement in the spring patient satisfaction scores that was unprecedented in the history of the medical center (Watson, 2009). This received the attention of executive leadership, and they began to explore to what these results might be attributed.

OPPORTUNITY

In 2007, Kaiser was opening a new medical center in the Diablo Service Area, much closer to where both Linda and I lived. The invitation to instill Caring Science as the foundation of nursing practice at a new medical center was irresistible for Linda and me. Esther joined; despite a long commute, she could not resist the opportunity to continue what we had started in Vallejo. In March 2007, Linda, Esther, and I transferred to the Antioch Medical Center (AMC), assisting to open a newly constructed 150-bed community hospital. Enlightened by our learnings at Vallejo, we set out to support the senior leader team.

We spent our first month orienting to the new facility, while orienting our colleagues and the senior leaders to Caring Science. Although supportive and engaged at the idea, the cost associated with opening was running above budget, and we were asked to delay bringing in Caring Science for 1 year. Esther, Linda, and I believed this would create the same situation we faced in Vallejo, having to overcome an ingrained culture versus setting the culture from the beginning. This was the reason we chose to transfer to the AMC. Committed to our vision, we cocreated a solution for an onboarding and orientation process that was cost neutral yet allowed us to educate the staff on the concepts and constructs of Caring Science.

The directors decided to incorporate content of Caring Science into every aspect of the organization, including the hiring and orientation process. We began intentionally hiring for compassion, creating standard questions to ask every applicant: from bedside nurses, nursing assistants, and respiratory care practitioners to our managers, assistant managers, and even our administrative staff. We developed the following questions (Foss-Durant & Kearn-Frolich, 2008):

- We aspire to create a compassionate, healing environment, centered around caring for the individual patient and family, congruent with their needs for comfort, safety, dignity, and respect, reflective of the patient's and family's culture and values.
  - How will you deliver this?

- The Kaiser strategic plan includes implementing a compassionate service culture.
  - How would you describe compassionate care? Can you give an example of a caring moment?

- At Antioch we are attempting to build a culture of excellence. We view care through the eyes of our patients.
  - How would you motivate your staff to focus less on the tasks and more on the "whole" patients? How would you handle resistance to this?

- Describe in detail a past work situation where your personal workload felt overwhelming and a peer asked you for help.
  - How did you handle it?

- Tell us about a work situation of which you are most proud. What determined your success?

Having developed a structure for the hiring process, we turned our attention to onboarding and orientation. There were several requirements that needed to be met for the hospital opening:

- Regulatory: Every staff member needed to be signed off on every piece of equipment, participate in emergency drills (code blue and fire), and be knowledgeable about workflows and policy and procedures.

- Way finding: Staff needed to learn how to navigate the facility and how to assist our patients, members, and visitors.

- Budget: Training needed to come in under budgeted hours.

- Time: Training needed to be completed by the end of October as we anticipated licensing survey the first week of November.

A simpler solution was to incorporate Caring Science language in our Policies and Procedures, specifically calling out the principles of the theory. We also knew staff needed to be able to speak the language we used. Thus, it was important to provide some basic education in Caring Science, sharing examples of how practice might look different when using the core concepts of Caring Science.

Rather than attempt to educate to the entire theory, the directors decided to begin by creating a progressive series of Caring Science modules, the first one introducing core concepts. We would develop annual content—this allowed us the time to more thoughtfully develop content and meet our needs in opening the medical center. We also believed we could achieve better understanding of the theory at the frontline staff level. Our first module used in orientation was limited to understanding three core concepts of Caring Science: authenticity, compassion, and Ethics of Face. We coined the term "Antioch Care Experience" Model or ACE. This module was introduced using a 2-hour leadership session during new employee orientation, highlighting the 12-year journey of the medical center from idea to construction, the promise to the community that they would no longer need to travel over "the hill" or bridge for healthcare, and an overview of each service line and the service line-specific commitment to patient-centric care. We designed a pin that was presented to each staff member who completed the leadership session. The orientation content was reviewed with the senior leaders, engaging them, insuring support, and providing opportunities to participate and share their views with the staff directly. AMC opened on November 7, 2007.

While we were in the process of opening AMC, the directors began participating in Caritas consortiums at the invitation of Dr. Watson. This was an opportunity for organizations working with Caring Science as a foundation for practice to come together and learn from each other. The group was small at that time. Consortiums were held in the fall and spring at hosting organizations. It was here that we met key partners who assisted us in future transformation and integration efforts: Jim D'Alfonso, Karen Drenkard, Linda Ryan, Barbara Brewer, and Lynne Wagner; these individuals became mentors and guides on our journey. We continued to keep in contact with Dr. Watson, updating her on our progress and methods as we were clearly "creating the road before us."

After well-deserved rest during the holiday season, we began 2008 with a continued focus on the need to enhance Caring Science education at AMC. We continued to use the ACE concepts and added content on creating healing environments at the unit level. Rather than delivering classroom-based content, we chose to create a competency for management: creating a healing environment for patients and staff. The competency included the following:

- Reading Chapters 1 and 2 of *Relationship-Based Care* by Mary Kolroutis (2012)

- Conducting an Appreciative Inquiry with staff

- Adjusting unit routines to provide a healing environment; for example, adjusting vital signs to reduce interruption allowing adequate rest for patients, handwashing rituals to provide space between patients, or pausing before entering a patient's room to let go and focus

- Submitting written documentation of the changes to the service director

The work we were doing was beginning to become evident in every aspect of our medical center. Our patient satisfaction, quality, and safety metrics were the top of the Northern California region that now included 21 medical centers.

We collaborated with other medical centers to share our journey and began presenting the work we were doing at various regionally organized management peer groups. It was unfamiliar for leaders to hear that Caring Science was a way of being, a personal and professional journey into which one entered, almost as if each person was creating a covenant with oneself. There was nothing concrete or prescribed to "give them"; it clearly was not the typical plan-do-study-act (PDSA) playbook implementation. We could simply "invite them" to participate in discovery and reflection and see where that would lead.

At AMC, we continued to evolve in Caring Science. Building upon the healing environment work in 2008, our focus in 2009 was exploring centering practices. Each unit was encouraged and supported to create a centering practice that frontline staff could use in daily practice. Units developed unique practices that were meaningful to them; these ranged from tea for the soul rituals to the creation of Caritas lounges for staff as well as for family members and visitors.

Early in the year, Dr. Watson and Robert Browning visited our leadership team, discussing their idea of developing an affiliation between HeartMath and Caring Science. I was very interested in supporting the use of HeartMath technology and science in the Caring Science journey. In August, HeartMath and Watson Caring Science Institute (WCSI) launched the Caritas HeartMath National Pilot at AMC. This was a gift to our staff who participated; the methodologies and tools shared for managing stress were relevant in not only the work setting but their personal lives as well. They truly felt appreciative that the organization took interest in them beyond their work and allowed them to attend the event.

As 2009 progressed, there was a need identified to create a deeper understanding of Caring Science for the individuals leading this work. The continued alignment of theory and practice required more expertise. Both Esther and I enrolled in the second cohort of the Caritas Coach Education Program (CCEP), a 6-month immersion in Caring Science offered by WCSI. The focus of my journey was on creating and mentoring Caritas leaders, whereas Esther focused on the importance of self-care: both concepts of equal merit when creating environments that support Caring Science practices at the bedside. After completing the CCEP in October 2009, I immediately went on to HeartMath Training in Boulder Creek, California. AMC now had two certified Caritas Coaches and one certified Heart-Math trainer.

AMC continued to perform exceedingly well in all areas of patient satisfaction. Typically, new hospitals experience exceptional performance for about 6 months, after which the newness wears off and performance begins to decline. AMC was setting a new trend. We began receiving invitations to present Caring Science to multiple audiences over the year—The Chief Nursing Officer Peer Group, Regional Executive Teams, and National PCS all had an interest in our journey. In October, Esther and I were invited to be CCEP Faculty and in November Esther joined the East Bay Service Area to bring Caring Science to the Oakland and Richmond Medical Centers.

The work continued at AMC; our plan for 2010 was to develop an understanding of the Caritas Processes®, having educated on authenticity, healing environments, and centering practices in the subsequent years. Each unit at AMC was assigned the task of reviewing the Caritas Processes, discussing how they are exemplified in practice, and then selecting one that best represented the work of the unit. Once identified, a poster was created to explain the process and how the process relates to the work of the unit. Our nursing leadership team scheduled Dr. Watson to visit in the latter half of the year to view the posters.

About this time, the Board of Directors began to ask why AMC seemed to be a positive deviant. They encouraged a deeper dive into what made AMC perform so well and established expectation that whatever the cause, Northern California was to begin spreading the process throughout the region. The diagnostic review determined that the only difference between AMC and the 20 other medical centers was the use of Caring Science to guide practice. In April 2010, AMC hosted the 12th WCSI International Caritas Consortium (ICC). Anita Zuniga, vice president of PCS in Northern California, was in attendance. ICC offered 2 days of inspiring speakers who reconnected each individual with the heart of his or her profession. Many of the Antioch staff attended. Anita left the event wanting each of the nurses in Northern California to have a similar experience. She worked with Sandy Small, senior vice president of Hospital Operations in Northern California, to plan a regional-wide implementation of Caring Science.

SYSTEM-WIDE IMPLEMENTATION

Following the Kaiser ICC, our regional president gathered all of the chief executive officers (CEOs), chief operating officers (COOs), and chief nursing officers (CNOs) from across the 21 medical centers for a full-day event to hear about Caring Science from Dr. Watson and Robert Browning from HeartMath. He formally announced the use of Caring Science as the foundation for professional nursing practice in Northern California, a significant statement and endorsement by the highest level of leadership in our Northern California Region. This full-day event was immediately followed by a 2-day immersion for the CNOs across Northern California in Caring Science and HeartMath. It was expected that the CNOs, as the leaders of patient care, would be accountable for embedding Caring Science in practice at the medical center level. I was offered the position of leading the integration of Caring Science across the Northern California region. It would be my role to provide consultation, education, tools, guidance, and continued learnings to guide and support their efforts.

"A Journey of a Thousand Miles Begins With One Step"—Lao Tzu

Leading the integration of Caring Science across 21 medical centers with 21 unique cultures in 19 different market areas presented a new set of challenges. There were no prior examples of a system-wide integration of Caring Science. The typical Kaiser Permanente, Northern California, methodology of improvement was to conduct iterative PDSA cycles, and develop a playbook with the expectation that each medical center implement the playbook without variation. We would track process and outcome measures and compare the medical centers to see which were the best performers. This process was not going to lend itself well to the integration of Caring Science—we needed a different approach. As Dr. Watson describes this work, it is a transformational process of being and becoming, not mandating and prescribing.

There were limited tools or defined processes for integrating Caring Science into practice. It was my vision that Caring Science become the fabric of the organization, that Caring Science become embedded in everything we do. When I transitioned into my role within regional PCS, I had the gift of working with Shawna, whose essence exudes Caring Science. Shawna, who had a nonclinical background in business administration and strategy consulting, was a key partner in developing the strategy and content for what became known as our Caring Science Integration program. We were committed to developing an organic approach, one that allowed medical centers to understand Caring Science and, on the basis of their inquiry, choose where to begin.

Our first phases provided opportunities for direct line management and educational teams to come together and develop an understanding of Caring Science from Dr. Watson and Robert Browning in management forums. Once the management forums were completed, we moved forward to staff forums aimed at educating and inspiring the direct care staff. At the end of each of the staff forums, the attendees were asked to share one word that best expressed how they were feeling about the journey to embed Caring Science within Kaiser. We used "wordles" (Figure 29.1) to understand the staff readiness for the Caring Science journey. Wordles captures the frequency of similar response; the larger and bolder a word appears in the cloud, the more frequently it was mentioned. A vast majority of staff felt hopeful and inspired, although some expressed frustration and concern about feasibility and level of leadership support.

To develop accountability at the medical center level, aligning strategic focus and encouraging the work, organizational performance goals were established in 2010 that

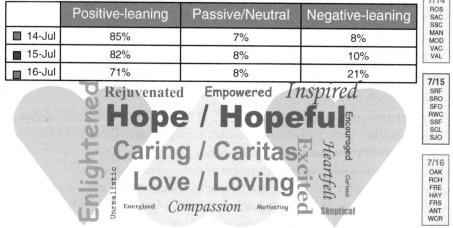

FIGURE 29.1 Staff RN forum—feedback.

supported Caring Science Integration. The goal explicitly required medical center leadership to do the following:

1. Schedule a medical center Caring Science kickoff by August 20 (I consulted with each CNO and assisted with the presentations for each of the kickoff meetings)

2. Add Caring Science questions to the standard interview questions for all PCS candidates by the end of third quarter (September 30); examples included:
   a. Please share an example of a "Caring Moment" you have experienced personally.
   b. Our vision for Patient Care is to create a "caring" experience for each and every patient in our hospital. How will you personally deliver this to ensure a "Caring Culture"?

3. Establish Caring Science Advisory Councils chartered to guide the integration process locally by the end of third quarter (September 30)

4. Have 30% of the inpatient units adopt at least one Caring Healing modality by the end of the year

5. Additional efforts were focused on creating local expertise by enrolling staff in the CCEP offered by WCSI or enrolling staff in a Level I HCP

The Level 1 HCP was a pilot developed in partnership with Jim D'Alfonso and WCSI faculty. I had reached out to Jim to discuss the need for an intermediate class, one that was less intensive than the CCEP and more advanced than the introductions to Caring Science we had been conducting. I was interested in using experiential learning methods. I had secured funding for a pilot program that would bring together four medical centers with a total of 60 participants, focused primarily on frontline RN staff. The objectives included providing more in-depth education on the broader scope of Caring Science and HeartMath, a practicum on how to apply caring healing modalities in their care setting, and a future planning session. We envisioned the staff who completed these sessions leading the integration efforts at their local medical centers.

In conjunction with WCSI, a 2.5-day HCP was developed and held in Oakland in September, with the opportunity to participate in ongoing webinar sessions for continued skill development and networking. Although our original pilot focused efforts on four of the 21 medical centers, the transformation felt by participants at a personal and professional level during these sessions was so dramatic that we were granted funds to conduct HCPs for all of the medical centers. To accommodate the remaining medical centers, three additional HCPs were conducted over the next 7 months (until April 2011).

As 2011 approached, we began framing Caring Science in the context of four key relationships: the traditional care relationship with the patients and their family members, the relationship with self, the relationship with the patient care team, and the relationship with the community or "communitas," as Dr. Watson would say. With the context of these four relationships, we created four leadership modules with the assistance of Trudy Triner, an Organizational Effectiveness, Learning, and Development specialist. It was one of our highest organizational priorities to support our first-level PCS managers in gaining greater awareness, comfort, and ability to lead from a Caring Science framework. Nurse managers and assistant nurse managers serve as the primary conduit for linking the efforts of front-line staff and executive leaders to create and sustain a Caring Sciences foundation. The outline of the four modules is as follows:

- Relationship With Self
  - Learn the background and content of Caring Science.
  - Understand the importance of Caring Science and its application to the future of Kaiser Permanente.
  - Understand the importance of the assistant nurse manager (ANM) and nurse manager (NM) roles and techniques for managing the transitions.
  - Gain awareness of the 14 attributes of a Caritas Leader.
  - Practice techniques for self-care.

- Relationship With Patient Care Team
  - Translate the principles of management and leadership into a Caritas Leader Framework.
  - Practice using authentic, heart-centered communications.
  - Create a compelling vision for your unit.
  - Practice using appropriate feedback to motivate and develop others.
  - Practice managing conflict effectively.
  - Develop an understanding of work style, your own and others, and the knowledge to adjust your style.
  - Develop comfort in discussing Caring Science with your team.

- Relationship With Patients and Family
  - Comfortably use rounding on patients to shape the care experience.
  - Listen authentically to patients and family.
  - Take specific steps when patient expectations are not met.
  - Recognize caring and uncaring behaviors and language.
  - Coach and mentor caring behaviors.

- Relationship With Medical Center Leaders and Community
  - Explore the roles of the ANM and NM as they relate to Medical Center Leadership and the communities we serve from a Caring Science/Caritas Leader framework.

Each module was accompanied by a reflective exercise using a set of guiding principles designed to allow participants to develop understanding of areas where they exemplified Caring Science in their administrative practice of nursing and to discover areas for growth. Specifically, four guiding inquiry questions were used to frame reflection and discussion:

- What does it mean to lead/practice with care?

- How do I align my actions and my words?

- How do I align mind-body-spirit and cocreate a healing environment?

- How do I communicate authentically and express my values and beliefs every day?

EARLY MEASUREMENT

We trialed three instruments in August 2010 as a baseline measure and again in August 2011 to obtain feedback from staff on the use of caring behaviors and the practice environment. The three tools were established survey instruments:

- Jan Nyberg: Caring Assessment Scale ("Nurse Manager Feedback")

- Eileen Lake: Practice Environment Scale of the Nursing Work Index

- Paula Stamps: Nurses and Work Satisfaction Index

Response rates were small (300), less than 10%. We stopped the surveys after 2011 because of the low response rate. There was a perception that the organization was creating "survey fatigue" as we were releasing three surveys across the region in the same time period. The comparative results of the Stamps survey depicted in Figure 29.2 are of interest.

For a detailed discussion on process and outcomes, I refer you to an article in the 2015 fall edition of the *Permanente Journal* titled "Transforming the Ethic of Caring-Healing Practice, Environment and Culture within an Integrated Care Delivery System" (2015).

DEVELOPING A PRACTICE MODEL

In 2012, I was urged to create a Caring Science Practice Model by the senior executives with the expressed intent to reinforce Caring Science expression in daily practice, action, and decision making. After multiple brainstorming sessions and attempts, we turned our

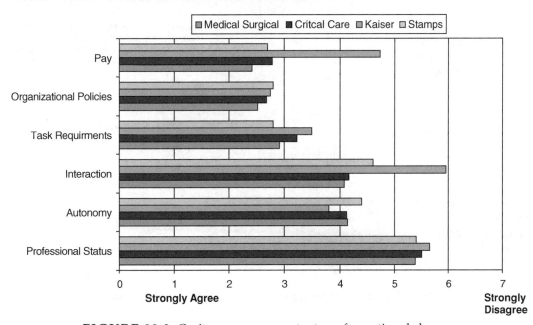

FIGURE 29.2 Caritas measurement—transformational change.

attention to the basis of nursing practice: the nursing process, taught by every school of nursing at every level of education. Once the decision to align with the nursing process was made, it was not difficult to interpret Dr. Watson's work through the lens of the Nursing Process. Examples of this work are found in Figure 29.3.

To assist nursing leaders at the medical centers to introduce the practice model, we created a series of concise and cohesive "Caring Science in Action" learning modules. These modules provided consistent content for educational sessions and dialogue with the direct care staff across the 21 individual sites. We began by reviewing the rationale for using theory in practice as an organizing framework that builds common terminology and provides language for describing and explaining nursing experiences. To engage the hearts and minds of staff, we created an acronym that articulated our commitment as nurses to be C.A.R.I.N.G.:

- **Compassionate**: We recognize and offer comfort to ease pain and suffering.

- **Authentic**: We act genuinely and maintain a calm presence.

- **Responsible**: We take accountability for our actions and honor our commitments.

- **Intentional**: We act with integrity and respond with respect.

- **Nurturing**: We demonstrate the capacity for understanding and kindness.

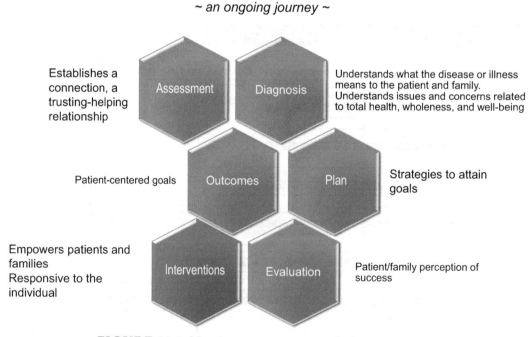

FIGURE 29.3 Nursing process as a guide for interactions.

- **Growth oriented**: We pursue self-development and lifelong learning and a corollary commitment to our patients—S.C.I.E.N.C.E.:
  - **Safe**: We take precautions to assure the prevention of falls, pressure ulcers, and hospital-acquired infections, and we are reliable in our adherence to medication safety, surgical safety, and workplace safety standards.
  - **Comfortable**: We create caring-healing environments; we are attentive to concerns; and we proactively and compassionately manage pain.
  - **Informed**: We engage in respectful dialogue at change of shift and at any time we review the plan of care and we take the time to check for understanding.
  - **Engaged**: We solicit in-the-moment feedback and involve our patients in the course of their care.
  - **Nurtured**: We cultivate a teaching and learning relationship to enhance their total health and work across teams to assure that the right level of care is received without delay.
  - **Connected**: We connect with our patients as individuals and serve as their voice when they are unable to speak for themselves with their loved ones and the caregiver team.
  - **Empowered**: We encourage and support our patients to get up and move, and to make decisions throughout their care journey that strengthen their mind, body, and spirit.

Each step of the nursing process was reframed from a Caring Science perspective; considerations were listed and a short narrative was added that provided an exemplar of Caring Behaviors. See an example in Figure 29.4.

MAKING CARING SCIENCE VISIBLE

As we cocreated the integration of Caring Science into the culture of Kaiser Permanente, Northern California, we recognized the power of creating touchstones, visible symbols, and language that aligned Caring Science with the vision, mission, and strategic goals of Kaiser Permanente, touchstones that resonated with all levels of the organization and more importantly were valued, inspired, engaged, and motivated. We began by intentionally shifting the language in the organization early in 2010, aligning more closely with the concepts and constructs of Caring Science. "Patient Satisfaction" and "Service" were reframed as "Care Experience," conversations around "throughput" now focused on the "patient's journey," and "staff satisfaction" discussions revolved around a "creating a highly skilled and motivated workforce."

We highlighted exemplars of Caring Science in our organization through the use of multimedia video that was widely shared and accessible. The first project was a Kaiser version that featured Jean Watson's "The Caring Moment" (companionarts.org/care-for-the-journey-1-landing.html), a spoken word piece (Stillwater & Malkin, 2009). We moved on to capture exemplars and inspirational messages from our senior leaders. In 2011, we asked each medical center to identify two caregivers who exemplified Caring Science and recorded their stories inspired by the format of StoryCorps stories that broadcast on National Public

Implementation: Link patient-centered goals and "Total Health"

- Partners with the patient and family to achieve
- Realizes new goals will emerge as they continue on the path of healing
- Role of the nurse as a health coach
- Communicates, through the Nursing Knowledge Exchange process, the goal of the day, what the patient and family can expect as well as eliciting the patients and families goal for the day
- Monitors progress and adjusts plan as needed

- Patient-and family-centered care
- Increased efficiency while decreasing cost through personalized care
- Leveraging our integration to meet the needs
- Providing the right level of care at the right time
- Honoring the wishes of the patient and family through advance care planning

His elderly mother was dying. There had been no catastrophic event but, she was slipping a little further away each day. She had prepared, declining interventions. In spite of her wishes, he just couldn't let go and struggled to keep her alive. He kept insisting we try to make her better. I spent a lot of time explaining what we were doing and why. When the time came to transfer her to a SNF, he actually put himself between the ambulance driver and her to keep them from taking her away. As I looked at him, he looked so sad and helpless. It dawned on me that this wasn't about him wanting to save her life. It was about him wanting to be a good son standing up for his mother as best he could. Once I understood this, the right words came easily. "You have been the best son your mother could have had. You loved her through all of this. There was nothing more that could have done." Suddenly he stopped resisting. It was almost as if he had been given permission to let go. He had done enough and someone had recognized this and acknowledged him for it (Genevieve Wright, Department Manager, Hayward Medical Center)

FIGURE 29.4 Caring Science informs and inspires the nursing process.

Radio (NPR). These Caring Chronicles audio files were available on Kaiser Permanente's intranet. Each subsequent year, we created video messages that exemplified Caring Science in Action; these premiered in conjunction with the regional Northern California Caritas Consortium that we organized (see the section "Sustainability").

To provide consistent messaging, we created templates for PowerPoint and internal communications. This extended to thank you notes that were used internally and externally. To reinforce the understanding that Caring Science Integration was foundational to achieving key operational and strategic goals within the organization, we created standard slides that demonstrated Caring Science alignment with key organizational initiatives (Figure 29.5). This was termed our "Convergence slide."

With the desire to further engage staff, managers, and leaders and to capture the value and inspiration of Caring Science Integration, we sought to develop a logo. The final graphic took two attempts to create and depicted how our Caring Science Practice Model supported the organizational goals. In our representational thinking of Caring Science Integration, the image of a tapestry kept coming to mind. We were fortunate to find someone who could translate our ideas into graphic form (Figure 29.6). We used this logo on all presentations and communications, and created lapel pins, glass etchings, and banners. We finally had a recognizable symbol or touchstone for our Caring Science work.

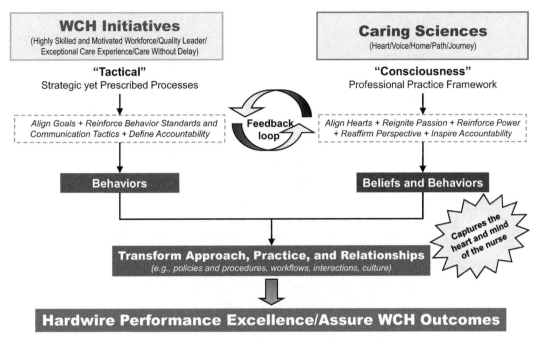

FIGURE 29.5 Integration—impact and influence.

SUSTAINABILITY

As we began this work, we intuitively knew we needed the ability to sustain the efforts, reconnect, and reenergize the hearts of those who were instrumental in driving forward the journey of transformation. This included building capacity by encouraging individuals to seek further development through HCP, CCEP, and HeartMath training participation, and provide opportunities for people to come together. We borrowed the idea of a consortium from Dr. Watson and in 2011, we hosted our first Caritas Consortium. We designed these events with the intent of driving dialogue and discussion at each medical center. Each day we had different participants with different keynote speakers, podium-sharing sessions, and breakout sessions. Our poster sessions, opening messages, music, and closing with Dr. Watson provided consistency across the days. Our assumption was that because the attendees knew each day was different, they would be motivated and encouraged to share their experiences when they returned to work, creating a dynamic dialogue within their medical center. The title of each consortium is listed as follows:

- 2011—Nurturing Hearts and Transforming Care

- 2012—Caring Connections, Catalyst for Change

- 2013—Holding Space for Human Flourishing

- 2014—Honoring Health, Healing, and Wholeness

- 2015—Journey to Shared Wisdom: Co-Creating Understanding

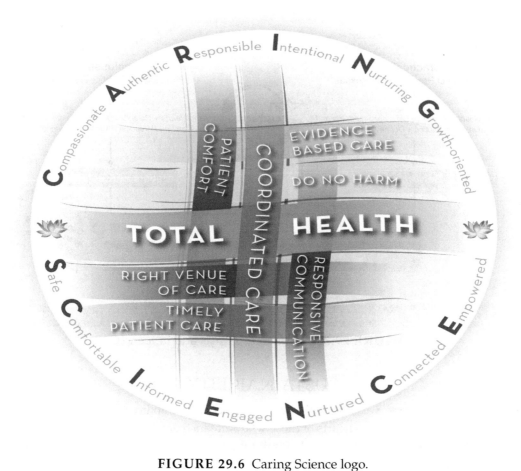

FIGURE 29.6 Caring Science logo.

CONCLUSION

"Just When I Think I Have Learned the Way to Live, Life Changes"—High Prather

Trudy retired in 2013 and joined her son, creating a team-building business; Esther retired in June 2014; in August of the same year, Shawna moved to the Pacific Northwest; Gwen retired in 2015; and I retired in July 2017. This leaves only one of the original codesigners of our Caring Science Integration effort, Linda Ackerman.

Jim D'Alfonso joined Kaiser Permanente, Northern California, in 2012 as an associate chief nursing officer and now serves as the executive director of the Nurse Scholar Academy. The Nurse Scholar Academy hosted the 2016 Caritas Consortium titled "Celebrating the Core of Caring in Practice, Quality, and Leadership." The format was a traditional single-day conference repeated over three sessions. Linda Ackerman has joined Jim's team and is leading Caring Science Integration in Northern California. Her focus has been on codifying and standardizing the Caring Science program, building consistency across the 21 medical centers.

It has been a several-year journey, and it has had some difficult starts and stops. When I look back at all that has been accomplished, the tangible and the intangible, and on how a handful of individuals with no additional funds changed the culture of an organization, I am truly amazed. Thank you for allowing me to be part of this journey.

NEXT ERA POSSIBILITIES

Education

- What is the power of education in realizing the post-2015 agenda? How are we preparing the leaders and staff?
- What is my role and what are the strategic actions I can take to impart evidence-based, dignified, and respectful education to the populations I serve?

Research

- What are the immediate areas for improvement on my street and in my town?
- How do we design or redesign healthcare to deliver focus on patient-centric total health promotion versus solely the treatment of illness?

Praxis

- How do the concepts of innovation, cultural humility, and a client-centered approach to intervention relate?

Theory and Knowledge Development

- How do we extend beyond our physical organizational boarders to improve the communities?
- Am I able to make the case between unsustainable practices and poor health outcomes?
- Is it my responsibility to address and work toward sustainable cities and communities for all?

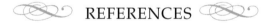 REFERENCES

Charon, R. (2008). *Narrative medicine: Honoring the stories of illness.* Oxford, UK: Oxford University Press.

Foss-Durant, A., & Kearn-Frolich, E. (2008) Caring science interview questions. Antioch Medical Center, Antioch, CA. Unpublished work.

Koloroutis, M. (Ed.) (2012). *Relationship-based care: A model for transforming practice.* Minneapolis, MN: Creative Health Care Management.

Stillwater, M., & Malkin, G. (2009). Care for the journey: Volume 1 [Audio CD]. Retrieved from http://companionarts.org/care-for-the-journey-1-landing.html

Watson, J. (2008). *Nursing: The philosophy and science of caring* (Rev. ed.). Boulder: University Press of Colorado.

Watson, J. (2009). *Assessing and measuring caring in nursing and health sciences.* New York, NY: Springer Publishing.

30

Nursing as Love: A Hermeneutical Phenomenological Study of the Creative Thought Within Nursing

Marlienne Goldin

CARITAS LITERACIES

By the end of this chapter, the caring-healing nurse will be able to

1. Link spirituality to nursing.

2. Identify physical touch as a form of communication.

3. Cite nurses' experience of love in their day-to-day clinical practice.

4. Give examples of nurses' feelings of connectedness with their patients.

5. Relate Caritas Caring to Agape Love.

I have observed nurses in practice for the past 35 years, caring for complete strangers, performing acts of caring in the most intimate way. I do not believe it is financial reward—there are plenty of jobs that pay far better. In fact, most people would not be able to provide care in the way nurses care, regardless of the financial reward. What is it that "drives" nurses? I believe it is a love of humanity. Compassion, duty to act, caring, tenderness, and love are all qualities associated with loving care that nurses provide. "Love" is a seldom-used word in nursing schools and in nursing practice. From my perspective, there is not an adequate term for the love exhibited daily by nurses for their patients. Rather than shrink from "love terminology," it is time nurses embraced and celebrated it. This chapter is about love, its attributes, and its connection to nursing.

ORIGINS OF LOVE

Many religious perspectives affirm in various and diverse ways that love is at the "heart of being" and that the ultimate reality or ultimate purpose of things is related to love. To explore this topic fully, there needs to be an inclusion in the discussion and research a broad range of concepts, including caring, agape and compassion, neurobiology, empathy, knowing, patience, honesty, and ethics. What part do these concepts play in nursing? Are they attributes of love? They certainly are embedded in nursing practice. What is the relationship of love to nursing? Is nursing a demonstration of agape love? According to Freud (1925), love is a need that is buried deep in the essence of human nature. Some would say it is the most important human emotion. The term "love" is used frequently in everyday language. It is difficult to define. As simple as the word may sound, its true meaning has been elusive.

"Altruistic love" is an ethical theory that regards the good of others as the end of moral action, by extension, the disposition to take the good of others as an end in itself. The term (French, *altruisme*, derived from Latin *alter*: "other") was coined in the 19th century by August Comte (1891) and adopted generally as a convenient antithesis to egoism. Altruism involves the unselfish concern for other people. It involves doing things simply out of a desire to help, not because one feels obligated to out of duty, loyalty, or religious reasons. The basic principle of altruism is that one has no right to exist for one's own sake, that service to others is the only justification for one's existence, and that self-sacrifice is one's highest moral duty, virtue, and value (Fitzgerald, 1998). Our heroes of the strength of altruistic love, Mother Teresa and Florence Nightingale, are people who have changed the world both dramatically and for the better. That is love; that is hope; and that is change. Other philosophers, Socrates, Plato, and Aristotle, argue that altruistic love is not really love at all, but a form of respect (Boeree, 2009). Respect is an attribute of love but does not automatically result in love.

NURSING AS CARING

Does choosing nursing mean that one chooses a profession of love toward humanity? The ethical and existential demonstration of unselfish love allows a nurse to come in right relationship with self and to live authentically. Eriksson (2002) puts forth three basic assumptions: (a) the basic motive for caring is the Caritas motive; (b) caring implies alleviating suffering in charity, love, faith, and hope; (c) a caring relationship forms the meaningful context of caring and derives its origin from the ethos of love, responsibility, and sacrifice (i.e., the Caritas ethic; Eriksson, 2002).

Agape, Caritas, and unselfish love have been used interchangeably in caring and nursing science. Love in a wider sense, like the unselfish agape and Caritas, has been marginalized in Western culture. The love from caregiver to patient has been misunderstood. Fitzgerald (1998) formed a thesis that human agape is what makes it possible to practice holistic caring, where caring is an art as well as a science. He concludes, "Rather than ignoring the concept of love and its relationship to the everyday practices of nurses, we should be embracing it" (Fitzgerald, 1998, p. 38). Nursing is directly related to caring for people, and it provides a perfect opportunity to practice the art of loving. "If one wants to become a master of any art, one's whole life must be devoted to it, or at least related to it" (Fromm, 1956, p. 86). If we believe that love is an essential ingredient in human existence, then demonstration of love in nursing practice is of critical importance.

LOVE'S ENERGY

Healers have said that love is a healing energy. In folklore and religious texts, the power of love to heal has been an accepted fact. Love is at the center of humanity. When one practices caring, one comes in contact with the core of one's spirit. The notion of caring as an expression of love and compassion is in direct correlation with ideas that have influenced caring for hundreds of years. Is caring a demonstration of love? According to Sister Simone Roach, "Caring is the human mode of being" (Roach, 2002, p. 23). Sister Roach believes that care is the fundamental and unifying force of nursing, and curing and healing cannot occur without care. Love is at the center of humanity. Caring is natural and is an expression of love. Love is not only the heart but also the force of caring. Caring requires us to act with unconditional love for another to help and heal. Most nurses will agree that caring for patients gives their own lives meaning. Does demonstrating love for patients promote nurses being in right relationship with self? The idea of caring as an expression of love and compassion fits in with ideas that have influenced caring for hundreds of years.

CARITAS CONSCIOUSNESS

The Mayo Clinic in Rochester, Minnesota, states, "Spirituality is an integral dimension of compassionate care and an important aid to healing for patients, their families and care givers" (Mayo Clinic, St. Mary's Hospital Sponsorship Board, as cited in Halifax, 2011, p. 147). Compassionate caregiving means listening with full attention. It is a shift in awareness and a developed skill to be authentically present in the moment. The care that the nurse offers is more intense, and more rewarding for the patient and the nurse. How can compassion be nurtured in nurses? Mindful focused attention, or as Watson (2008) refers to it "Caritas Consciousness" (p. 78), enables the nurse to form a spirit-to-spirit connection with the patient. Compassion is considered one of the qualities of an exemplary nurse (Kret, 2011). Understanding the meaning of compassion is crucial to nursing professionals. It is a core value.

A HERMENEUTICAL PHENOMENOLOGICAL STUDY

This author conducted a research study using hermeneutic phenomenology in an attempt to understand and interpret the essence of love as manifested in the day-to-day practice of nursing. The core of the theory of human caring is about human-caring relationships and the deeply held beliefs of human experiences of life itself, not just health illness phenomena as traditionally defined within medicine (Fawcett, 2002). Traditional quantitative methodologies are not well suited for studying the theory of human Caring Science because they cannot answer questions regarding the meaning of something to a human being. "As nursing continues to advance as a human Caring Science through theory and research, it is called to continue to question its old dogmas, transcend its existing paradigms and refocus its scientific attention to human phenomena that are consistent with the nature of nursing and preservation of humanity" (Watson, 2012, p. 29). This research was based on the commitment to human phenomena.

INTERPRETIVE PARADIGM

"Conventional science is thought to be value-neutral; but it is not. Conventional science values objectivity" (M. Hills, personal communication, 2014, doctoral seminar, Watson Caring Science Institute [WCSI]). "Caring Science is also value-laden, and it is philosophically grounded in values of relationship, context, meaning, and subjective views of reality—acknowledging, but not limited to, empirical-objective physical phenomena alone" (Watson, 2008, p. 115). The interpretive paradigm allows the researcher to look at the world through the perceptions and experiences of the study participants. In looking for the answers, the researcher using the interpretive paradigm uses the participants' experiences to build and translate his or her understanding from the collected data.

HERMENEUTIC (INTERPRETIVE) PHENOMENOLOGY

The goal of this research study was to understand a human phenomenon, love in nursing, and practitioners' experiences of this phenomenon. The goal is always to learn more about the human experience and what it means to be human, or, in the case of this study, what it means to be a nurse in practice. Hermeneutic phenomenology is a qualitative research methodology. Creswell (2009) states, "Qualitative research is a means for exploring and understanding the meaning individuals or groups ascribe to a social or human problem" (p. 4). Using a hermeneutic phenomenological research methodology was appropriate as the focus of this research study to attempt to understand and interpret the essence of nurses' experiences with the manifestation of love in their day-to-day practice. Hermeneutic phenomenological research helps us to learn through the lived experience of others. We learn what it means to be human through the experience of others. Communication and language are intertwined and hermeneutics offers a way of understanding such human experiences captured through language and in context (van Manen, 1997). The research question leads the researcher to reflect and implement hermeneutic inquiry to clarify the meaning of the experiences and address the research question, How does love manifest itself in the day-to-day practice of nursing? The purpose is to understand this experience or phenomenon of love (Creswell, 2003).

RECRUITMENT

With approval of the institutional review board, the researcher solicited by email 70 nurses in three critical care departments, requesting participation in a 45- to 60-minute interview. Ten nurses replied and eight initially committed and appeared for interviews. This research study used volunteer registered nurses (RNs). Informed consent forms were emailed to each participant with a letter of introduction to the study. Each participant was asked to sign the consent form and bring it with him or her to the interview.

All eight participants were in practice at least 2 years, with the average being 22.5 years. The participants were experienced critical care nurses who volunteered to be interviewed. Participants selected the time and location of the interviews. Seven of the participants were critical care RNs working in three separate specialized intensive care units (ICUs), medical-surgical ICU, thoracic surgical ICU, and cardiac ICU. Seven RNs were used by a healthcare system in a southeastern U.S. city. One nurse, in private practice, who heard about the study, requested to be included as a participant. The RN in private practice had been in nursing for 44 years.

Data Collection

In hermeneutic phenomenology, the interview serves very specific purposes. First, it is used as a means for exploring and gathering narratives (or stories) of lived experiences. Second, it is a vehicle by which to develop a conversational relationship with the participant about the meaning of an experience. Interviews allowed participants to share their stories in their own words.

In phenomenological research, the importance is always on the meaning of the lived experience. We want to know what this experience is like for the study participants. The researcher for this study obtained multiple perspectives to obtain rich and unique stories from the participants that allowed for a clear interpretation of experiences and the value of their meanings.

When someone talks about his or her lived experience and it is captured and recorded accurately, he or she is saying this is what it is like to be me. The reader of the research data sees the meaning of life through another's eyes.

Findings and Discussion

The researcher interpreted a number of themes, or meanings, from the question of how love is experienced in day-to-day practice from all participants. The main themes that emerged were the following: Spirituality, Oneness/Unity of Being, Knowing, Touch, Diversity, and Love.

Spirituality/Religion

Although value judgments should play no role in the distinction between spirituality and religion, there are those who may see one as preferable to the other. For this study, no preference is given to either, hence the use of both terms together. Debate continues about the definitions of both terms. As Anandarajah and Hight (2001) explain, spirituality includes such areas as the cognitive or philosophic, the experiential and emotional, and the behavioral. The range of spirituality and religion along with a lack of clarity and agreement on definitions further complicate efforts to classify an approach to assessment and to research. Sometimes both terms are used interchangeably. Some see religion as the manifestation of one's spirituality, yet a person can be spiritual without being religious. A person can also be outwardly "religious" in performing certain actions, and yet not focus on the underlying principles of spirituality.

All nurse participants had a strong connection to spirituality in their practice. The process of ongoing spiritual growth is the foundation for caring, empathy, and transpersonal human-to-human connection with another (Watson, 2008). The responses were evenly distributed between God either directing them or working through them, prayer, and spirituality not connected to religion. Some referred to it in the form of religion, referencing how God works through them. One referred to God guiding her to nursing. Some mentioned God, and others mentioned soul or spirit. For example, one participant stated, "Thank the Lord, He led me to choose nursing. I could be working in a bank, instead of helping people get well." Another participant referred to a soul-to-soul, heart-to-heart connection and stated, "The easiest patients to love are the ones you make a soul to soul connection with." Some nurses referred to there being one Creator of all people. "I had a really critical patient who was Muslim, and he was dying. His children were at the bedside. I know we prayed differently but I know we pray to the same God." One participant with 44 years of nursing experience replied, "In my first face to face encounter I recognize the divinity in each of the people that I care for."

All participants agreed that they practiced in a sacred environment and nursing was a spiritual profession. One of the younger participants said, "God has given me a spiritual gift to give my patients. I guess you could say I try and have a spiritual relationship with all my patients."

Quinn (1992) talks about the nurse creating the patient's environment and nurses working in a sacred space. One of the participants said, "I try connecting with patients on a deep level, almost spiritual I would say … We work in a sacred space with patients. Going into a patient's room is like entering a sanctuary." Quinn posits that we are connected to all of life and can repattern and heal ourselves and others through the intentional use of our consciousness. Nurses know that they are not in charge of healing the patient, but by holding sacred space with them, the healing process can occur. By creating a safe and supportive environment, healing can progress. A nurse with 44 years of experience said, "I have to clear my own field so that I can be spiritually present for my patients." He went on to say, "Each patient has a uniqueness; each soul is special."

Mindful focused attention, or as Watson (2008) refers to it "Caritas Consciousness" (p. 78), enables the nurse to form a spirit-to-spirit connection with the patient. A participant replied, "I love connecting with people, that's the beauty of nursing. You can't just connect on a superficial level. You have to go deeper into a person's soul." Spirituality is a strong component of many modern-day nursing theories. A nurse spoke the following, "My patients need me; I can't explain it in words, but I feel it's my purpose to ease their pain, help them heal or even die peacefully. It's holy work, what we do every day." One participant compared nursing as doing God's work. "I work weekends only, and many people comment that I don't attend church. I tell them I'm in church doing God's work every weekend when I'm taking care of the sick and injured patients in the hospital. You can honor God in many ways outside of church. Didn't God say, 'Love one another'?" One of the participants included prayer in her response. "Critical care gave me new purpose; I could partner with the patient and make a real spiritual connection, not just with the patient but with the family as well." She went on, "I pray for, and with, my patients. I take their lead. If they ask me to pray with them, I do; but whether or not they ask me, I always pray for them."

Oneness/Unity of Being

Most participants felt that there was a unity among themselves and the patients, a collective oneness. One nurse said, "Every patient has a story, and in some ways they are all the same story." This tied into the spirituality theme of all human beings belonging to the same human race, one creator. A nurse in practice for 22 years said, "Nursing reminds me that we are all connected. We are one human race, regardless of everything else." Some said that they saw themselves, or their loved ones, in their patients. A participant replied, "I look at a patient and think it could be me in that bed. Their story could be my story." Two nurses even referred to themselves as being in the patient's condition one day in the future. One said, "When I go home at night and walk out of the hospital, I always remember that some of the patients will never walk out of the hospital, and someday I will be one of those patients, being carried out."

The connection between nurse and patient appeared frequently in the responses. A nurse with 15 years of experience said, "We were all created the same. It is easy to care for patients if you keep that in mind." She went on to say, "I like to think I leave a little bit of my spirit with each patient, a little of me because I know I take a little bit of them into my spirit." Another participant said, "I was a hospice nurse before going into critical care. With each patient's death, some of me died along with them." She continued, "Part of my spirit died each time. There are some patients you never forget; they leave an imprint on your soul."

The concept of interconnectedness is rooted within science, especially complexity science, and has been described in many ways: for example, Ochs (1986) said, "We are all connected to everything" (p. 121). According to Watson (2008), "We realize that what we do for ourselves benefits others, and what we do for others benefits us" (p. 10). The nurse with 40 years' experience said, "The same creator brought all of us into being. What I do for someone else I'm also doing for me." The prayer of St. Francis of Assisi says that "it is in giving that we receive." Two of the participants' responses related to that concept. They felt rewarded for caring for their patients. One reported, "I feel blessed that they trust me." Another said, "My greatest joy is seeing a patient get well." The unity of life is a spiritual principle as well as a scientific one. There were many responses from participants talking about identifying with their patients. One said, "I look at each patient as my family member; it could be my Dad, my Mom, my sibling, whoever. I try and take care of them as if they were my family member." She continued, "After all, aren't we part of one family, the family of man? If we all thought like that there would be no war, because we are all part of one human race."

The spiritual principle of the unity of life says that all things are interconnected because at its deepest level creation is indivisible (Easwaran, 1989). According to him, the reality exists at the core of all life whether we call it the divine spark or the divine within. One of the most experienced participants said, "Seeing the divine in each one of my patients connects me to them. The Divine is in each of us, and it is reflected back."

A few of the participants referred to the patient and themselves as a team, working together as one. A participant went on to say, "It's much more than a paycheck. I'm connected to my patient. When the patient does well, I feel it's because we've worked together; we are working for the same outcome. We have the same goals. We set them together every day, if the patient is able. It may just be getting out of bed to chair, but when it happens it is both our success." Another said, "My patient and I are a team; each milestone is a win for both of us. We work together as a unit." One participant continued the thought of oneness and spoke about the end of her patient's life. "Back when I worked in hospice, the patient and I were a team then too, but the only win for us was a peaceful easy death. We set that goal together too."

Across time, cultures, and religious traditions, the spiritual principle of unity, or connectedness, can be found in simple and familiar statements. "Do unto others as you would have them do unto you." "Love your neighbor as yourself" (The Bible, Matthew, 22:39). The message of all great religions is the same: "Regard everybody as yourself, because everybody is you" (Easwaran, 1989, p. 236). If we practice seeing ourselves in all, we will ensure a peaceful world. According to Watson (2008), Caring Science makes more exact that unity and connectedness exist among all things in the circle of life: change, sickness, grief, death, and rebirth. Caring Science moves humanity closer to peaceful relationships.

Knowing

Nurses described knowing their patients as one of the most important aspects of their job. Most of them said that it required effort but could make caring for the patient so much easier. From the responses, the researcher interpreted that many nurses felt that it was a moral responsibility that preserved the patient's dignity. One nurse said, "Not seeing the patient as a person diminishes him." She continued, "I treat my patients as human beings not just as units of work to care for." Dr. Jean Watson referred to the concept of seeing and relating to the patient as a person and not a disease or illness as far back as 1985 (Watson, 1985).

All participants said that to best help the patients, the nurse must know them as people, not just as patients. Every participant mentioned the importance of knowing the patient. One participant stated, "I have to get to know my patient to really find out what's important to him." All agreed that one has to look beyond the disease process to see the person. Another participant answered, "I have to see him as a person, not a patient." Still another said, "You have to get to know him as a person. Listening is important; it's how I get to know my patients." She continued, "I get to know what's important to them, how their illness impacts their life." Another participant replied, "I get to know what's important to them, whether it's being able to coach their son's team, or play with their grandchild, or even live long enough to see a child get married. When I know what matters to them I can help them set realistic goals."

Most agreed that knowing the patient took time, and could not be rushed. I interpreted this as being fully present to the patients. The nurses frequently referred to the patient as a person, seeing beyond the disease. All of them agreed that it was important not to be rushed at the start of the shift, so they could really meet with the patient. A nurse with 15 years' experience said, "You can't get to know a patient with the computer screen between you and the patient." She continued, "You have to look into a person's eyes and really listen to them in order to get to know them. Patients appreciate when you take the time to get to know them, and it makes caring for them much easier." The report from the off-going nurse was not sufficient for them to know the patient. The researcher interpreted this as the art of knowing that the patient was just as important as the science and technology.

All participants talked about how knowing the patient can ease goal setting. It also put the nurse in a position of being the patient's advocate. A nurse with 22 years' experience told the following story: "I had a patient who was refusing to take his medication. I realized after I got to know him that he wasn't just a non-compliant patient. The medication produced bad side effects that were very unpleasant, and effected his getting up for work in the mornings. If I hadn't gotten to know him, I could have written him off as non-compliant."

I interpreted the nurses' importance of knowing the patient to be distinctly related to good nursing judgment and care. An experienced nurse made the following statements: "Listening to the patient can make a nurse's job so much easier. They'll tell you which is their good vein for drawing blood. They'll tell you how to move them or what works best for them. They will give you the answers if you take time to know them." She continued, "Nine times out of ten if you ask the patient questions and really listen to him, he'll give you the answers. Getting to know him helps you to figure out what is really going on with him physically."

As the nurse finds out more about the patient, he or she finds more about himself or herself. An experienced cardiac nurse made the following comments: "I have learned so much from making the effort to know my patients. By listening I learned the important things in life … I've taken care of Holocaust survivors, I listened to their story." She continued, "I've learned so much from knowing who my patients are. I learn from each patient. How can you learn from them if you don't take the time to know them?"

According to Tanner, Benner, Chesla, & Gordon. (1993), knowing the patient is very different from the formal scientific knowing, but she noted that it was a core element of clinical judgment. In the Tanner study, which included 130 nurses, the language the nurses used to describe knowing the patient was strong, direct, and clear. Implanted in the interviews of knowing the patient is the significance that knowing was essential to nurses' practice, getting a grasp of the patient, getting situated, and understanding the patient's situation in context with their condition, nuances, and qualitative distinctions. The nurses frequently described knowing the patient as a person. They described knowing the patients' patterns and responses. Two broad categories of knowing the patient emerged from this study: nurses knowing their patient's pattern of responses and knowing the patient as a person.

Knowing the patient is at the center of clinical judgment and is more comprehensive than what is captured in formal assessments of body systems. One of the younger, less experienced nurses said, "I love putting the pieces of the patient puzzle together to get the answers." Many of the nurses mentioned that taking the time to know the patient made their jobs easier. A participant said, "I have to know their strengths and their weakness so I know what I have to overcome to help them get well. If nurses took the time to get to know their patients they would have an easier time teaching them." All participants spoke of knowing the patient as a positive aspect of their work. One said, "I like to look behind the patient's disease. What does, or did, he do for a living. What are his hobbies? What are his goals, and how can I help him achieve them?" Another replied, "I want to know their story. How can you experience love if you don't get to know your patient?"

Knowing the patient is essential to the patient feeling he or she is cared for. In an empirical study of patients' experiences of feeling cared for, Brown (1986) discovered that patients placed caring acts at the top of their list, not being just another case, but that their care was personalized and not routine. Similarly, from a series of studies, Swanson (1991) described knowing as one of the five dimensions of caring, defining it as "striving to understand the meaning an event has in the life of another."

Touch As Communication

Touch is an integral aspect of nursing care. It is the most powerful of all senses. Of all the human senses, touch is the one that initiates us into relationships with each other. From birth to death, people use touch to communicate with their environment and each other.

We manifest friendly intentions by touching a stranger in greeting with a handshake; we sooth babies by holding them; and we ease suffering by reaching out to touch a hand. It is generally acknowledged that human touch is essential for human survival and growth. Nurses use touch to help establish rapport and to convey a sense of caring and human concern that words alone cannot always accomplish. A nurse with 22 years' experience said, "I try and sit at the bedside and rest my hand on the patient when I'm explaining something to him. I think when I touch him as I'm teaching, it sinks in better ... you know like osmosis!" Another participant replied, "Tucking a warm blanket around the patient gives me satisfaction."

In this study, the researcher interpreted that touch was a means of communication between nurse and patient. A nurse stated, "Sometimes just a touch on their arm helps make the connection." The researcher interpreted that for some nurses it was a way of showing compassion and caring. One of the participants replied, "Sometimes all you can do to offer compassion is to pat a grieving family member on the back. I hugged his wife and cared for her. How she wanted to be cared for!" One participant observed a difference in the patient's anxiety level when she held his arm. She said, "A touch on the arm and sitting quietly for a few minutes can calm the most anxious patients."

This researcher interpreted physical touch as form of communication without words between patients and their nurses. A participant said, "We touch patients a lot in healthcare, and not all of it is gentle, or caring." All mentioned it as being an important aspect of building a relationship with the patients. The nurse in private practice mentioned, "I make sure when I introduce myself to my patients that I extend my hand. It starts us off as equals in the healing process." He went on, "I like to partner with my patients ... Starting every appointment off by shaking hands makes the connection between us. It levels the playing field; we're in this together." Another nurse replied, "One of my greatest joys is giving a patient a back rub. Caring, touching, and bathing patients ... that's what nursing is all about."

Although these were all experienced nurses, science and technology were rarely mentioned in their responses. An experienced nurse observed, "Maybe it takes time and practice for new nurses to realize that hand holding is just as important to the patient as the CT scan is." She went on, "Having a patient squeeze my hand makes my day."

The use of touch is a basic part of nursing practice that is frequently overlooked as a means of communication. As humans, we are programmed to form bonds that strengthen relationships. From this study, we can conclude that not only is touch a form of nonverbal communication but also it provides comfort and helps build the healing relationship between the patient and the nurse.

Diversity

Nurses provide patients with interpersonal encounters that convey unconditional acceptance. This enables patients to believe in their worth as human beings. Each person's health encounter should be unique, and it seemed that the nurses felt the same way. A participant responded, "I learn something new from each patient. No two patients are alike. I love having different kinds of patients." Diversity of patients and their conditions seemed to play a big part in nurse satisfaction with their professional role. One participant said, "Critical care is similar to working in the emergency department (ED); you never know what kind of patient you'll get next. There is no such thing as a routine patient in our critical care department." Another said, "You never know what a patient will tell you. Even after you've been treating her, or him, for years, there are always surprises."

From the interview responses, the researcher interpreted that the critical care nurses thrived on the diversity and unpredictability of the work environment. A nurse with 15 years' experience said, "Keeps my brain working and keeps me on my toes. You can't ever have a boring day, jumping from one crisis to another." Diversity and unpredictability also seemed to give the nurses an opportunity to continually learn. A participant said, "You can never know it all; each patient is a new lesson." The researcher interpreted from the following responses that the nurses thrived on challenges. An experienced nurse said, "In nursing school you concentrate on one thing at a time; in work everything comes at you all at once." She went on, "The technology is easy, the human beings are the challenge. Every cardiac patient reacts differently to the same procedure. Every patient needs something to help recover, I just need to find out what works for him." She continued saying, "The longer you're in nursing, the more you can sort of project what some people are going to be like; but there is always that person, even now, where you say, 'Oh I was wrong.'"

The critical care nurses spoke of no two patients being alike, and not knowing what was going to come at them next. A participant answered, "What works for one patient doesn't always work for another." He continued, "Each patient is different, and learns differently. Diversity was definitely a positive in the critical care nurse environment. Diversity of patients and their diseases may be why critical care nurses have less turnover than medical-surgical nurses."

Love

When asked, "How do you experience love in your day-to-day practice?" each nurse shared experience of love in practice in very personal ways. Response of some of the nurses to that question was, "When I come into a patient's room and he smiles at me." A participant answered, "When he thanks me for giving him a back rub." Another said, "Just by being present for my patient," and yet another nurse said, "Holding a hand and sharing the bad news." Yet another replied, "Everyday from the time I walk on the unit, or remember a special patient, or occasion, or have a patient squeeze me hand, or cry with a patient's family member." One nurse replied with a few examples, "Helping people maneuver through the healthcare system. Guiding their decision making." Still another said, "Supporting and giving them strength." He continued, "Just sitting and listening to their fears. Answering the same questions, no matter how often the patient asks."

Many of the responses seemed to center around patient or patient's family interactions. A participant answered, "When I bring the worried husband a cup of coffee. Helping the family say goodbye, sharing in their sorrow." She continued, "Being thanked for caring. Being joyful with a patient is experiencing love."

Some of the participants used the word "love." One answered, "Once you know them and build a relationship, you sort of have to love them." Another replied, "I hold hands, I sit, I cry, and yes I even hug." An experienced nurse of 22 years reported, "I truly love them. Nursing is the giving and receiving of love." Another participant answered, "When I make the soul to soul connection, that's when I really experience it. Nursing comes from your heart, the same place love comes from, and it's who you are."

From shaking hands when greeting the patient at the beginning of the shift to helping patients die with dignity, and almost any action in between, were interpreted as expressions of love in nursing practice. One nurse said, "Giving comfort is how I express it. Celebrating a good surgical outcome." Another replied, "To deeply care, as a parent does in the neonatal intensive care unit , it's how I feel about my patients." Still another said, "When I have a deep heart to heart connection, I'm really content." One participant gave a number of examples, "Sharing life similarities. Preserving their dignity. Being sensitive to their needs. Sharing in our humanity." A participant answered, "Helping people die with dignity."

Seeing patients recover or improve was a common response. This was interpreted as pride in doing a good job. A nurse gave the following examples, "Teaching my patients and impacting their future. Discharging them home. When I transfer a patient out to the floor, and he's so much better than he was when he came in." The least experienced of the participants replied, "When a bad TBI [traumatic brain injury], comes back a year later, walking and talking to thank me, and he has no recollection whatsoever of being on my floor." Another nurse said, "I want to be there for them; I want to meet their needs, physically, emotionally, and spiritually."

Acting in the patient's "best interest," whether enforcing rules or breaking them, was considered expression of love by the researcher and the participants. As one participant said, "Bending the rules is sometimes showing love." In contrast, another participant stated, "Setting limits when it's in the patient's best interests."

Although the word "love" was not used frequently by the study participants, examples of nursing caring actions were interpreted as love on the part of the nurse. For example, one participant said, "When I advocate for the patient with the physician, and I refuse to back down … and finally get an order for what the patient needs."

A few nurses mentioned coming to work, or just being in the nursing profession. One said, "When I get up in the morning and know I'm going to make a difference in someone's life today." Another said, "The team working together, to help someone heal, it's an expression of love. It's worth more than my paycheck." Still another replied, "The complexity of the human body, it's an amazing creation. Never forgetting the real art of nursing, caring, and touch." The final interview participant said, "Being needed by someone." These findings reinforce that "Love is the underlying healing power behind a nurse's duty to care" (Watson, 2003).

From walking into work in the morning to leaving the building at the end of the day, and all the caring moments in between, it seems that all of the nurses in the study found joy and love in their day-to-day exchanges with their patients.

Caring As Precursor of Love

Caring has long been recognized as central to nursing practice. This study reinforces the connection between love and nursing practice. Sister Simone Roach (2002), a nurse researcher, says that Human Caring is about love. The desire to love and be loved is at the heart of the human condition. Nursing has an ethical moral responsibility to preserve the dignity of the patient. When nurses confirm the patient's dignity, they confirm his or her worth as a human being. This enables the nurse to establish a transpersonal relationship. Ray (1997) said, "Dwelling deeply with love as the motive of caring as a way of being in nursing and communicating its inner structure, illuminated its meaning as spiritual, a sacred art" (p. 174).

Katie Eriksson (2007) in her Theory of Caritative Caring says, "Caring's essence can be summarized as an ethos of love, a message of daring to believe in the possibility of love" (p. 201). Caring has always been at the core of nursing. Watson's Theory of Human Caring (2002) places emphasis on the importance of the caring relationship.

> When the universal energy of love, of caring, healing, wholeness, connectedness and compassionate human service honors the evolving human spirit and infinite field of creativity and visionary moral ideals for humanity, nursing is then contributing to self, other, society, the planet Earth … the very universe. (Watson, 1985, p. 228)

CONCLUSION

This study not just reinforces Caring Science, it also surpasses Caring Science and takes it to a deeper level. It becomes more than another form of Caring Theory. It is a dynamic human energy, which touches soul and spirit of both the patient and the nurse. Omitting love from human caring threatens the very foundation of the nursing profession. It is time nursing embraced and celebrated love.

NEXT ERA POSSIBILITIES

Education
- If caring and love are central to the practice of nursing, should caring and love be included in nursing curricula?
- In what ways do nursing curricula need to be expanded to include caring and love?

Research
- Do high staff satisfaction and engagement scores result in improved patient outcomes?
- What are the necessary behaviors and skills on the part of nursing administrators that increase staff nurse satisfaction in the workplace?

Praxis
- Can a caring and loving nursing practice exist in today's healthcare environment?
- Can a nursing director who practices loving kindness toward staff increase nurse recruitment and retention?
- Is it possible for medical-surgical nurses, with five or six patients, to create loving caring relationships with patients?

Theory and Knowledge Development
- Love has been included in many nursing theories and it is central to nursing practice. Does omitting love from human caring threaten the foundation of nursing practice?

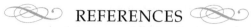

REFERENCES

Anandarajah, G., & Hight, E. (2001). Spirituality and medical practice: Using the HOPE questions as a practical tool for spiritual assessment. *American Family Physician, 63*(1), 81–89. Retrieved from https://www.aafp.org/afp/2001/0101/p81.html

Boeree, G. G. (2009). *The Ancient Greeks Part II.* Shippensburg, PA: Shippensburg University.

Brown, L. (1986). The experience of care: Patient perspectives. *Topics in Clinical Nursing, 8*(2), 56–62.

Comte, A. (1891). *The catechism of positive religion.* London, UK: Trubner.

Creswell, J. W. (2003). *Research design: Qualitative, quantitative, and mixed methods approaches* (2nd ed.). London, UK: Sage.

Creswell, J. W. (2009). *Research design: Qualitative, quantitative, and mixed method approaches* (3rd ed.). Los Angeles, CA: Sage.

Easwaran, E. (1989). *The compassionate universe: The power of the individual to heal the environment.* Tomales, CA: Nilgiri Press.

Eriksson, K. (2002). Caring science in a new key. *Nursing Science Quarterly, 15*(1), 61–65. doi:10.1177/089431840201500110

Eriksson, K. (2007). The theory of carative caring: A vision. *Nursing Science Quarterly, 20*(3), 201–202. doi:10.1177/0894318407303434

Fawcett, J. (2002). Scholarly dialogue, the nurse theorists: 21st century updates–Jean Watson. *Nursing Science Quarterly, 15*(3), 214–219. doi:10.1177/089431840201500307

Fitzgerald, L. (1998). Is it possible for caring to be an expression of human agape in the 21st century? *International Journal for Human Caring, 3*(1), 32–39.

Freud, S. (1925). *Civilization and its discontents.* London, UK: Penguin Books.

Fromm, E. (1956). *The art of loving.* New York, NY: Harper & Row.

Halifax, J. (2011). The precious necessity of compassion. *Journal of Pain and Symptom Management, 41*(1), 146–153. doi:10.1016/j.jpainsymman.2010.08.010

Kret, D. D. (2011). The qualities of a compassionate nurse according to the perceptions of medical-surgical patients. *Medsurg Nursing, 20*(1), 29–36.

Ochs, C. (1986). *An ascent to joy: Transforming deadness of spirit.* Notre Dame, IN: University of Notre Dame Press.

Quinn, J. F. (1992). Holding sacred space: The nurse as healing environment. *Holistic Nursing Practice, 6*(4), 26–36. doi:10.1097/00004650-199207000-00007

Ray, M., & Roach, M. S. (1997). *Caring from the heart: The convergence of caring and spirituality.* Mahwah, NJ: Paulist Press.

Roach, M. S. (2002). *Caring: The human mode of being* (2nd ed.). Ottawa, ON, Canada: Canadian Hospital Association Press.

Swanson, K. (1991). Empirical development of a middle range theory of caring. *Nursing Research, 40*(1), 161–166. Retrieved from https://journals.lww.com/nursingresearchonline/Abstract/1991/05000/Empirical_Development_Of_a_Middle_Range_Theory_of.8.aspx

Tanner, C. A., Benner, P., Chesla, C., & Gordon, D. R. (1993). The phenomenology of knowing the patient. *Journal of Nursing Scholarship, 25*(4), 273–280. doi:10.1111/j.1547-5069.1993.tb00259.x

van Manen, M. (1997). From meaning to method. *Journal of Qualitative Health Research, 7*(3), 345–369. doi:10.1177/104973239700700303

Watson, J. (1985). *Nursing: The philosophy and science of caring.* Niwot: University Press of Colorado.

Watson, J. (2003). Love and caring: Ethics of face and hand—An invitation to return to the heart and soul of nursing and our deep humanity. *Nurses Administration Quarterly, 27*(1), 197–202. Retrieved from https://journals.lww.com/naqjournal/Abstract/2003/07000/Love_and_Caring__Ethics_of_Face_and_Hand_An.5.aspx

Watson, J. (2008). *Nursing: The philosophy and science of caring.* Boulder: University Press of Colorado.

Watson, J. (2012). *Human caring science: A theory of nursing.* Sudbury, MA: Jones & Bartlett.

VIII

Global Caring Science

31

The Essential Nature of Caring Partnerships: Contextual Relevance and Cross-Cultural Ethical Considerations

Michele J. Upvall, Diane L. Gullett, and William Rosa

CARITAS LITERACIES

By the end of this chapter, the caring-healing nurse will be able to

1. Identify the characteristics of partnership inherent to the role of the Caritas nurse.

2. Explore the process and intermediating factors affecting caring partnerships from the perspective of guest and host partner.

3. Analyze potential ethical challenges to developing and sustaining caring partnerships.

4. Apply key elements of the partnership process to transnational exemplars at the individual and organizational levels of care.

Partnership begins with relationship to self and extends to others, but how these partnerships are expressed may differ according to context and cultural background of the participants. This chapter addresses partnerships manifested at the global level, although the approach to global partnership and lessons learned from our global partners may also be relevant to partnerships within our own diverse communities. Regardless of borders, we share a common humanity with varying expressions of caring and manifestations of partnership, but all are grounded within Watson's Caritas Processes® (n.d.).

Caring partnerships begin with the first Caritas of *Embracing altruism and practicing loving-kindness toward the self and others*. Intention to help others begins with loving-kindness to self, radiating to others. In this perspective, loving-kindness is not necessarily an action but an attitude or a position the Caritas nurse embraces that will guide action in context (Sitzman & Watson, 2014). Why is it so important to begin the discussion of partnerships with this first Caritas, the concepts of altruism and loving-kindness? Simply stated, nursing, especially within the context of partnerships, is hard work. Without loving-kindness, compassion fatigue can prevail, but an attitude of loving-kindness can promote resiliency in partnerships. Carter and Saltee (2015, p. 6) remind us to take care of the self in partnership through the acronym:

- **P**ause and be still

- **A**ppreciate

- **R**est

- **T**ake your time

- **N**ourish

- **E**njoy

- **R**estart

Integrating these practices into caring partnerships can provide the self-renewal necessary for the hard work of partnership in any context.

The fourth Caritas Process, *Developing and sustaining loving trusting-caring partnerships* (Watson, n.d.), provides the foundation for the remainder of this chapter as we explore the meaning, characteristics, process, and ethical foundations of partnership across cultures and boundaries through the lens of the Caritas nurse. Being present, authentic, and genuine in caring partnerships shifts the dynamic of "me" and "you" in partnership to "we" and "us" (Sitzman & Watson, 2014). As the caring partnership is nurtured into one of inclusiveness, power disparities among the partners fade. Courage in partnership is required to sustain this level of authenticity and can be realized only as all individuals confront issues potentially facing the partnership, issues of the following: What are my personal biases and how do I manage them? Who has the resources? How are resources distributed? Addressing these questions within the context of a caring partnership requires an inner strength and the courage to confront the questions (Upvall, 2014), but from a position of loving-kindness.

PRINCIPLES OF PARTNERSHIP

The context of any partnership begins with the self, entering into the partnership dynamic as a guest (Milton, 2012) with an invitation, either spoken or unspoken, to enter into the partnership. Reverence, a deep appreciation for the other without judgment, allowing the caring partnership to unfold in a context of uncertainty and without judgment provides the basis for a caring partnership and is the first principle for establishing caring partnerships (see Box 31.1). This reverence is a simple, "… *abiding with another* as a deep appreciation unfurls in the moment for the opportunity to be with another …" (Milton, 2016, p. 275) that can continually be transformed throughout the life of the partnership.

BOX 31.1

Principles for Partnerships

- Approach partnerships with a spirit of reverence.
- Foster mutuality among all partners throughout all phases of the partnership.
- Share responsibilities, expecting to be accountable to all partners.
- Promote mutual learning to build capacity of all partners.
- Maintain continuity of the partnership, allowing for variability over time.

(Lasker, 2016; Swiss Commission for Research Partnerships with Developing Countries, 2014)

In a cross-cultural context, maintaining reverence may be the most significant principle to observe throughout the partnership. Setting aside judgment, allowing the partnership to unfold and be shaped in the moment assumes a flexibility that can be a personal challenge in Western, individualist societies that value achieving objectives and making "progress" the pinnacle of success.

The second principle, fostering mutuality, connotes equity among all partners and reduces the potential for power differentials within the partnership. Mutuality is realized through the process of collaboration beginning with simple coordination of activities through close collaboration over time. In this perspective, close collaboration is manifested by "… states of mind and spirit that are open—open to self-examination, open to growth, open to trust, and open to mutual action" (Lehman as cited by Rosenberg, Hayes, McIntyre & Neill, 2010, p. 7).

Shared trust and mutual action leading to solidarity and equity in a partnership are possible when responsibilities are also shared among the partners and all are accountable for the results. This shared responsibility and accountability constitutes the third principle of partnership and leads to mutual ownership of partnership outcomes. Sharing responsibility begins with setting goals for the partnership together regardless of the type and amount of resources brought to the partnership by any of its members. The caveat to sharing responsibility and accountability is recognizing that individuals bring different skills and competencies to the partnership. These knowledge differences become learning opportunities among the partners when they are acknowledged and actively pursued.

Promoting mutual learning, the fourth principle of partnership, leads to ongoing development of all partners in the relationship. Mutual learning is more than simple inquisitiveness and superficial understanding gained from library searches and textbook knowledge. Learning from each other begins with respecting and understanding the context of the partnership and the system in which the partnership resides as well as the knowledge base of all partners. Reflecting on learning and sharing insights through respectful dialogue among partners promotes mutual learning. The question of "What have we learned?" is more powerful than "What have I learned?" and leads to capacity building among all partners.

In a partnership on the basis of the Caritas Processes, capacity building begins with the "we" of mutual learning. Previous conceptualizations of capacity building focused on what "I" could bring to the relationship. Traditionally, knowledge and resources were provided to develop the capacity and skills of the "other," encouraging a dependent relationship with significant power imbalances. When mutual learning is emphasized, the knowledge gained from the partnership provides synergy for ongoing growth and development, developing the capacity of all partners.

The final principle of partnership, continuity, moves the relationship from an in-the-moment experience to a relationship where new opportunities for growth among the partnerships are encouraged. As mutual goals are achieved, new goals can be developed with new ideas and projects emerging. Unfortunately, there are numerous stories of organizations providing sporadic services in global health literature. Ultimately, these organizations not following principles of partnership can cause more harm, creating dependency and unrealistic expectations. Lasker (2016) documents many of these stories from across the globe emphasizing that outcomes of partnerships must be sustainable, lasting beyond the life of the partnership. Mutuality and continuity according to Lasker (2016) are not exclusive to each other. A strong partnership based on shared mutuality fosters continuity.

FROM GUEST TO PARTNER: THE PROCESS OF PARTNERSHIP

Partnership implies a shared understanding, achieving mutual goals through collaboration (World Health Organization [WHO], 2010), but what is the genesis of these partnerships and how are they developed (see Figure 31.1)? Caring partnerships begin gently as strangers come together for a common purpose. Again, the metaphor of guest (Milton, 2012) provides a starting point in the partnership process. Being a guest implies that an invitation has been extended with a desire for working together.

In a guest/host relationship, the partners are beginning to know and understand each other albeit at a superficial level. Rules for being a "good" guest include respecting the beliefs and norms of the host and sharing information to expand the relationship. Outcomes or goals may not necessarily be fully known or explicated during this phase of the partnership,

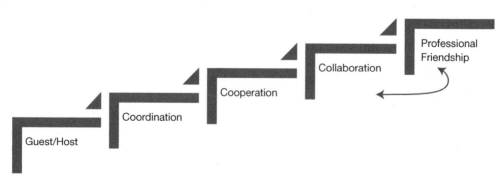

FIGURE 31.1 The process of partnership.

but are clarified as the partnership moves from guest status to coordination of activities to meet goals.

Coordination begins once mutual goals are identified. Sharing information in an open, empathetic environment where power differentials are recognized and addressed facilitates mutuality, ensuring that all partner goals are included. Often, these power differentials are linked to the type and amount of resources brought to the partnership. For example, in a joint research project, the partners collecting data may acquiesce to the opinions of the principal investigator who controls the funding. Or one of the partners may feel he or she lacks experience or credentials to provide meaningful feedback and, so, remains silent. Mutuality cannot exist where issues of power undermine the partnership. In a partnership based on caring, power differentials are assessed and directly confronted, moving the partnership from coordination to close collaboration where all partner efforts are aligned (Rosenberg et al., 2010).

Professional friendships can enhance collaboration or be the result of collaboration (Barnes, Brown, & Harman, 2016; Beran et al., 2016). Too often, the informal aspects of partnership are ignored or not given any credit toward goal achievement. Yet, this informal sphere of partnership creates the space to define success of the partnership and give meaning to the partnership even when the original goals were not met. New initiatives may be identified or changes to the existing partnerships goals may be more readily embraced. Friendships are built on trust and credibility among the partners requiring continuity, unbound by time constraints.

ETHICAL FOUNDATIONS OF CARING PARTNERSHIPS

Relationships founded upon the elements of respect, trust, and mutuality can be considered "good" relationships, but the complexity partnerships require an additional lens for understanding. Relational theory offers "… a reflexive process where one is always assuming and looking for the ways in which people, situations, environments, and processes are integrally connecting and shaping each other" (Doane & Varcoe, 2013, p. 209). There is recognition that our partnerships are shaped by context and all partners enter partnership with their unique sociocultural, historical, and political perspectives. Our responses to each other continually shape ourselves and the partnership as a whole, creating synergy among the entities.

The framework, *The Ethics of Engaged Presence* (Hunt, Schwartz, Sinding, & Elit, 2014), extends relational theory to global health. Although Hunt et al. intended the framework to be used from the perspective of a healthcare provider rendering assistance to another country as an expatriate, the framework can be extrapolated to all individuals embodied in a caring partnership. In this framework, there is recognition of a shared humanity and vulnerability that promotes solidarity among the partners. There is a sense that all are "in this together," manifested as a commitment to the partnership. The second element of the framework is acknowledging limits and risks. No one in the partnership can have all the answers and there should be no expectations among the partners that perfection can be achieved. As goals of the partnership are achieved, the potential risks and consequences, positive and/or negative, should be anticipated and openly acknowledged. The third and final element of the framework, providing competent, practical assistance, cautions all partners to work within their areas of skill and expertise. Although mutual learning is expected throughout the partnership, each partner should be aware of his or her capabilities at the start of the relationship.

Elements of engaged presence are supported first, by the orientation of introspection and reflective practice, followed *by ongoing collaboration and partnership building.* All partners need to have an awareness of their contribution to the partnership, understanding how they as individuals shape the partnership as well as the contextual factors that impact the partnership. That is, "… continually think through not only what it is we are doing, but also what it is that is shaping and influencing what we are doing" (Doane & Varcoe, 2013, p. 214).

EXEMPLARS OF CARING PARTNERSHIPS

INDIVIDUALS ACROSS BORDERS: CARING THROUGH NURSING PARTNERSHIPS IN BONDEAU, HAITI (DIANE L. GULLETT)

Forming global partnerships grounded in caring, cultural humility, and compassion remains the foundation by which nurses can impact the health of global communities. My unfolding transcultural journey in understanding the lived meaning of nursing as caring through global partnerships begins with my work in Bondeau, Haiti. My doctoral work was on the lived experience of suffering through the 2010 earthquake in Haiti. As a way to inform this doctoral work, I was invited to join my dissertation chair, "Dr. B," on her trip to Haiti. Dr. B, faculty at Florida Atlantic University's College of Nursing (FAUCON), was a board member of the South Florida Haiti Project (SFHP) in the capacity of assessing the health needs of the local community in Bondeau, Haiti. A community assessment revealed the need for a school-based health program.

The SFHP was formed in 2010 to advance the work started by St. Gregory's Episcopal Church in 2003 to improve the living conditions of a rural community in Bondeau, Haiti. As part of this expanded mission, the SFHP recognized the need for a school-based health program. The SFHP believes in forging meaningful and sustainable relationships with the communities they serve. Providing aid is not simply a matter of building a school or establishing a food program and then moving on; rather, it means establishing ties, staying in the community, and forming lasting bonds (SFHP, 2018).

The philosophy of the SFHP mirrored both Dr. B's and Florida Atlantic University's philosophy of community engagement. The SFHP mission to improve the living conditions of people living in Bondeau through the creation of a school-based health program also aligned with FAUCON's research priority area of Health Equity focused on clarifying disparities associated with human uniqueness, such as ethnicity, race, socioeconomics, gender, and age. From the start, this community health nursing project to bring a sustainable school-based health program to Bondeau, Haiti, was grounded in the values of respect, wholeness, and caring as a way to promote community participation and intersectoral collaboration framed within Parker and Barry's (1999) Community Nurse Practice Model (CNPM).

Dr. B was already familiar with the Bondeau community and had completed a needs assessment on an earlier visit. Dr. B wished to focus this community assessment specifically on the health needs of the women and children and was eager to begin with a focus group. Having no formal way to contact local community members for a focus group, the local pastor sent word and arranged a meeting in 2 days' time at the church rectory. We were stunned to walk into a "focus group" of approximately 80 women and children! I asked myself, What are we going to do for all of these women and children? After all, we had been expecting perhaps 15 people at most. We had not come with medications or supplies of any sort, only ourselves. The whole experience, for me, transformed understanding of nursing as a practice of nursing to caring and growing through nurturing others from a classroom concept to a genuinely lived one.

I watched with fascination as the two faculty members walked to the front of the rectory, in about 90°F weather, with no fans, and started to address the group collectively with a simple hello, "Bonjour." Through the assistance of language facilitators, we began to explain the purpose of the meeting and asked the simple question: "What can we do to be helpful to you?" and "What do you care most about for yourself, family, or community?" (Barry, King, Goodman, Grumme, & Gullett, 2016, p. 424). People shared their stories and concerns and not one person left without feeling as if his or her story had not been heard. What was anticipated to last an hour turned into a 3.5-hour session in which the community lifted their voices and with this, a sense of trust and shared responsibility emerged between the women and children and ourselves.

Through authentic presence, active listening, and reverence, we, as nurses, entered the world of those women and children in Bondeau. Calls for nursing are heard and nursing responses are developed from the community's hopes and dreams (Barry et al., 2016). In that moment, we heard the community's calls for nursing and, through our knowledge of nursing as caring, were guided to identify and respond to these calls (Boykin & Schoenhofer, 1993, 2001). Through a genuine willingness to come to know the community and acknowledge the cocreating of the moment, not through a prescribed categorization of what it "should be" but rather "what it was," mutuality was created through shared responsibility and accountability. The flexibility and openness by which the nursing situation was embraced and allowed to unfold shaped a moment in time that remained free of assumptions. In that moment, as a lived experience of caring, space was created in which openness to come to know the other was created and allowed for mutual learning to occur between all who were present.

The overall experience, for me, presents itself in the form of a double helix of shared caring partnerships. One strand of the helix represented the caring partnership between the FAU nurses and community of women and children in Bondeau. The other strand of the helix were those global partnerships formed between FAU and the other partners working for the community in Bondeau including local partners familiar with available resources.

The essence of reverence between the FAU nurses and community was evident in the deep appreciation shared among all the participants and the nurses without judgment, fostering mutuality. Collaboration manifests with the dialogue between the women and the nurses regarding their health concerns and cocreates a sense of shared risk through open communication among both community members and nurses. Shared responsibility and accountability became evident through a shared understanding of the unique skills and competencies all brought to the project. The community shared their knowledge of culture, health beliefs, and hopes and dreams for their well-being, whereas the nurses shared their professional knowledge. Mutual learning was evident in open dialogue about local living and health conditions that informs nursing knowledge about mutually agreed-upon solutions to identified health problems. Continuity occurred by using the knowledge gained from the community health assessment to develop mutual goals and realistic solutions to address identified needs.

The other strand of the helix representing a broader perspective of the community recognized reverence through appreciation of each other's contributions toward a shared goal grounded in loving-kindness. Shared mutuality became evident in the collaboration and coordination over time and through a process of achieving the mutually agreed-upon goal. In this exemplar, the need for a school-based health clinic and a nurse to coordinate and address the health of the children and the Bondeau community emerged. The Collaboration needed to address this need in a "real" manner and required a sense of shared responsibility and accountability among all partners to determine how to achieve this common goal, with each partner having a stake in the outcome.

The recognition of a need for a school health nurse to manage the health clinic generated new opportunities for growth while simultaneously creating a set of challenges requiring problem solving among all involved partners. An understanding of the capacity of all the partners involved is required to do so. Recognizing and building the capacity of all partners led to a delegation of tasks and roles that would help to achieve the shared goal of all partners. The SFHP through St. Gregory's began fundraising necessary to pay the salary of a local school health nurse. The FAU faculty started building relationships with schools of nursing in Haiti to find a nurse who would best meet the needs of the local community and other partners. In addition, outlining the role of the school health nurse was essential to meeting the needs and expectations of all involved partners. The first step to addressing global health inequity in Haiti begins with global caring partnerships capable of working "with the Haitian people, listen to their demands and give them the control over the reconstruction of their own country" (Edmonds, 2012, p. 450).

The caring partnership between Dr. B, FAUCON, the SFHP, and the community of Bondeau, Haiti, is a continuing collaboration and evolving global caring partnership. It has been a journey for me in learning to live the reality of nursing as caring as a doctoral student, as a nurse, and as a person. I am humbled every day at the power of genuine kindness and authentic caring to make a difference in the lives of people and communities locally and globally. This exemplar illustrates the power of global caring partnerships to build the capacity of local people as a way to strengthen and build sustainable communities.

ORGANIZATIONS ACROSS BORDERS: THE RWANDA HUMAN RESOURCES FOR HEALTH PROGRAM (WILLIAM ROSA)

For organizations and their initiatives to engage in caring partnerships, caring, as well as the ethics of inclusivity and mutuality, must be at their foundation. If organizational leaders are unable to role model caring behaviors, there will likely be a trickledown effect: the message being "Caring is not our value." Similarly, if caring is not integrated into the recruiting, training, and hiring process, the workforce sustaining the organization will likely fall short of delivering services reflective of human caring ideals. Beyond the outcomes organizations hope to achieve, there must also be an ethos of caring within a particular work culture that assures employees they are cared for by leaders, and, in turn, that employees demonstrate high caring regard for the goals and infrastructure of the organization.

In the summer of 2015, I moved to Kigali, Rwanda, as U.S. faculty (USF) for the Human Resources for Health (HRH) Program. HRH had evolved from the vision of the former Rwandan minister of health (MOH), Dr. Agnes Binagwaho, in 2011. Binagwaho was able to rally the support of major U.S. academic medical centers, as well as schools of nursing, public health, and dentistry, to partner on a 7-year initiative that intended to change the landscape of healthcare in Rwanda. In August 2012, the HRH Program was started with goals of improving the quality of healthcare education for the healthcare workforce, increasing local healthcare worker autonomy, and steadily decreasing dependence on foreign assistance (Binagwaho et al., 2013). Central to the program's evolutionary design was the use of a "twinning model"—the assignment of one USF member to a Rwandan faculty (RF) member for the benefit of skills transfer (Ndenga et al., 2016).

Nursing development was a substantial focus of the HRH Program, and objectives sought to advance the profession in practice, research, education, policy, and leadership arenas, with the most substantial project being the implementation of Rwanda's inaugural graduate nursing program (Uwizeye et al., 2017). Although USF and RF were "twinned," endless opportunities arose to explore cultural differences, similarities, values, priorities, and each culture's views on what was meant by "partnership." It slowly became clear that USF tended to be more focused on the achievement of objectives, the science of implementation, and evaluation, meeting requirements put forth by U.S. academic institutions, publishing findings, and using a Western-based evidence-based model. RF more often focused on the quality of working relationships, developing "friendships" with USF to more effectively collaborate, seeking out fairness in workload and responsibility, moving cautiously to ensure all project details met local standards, and integrating the Rwandan context and cultural/traditional ways of knowing into program design.

In this partnership, opportunities often needed to be created to promote caring communication, deep listening, and reflective environments to ensure progress and sustainability. In the HRH model, faculty on the ground often felt they were the proxies of larger organizations at play. For example, USF were employees of various academic institutions, and RF were the representatives of the MOH (and the ones who would be responsible for maintaining the programs left behind after the HRH program was finished). Faculty on both sides needed to find ways to ensure organizational goals were met, while ensuring their twins and fellow colleagues were cared for in the process. This was at times challenging, but also deeply rewarding when it came to fruition. This work was a reminder that caring happens in small moments, and that we are very often perceived as organizational representatives by the nature of our work; our organizational culture always follows us. This gives us all the more reason to ensure the organizations for which we work are invested in caring behaviors and that outcomes are attained through attention to humanistic values.

One of my greatest joys while working for the HRH Program was the ability to align the students of the graduate program with the American or international professional associations respective to their specialty to create new partnerships. As there are currently no specialty nursing associations within Rwanda, relationships with these organizations gave the students access to resources, a global networking platform, educational opportunities, and scopes and standards of practice that they would be able to contextualize for their practice on graduation (Mukamana, Karonkano, & Rosa, 2016; Mukamana, Niyomugabo, & Rosa, 2016; Mukamana et al., 2016). The cornerstone of the association–student partnerships was based on an ethic of caring. Organizations, such as the Association of periOperative Registered Nurses, American Nephrology Nurses Association, American Association of Critical-Care Nurses, Academy of Medical-Surgical Nurses, and the Oncology Nursing Society, stepped forward to ask, "What can we do? How can we help?" They realized that the global community of nurses extended beyond their membership and included millions of nurses in resource-constrained settings whom they may never meet or know. But the Rwandan nursing students felt seen and acknowledged, re-energized to advance the status of their profession locally knowing they had the support of international colleagues who cared.

The HRH Program was a new model in global health education but, for me, it was also an emergent structure for how organizational caring is demonstrated and lived. Several organizations at a multitude of levels were invested in the betterment of the Rwandan people and the improvement of healthcare in Rwanda and East Africa. HRH Rwanda leaves countless lives touched and inspired for the better.

CONCLUSION

Caring partnerships are complex and applying the principles of partnership is a fluid process that challenges us at both individual and organizational levels to be patient and caring toward ourselves as well as each other. The exemplars of Haiti and Rwanda, two vastly different countries, demonstrate Caritas Processes in action. Choices were made in Haiti when 80 people instead of 15 people elected to participate in the beginning of a community change process. Caring opportunities were created in Rwanda that would benefit all partners representing large organizations that spanned the globe. In both exemplars, caring was rooted in the individual but impacted an entire community and even nations. Caring partnerships begin with each of us as fully committed individuals who practice our altruism through kindness and caring.

NEXT ERA POSSIBILITIES

Education
- How do I role model a caring partnership for those with whom I work and interact on a regular basis?
- How can I incorporate the precepts of caring relationships into nursing curricula?
- What is the optimal approach I should use in teaching nursing students, new graduates, and experienced nurses?

Research
- What research questions need to be addressed to further my knowledge of caring partnerships?
- How can I integrate multiple research methods to develop an understanding of the art and science of partnerships?

Praxis

- How can I incorporate the concepts of a caring partnership into my practice?
- What am I doing now to promote caring partnerships in my practice and how can I sustain these practices?

Theory and Knowledge Development

- What additional conceptual analyses do I need for constructing a comprehensive definition of a caring partnership?
- How can I include all partner perspectives when developing and sustaining a caring partnership?

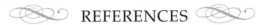 REFERENCES

Barnes, A., Brown, G. W., & Harman, S. (2016). Understanding global health and development partnerships: Perspectives from African and global health system professionals. *Social Science & Medicine*, *159*, 22–29. doi:10.1016/j.socscimed.2016.04.033

Barry, C. B., King, B. M., Goodman, R., Grumme, V., & Gullett, D. (2016). Coming to know a community: A community assessment in rural Haiti. In M. A. Ray (Ed.), *Transcultural caring dynamics in nursing and health care* (pp. 420–430). Philadelphia, PA: F. A. Davis.

Beran, D., Aebischer Perone, S., Alcoba, G., Bischoff, A., Bussien, C. L., Eperon, G., … Chappuis, F. (2016). Partnerships in global health and collaborative governance: Lessons learnt from the Division of Tropical and Humanitarian Medicine at the Geneva University Hospitals. *Globalization and Health*, *12*, 14. doi:10.1186/s12992-016-0156-x

Binagwaho, A., Kyamanywa, P., Farmer, P. E., Nuthulaganti, T., Umubyeyi, B., Nyemazi, J. P., … Goosby, E. (2013). The human resources for health program in Rwanda: New partnership. *New England Journal of Medicine*, *369*(21), 2054–2059. doi:10.1056/NEJMsr1302176

Boykin, A., & Schoenhofer, S. (1993). *Nursing as caring: A model for transforming practice*. New York, NY: National League for Nursing.

Boykin, A., & Schoenhofer, S. (2001). *Nursing as caring: A model for transforming practice* (2nd ed.). Sudbury, MA: Jones & Bartlett.

Carter, S., & Saltee, S. (2015). The inner work of partnership: Tools for making the personal shift from domination to partnership. *Interdisciplinary Journal of Partnership Studies*, *2*(2). doi:10.24926/ijps .v2i2.110

Doane, G. H., & Varcoe, C. (2013). Relational practice and nursing obligations. In W. Cody (Ed.), *Philosophical and theoretical perspectives* (5th ed., pp. 201–219). Burlington, MA: Jones & Bartlett.

Edmonds, K. (2012). Beyond good intentions: The structural limitations of NGOs in Haiti. *Critical Sociology*, *39*(3), 439–452. doi:10.1177/0896920512437053

Hunt, M. R., Schwartz, L., Sinding, C., & Elit, L. (2014). The ethics of engaged presence: A framework for health professionals in humanitarian assistance and development work. *Developing World Bioethics*, *14*(1), 47–55. doi:10.1111/dewb.12013

Lasker, J. N. (2016). *Hoping to help: The promises and pitfalls of global health volunteering*. Ithaca, NY: Cornell University Press.

Milton, C. L. (2012). Teaching-learning in community: The metaphor of nurse as guest. *Nursing Science Quarterly*, *25*(2), 137–139. doi:10.1177/0894318412437959

Milton, C. L. (2016). Abiding with reverence in nursing practice. *Nursing Science Quarterly*, *29*(4), 275–276. doi:10.1177/0894318416660538

Mukamana, D., Dushimiyimana, V., Kayitesi, J., Mudasumbwa, G., Nibagwire, J., … Rosa, W. (2016). Nephrology nursing in Rwanda: Creating the future through education and organizational partnership. *Nephrology Nursing Journal*, *43*(4), 311–315.

Mukamana, D., Karonkano, G. R., & Rosa, W. (2016). Advancing perioperative nursing in Rwanda through global partnerships and collaboration. *Associastion of periOperative Nurses (AORN) Journal, 104*(6), 583–587. doi:10.1016/j.aorn.2016.10.006

Mukamana, D., Niyomugabo, A., & Rosa, W. (2016, June). Global partnership advances medical-surgical nursing in Rwanda. *Med-Surg Nursing Connection*, 1–5. Retrieved from https://www.amsn .org/sites/default/files/documents/articles-events/amsn/msnc0616.pdf

Ndenga, E., Uwizeye, G., Thomson, D. R., Uwitonze, E., Mubiligi, J., Heat-Gauthier, B. L., … Binagwaho, A. (2016). Assessing the twinning model in the Rwandan Human Resources for Health Program: Goal setting, satisfaction and perceived skill transfer. *Globalization and Health, 12*, 4. doi:10.1186/s12992-016-0141-4

Parker, M. E., & Barry, C. D. (1999). Community practice guided by a nursing model. *Nursing Science Quarterly, 12*(2), 125–131. doi:10.1177/089431849901200211

Rosenberg, M. L., Hayes, E. S., McIntyre, M. H., & Neill, N. (2010). *Real collaboration: What it takes for global health to succeed*. Los Angeles: University of California Press.

Sitzman, K., & Watson, J. (2014). *Caring science, mindful practice: Implementing Watson's Human Caring Theory*. New York, NY: Springer Publishing.

South Florida Haiti Project. (2018). About us. Retrieved from http://www.southfloridahaitiproject .org/home/come-on-a-pilgrimage

Swiss Commission for Research Partnerships with Developing Countries. (2014). *A guide for transboundary research partnerships* (2nd ed.). Retrieved from https://naturalsciences.ch/service/ publications/9505-a-guide-for-transboundary-research-partnerships-2nd-edition---2014-

Upvall, M. J. (2014). Nurse and visiting organization factors for global partnership. In M. J. Upvall & J. Leffers (Eds.), *Global health nursing: Building and sustaining relationships* (pp. 51–61). New York, NY: Springer Publishing.

Uwizeye, G., Mukamana, D., Relf, M., Rosa, W., Kim, M. J., Uwimana, P., … Moreland, P. (2017). Building nursing and midwifery capacity through Rwanda's Human Resources for Health Program. *Journal of Transcultural Nursing, 29*(2), 192–201. doi:10.1177/1043659617705436

Watson, J. (n.d.). 10 Caritas Processes. Retrieved from https://www.watsoncaringscience.org/jean-bio/ caring-science-theory/10-caritas-processes

World Health Organization. (2010). Framework for action on interprofessional education and collaborative practice. Retrieved from https://www.who.int/hrh/resources/framework_action/en

32

Scandinavian Caring Sciences

Charlotte Delmar

CARITAS LITERACIES

By the end of this chapter, the caring-healing nurse will be able to

1. Discuss the lineage of Caring Science in Scandinavia.

2. Identify how care ethics and various philosophies of caring influence the ongoing development of Caring Science scholarship.

3. Summarize the components of the Theory of Relational and Existential Life Phenomena.

༺སོ༻

The development of Caring Science and the body of caring knowledge in Scandinavia took its departure in the beginning of 1970, notably influenced by Norwegian nurse and philosopher, Professor Kari Martinsen, and Finnish/Swedish nurse and philosopher, Professor Katie Eriksson, as the pioneering caring scholars. They advocated that care is and should be a prerequisite for good nursing and the pivotal point is the ontology of the ethical foundation and the meaning of love and mercy or Caritas by Eriksson (1987a, 1987b).

THE PIONEERING CARING SCHOLARS

Professor Eriksson, born in 1943, is known as the founder and chair of Caring Science at the Institutionen för Vårdvetenskap (IV), Åbo Academy, in Vasa, Finland, established in 1987. Already in 1974 she wrote about *vårdprocessen* (the nursing care process), first in a compendium and later as an approach to curriculum construction within nursing education (Eriksson, 1974, 1981). The necessity of a humanistic-oriented Caring Science was pointed out in the Nordic countries as well in the United States (Parse, 1981; Watson, 1988). To shape

---

BOX 32.1

Basic Assumptions of Eriksson's Theory

---

1. The human being is fundamentally an entity of body, soul, and spirit.

2. The human being is fundamentally a religious being, but all human beings have not recognized this dimension.

3. The human being is fundamentally holy. Human dignity means accepting the human obligation of serving with love, of existing for the sake of others.

4. Health means a movement in becoming, being, and doing, and striving for integrity and holiness that is compatible with bearable suffering.

5. The basic category of caring is suffering.

6. The basic motive of caring is the Caritas motive.

7. Caring implies alleviating suffering in charity, love, faith, and hope. Natural basic caring is expressed through tending, playing, and teaching in a sustained caring relationship.

8. Caring relationship forms the meaningful context of caring and derives its origin from the ethos of love, responsibility, and sacrifice, that is, a caritative ethic.

Source: Eriksson, K. (2002). Caring science in a new key. *Nursing Science Quarterly, 15,* 61–65. doi:10.1177/089431840201500110

---

the meaning of caring, the first Caring Science research program at the IV was focused on the whole human being, health and suffering, love, mercy, and care (Eriksson, 1987a, 1987b).

Although Eriksson has published journals in English and many books in Swedish and Finnish, *The Suffering Human Being* (2006) is the first and only book published in English as a translation of a work written in Swedish in the early 1990s (Eriksson, 1993, 1994). It is an important contribution with "suffering" as the basic category of Caring Science; Eriksson identified several dimensions of the concept. She revealed that to suffer may imply a semblance of power; the experience of suffering may hold a meaning of sacrifice. Furthermore, Eriksson provided a position model outlining the difference between good and evil suffering and she described three intertwined kinds of suffering: suffering of illness, suffering of care, and suffering of life.

The basic motive of caring is the Caritas motive, understood as a genuine desire to alleviate suffering. The Caritas motive is the unselfish and deepest ethical motive, the idea of love and compassion with respect to the absolute dignity of the human being. To give the reader an overview of the ontology and leading ideas in Eriksson's theory, the basic assumptions are described in Box 32.1.

As an academic discipline, Eriksson thought that you have to look for international relationships. It was the International Association for Human Caring (IAHC) that became the place of union for further discovery and dissemination of Caring Science.[1] A lecture at the

---

[1] The Nordic College of Caring Science (NCCS), established in 1981, also shared and developed the body of caring knowledge. In 2011, professor Eriksson and professor Martinsen became honorary members of NCCS. Today both of them hold emerita positions.

13th IAHC conference in April 1991 in Rochester, New York, was the beginning of many years of acquaintance (Eriksson, Lindström, & Nyström, 2012, p. 92). But the absolute climax was the Nordic conference titled "Carita et Passio," in Vasa in May 1991. The meeting with Professor Jean Watson, University of Colorado, encouraged both of them to deliver a keynote presentation together in 1992 in Melbourne, Australia. The title was "Human Caring: A Global Ontology for the Discipline of Nursing."

Care ethics plays a prominent role in understanding the ontology and essence of caring. That is why Eriksson and her colleagues have collaborated with Umeå University, Sweden, especially professor Astrid Norberg, the first professor in nursing research in Sweden, whose research area has been dementia and ethical reflections. But over the past 35 years, it is professor Martinsen from Norway who has been in multiple care ethics and academic dialogues with professor Eriksson. They have traveled to many of Scandinavia's different universities and visited several diverse groups of nurses.

Professor Martinsen, born in 1943, is known as a Norwegian/Danish leader within caring philosophy and diaconal nursing history. At the same time when Eriksson (1974) wrote about the nursing care process, Martinsen (1975) wrote about the connection between philosophy and nursing. It would be difficult to point to one main work by Martinsen, as her writing and understanding involve a continuous, moral, philosophical development of care in nursing (Martinsen, 2012). Martinsen's philosophy of care is not a logical construction of concept and theory, but instead a continued phenomenological unfolding of care and ethics to be understood as a framework to reflect and connect to its impact on nursing. Put very briefly, relationship-based caring, grounded in love and trust, is the essence of a good nursing practice. The following is a focused overview of the ontology's selected meanings concerning the essential meaning of the relations, and moral and practical care, understood in light of each other.

The Relations

The relations are grounded in the ontology of interdependence; in the words of Løgstrup (1956/1986, 1997), interdependence is the fact that we fundamentally are dependent on each other. It means that we cannot meet each other without being in mutual relationship, where we mutually hand ourselves to each other. In *The Ethical Demand* (1956/1986, 1997), Løgstrup has a phenomenological analysis of the origin of the ethical demand, which is precisely that a person has his or her reality together with other people and that we give each other reality. Thus, the individual person belongs in a world where he or she has something of the other person's life in his or her power. This basic assumption and a responsibility for the weak and vulnerable is, according to Martinsen (1993, 2006), the most fundamental ethical principle; you cannot question human worth. *Care and vulnerability* (2006) is the first and only book written in English at the same time Eriksson published *The Suffering Human Being* (2006).

Moral Care

Love and trust in a situation are important sources of moral care. Martinsen's philosophy follows from the perspectives of the universal human being's understanding of love and trust. The ethical demand is love (Martinsen, 1993, p. 72) because in the interdependency, we are reaching out to each other. The other makes an impression on me and I am moved sensuously, bodily, and in impression; there is an appeal to take care of the other's life and to act for the good of the other (Martinsen, 1993, p. 19, p. 57). The appeal of love is silent, unspoken, quiet, and invisible, and hidden in the situation. But love has two sides.

Love is spontaneous and universal; the modesty of the ethical demand—or love—is an idea. That love is spontaneous and universal means that love shows itself as an altruistic act, which takes us by surprise before we know it (Martinsen, 1993, pp. 74–78). In the spontaneity, a universal feeling is expressed, a possibility of life directed at the other, for the other's sake, beyond oneself. That love is an idea means that when love is in hardship, arguments, rules, and principles can step in, to preserve love. Love as an idea is a normative morale created by society, which can intercede, if there is a conflict between selfishness and the other or if the situation is complicated (Martinsen, 1993, p. 77). In the mutual dependence on each other, it is an ethical demand to take care of the life that trust put in our hands. Trust is always present in our lives. But we can destroy trust, so that mistrust appears (Martinsen, 1993, pp. 60–61). When a person trustingly exposes himself or herself, mutuality is vulnerable.

PRACTICAL CARE

Moral practice is also a practical issue where the activity unfolds itself in concrete situations. The ethic shows itself through actions in concrete situations, and understanding a situation is necessary to manage power in the relationship.

SCANDINAVIAN CARING SCIENCE: CONTINUED EMERGENCE

From 1990 to 1995, Martinsen was employed at Aarhus University, Denmark, to build up a master of science degree in nursing and caring. She has had a great impact on Danish nursing and inspired me to continue to unfold and develop the ontology, epistemology, and methodology of a Caring Science in nursing. Since being her graduate student in 1992, we have collaborated in a number of ways.

With great respect for Dr. Eriksson and Dr. Martinsen as the first generation of caring philosophers and theorists, I am honored to be one of the next generation, developing and expanding Caring Science. The emerging theory of Caring Science is continuing, and especially the many years of collaboration with Dr. Martinsen have inspired me to develop a combined Ethical Demand Model and Theory of Relational and Existential Life Phenomena. The development of the model emanates from an intertwined approach between a philosophy of care and empirical research from a patient's perspective in clinical nursing practice. The philosophy of the late Danish philosopher K. E. Løgstrup is the underlying ontology (Løgstrup, 1956/1986, 1997). Last but not the least, the empirical nursing research, in which I have been involved over the past 20 years, also forms an essential part of the model and the theory.

To give the reader an overview, I first present the entire Ethical Demand Model as basic assumptions (Box 32.2). It is important to make clear from the beginning that the model is a "thinking horizon" that comes into play only in the specific situation as an ethical demand. Subsequently, I choose essential keywords that have emerged in my work and give them special attention by unfolding the meanings of caring. The keywords are "Autonomy and

---

BOX 32.2

The Ethical Demand Model

---

1. A care ethic is based on **interdependence**, a relational philosophy of life in contrast to an individualist, liberalist philosophy of life. The fact is that we fundamentally are dependent on each other. It is so fundamental that we do not think about it. It is a way of being in the world (Delmar, 1999/2006, 2013a; Løgstrup, 1956/1986, 1997; Martinsen, 1993, 2006).

2. A care ethic is expressed in a moral practice and concerns **trust and power**. It concerns the way in which power is shaped so that trust in relations is maintained (Delmar 1999/2006, 2012, 2013a; Martinsen, 1993, 2006).

3. A care ethic is helping without infringing. It is the preservation of the patient's **dignity** (Delmar, 1999/2006, 2012, 2013a; Martinsen, 1993, 2006).

4. A care ethic involves attending to the **other** so that his or her life-conducive possibilities are expanded (Delmar, 1999/2006, 2012, 2013a; Martinsen, 1993).

5. A care ethic involves an attention toward **life phenomena** and acting on this (Delmar, 1999/2006, Delmar et al., 2005, 2006, 2013b).

6. A care ethic presupposes the nurse's development of **courage** and mindful, contextual attention (Delmar, 1999/2006, 2004, 2008).

7. A care ethic presupposes professionalism in nursing, using the profession's total body of knowledge, reflected and shaped in the concrete **situation** (Delmar, 1999/2006, Martinsen, 1993).

---

dignity in the light of interdependence" and "trust and power" discussed in the following text; "life phenomena" and "courage" are discussed at greater length in the section "The Theory of Relational and Existential Life Phenomena." This work also demonstrates how a caring consciousness and a commitment to care ethics can transform nursing actions into concrete practices.

Autonomy and Dignity in the Light of Interdependence

In Scandinavian nursing, there is the tendency to leave the sick and vulnerable to the care of family to await the emergence of self-management. It is time to ask the following questions: Will the world be only for the strongest and survivors? What about the weakest persons, those whose state of health is beyond their control, who are frail, elderly, afflicted with mental illness, or with limited resources? In our society in general, independence of others' help, self-care and self-determination, and the opportunity to choose and take responsibility for one's own life are dominant values called "autonomy" or "self-managing" (synonyms). It is documented (Delmar, Alenius-Karlsson, & Mikkelsen, 2011) that the fear of becoming dependent on others' help is firmly rooted in the philosophy that informs an individualist society where the original meaning of "autonomy" relates to independence (van Thiel & van Delden, 2001). In other words, every person is the architect of his or her own fortune. In an individualist society, dignity is closely connected with the ability to manage and with being independent of others' help. The values associated with self-management that support self-care and self-determination and taking responsibility for one's own life are in many ways vitalizing; the nurse is constantly obliged to take care not to patronize patients by usurping their responsibilities and not to give the chance to cope on their own. The patients should be their own masters. The problem, however, is that this perspective on dignity and autonomy seeking may become so dominant that it may affect dignity and become a barrier to seeking help when needed. When help is needed, there is a risk that the individual will feel inadequate, even guilty. Thoughts of guilt and punishment walk hand in hand with the responsibilities connected with self-management and self-care.

Dignity is associated with being respected as a human being with a life to be lived and choices to be made. It is associated with being able to cope and being independent of others' help. Dignity is associated with integrity. Independence of others' help in combination with self-determination and the opportunity to choose and take responsibility for one's own life represents the self-managing philosophy of life (Delmar, 1999/2006; Eriksen, 2003). Such self-managing values maintain that dignity is preserved and we as human beings are respected as the masters of our own lives. This philosophy of life is meaningful for health and well-being of people, because as human beings we want to take control over our own lives. But the existential question is: What happens when people become sick, suffering, and vulnerable? How can self-care and self-management preserve dignity in such life situations? An empirical study documents that apparently self-managing orthopedic patients can have problems by mastering their own situations, and actually independent of age. A young (24-year-old, soldier), male patient says:

> … there are some nurses who tend to be a bit too quick getting out [of the door] when you're wheeled to the toilet. They may think: 'He's young; he can handle it on his own.' But what if there is a problem? … There could be something—they ought to make sure you're OK, but they don't take the time for that, I think. They may think you're young, so you're fine, you can cope [on your own]. That may be true, but on the other hand, I could have had trouble dealing with something, right? (Delmar 1999/2006, p. 128)

Another empirical study among chronically ill patients shows how there is a risk in being overwhelmed by feelings of insufficiency, guilt, and shame. A patient with diabetes thinks about the complications of the disease: "You think about it each time, you know. For example, what if you have some shoes on which are a bit too tight, you know? Well, have you now destroyed something for yourself, right?" (Delmar et al., 2006) As it is shown in findings, the quotation raises the question about the self-blame aspects from recognition of powerlessness in coping with the demands of constant self-responsibility and self-control. Self-management as the goal of nursing may give the nurse inappropriate conceptions about patients who will *always* be active and self-managing. There is a risk that the nurse may leave too much in the hands of the patient and thereby lose control of the situation with consequences for the dignity of the patient. This may also be the case for patients who lack the capacity to make what are often difficult choices related to their own lives, or who may not possess the strength and drive to cope on their own. It is conceivable that even those patients who appear to be self-managing may not have a sense of mastering their lives because the insecurity fostered by the volatility of their situation is ever present.

Nurses have learned, and are still being taught, the merits of the self-managing values. In many ways, this is also a stimulating way of thinking, but research demonstrates the risk of placing the values of self-management and independence into the philosophical foundation of nursing. This may inspire an unfortunate conception of patients as being *always* active and self-managing—*always* capable of making the right choices (Delmar, 1999/2006; Delmar et al., 2005, 2006). In such cases, the liberal, individualist philosophy of life and human nature has suppressed the foundation of helping in such ways that patients retain their dignity and integrity (Delmar, 1999/2006; Martinsen, 1993). When this occurs, independence, self-care, and self-management have become such dominant values that we risk abandoning the patients so that their dignity and integrity is affected. At the same time, it represents the health professionals' failure to fulfill their professional responsibilities, and unnecessary suffering through the care may be the result (Eriksson, 1994). Including other people into one's life situation can be an important sign of self-management. However, empirical research (Delmar et al., 2006) shows that it is the view of the human being that determines whether help from others and self-managing on one's own can be combined. With a relational view of the human being, that is, the basic condition that people always enter into relations of dependence, there is no contradiction between interdependence and autonomy/self-management. In contrast, an individualist, liberalist view of the human being promotes an attitude of blaming oneself with the potential for feelings of inadequacy and guilt.

TRUST AND POWER

Relational philosophy holds the view that the development of autonomy/self-management and room for action and life-conducive possibilities takes place in the mutual influences to which individuals are subjected. We are born into a society in which we, either in our thinking or in action, are influenced by each other. One needs only reflect on the strong influence that other people's moods, whether happy or irritated, have on our own frame of mind and our desire for self-expression. It is in this state of mutual influence that life-conducive possibilities may be expanded or constrained. Attending to the patient to expand life-conducive possibilities, the nurse has to be aware of her or his role in the asymmetrical nurse–patient relationship (Delmar, 2012). The nurse should keep in mind that interactions between nurse and patient are based on a power relation that constitutes a different relationship than is found between two friends whose connection is fully voluntary and reciprocal. In the asymmetrical, professional relationship, the nurse must be able to move freely between closeness and distance.

Trust is a so-called life manifestation (a relational, ethical life phenomenon); as such, trust is a given in our lives. But trust is vulnerable and we may undermine it, with the result that, in the worst case, mistrust takes its place (Løgstrup, 1956/1986). In our interdependence and in the act of surrendering ourselves to one another, power will always be in play. A receptive attitude may expand the other's room for action by making the other's world light, diverse, and safe. A rejecting attitude reflects a conquering and domineering way of thinking, which can destroy the other by rendering her or his world narrow, dark, tedious, and menacing. A morally responsible exercise of power is to act in such a way that the other's room for action is expanded. In the trusting relation, there is an expectation that the other receives the trust proffered and responds to it. But the risk of rejection is always present. The reason is that in human relationships, we are always subject to power as it plays a role in the way we express ourselves (Løgstrup, 1972/1976). The crux of the matter is how power is exercised between closeness and distance.

When closeness stands alone, one may say that care becomes overprotective. This happens if the nurses' emotions become private and self-centered so that nursing fossilizes in sentimental, overprotective care, or if the nurses have misconceived sympathy for the patient, and also if the nurses distance themselves by objectifying the patient with a know-it-all attitude, or they are more preoccupied with principles, regulations, or standards than with the concrete situation; all of these lead to the loss of the decisive moment. Nursing care stagnates in a domineering way of thinking and in the suppression of the patient, who is per se the "asking for help" party. One may also call it "paternalism" when a nurse rejects embracing his or her own vulnerability and elects to keep a protective distance. Overprotective care and paternalistic care are of the same ilk in that both of them lead to a situation where care becomes laissez-faire. Passivity results in a lack of person-centered attention, thereby constraining or destroying altogether the patient's life-conducive possibilities.

Another aspect that may create distance between nurse and patient and create paternalistic care is reducing "care" merely to the technical. The result seems to be that patients are not given the chance to talk with a nurse about deeper issues of suffering and illness. Anxiety, grief, hope, loneliness, and worries about the future are some of the existential life phenomena that are experienced in connection with suffering (Delmar, 2006). I use the term "instrumental oriented" for nurses who thus overlook or disregard patients' suffering and the life phenomena that become more prominent in the course of an illness. Among nurses themselves, the colloquial phrase is "they *only* do what's absolutely necessary" about such nurses. One nurse said:

> ... sometimes I'm thinking that there are some nurses who are a bit superficial—doing *only* the necessary ... what has to be done, without getting down to the [patients'] problems. Like washing the patients, and then perhaps giving them something to drink—and that's bad nursing .... (Delmar, 1999/2006, p. 111)

If the nurse takes care only of the patient's basic needs and overlooks the real problems in the suffering, there is a risk of creating a distance that may restrict the patient's room for action. In navigating between closeness and distance in the asymmetric power relation, courage seems to play a significant role in a nurse's ability to engage in care (Delmar, 2004; Thorup, Rundqvist, Roberts, & Delmar, 2012).

THE THEORY OF RELATIONAL AND EXISTENTIAL LIFE PHENOMENA

Patients have to be given the chance to talk with a nurse about phenomena that occupy them in relation to their suffering. Care ethics involves an attention toward life phenomena and acting on this. "Life phenomena" is a general term for the various relational-ethical and individual-existential phenomena that are a given in our lives (Delmar, 2013b; Box 32.3).

BOX 32.3

Examples of Relational-Ethical and Individual-Existential Phenomena

---

- Ethical life phenomena (relationship-based): Interdependence, trust, interpersonal power, hope, compassion, charity, universally human vulnerability, and harmony
- Existential life-conducive life phenomena (based on the individual): Life courage, joy of life, hope, longing, security, happiness, and harmony
- Existential life-constraining life phenomena (based on the individual): Hopelessness, loneliness, powerlessness, longing, despair, guilt, shame, and vulnerability

---

The Danish/Norwegian and German life philosophical traditions view phenomena in terms of a more ethical nature: some as existentially life-conducive, and others as existentially life-constraining. Both ethical and existential life phenomena are essential life phenomena in their own right, and of separate value, but it is the combination of the two phenomena (ethical and existential) that creates the whole person.

Some of the life phenomena are mentioned under more than one heading in Box 32.3. This goes to show that it is not a categorical division or a checklist. Whether a life phenomenon such as longing is conducive to life or life-constraining depends on the circumstances and the specific situation in which that longing is expressed. Longing reminds us of universal interdependence and is in this way life-conducive. On the contrary, if a spouse suddenly dies, the longing can be so existentially intense that it constrains the room for action for the surviving person. The same may be said about human vulnerability as an ethical phenomenon, which can be existentially life-constraining in certain situations (Delmar, 2013b).

What matters for patients is that nurses support that which is ethically dignified and existentially life-conducive. By linking to patients' individual experiences of their suffering and the way it interferes with the existential qualities of life, we can explore the implications of life phenomena. Research from the Scandinavian countries shows that patients want nurses who are trained in helping ill and vulnerable people with their despair, insecurity, hope, and suffering (including Delmar et al., 2005, 2006; Delmar, Rasmussen, & Dolmer, 2009). But it seems to be true that these most basic phenomena of life are those that nurses become aware of only late in the caring process, and with the greatest difficulty, as discussed in the following text.

Hope, doubt, and hopelessness are universally human life phenomena, which become more evident when one's life situation changes. Life phenomena are not static, but in constant movement. In moving toward hope, one's life courage will also grow, but doubts can come to the fore and shake the hope, setting in motion a swing toward hopelessness and despair. As hopelessness and despair are not conducive to the patient's healing and rehabilitation process, it is essential for nurses to learn more about how hope and life courage impact a patient's efforts to take the changes that have occurred in the patient's life into account.

The meanings and nuances of hope, doubt, and life courage are exemplified through qualitative interviews with chronic sufferers (Delmar et al., 2005, 2006). The study shows how patients constantly fluctuate between hope, doubt, and hopelessness. There were periodic swings between self-control and loss of control, and this brings with it uncertainty, frustration, and difficult choices in a process where patients eventually experience a collapse of meaning. Contracting a chronic disease is a shattering experience—and the life phenomena are awakened and come to expression. In the interviews, several of the patients expressed their hopes and wishes for the future: hope for healing, hope that the disease would pass, hope that a new medicine or technology would appear, hope of living a "normal" life again. Hope enables people to cope with difficult situations in life such as loss and suffering. Hope and life courage are closely knit, and it is definitely one of the nurses' primary tasks to further the patient's life courage amid the suffering. Where there is hope, life courage can blossom. Hope thus supplies the energy for life courage and self-realization to grow. Hope looks to the future and entails the wish that one's life situation can change, which gives an experience of feeling a sense of freedom and of having control over one's life—a control that was momentarily lost. There is no precise definition of hope, and it is important to be aware that hope is expressed in so many ways.

Denial as a psychological defense mechanism can help the patient through difficult times. But repression can also appear as a kind of self-deception, with the result that recognition of the suffering and illness fails, and the patient does not achieve harmony with himself or herself and his or her new situation. This makes it important for the nurse to be aware that it is not always a case of psychological repression. "Forgetting" and pushing away the fear of, say, late complications can help the patient edge back to gaining life courage—one of the life-conducive life phenomena. What at first glance may appear to be a psychological defense mechanism may have the effect of giving relief and supporting the retention of the existential hope that is absolutely decisive for the patient's life courage and for the opportunities that appear along the road through life with the chronic illness. So, the message to the nurse is: Be aware of the various expressions that hope can take, and examine closely if this is a case of psychological defense mechanism or an expression of relief and the existential life conducive—hope. Where there is hope, there is also room for doubt.

Both hope and doubt are inconstant companions, and to help the patient in the battle between the two, it is the nurse's task to be aware that the patient may swing between hope and doubt—for instance, in connection with visits to the outpatient clinic, readmission, or when the patients is confronted with the fact that the illness is chronic. It is important to be aware of the existential qualities in patient suffering because life-conducive phenomena enable patients to cope with difficult situations.

But there is a risk that the biomedical explanation model and theories about needs will dominate the nursing offered. This example concerns a 40-year-old family father, who had suffered a blood clot in the heart and completed a rehabilitation program (Delmar et al., 2005, 2006). The rehabilitation program was based, in particular, on health professionals' knowledge and ideas on patients' general needs for information— about the effects of smoking, diet, and exercise, and anatomical and physiological information on blood clots in the heart, in other words, the kind of general information about the disease. The bodily, physiological needs are given special attention, and the man no longer *has* a blood clot in the heart—he no longer *has* the diagnosed illness. That belongs to the past. But it turned out that every day, this family man would be thinking of life and death as something that was and is interwoven with the fear that it will happen again. He was constantly pondering the question of what it means to *be* a person, a spouse, and a father. There was the constant, lurking fear that could become a life-constraining life phenomenon that would disturb his ability to achieve harmony with himself and his new life situation.

If nursing patients who have had a blood clot in the heart is to be concerned not only with smoking, diet, and exercise, then nurses need to give attention to life phenomena, both in daily clinical practice and in nursing research and science. There is a need to know the nuances and multiple ways that a life phenomenon such as fear can influence our lives. So life and in particular *being* a person with an illness takes more than meeting general needs for information concerning lifestyle changes. When nursing is driven solely to satisfy needs, there is a risk that the life phenomena become invisible.

So what is the future challenge for care ethics focusing on life phenomena? The development of the theory and new heuristic insights to the complex field of nursing theory goes beyond the human activity or drive to satisfy needs. To add a deeper understanding of the existential meaning of being a person with an illness, the following sections focus on essential distinctions in relation to needs.

GRATIFICATION

Needs will seek gratification, whether they are bodily, physiological, or cultural. Their fluctuation creates inner tensions that strive for release. Needs will rise and seek gratification. Their expression is rhythmical, intensifying until satisfaction and a new cycle begins (Delmar, 2013b); for example, the need for food. You get more and more hungry until you get the food. And it starts all over again. But existence also embraces phenomena that have nothing to do with needs and gratification. Life phenomena do not have such rhythms. They do not have phases; they are not cyclical—but rather fluctuate between opposite poles, such as hope and doubt (Delmar, 2013b).

RATIONALIZATION AND REPRODUCTION

Technology and industrial production make a business of gratifying human needs. For instance, there is a risk that developments in health technology may create a vicious circle where the need for even more advanced methods capable of accomplishing more and more will only stimulate the growth of further needs for more technology. Or it could happen at the expense of others' needs—such as those of the homeless, the mentally ill, the elderly, and underprivileged patients—or at the expense of the individual's lifeworld.

Life phenomena are not a question of the inexhaustible satisfaction of growing individual needs in a constant process of refinement. A life phenomenon is either present or absent. Life phenomena cannot be refined and diversified, whereas they become more evident when illness intrudes. Life phenomena have their origin outside the realm of technological and industrial solutions. They are not about solving problems, but about embracing the existential. Helping the patient in such matters means helping him or her to understand the various expressions of life phenomena to make space for those that are ethical and life-conducive rather than life-constraining (Delmar, 2013b).

CONSCIOUSNESS AND ATTENTION

Needs are consciously registered as the experience of want, and the longer gratification is deferred, the stronger the experience of need becomes. The more vital a need is, for example, thirst and hunger, the stronger our awareness of it will be, and we will direct our attention toward fulfilling the need through goal-directed activity (Delmar, 2013b). In general, needs can be gratified only through directed activity, such as providing food and drink, or dedicating a large part of existence to work—something that does not necessarily entail self-actualization, but whose only merit is to provide the means for acquiring things and material possessions to gratify one's needs.

Problems may occur in the pursuit of gratifying those needs. They can detach themselves, become independent, and determine the person in such a way that they will dictate what he or she does in the world. If, for example, one lives a life where needs govern all human intercourse and interaction, relationships will be governed by the experience of need. This view will serve an individualistic philosophy of human nature characterized by egotistically motivated human intercourse and the exploitation of others for the gratification of one's own needs.

But an active engagement and receptive directedness is not always structured by needs as exemplified by the ethical life phenomena such as compassion and trust. The nurse who has true compassion is not aware that he or she is compassionate; the trustful does not know that he or she is trustful. If someone is consciously trying to be compassionate, the attention is directed at oneself, and the focus of attention is one's own rather than the other's situation. Life becomes self-centered, circling around the gratification of one's own needs (Delmar, 2013b).

CONCLUSION

Because there is no recipe for good nursing care, literacy development beyond sensuous contextual attention is required. Furthermore, it is essential to vocalize the Ethical Demand Model as a basis for nurses' actions and clinical decisions. The model has to be understood as a framework directed toward the patient and family in an attempt to find out for what help the patient is expressing a need. The framework is not a set of rules but a mind-set to become more conscious and mindful in concrete practice and to become more visible in the political context nurse theorists have to collaborate with clinical nurses with the purpose to make values, philosophies, and theories explicit.

NEXT ERA POSSIBILITIES

Education
- How can the Ethical Demand Model be integrated into curricula across settings as a vehicle for embodying Caring Science values?

Research
- What research methods could be ideally used to explore life phenomena as discussed in this chapter?

Praxis
- What keeps nurses from skillfully navigating the more challenging and vulnerable human phenomena related to hope and hopelessness earlier in the caring process?

Theory and Knowledge Development

- What are my own thoughts on the Theory of Relational and Existential Life Phenomena, and what developments do I foresee?

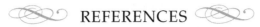 REFERENCES

Delmar, C. (2004). Development of ethical expertise: A question of courage. *International Journal for Human Caring*, 8(3), 8–2.

Delmar, C. (2006). The phenomenology of life phenomena–in a nursing context. *Nursing Philosophy*, 7(4), 235–246. doi:10.1111/j.1466-769X.2006.00282.x

Delmar, C. (2006). *Tillid og magt–en moralsk udfordring*. Copenhagen, Denmark: Munksgaard. (Original work published 1999)

Delmar, C. (2008). No recipe for care as a moral practice. *International Journal for Human Caring*, 12(4), 38–43.

Delmar, C. (2012). The excesses of care: A matter of understanding the asymmetry of power. *Nursing Philosophy*, 13(4), 236–243. doi:10.1111/j.1466-769X.2012.00537.x

Delmar, C. (2013a). Becoming whole: Kari Martinsen's philosophy of care: Selected concepts and the impact on clinical nursing. *International Journal for Human Caring*, 17(3), 20–28.

Delmar, C. (2013b). Beyond the drive to satisfy needs—in the context of health care. *Medicine, Health Care & Philosophy*, 16(2), 141–149. doi:10.1007/s11019-011-9362-8

Delmar, C., Alenius-Karlsson, N., & Mikkelsen, A. H. (2011). The implications of autonomy: Viewed in the light of efforts to uphold patients' dignity and integrity. *International Journal of Qualitative Studies on Health and Well-Being*, 6(2). doi:10.3402/qhw.v6i2.6045

Delmar, C., Bøje T, Dylmer, D., Forup, L., Jakobsen, C., Møller, M., ... Pedersen, B. D. (2005). Achieving harmony with oneself: Life with a chronic illness. *Scandinavian Journal of Caring Sciences*, 19(3), 204–212. doi:10.1111/j.1471-6712.2005.00334.x

Delmar, C., Bøje, T., Dylmer, D., Forup, L., Jakobsen, C., Møller, M., ... Pedersen, B. D. (2006). Independence/dependence–a contradictory relationship: Life with a chronic illness. *Scandinavian Journal of Caring Sciences*, 20(3), 261–268. doi:10.1111/j.1471-6712.2006.00403.x

Delmar, C., Rasmussen, B., & Dolmer, I. (2009). Staying in "the stream of life": Rehabilitation of older people in their own homes following total hip replacement. *International Journal of Older People Nursing*, 4, 272–279. doi:10.1111/j.1748-3743.2009.00174.x

Eriksen, C. (Ed.). (2003). *Det meningsfulde liv* [The meaningful life]. Århus, Denmark: Århus Universitetsforlag.

Eriksson, K. (1974). *Vårdprocessen (kompendium)* [The care process (compendium)]. Helsinki, Finland: Helsingfors svenska sjukvårdsinstitut.

Eriksson, K. (1981). *Vårdprocessen—en utgångspunkt för läroplanstänkande inom vårdutbildningen* [The care process—a starting point for curriculum thinking in health education] (Unpublished doctoral dissertation). Helsinki University. Pedagogiska Institutionen, Helsinki, Finland.

Eriksson, K. (1987a). *Vårdandet idé* [Caring idea]. Stockholm, Sweden: Almqvist & Wiksell. (Suom 1987. Hoitamisen idea. Sairaanhoitajien Koulutussäätiö, Helsinki).

Eriksson, K. (1987b). *Pausen* [The pause]. Stockholm, Sweden: Almqvist & Wiksell. (Suom 1989. Hoitamisen idea. Sairaanhoitajien Koulutussäätiö, Helsinki).

Eriksson, K. (1993). *Möten med lidanden* [Meetings with suffering]. Vårdforskning 4/1993. Åbo Akademi, Vasa: Institutionen för vårdvetenskap.

Eriksson, K. (1994). *Den lidande människan* [The suffering man]. Stockholm, Sweden: Liber utbilding.

Eriksson, K. (2002). Caring science in a new key. *Nursing Science Quarterly*, 15, 61–65. doi:10.1177/089431840201500110

Eriksson, K. (2006). *The suffering human being*. Chicago, IL: Nordic Studies Press.

Eriksson, K., Lindström, U., & Nyström, L. (2012). *Jubileumsskrift 1987–2012* [Jubilee script 1987–2012]. Enheten för vårdvetenskap, Åbo Akademi, Vasa.

Løgstrup, K. E. (1976). *Norm og spontanitet. Etik og politik mellem teknokrati og dilettantokrati* [Norm and spontaneity. Ethics and politics between technocracy and dilettante meritocracy]. Copenhagen, Denmark: Gyldendal. (Original work published 1972)

Løgstrup, K. E. (1986). *Den etiske fordring* [The ethical demand] (11th ed.). Copenhagen, Denmark: Gyldendal. (Original work published 1956)

Løgstrup, K. E. (1997). *The ethical demand*. Notre Dame, Indiana: University of Notre Dame Press.

Martinsen, K. (1975). *Filosofi og sykepleie: Et marxistisk og fenomenologisk bidrag* [Philosophy and nursing: A Marxist and phenomenolgoical contribution]. Filosofisk Institutes stensilserie nr. 34. Bergen, Norway: Universitetet i Bergen.

Martinsen, K. (1993). *Fra Marx til Løgstrup. Om etikk og sanselighet i sykepleien* [From Marx to Løgstrup: About ethics and sensibility in nursing]. Oslo, Norway: Tano A/S.

Martinsen, K. (2006). *Care and vulnerability*. Oslo, Norway: Akribe.

Martinsen, K. (2012). *Løgstrup & sygeplejen* [Logstrup & nursing]. Aarhus, Denmark: Forlaget Klim.

Parse, R. R. (1981). *Man-living-health: A theory of nursing*. New York, NY: John Wiley & Sons.

Thorup, C. B., Rundqvist, E., Roberts, C., & Delmar C. (2012). Care as a matter of courage. Vulnerability, suffering and ethical formation in nursing care. *Scandinavian Journal of Caring Sciences, 26*(3), 427–435. doi:10.1111/j.1471-6712.2011.00944.x

van Thiel, G. J., & van Delden, J. J. (2001). The principle of respect for autonomy in the care of nursing home residents. *Nursing Ethics, 8*(5), 419–431. doi:10.1177/096973300100800506

Watson, J. (1988). *Nursing: Human science and human care. A theory of nursing*. New York, NY: National League for Nursing.

33

Caring Practices in an Era of Conflict: Middle East Nurses*

Julie Benbenishty and Jordan R. Hannink

CARITAS LITERACIES

By the end of this chapter, the caring-healing nurse will be able to

1. Describe ways in which Caritas nurses serve as peacemakers.

2. Explore continuity of care in the context of healthcare systems in the midst of communal conflict.

3. Extend kindness and humanity.

4. Promote actionable research and cultural safety within a Caring Science framework.

⟡

Although the experience of conflict is not universal, we offer this chapter as a framework for looking at the ways in which conflict invades the healthcare system. Our hope, in doing so, is that nurses globally can apply key concepts to their own unique political and social landscapes. In recognizing that conflict exists in different forms, we chose to focus on Israel and Palestine, to achieve the depth necessary in applying theories of "peace through health" (Arya & Santa Barbara, 2008). We draw particular attention to hospitals in multicultural areas that receive high levels of traffic from all sects of society and clinics that are relatively homogenous.

---

*This chapter is reprinted from Benbenishty, J., & Hannink, J. R. (2017). Caring practices in an era of conflict: Middle East nurses. In S. Lee, P. A. Palmieri, & J. Watson (Eds.), *Global advances in human caring literacy* (pp. 199–208). New York, NY: Springer Publishing.

In Israeli hospitals, political conflict often plays out between hospital staff and the patient/family population. Ethnic, religious, and citizenship diversity among healthcare professionals, patients, and their families reflects the region's population, creating the potential for the hospital to work as a bridge to peace or as a powder keg.

Nurses are peacebuilders at the cellular level of disease and injury, like armies. They are in charge of organizing the chaos of disease and "battling" accordingly. In addition to medical intervention, the nurse must assess the patient's mental state, ensure proper nutrition and hydration, and work toward mobility. Yet, the disease army does not operate without external allies and battlefield conditions. The nurse must consider the patient's identity, position in the family, and position in society. After initial assessment, nurses have to direct patients and their families on what the "new normal" will be. This may include extended time in the hospital or necessary accessibility changes that will need to be made indefinitely. The nurse then coordinates with a multidisciplinary team to streamline the patient's care plan with consideration for elements of holistic health that biomedical systems may ignore.

Simultaneously, nurses' care is inherently part of political and social conflict. Nurses are representatives both of the health system and of their individual identities. In cases where conflict permeates society, such as in Israel and Palestine, identity becomes a central factor for health workers, patients, and families. Rather than personal identity being "separated" from profession, nurses are aware of their identity and the identity of others, and find ways to mitigate potential problems. In other words, although systems of conflict enter the hospital, nurses create an atmosphere of new norms and values that leads to multicultural coexistence within the hospital (Goffman, 1961).

CROSSING THE BORDER: ISSUES OF MULTICULTURAL CARE

AA is a 45-year-old truck driver living in Hebron, West Bank. While driving a truck in Israel, he was involved in a head-on collision with another truck. He arrived at an Israeli hospital with life-threatening injuries.

During AA's hospitalization, Israeli authorities issued passes for his family to visit between West Bank and Israel, and his youngest brother was by AA's bed constantly. This brother spoke only Arabic and a little English, which limited communication between him and the healthcare team; however, he was included in discussions regarding AA's care.

After 3 weeks in an ICU, AA recovered for another 2 months in the surgical department. During this time, AA was asked what he remembered about the accident and his ICU care. An Arabic-speaking nurse translated:

> I don't remember the accident at all. I do remember my dreams and nightmares during the time I was in ICU. I dreamt I was finally going to Hajj Pilgrimage to Mecca (Pilgrimage—A journey made for spiritual reasons, often to a place of special religious significance). I spent months planning my trip delving into every intricate detail. I was very excited; a life dream was coming true. The week preceding my departure I spent hours with my wife planning the farewell dinner; we would sacrifice a lamb, grill the meat; there would be the best salads with the freshest vegetables, spicy rice, stuffed vegetables, and the most extensive honey-coated baklava desserts filled with

varieties of nuts. It is very traditionally significant that we have this family gathering. In ancient times those who set out for the Hajj had many hardships to overcome in order to travel to Mecca, and many did not return. This was a true farewell dinner. Friends close and distant relatives were all notified weeks before. We spent the entire day setting the table and arranging space for everyone to sit. We waited impatiently for our guests to arrive. No one came. I will certainly die on my Hajj. (AA)

AA reported this delirious dream signifying many cultural aspects of this particular patient. His unconscious was plagued by worries that he would die in the ICU.

In addition, one can understand from this dream that AA felt socially isolated during his time in the ICU, which was triggered by the physical distance of his mother, wife, children, and extended family members. The importance of family in the Arab context intensifies the need of the family's presence for patient well-being.

After 3 months of total hospital length of stay, AA was ready to be released. His postdischarge treatment included care of his amputated stump, stoma care, remobilization, physical therapy, occupational training, and community reintegration, among other issues associated with posttraumatic return to life outside the hospital. Ideally, these ongoing medical concerns would be treated by therapists, nurses, and doctors in the community. These healthcare workers would have a full report on AA's case, understand the needed care, and be able to ask questions during a nurse-to-nurse handover.

This is not the case, however, in Israel/Palestine. Whenever patients have to be transferred for continued care in the Palestinian Authority or Gaza Strip, medical teams do not have the luxury of communicating with the next care team. AA's treating nurse, JB, did not know where to turn: She spoke with her Arab colleagues who worked in Israel but lived in the West Bank to attempt to establish contact with AA's next care team. She tried contacting nurses at a large hospital in the West Bank, and the Ministry of Health liaison; none of these efforts were successful. Unsatisfied with sending AA back into the world without ensuring continuity of care, JB attempted to maintain contact with the patient's brother and transmit medical information by phone through a translator.

The preceding case highlights several of the issues that arise as hospitals serve transnational patients. Differences in language, culture, and conflict experience require careful navigation by individual nurses and the nursing team. This example represents challenges in caring practices in areas of political conflict.

CROSSING THE BORDER: LANGUAGE

Although only context can affirm these numbers, communication psychologists often rely on the 55/38/7 formula, stating that 55% of communication is body language, 38% is tone of voice, and 7% is the actual words spoken (Mehrabian & Wiener, 1967; Newcomb & Ashkenasy, 2002). Nonverbal communication is essential in creating the nurse–patient relationship, rooted in the establishment of trust. It can be either intentional or unintentional. Although intentional nonverbal communication conveys conscious thought, unintentional nonverbal communication often reveals subconscious thought. Unintentional nonverbal communication, such as hands on the hips, failure to make eye contact, or looking at your watch, can imply absence from the patient, which is detrimental to trust building (Benbenishty & Hannink, 2015). In a recent study at a Jerusalem hospital, a Jewish nurse stated:

> Because I don't think that language is a barrier—the barrier is if you are blinded by your own fears. And when you discover that the person in front of you is the same human being as you—the same needs, the same hopes, so this is how I think we could—and should—begin to live together.

This example reflects the caring creative practice nurse[s] use to overcome and prevent conflicts when there are language barriers. (Jewish nurse, in Benbenishty & Hannink, 2015)

CROSSING THE BORDER: RELIGION AND TRADITION

There is a professional requirement for nurses to achieve competence in the delivery of spiritual care and to assess and meet the spiritual needs of their patients. Recently, the area of spirituality has come under criticism, bringing into question the role of the nurse with regard to the provision of spiritual care. If one traces the antecedents of nursing and healthcare, it is evident that these had a strong religious (Bradshaw, 1994) and spiritual heritage (McSherry & Jamieson, 2011).

Koenig and Larsen (2001) describe that it was religious communities that cared for the sick, destitute, and dying in a holistic integrated way. The findings imply that nurses, with or without a religious belief, consider providing competent spiritual care to be an integral part of their role. There seems to be an acceptance that, irrespective of one's own personal belief, there is a fundamental need to support patients to meet their spiritual needs (McSherry & Jamieson, 2011).

In our qualitative study of a Jerusalem hospital, an Arab nurse asserted:

> For example, I came to a patient to give him medication, and he said, "for the moment, I want to pray." So I said, 'Okay, when you finish, tell me.' I understand the importance of praying, so yes I pay attention to give respect to every culture and to respect religion in the hospital. But, in my opinion also, if it is an emergency, I will not wait until he prays. I explain to him, I will tell him that it is an emergency and I have to take care of him and after he can pray. Somebody who is calm, stable[,] I can tell him 'Okay, you can pray, and after I can take care of you.' It's a prioritization of what he needs, but it's important to me to give respect to all culture and all religion. (Arab nurse, in Benbenishty & Hannink, 2015, p. 1359)

Respecting religious practices is another manner in which nurses mitigate the potential clashes that may arise in the healthcare setting.

EAST MEETS WEST: UNDERSTANDINGS OF "HEALTH"

Conflicts are likely to occur whenever patients' health practices and beliefs differ from conventional Western care. For example, in the wave of Ethiopian immigration to Israel, Ethiopians held different beliefs on how the body functions. Similar to beliefs in the Evil Eye and other spiritual elements that create physical ailment, Ethiopian Jews hold different understandings of how disease enters the body (Hodes, 1997). In the case of a woman with hepatitis C, the nurse told her that her blood test reflected that her liver was diseased and required treatment. The patient asked, "What does my blood have to do with my liver?" Although the initial reaction of medical professionals may be to explain their understanding of the body, it is more important to have the patient tell nurses and doctors how he or she understands his or her body. In doing so, disease, treatment, and healing options can be explained within the context that the patient understands.

Health education is dependent on cultural belongings. As we continue to globalize, Western medicine is either blended with or in opposition to traditional understandings of health and the body.

As the ideal marriage type in Arab Muslim society is between paternal first cousins (25%) and 75% of Palestinians marry some family relation, this results in an abnormally high rate of autosomal recessive disorders. One of these is Krabbe disease, which destroys the protective coating of the nerve cells in the brain and throughout the entire nervous system (Mayo Clinic, n.d.). The young infant is relatively normal, but around 6 months of age, feeding difficulties, unexplained crying, fever without infection, decline in alertness, delay in typical development milestones, muscle spasms, loss of head control, and frequent vomiting develop. The disease quickly progresses to include seizures, loss of developmental abilities, progressive loss of hearing and sight, rigid/constricted muscles, fixed posture, and progressive loss of the ability to swallow and breathe. Krabbe is incurable and treatment focuses on symptom relief. Most babies with Krabbe die before age 2, typically because of respiratory failure or complications from immobility.

The experience of having a sick child is draining on the mother in Arab society, where women are considered the caregivers. The frequent hospital stays, medication, additional health needs, and demand for constant care place a heavy financial and emotional burden on families. In addition to caring for a progressively disabled child, women are often blamed for their child's disease, as the disease is seen as passing from mother to child while in utero. In one case, a mother gave birth to three children with Krabbe, all of whom died before the age of 2. The woman's husband took a second wife, as his first wife's womb was cursed by the Evil Eye placed on the woman by jealous neighbors. In other cases, women were divorced after singular or multiple Krabbe births, because the women were seen as having "bad wombs."

Healthcare interventions in such cases require a refined cultural competency to provide the best care for each patient within the confines of tradition. Ultimately, a community nurse in one of the Israeli/Palestinian villages with a high rate of Krabbe worked with local clinics, nurses, imams, and higher Islamic authorities to advocate for abortion for babies diagnosed with Krabbe (earlier than 10 weeks). In more preventative measures, the local imam refused to marry anyone who had not been genetically tested or had high genetic probabilities of producing a Krabbe baby. Since this intervention 6 years ago, there has not been a single, new Krabbe case in this village.

In the same way that culturally competent care can relieve medical and social ills, poor cultural competency reproduces stereotypes and may lead to further micro-level conflict. The aim of cultural safety is to create an environment in which members of different groups feel safe to express and discuss their identity (Richardson & Carryer, 2005; Spence, 2005). However, the very act of raising issues that are connected with cultural safety can cause members of all groups to feel unsafe.

A study conducted on a mixed group of Arab and Israeli nursing students was a formative evaluation, using action research, of an academic nursing program in Israel. Part of this research was related to the integration of cultural safety education into the curriculum. The findings of the study showed that making it safe for minorities to present their culture to the majority group, dealing with the tendency of groups to deny the existence of conflict, making dynamics of oppression discussable, and creating conditions in which people can freely choose their individual and group identities were central challenges to be addressed in cultural safety education. The findings indicate that cultural safety education may engender painful issues that may make people feel unsafe. This does not imply that cultural safety education is not an important goal. On the contrary, the challenges that are described in this paper show how meaningful ethnic, national, and political identifications are for nursing students. It therefore indicates the importance of implementing cultural safety education in the nursing curriculum (Arieli, Friedman, & Hirschfeld, 2012). Understanding others and respecting traditional beliefs is yet another mode in which nurses mitigate conflicts before they erupt.

EDUCATED AS ENEMIES: OVERCOMING STEREOTYPES

Conflict in the Middle East is complex and requires more diligent research to fully understand its context than what can be offered here. Despite being political enemies, the Syrian Civil War and its proximity to Israeli hospitals compelled the State of Israel to accept those wounded by war into the care of Israeli doctors and nurses. Having Syrian patients was complicated by language, but more so by the two countries having a history of political animosity, raging wars, and constant hostility between them. Syrian patients, unlike Palestinians, had not had any contact with Israelis outside of stereotypes and media portrayals. Similarly, Israeli healthcare professionals were unaccustomed to treating Syrian patients.

In an Israeli hospital close to Syria's border, a nurse made the following observation:

Years of bloody civil war has caused thousands of Syrians to flee from their homes, and a few people caught up in the conflict and suffering found themselves in my country. Israel has considerable experience in dealing with the casualties of war and providing medical care for enemy soldiers. Syrian civilian casualties, however, are a new experience for the Israeli health service. One of our Syrian patients, Muchamed[,] is already acquainted with the staff of the internal medicine department. He has learnt all our names. His questioning eyes search our faces but we have no answers. We feel his anxiety. The complexity of life in the Middle East has brought us together. While the distances are small, we have grown up worlds apart. Now his loneliness and the tragedy of his diagnosis have connected us. The connection is a sincere one. We care about him, and we want him to mend and heal. Nursing and caring for the sick and wounded extend far beyond borders. In Israel, medical and nursing teams are ready and waiting at a second's notice to absorb and treat the wounded from Syria. We are willing and prepared to do what we can to meet their needs and ease their suffering. Our relationship, perhaps improbable, is, after all, a human one. Humanity seeks to restore peace where there is anxiety, kindness where there is cruelty, and boundless love and care where there is desolation and despair. Nurses are the true ambassadors of peace. (Israeli nurse, in Eisenberg & Benbenishty, 2013, p. 543)

Frequent interaction between Syrian patients and Israeli Jews created trusting bonds, despite what politics, nationality, and religion dictated. Through trust building, the patient and the nurse were able to see each other as human beings in need of the same resources to maintain a good quality of life. Rather than being enemies, both leave the hospital with a greater understanding of that which is similar being more important than that which is different. Overcoming decades of enemy camps illustrates another aspect on a national/ international level in which nurses demonstrate, in their role modeling, caring practices to calm conflicting stereotyping.

PRACTICAL APPLICATIONS OF CARING PRACTICES

Nurses, by making order out of the chaos of disease, have acted as conflict mitigators since the beginning of the profession. Practical applications for mitigating conflict through nursing comprise two parts—the first clinical and the second toward social justice. Although both are patient-centered, they can also serve as models for interhealthcare conflict.

In clinical settings, the nurse's presence sets the tone for relationship building or interpersonal conflict. When this coincides with caring across identity marker boundaries, either it can open conversations, expose vulnerability, and lead to trust or it can reinforce stereotypes, which are detrimental to the nurse–patient relationship, patient healing, and relationships with greater society. Cognizance of presence on behalf of nurses includes reflecting on body language, tone, and acting with cultural competency. Although we cannot assert nurses are not allowed "off-days," we advocate for nurses reflecting on how their physical and emotional presence may affect others.

Structurally, healthcare settings can facilitate nurses' dual role as conflict mitigator by caring for nurses, providing burnout prevention, providing self-care rooms and staff support, and offering frequent debriefing with the aid of holistic healers, chaplains, and social workers. In the United States, some hospital staff members refer to the self-care process described as a "Code Lavender," which is used whenever a nurse has experienced a resuscitation or death during her shift. Rather than expecting nurses to continue healing other patients while pushing their own emotional wounds aside, a Code Lavender creates the space to recognize human emotions implicit in healing work. Hospitals could also offer resources for continuing education concerning cultural competency. Departmental nurses, for example, who specialize in cultural competency could be available for consultation, where medicine meets culture. Experts should be consulted on hospital decisions that have implications for diversity and on call to mediate conflicts between nurses and patients or between the hospital staff. Maintaining cultural competency teams allows nurses to apply their conflict mitigation skills without involving representatives from different strata of the healthcare hierarchy. Other interventions are nurse leadership training, focusing on team building in multicultural staffs, and arranging staff recreation and outings.

In our research, we found that the head nurse and nurse administrators are instrumental in creating space for multicultural staffs to flourish. Conversely, nurse leadership can isolate or cluster nurses on the basis of identity, which results in distrusting relationships between nurses. By continuing to train nurses in leadership positions about multicultural team building, hospitals themselves demonstrate the possibilities for coexistence and partnership in larger society.

Nurses are also political actors outside of the hospital, with the potential to influence policy and social norms. As role models, nurses are obligated to have a code of behavior conducive to their profession. Some go beyond this call to try to challenge systems that produce negative health outcomes, which include war, violence, abuse, and injustice (Arya & Santa Barbara, 2008). In the spirit of improving quality of life for all, a team of nurses from the Jerusalem area (including Hebron, Bethlehem, East Jerusalem, and West Jerusalem) has assembled with the goal of advancing patient outcomes across political and social borders. Nurses in the Middle East, a nonprofit organization, operates on the tenet that mutual caring has the potential to mediate the ways political oppression determines life chances and health outcomes. By working together on projects such as genetic disorder testing, early childhood injury, and alleged mistreatment of prisoners and terrorists in hospital settings, nurses involved have become not only colleagues but also friends while bettering patient treatment and outcomes. As a young organization, its members have already made an impact on the face of the Israel/Palestine healthcare world, and intend to continue. Although recognizing their efforts may not solve the political conflicts, they maintain the potential for changing the ways the populations perceive each other. For the past 4 years, Dr. Jean Watson has supported the Nurses in the Middle East by providing financial support for nurses from low-resource areas to attend the annual conferences. The mission statement of this nonprofit group is based on the Watson Caring Theory: Mission—"Middle Eastern Nurses Uniting in Human Caring promotes the practice and application of Caring Science/Caring theory for translating theory into concrete evidence-based approaches for self and others."

CONCLUSION

In this chapter, we have offered a new perspective for conflict mitigation. In our experiences as researchers, nurses often fail to recognize the magnitude their care has toward mediating conflict on personal and societal levels. Not recognizing such actions speaks to the ways that power and powerlessness have been reproduced in health hierarchies—because nurses are predominantly women and politicians predominantly men, nurses understand their potential for political impact through the lens of structural patriarchy. It is our intention that writing against this system of gendered oppression will encourage nurses to own their conflict mitigating powers from the cellular to global level. Second, we advocate for scholars to research nurses as essential to any political or social conflict resolution strategy. On an even larger scale, we aspire that soon nurses will not only have a place at the negotiation table but also change the table altogether.

NEXT ERA POSSIBILITIES

Education
- What Caritas literate teaching–learning strategies support the development of conflict mitigation powers?
- Why are pedagogies that include critical and emancipatory reflection necessary for nurses and other healthcare professionals to address inequities and eradicate barriers to healthcare?
- How does the creation of safe learning environments for students facilitate the development of safe healthcare settings for nurses and patients?

Research

- What research questions related to nursing leadership need to be answered to ensure safe multicultural spaces for nursing students and practicing nurses to flourish?
- What are the prospects for discovering new ways of knowing when we expand our ideas of what counts as meaningful data for informing and challenging systems to create positive health outcomes?

Praxis

- How does Caring Literacy compel respect for religious practices, cultural safety, and caring practices in areas of political conflict?
- How does Caring Science praxis advance peacemaking and extend kindness and compassion for all humanity?

Theory and Knowledge Development

- What global health paradigms complement Caring Science and through their synthesis expand ways of knowing?

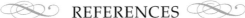 REFERENCES

Arieli, D., Friedman, V. J., & Hirschfeld, M. J. (2012). Challenges on the path to cultural safety in nursing education. *International Nursing Review, 59,* 187–193. doi:10.1111/j.1466-7657.2012.00982.x

Arya, N., & Santa Barbara, J. (2008). *Peace through health: How health professionals can work for a less violent world.* Bloomfield, CT: Kumarian Press.

Benbenishty, J. S., & Hannink, J. R. (2015). Non-verbal communication to restore patient–provider trust. *Intensive Care Medicine, 41,* 1359–1360. doi:10.1007/s00134-015-3710-8

Bradshaw, A. (1994). *Lighting the lamp: The spiritual dimension of nursing care. Royal College of Nursing Research Series.* Harrow, UK: Scutari Press.

Eisenberg, S., & Benbenishty, J. (2013). Milk and rice. *International Nursing Review, 60,* 543–544. doi:10.1111/inr.12067

Goffman, E. (1961). *Asylums: Essays on the social situation of mental patients and other inmates.* New York, NY: Anchor Books/Doubleday.

Hodes, R. M. (1997). Cross-cultural medicine and diverse health beliefs: Ethiopians abroad. *Western Journal of Medicine, 166,* 29–36.

Koenig, H. G., & Larsen, D. B. (2001). Religion and mental health: Evidence for an association. *International Review of Psychiatry, 13*(2), 67–78. doi:10.1080/09540260124661

Mayo Clinic. (n.d.). Krabbe disease. Retrieved from https://www.mayoclinic.org/diseases-conditions/krabbe-disease/symptoms-causes/syc-20374178

McSherry, W., & Jamieson, S. (2011). An online survey of nurses' perceptions of spirituality and spiritual care. *Journal of Clinical Nursing, 20,* 1757–1767. doi:10.1111/j.1365-2702.2010.03547.x

Mehrabian, A., & Wiener, M. (1967). Decoding of inconsistent communications. *Journal of Personality and Social Psychology, 6,* 109–114. doi:10.1037/h0024532

Newcomb, M., & Ashkenasy, N. (2002). The role of affect and affective congruence in perceptions of leaders: An experimental study. *Leadership Quarterly, 13,* 601–614. doi:10.1016/S1048-9843(02)00146-7

Richardson, F., & Carryer, J. (2005). Teaching cultural safety in a New Zealand nursing education program. *Journal of Nursing Education, 44,* 201–208.

Spence, D. G. (2005). Hermeneutic notions augment cultural safety education. *Journal of Nursing Education, 44,* 409–414.

34

Caritas, Peace, and Change in Japan*,**

Mayumi Tsutsui, Rina Emoto, and Jean Watson

CARITAS LITERACIES

By the end of this chapter, the caring-healing nurse will be able to

1. Describe the historic background of major Japanese Caring Science initiatives, programs, and projects.

2. Recognize the value of personal/professional Caring Science developments in Japan.

3. Provide exemplars of Japanese initiatives and scholarship that build Caring Literacy.

This chapter highlights some of the elements of Caritas Literacy in Japan that were introduced over 20 years ago. A backdrop of developments in Japanese Caring Science Theory, including programs and activities, is offered as a historical context, reflecting devoted Japanese scholarship in Caring Science Theory since the mid-1980s. Next, the chapter emphasizes the more recent caring and peace initiatives beginning with the First International Hiroshima Caring and Peace Conference, held in Hiroshima at the Red Cross Hiroshima College of Nursing, March 2012. The final section summarizes two Caring Theory–guided research studies that provide a pattern for Caritas Literacy in relation to the caring environment.

*For more information on global activities in Japan and elsewhere, visit Jean Watson and the Watson Caring Science Institute (www.watsoncaringscience.org)—the site includes videos of the International Hiroshima Caring and Peace Conference.
**This chapter is reprinted from Tsutsui, M., Emoto, R., & Watson, J. (2017). Japanese caritas for peace and change. In S. Lee, P. A. Palmieri, & J. Watson (Eds.), *Global advances in human caring literacy* (pp. 209–216). New York, NY: Springer Publishing.

JAPANESE CARITAS FOR PEACE AND CHANGE

As early as 1989, Dr. Watson was invited to keynote the First Scientific Nursing Research Conference in Tokyo, Japan. This event, along with caring theory books being translated into Japanese and annual student/faculty visits to the University of Colorado to meet Dr. Watson and others from the mid-1980s, is reflective of early interest in caring theory and Watson's Caring Science. In December 2000, Dr. Watson was invited to once again present the keynote presentation to 3,000 Japanese scholars attending the 28th Academic Conference of the Japan Academy of Nursing Science under the leadership of Dr. Yasukata.

In 2012, immediately prior to and coordinated with the International Hiroshima Conference on Caring and Peace, the Japanese Red Cross College of Nursing (in Tokyo) hosted a formal presentation during which Dr. Watson was awarded an honorary doctorate. This occasion was a reflection of the more than 20-year history of Japanese Nursing and Red Cross Colleges' (in both Hiroshima and Tokyo) commitment to the development of knowledge, values, philosophies, theories, and practices of human caring. Dr. Fumiaki Inaoka; his wife, Mitsuko Inaoka; and Ms. Michiko Tomura were translators of the first Japanese edition of Watson's original theory book: *Nursing: Human Science and Human Care: A Theory of Nursing* (1985). Dr. Tsutsui translated Watson's *Assessing and Measuring Caring in Nursing and Health Sciences* (2001).

Adoption and implementation of Caring Science is ongoing in Japan. Examples include formal Caring Science curricula, pedagogies, research, creative scholarly projects, conferences, and research. Of note, a Center for Human Caring was created in the Hiroshima Red Cross College of Nursing as early as 2000. Watson's books—*Measuring Caring, Postmodern Nursing*, and the original and revised *Human Caring Science* texts—have been translated into Japanese since the mid-1980s, reflecting a more than 30-year interest and collaboration in Caring Science. Dr. Watson was invited to present the inaugural keynote address at the establishment of the Japanese Red Cross Hiroshima College of Nursing in 2000.

Since the 2012 International Hiroshima Conference on Caring and Peace, a new International Collaborative Center has been created at the Japanese Red Cross College of Nursing (in Tokyo). It is led by Dr. Mayumi Tsutsui, who is a Caring Science scholar and regular participant in Caring Science programs in the United States and throughout Japan. Dr. Watson returned at the request of Japanese nurses to deliver a second keynote address at the Second International Conference on Caring and Peace, November 2015. (The Third International Conference on Caring and Peace was held on March 25–26, 2017.)

More recently, in 2016, a new International Society of Caring and Peace has been established, with Dr. S. Shindo as the new president/chair (Dr. Jean Watson, honorary chair emerita) providing continuity from the 2012 Conference, where Dr. Shindo served as conference moderator and chair. These personal/professional connections and formal scholarly Caring Science occasions have continued since 1989 to the current moment.

The newest innovation extends the collaboration between Dr. Watson and Japanese nurses. Japan was one of the first countries in the world to be designated a Watson Caring Science Global Associate, Japan International Society of Caring and Peace, with participation in the cocreation of Watson Caring Science—World Portal Program Development (2016–2018, www.watsoncaringscience.org).

EXEMPLARS OF JAPANESE SCHOLARSHIP AND CARING SCIENCE LEADERSHIP

With this background of personal/professional history of Japanese Caring Science scholarly evolution, the section "International Hiroshima Caring and Peace Conference—March 2012" emphasizes the caring and peace global conferences and continuing commitment to caring and peace.

INTERNATIONAL HIROSHIMA CARING AND PEACE CONFERENCE—MARCH 2012

The early leaders for the 2012 Caring and Peace Conference include Dr. Shindo, president of the Japanese Red Cross Hiroshima College of Nursing at that time; and Dr. Inaoka, former inaugural president of the Japanese Red Cross Hiroshima College of Nursing and moderator–host of the Watson Caring Science Institute, First Asian Pacific International Caritas Consortium prior to the Caring and Peace Conference; it is also imperative to acknowledge and name Ms. Michiko Tomura, devoted Caring Science faculty member in the Japanese Red Cross Hiroshima College of Nursing, a major leader with all the evolution of Caring Science in Japan, and currently a doctoral student in the United States.

SUMMARY OF 2012 CONFERENCE—ADVANCING CARITAS LITERACY IN RELATION TO PEACE

This 2012 International Hiroshima Conference on Caring and Peace brought forth new intellectual–experiential scholarly connections between human caring and peace, that is, invoking a Caritas Literacy consciousness that practices of human caring are indeed practices of peace.

The ancient land of Japan and Hiroshima, the city of world peace as well as the site of the Hiroshima Peace Memorial Museum, provided a perfect setting for this first of its kind conference. Here, the conference opened by fire from the sacred mountain on the Island of Miyajima, radiating the light of caring and peace to all present and to all caring practitioners around the world.

The Caritas Literacy rhetorical questions, which arose from the opening conference keynote—*Touching the Heart of Our Humanity: The Caritas Path of Peace* (Watson, 2012)—were as follows:

- What is peace?

- What is the origin of peace?

- What is inner peace? How do we obtain it?

- How do we manifest and sustain human caring and peace in our hearts, minds, and daily acts?

- Is there a connection between inner peace and outer peace?

- How do we offer up our hearts to caring and peace when there is so much pain in our hearts and in our world?

The approach to these rhetorical yet universal Caritas Literacy questions was addressed through philosophical–ethical and practical ideals from the Latin notion of Caritas and Caring Science (Watson, 2012):

> We as nurse and health professionals know, that when we step into the theories and philosophies of human caring, we step into a deep ethic and life practice that connects us with the heart of our humanity, of healing the whole; it is here in this connection, we touch the mystery of inner and outer peace that unites humanity across time and space around the world.

Indeed, this Japanese conference affirmed that Caritas Literacy, as addressed in this book, includes human dignity, basic civility, and humanity, which is peace in action.

This Hiroshima conference created Caritas Literacy experiences, space, and intellectual discourses whereby the audience engaged in awakening of Caritas consciousness—awakening to the reality that when we offer our own lives, one person to another, finding more conscious intentional ways to live, gestures of peace within and without, we become caring/we become peace/we are peace. We become a living beacon of hope and action for Caritas Literacy in relation to caring and peace for our world. Living and speaking Caritas Literacy generate peace from within. As such, this 2012 Japanese conference laid the global foundation for nurses to participate in cocreating a moral community of caring and peace for our world.

JAPAN—CONTINUING CARITAS

The 2012 International Hiroshima Conference on Caring and Peace was a prelude to the more recent works in Japan including the new international society and projects. The Caring Science Institute has supported the creation of an ethical–scholarly professional community of caring scholars and practitioners. For example, Japan held its Second International Conference on Caring and Peace in the fall of 2015, and the third one was held in March 2017.

A continuation of these global Caritas Japanese activities includes the 2016 creation of the International Society of Caring and Peace, formally extending Caritas into the Asia Pacific and beyond. Dr. Mayumi Tsutsui, coauthor of this chapter, is a founding member of the new International Society of Caring and Peace, allowing this momentum to live on.

In summary, these grassroots Japanese efforts continue to attract nurses and health professionals from around the world; together, they stand as beacons for global initiatives, reflecting the Caritas Literacy initiatives informing this book. For more information on both the Japan conferences, go to www.watsoncaringscience.org under Global Programs. In the following section, we provide two exemplars of Caritas scholarship in Japan.

CARITAS LITERACY RESEARCH EXEMPLARS

JAPANESE RED CROSS COLLEGE OF NURSING—TOKYO RESEARCH PROGRAM: INTEGRATIVE REVIEW

Drs. Tsutsui and Emoto and their colleagues from the Japanese Red Cross College of Nursing conducted what may be considered first-generation Japanese research on Caring Science. This Caring Theory–guided Japanese research study was conducted in two

phases. In the first phase, the authors conducted an integrative review focusing on literature relating to Watson's Caring Theory (Tsutsui, 2011).

Cumulative Index to Nursing and Allied Health Literature (CINAHL), Full Text, and
ICHUSHI (Japan's medical databases) were searched from 2000 to July 2010. The studies
of human caring were examined carefully for fit with the intended purposes of this
project. Thirty-two studies were relevant to the assessment made through methodological qualitative–quantitative inquiry of the caring environment. The findings identified
four steps of creating an environment for caring and substantiated several aspects of
Watson's theory:

- A nurse or nurse student must first treat self with gentleness and dignity prior to
caring for patients, families, and communities.

- Nurses benefit from participation in a Watson theory session, offering intensive,
purposive support to translate theory into daily clinical nursing practice.

- The caring theory intensive may be a contributing factor to a patient's perceptions of
nurses and satisfaction with healthcare services.

- Even though technology has advanced, caring is the value that inspires nursing and
development of patient care with the team.

In the second phase, the authors explored a synthesis of Watson Caring Science as a
guide to creating–healing environments on pediatric wards in a medical setting and was
approved by the Japanese Red Cross College of Nursing Ethics Committee. The focus of
this inquiry was to assess what aspects of Watson's Theory of Human Caring create an
environment for caring (Tsutsui, 2010).

JAPANESE RED CROSS COLLEGE OF NURSING—TOKYO RESEARCH PROGRAM: CREATING A CARING ENVIRONMENTAL MODEL

The results of the integrative review yielded the four steps mentioned earlier to creating
a caring environment. Next, the researchers conducted a study using a participatory
action research (PAR) intensive designed to help nurses explore the Caritas Processes®
and their effects on the nurse, the child, and the healthcare experience (Emoto, Tsutsui, &
Kawana, 2015).

The background of this work is based on cultural norms. In Japan, even though people
may have a need to ask questions, they may be hesitant to do so, because they are likely to
believe that it can affect their relationships with others by being perceived as burdensome
or overly assertive. Because harmonious interpersonal relationships are highly valued,
direct confrontation is avoided whenever possible. There is a reliance on the sensitivity of
the other person to pick up the point of the conversation.

The pediatric ward is very busy. As children's verbal and cognitive abilities are in the
process of development, assessment of the child's condition is very difficult. Caring for
children takes more time than for adults, accounting for time to explain and engage

children in the various treatments. At the time of the PAR, Japanese nurses discussed patients and families in care conferences; however, there was no opportunity to discuss professional practice issues that impacted their confidence in caring for children. As a result, clinical and practice challenges remained "buried," sometimes negatively impacting nurses' satisfaction with their own performance and their jobs.

The researchers conducted PAR in six hospitals in Japan in six pediatric wards and one pediatric outpatient department. The study was approved by the Ethics Committee of the Japanese Red Cross College of Nursing. The researchers recruited six master's-prepared clinical nurse specialists with greater than 5 years of experience as coresearchers. In turn, the coresearchers recruited nurse members; together, they designed the research collaboratively. The groups held discussions and data were used from the narrative discussions and other sources. The data were rich descriptions of nurses' clinical challenges. The discussions identified issues that nurses were facing silently because of cultural norms. For example, one pediatric nurse received harsh words from a pediatric patient and family. Although she wondered what she did to deserve being treated in such a way, she suppressed her feelings and continued to provide care. The nurse who was hurt by the patient's/family's harsh language had difficulty talking about the experience because she believed that telling about feeling hurt "would result in being labeled as being an incapable nurse," and "revealing my true feelings and saying something improper is not what a good nurse is supposed to do." She eventually began talking and revealed that she had tried to maintain a distance from the child and the family but that her work motivation diminished. The session resulted in peers sharing similar experiences and feelings. They empathized with her feelings without denying them and helped her regain the motivation for providing care. After 8 months, the healing experience of nurses resulted in improvements in care among children and families.

We need to care for ourselves, without being held back by fixed ideas such as what a nurse *should be*. Participating in PAR provided ongoing opportunities in which nurses could talk about their feelings without hesitation. Nurses found these sessions invaluable. They felt cared for by their superiors and the organization. They felt more able to care for patients/families in ways that could facilitate health and healing.

The results of ongoing dialogue about challenging situations allowed nurses to share negative experiences that were undermining their confidence. To improve the situation, nurses were given mutual understanding between staff nurses. As a result of dialogue, nurses were released from negative experiences. Identity crises were changed to competencies and nurses expressed more passion for nursing. The model that was developed as a result of this research showed an iterative relationship between the Caritas Processes, healing nurses, redefining existing problems, and disclosing hidden problems.

This action research was supported by one of Dr. Watson's Carative Factors, "the provision for a supportive, protective, and (or) corrective mental, physical, sociocultural, and spiritual environment" (Carative Factor #9) and was found to be key to a secure and safe caring environment for the care provider. This study was supported by the Grant-in-Aid for Scientific Research from the Ministry of Education, Culture, Sports, Science, and Technology for the fiscal years of 2007 to 2010. Dr. Watson served as a research mentor in these studies.

CONCLUSION

This chapter has provided a historical overview of Japanese developments and interest in Caring Science and Theory of Human Caring over the past 30 years. For example, the first foreign translation of Watson's *Theory of Human Caring* was in Japanese (translated by Fumiaki Inaoka [Watson, 1985]). Japanese nursing has been a leader in academic–research scholarship as well as projects and programs in Caring Science Theory. Another example is that the Japanese Red Cross Hiroshima College of Nursing was inaugurated with Caring Science Theory as the basis of its curriculum and Dr. Watson was the inaugural keynote speaker. This was followed by the establishment of the Japanese Red Cross Hiroshima College of Nursing Center for Human Caring, which was modeled after the Center for Human Caring, University of Colorado, in the 1980s.

As the focus on Caring Science advanced in Japan, the first Japanese research conferences included a Caring Science Theory focus and featured Dr. Watson as a keynote speaker (1989). This culminated in the Japanese Red Cross College of Nursing (in Tokyo) awarding Dr. Watson an International Honorary Doctorate (2012), followed by the Japanese Red Cross Hiroshima College of Nursing sponsorship of the First Asian Pacific International Caritas Consortium and the First International Hiroshima Caring and Peace Conference.

These historic beginnings are continuing up to the current time, embracing the Second International Conference on Caring and Peace, Tokyo (2016), held in March 2017. (The conference continues in September 2019.) Finally, the chapter closes with an overview of extant caring theory research, which provides some guidelines for Caritas Literacy—Japan, in relation to the caring environment. The PAR was an important milestone in Japan, helping nurses care for each other, thus creating a caring-healing environment for all.

NEXT ERA POSSIBILITIES

From reading and reflecting on the scholarly evolution of the Japanese path to Caritas for peace and change, contemplate the following:

Education
- What does the 2012 International Hiroshima Conference on Caring and Peace teach about the value and significance of learning in context?
- How does context create a palate for the exploration of human caring and peace?
- What current contexts provide a palate for critical reflection on caring, peace, and Caritas Literacy?

Research
- How do findings from the integrative review on Watson's Caring Theory inform future directions for research?
- On the basis of the study on cultural norms described in this chapter, what studies need to be carried out within your culture to encourage Caring Literacy?

Praxis
- How do I radiate gestures of peace from within and without?
- How do findings from the integrative review described in this chapter guide praxis-based scientific knowledge?

Theory and Knowledge Development
- How do cultural norms inform middle-range theory development in Caring Science?

 REFERENCES

Emoto, R., Tsutsui, M., & Kawana, R. (2015). A model to create a caring and healing environment for nurses in child and family. *International Journal for Human Caring, 19*(1), 8–12. doi:10.20467/1091-5710-19.1.8

Tsutsui, M. (2010). *Environment creation of caring and healing in pediatric nurses: Nursing action research* (Research Report of 2007–2010). Grant-in-Aid for Scientific Research, Ministry of Education, Culture, Sports, Science, and Technology, Tokyo, Japan.

Tsutsui, M. (2011). Caring in nursing: Its trends and perspectives. *Journal of Nursing Research, 44*(2), 115–128.

Watson, J. (1985). *Nursing: Human science and human care: A theory of nursing* (F. Inaoka and M. Inaoka, Japanese Trans.). Sudbury, MA: Jones & Bartlett.

Watson, J. (2001). *Assessing and measuring caring in nursing and health sciences* (M. Tsutsui, Japanese Trans.). New York, NY: Springer Publishing.

Watson, J. (2012, March). *Touching the heart of our humanity: The Caritas path of peace* [Keynote address]. International Hiroshima Conference on Caring and Peace, Hiroshima, Japan.

35

Caritas Nursing and Professional Practice in Peru*

Patrick A. Palmieri

CARITAS LITERACIES

By the end of this chapter, the caring-healing nurse will be able to

1. Describe the state of Caring Science nursing practice in Peru.

2. Discuss how performance improvement initiatives contribute to the success of advancing nursing as a caring discipline.

3. Advance the notion that Caritas nursing can develop nursing knowledge and informed practice.

Peruvian nursing, or *enfermería peruana*, has evolved as a vocation and somewhat apart from the international nursing community. The focus of many Latina scholars is to advance enfermería peruana from a vocation to a theoretically guided discipline with an established science. This chapter is the narrative, lived experience of a Peruvian American nurse who reflects on a 10-year journey to create space for the emergence of postmodern nursing in Peru. I comment on the state of the science and proposes a new future that is guided by Caring Science. To build South American communitas, I along with others have worked to establish Sociedad de Watson, a Watson Caring Science Global Associate that links enfermería peruana to global Caritas, as described in other chapters in this book, that will build Caring Literacy through the translation of texts, the development of Caritas curricula for Latin American schools of nursing, and links to global Caring Science scholars.

---

*This chapter is reprinted from Palmieri, P. A. (2017). The co-emergence of caritas nursing and professional nursing practice in Peru. In S. M. Lee, P. A. Palmieri, & J. Watson (Eds.), *Global advances in human caring literacy* (pp. 71–88). New York, NY: Springer Publishing.

Peruvian nursing, or enfermería peruana, is perceived as a vocation. Since the early 2000s, there has been increasing awareness of grand theories and a distinct disciplinary body of knowledge, but this is not yet widespread. Clinically, nursing's primary role is to carry out medical orders. The educational preparation consists of 5 years at the university; however, there are neither competency-based licensure examinations nor competency-based specialty certifications. The advanced practice role is currently being developed.

Nursing science in Peru is underdeveloped and often based on principles and methods borrowed from public health. In fact, most doctorally prepared nurses study public health rather than nursing theory and science. The situation in Peru is similar to Haynes, Boese, and Butcher's (2004) description of American nursing in the 1970s as evolving from a vocation to a profession grounded in a discrete and defined disciplinary knowledge. But this can be partially explained by the 1978 creation of the Colegio de Enfermeros del Perú (National Board of Nursing) and the 2002 law to create the Peruvian nurse practice act (Ministerio de Trabajo y Promoción del Empleo, 2002). In reality, enfermería peruana is young and immature but ready to grow with nurturing knowledge from the international nursing community.

Importantly, there is a proud nursing tradition in Peru, but this contributes to a partial disconnect of enfermería peruana from the global nursing community. For example, the nursing color in Peru is turquoise rather than purple (Rogerian) or white (sterile), the nursing day is celebrated on August 30 instead of May 12 (Nightingale's birthday), and the Catholic Saint of Nursing is Saint Rose of Lima, not Saint Camillus de Lellis (International Red Cross founder and official Vatican Saint of Nursing). There are no Sigma Theta Tau International (STTI) chapters in Peru, and there is no representative organization for enfermería peruana at the International Council of Nurses (2015). Overall, enfermería peruana is remarkably different than North American nursing and somewhat apart from the international nursing community.

This chapter describes my lived experience and professional reality as a Peruvian American nurse. These comments might seem ethnocentric, but I hope they may shed light on the current evolution of nursing in Peru. I speak about my lived experience as a relatively young male nurse, educated in the best American and British universities, mentored by exceptional scholars in multiple disciplines, including nursing, management, education, and evidence-based healthcare, transitioning from an intellectually stimulating and beautiful Duke University campus to live and work in the exciting capitol of Lima, Peru. At the time and still true today, my relocation was motivated by my two loves in life: my new Peruvian wife, an accomplished economist and bank leader, and our nursing profession.

DEVELOPMENT OF GLOBAL NURSING KNOWLEDGE

The North American nursing tradition, with a remarkable history, evolved with the contributions of notable nursing scholars, including theorists, researchers, and practitioners. The discipline continues to gain strength and expand in visibility. From England, Florence Nightingale provided our initial call to action when she prepared women to care for the wounded and to comfort the dying soldiers during the Crimean War (Cook, 1913). Nightingale (1859) then emancipated our noble profession, stating:

> I use the word nursing for want of a better. It has been limited to signify little more than the administration of medicines and the application of poultices. It ought to

signify the proper use of fresh air, light, warmth, cleanliness, quiet, and the proper selection and administration of diet—all at the least expense of vital power to the patient. (p. 2)

Continuing Nightingale's work, American nursing scholar Virginia Henderson (1966) further defined contemporary nursing for the International Council of Nursing, stating:

The unique function of the nurse is to assist the individual, sick or well, in the performance of those activities contributing to health or its recovery (or to peaceful death) that he would perform unaided if he had the necessary strength, will or knowledge. And to do this in such a way as to help him gain independence as rapidly as possible. (Tomey & Alligood, 1998, p. 102)

Over the next 50 years, the nursing profession rapidly advanced. Importantly, the discipline emerged with the introduction of theories, matured with the synthesis of concepts, and the result is our theory-infused and informed practice (Meleis, 2007), the nursing praxis. This evolution emancipated nursing as a legitimate discipline, a carative health profession complementary to the curative medical partner (Watson, 2008).

Henderson introduced the Science of Unitary Human Beings (Rogers, 1980), which was then advanced by Dr. Jean Watson to the Theory of Human Caring, to "explicate a distinct unitary view of human with a relational caring ontology and ethic that informs nursing as well as other sciences" (Watson & Smith, 2002, p. 461). The major elements contextualizing her theory to inform nursing practice include the Carative Factors, the transpersonal caring relationship, and the caring occasion/caring moment (Watson, 2001).

From Nightingale to Henderson, from Rogers to Watson, the North American nursing renaissance is expanding and informing the global nursing community. The renaissance is evidenced as Gallup (Saad, 2015) again reported nursing as the most trusted profession, for the 14th consecutive year, noting, "With an 85 percent honesty and ethics rating—tying their high point—nurses have no serious competition atop Gallup ranking this year [2015]" (para. 5). I believe Dr. Watson is largely responsible for the American public's confidence in nursing. Dr. Watson (2012) believes that nursing has evolved to advance positive social change from the individual to the global community:

Nursing has consistently been affirmed by the public as ethical and worthy of public trust. Nursing's evolving science, theories, methods, and practices are expected to adhere to this public vision and hope for survival with integrity and purpose for this century and beyond. (p. 30)

For nursing to be defined in parsimonious worldview (Fawcett, 1993), we need a discrete and identifiable body of knowledge with theories and concepts constructed (Daly, 1997) to inform and guide nursing practice (Mitchell, 2002). Caring Science will inform this parsimonious worldview, including South America. Although nursing in South America has evolved as a discipline, nurses do not have enough knowledge to advance further (Mujica, 1982; Urra, 2009). My work is dedicated to my profession in Peru, to help my Peruvian colleagues achieve the public trust through advancing this worldview.

TRANSITIONING CARING TO SOUTH AMERICA

Despite the North American nursing renaissance, there are many countries in which the nursing discipline is underdeveloped and, the practice is neither informed by the robust disciplinary knowledge nor theoretically driven by scientific inquiry. This is especially true in South America (Urra, 2009), where nursing struggles to emerge with a well-defined identity, literally fighting the suppressive *sociomedico* model. But, for the sake of their patients, Peruvian nurses may create their own road map, references from the North American caring–loving–healing tradition and knowledge. Advancing nursing from a vocation to a profession to a theoretically guided discipline with an established science is indeed the focus of many Latina nursing scholars. The Theory of Human Caring is a way for enfermería peruana "to see" (Watson, 2008), to know, to reflect, and to understand (Carper, 1978). This is where I transition from the context into my personal story as I relocated to Peru to live and work nearly a decade ago, became a Peruvian citizen on July 4, 2012, and then met my mentor, Dr. Jean Watson.

In this chapter, I speak for the first time about my lived experience as a nurse working in the Andean region (Bolivia, Chile, and Peru) of South America. In particular, I focus on my new country, Peru. Cultural context is essential to explain how Caring Science and the Caritas Processes informed my leadership practices and provided me with the continued strength and courage to advance contemporary nursing knowledge in Peru. The word "Caritas" is especially meaningful to describe the way nurses bring caring, loving, and heart-centered care to patients and their families through their practice as well as accepting the same self-care into their personal lives (Watson, 2009).

Enfermería peruana is poised to enter a new phase in development and could benefit from mentorship from academics, theorists, administrators, and advanced clinicians from other countries. With global nursing knowledge as the compass and the North American road map as a reference for the journey, the Caritas-informed nursing renaissance can be replicated in Peru. However, the discipline of nursing, as women's work, mimics the female role in society, which is explained in the following section.

PATERNALISTIC SOCIOMEDICAL CULTURE

The Peruvian health sector is especially challenging for nurses to navigate and disabling for nurses seeking to professionally advance as leaders. First and foremost, *enfermeras peruanas* (Peruvian nurses) are largely women working in a male-dominated and -directed environment. The general Peruvian "machismo" culture extends with more purpose, a harsher reality, and nearly dictatorial style as traditionally male physicians control the healthcare sector. As a former health insurance executive responsible for the creation of the largest privately owned health system in Peru, I experienced working as a corporate and sector leader. My belief is that the Peruvian health sector not only is dominated by a "machismo" philosophy but also overlaps with a paternalistic sociomedical culture. But we need to heed the words of Nightingale (1859) as, "No man, not even a doctor, ever gives any other definition of what a nurse should be than this—devoted and obedient. This definition would do just as well for a porter. It might even do for a horse. It would not do for a policeman" (p. 200).

In this health sector culture, women are marginalized, including female patients, and often mistreated and sometimes harmed, emotionally and physically. Enfermeras peruanas are responsible for implementing physician orders and expected to comply without exception to directives issued by the "white jackets." These are the male physician hospital leaders who literally wear formal white blazers at work, a symbol of their power and sector status. With frequency, I observe nurses giving their chairs to physicians and I listen first-hand to accounts of sexual harassment and other injustices. Furthermore, I have witnessed instances of physical and verbal abuse against nurses in hospitals, including screaming, grabbing, and throwing objects. Finally, nurses work in unsafe and stressful environments. On the typical medical–surgical unit, the nurse-to-patient ratio ranges from 1:20 to 1:40; in the emergency department (ED), the ratio is as high as 1:20. This reality begs the question whether enfermeras peruanas can engage in informed and reflective practice. The ratios, however, further evidence the lack of respect and concern for enfermería as an important Peruvian health profession.

SITUATIONAL ASSESSMENT

Watson (1999) suggests that nurses need to assess and critique their situations and see where or how they are in their environment, and then locate themselves within the framework of the emerging ideas in relation to their own paradigm of a caring professional nursing practice, including the relevant theories and philosophies. Furthermore, Watson (2001) states:

> If one chooses to use the caring perspective as theory, model, philosophy, ethic or ethos for transforming self and practice, or self and system, the following questions may help: Is there congruence between (a) the values and major concepts and beliefs in the model and the given nurse, group, system, organization, curriculum, population needs, clinical administrative setting, or other entity that is considering interacting with the caring model to transform and/or improve practice? Are those interacting and engaging in the model interested in their own personal evolution? Are they committed to seeking authentic connections and caring-healing relationships with self and others? Are those involved "conscious" of their caring-caritas or non-caring consciousness and intentionally in a given moment and at an individual and system level? Are they interested and committed to expanding their caring consciousness and actions to self, other, environment, nature and wider universe? Are those working within the model interested in shifting their focus from a modern medical science-technocure orientation to a true caring-healing-loving model? (pp. 349–350)

As such, enfermeras peruanas need to recognize their current practice environment, which negatively impacts their nursing work and their being. Furthermore, enfermeras peruanas can create the space to transform and improve their practice and their own personal development. Finally, through the Caritas, enfermeras peruanas can expand their own consciousness and shift the current paternalistic sociomedical orientation to embrace a nursing practice premised on caring–healing–loving relationships.

CONTEXT FOR CHANGE

Advancing enfermería peruana from vocation to profession requires the nursing practice to be informed by the disciplinary knowledge derived from Caring Science. When enfermeras peruanas receive international support and scholarly guidance, they can consciously shift their paradigm from the curative medical model to the carative nursing orientation, to practice caring–loving–healing. Through Caring Science, they can overcome mere compliance with the antiquated machismo sociomedical culture, displacing the medical ego, by engaging in reflective and Caritas-informed practice. As enfermeras peruanas increasingly understand the disciplinary knowledge offered by the Theory of Human Caring, they will embrace their new Caring Science paradigm and implement the Caritas into their daily self-care and patient care.

An assumption for intentional caring-loving-healing–informed practice is the presence of a "safe space (sacred space) for people to seek their own wholeness of being and becoming, not only now but in the future, evolving toward wholeness, greater complexity and connectedness with the deep self, the soul and the higher self " (Watson, 1999, p. 102). When enfermeras peruanas establish their space, they can separate their identity from medicine by consciously and independently existing, developing, advancing, and achieving the wholeness in their caring-loving-healing practice, for self as well as others. When enfermeras peruanas establish their unique identity from medicine, their caring-loving-healing environment with a Caritas-infused practice, enfermería will become relevant to the health sector. Healing is an essential human attribute need that nurses offer to the public through their sacred practice.

Aware of the success with advancing hospital nursing through implementing nurse caring models grounded in Caring Science with Caritas-informed practices (Watson & Foster, 2003), from about 2007 to 2012, I led an ambitious agenda to clear a space for nursing with three strategies: (a) Develop nurse-led projects specific to quality improvement, patient safety, and risk management; (b) advance contemporary Caritas-informed practice by mentoring young and dynamic nursing leaders; and (c) exercise a new voice for nursing through public policy and political action. Then, in 2012, immediately after leaving the health system to focus on advancing enfermería peruana, my work sought to redefine nursing as a profession rather than a vocation with an established discipline defined by nursing knowledge instead of the legal constructs intended to restrain nursing. About a year after undertaking this work, I encountered resistance and experienced many failures. These experiences prompted extensive reflection and my return to reviewing the nursing literature and engaging in self-learning.

HOW I CAME TO BEING WITH CARING SCIENCE

In early 2014, I was frustrated with the many barriers my Peruvian colleagues were facing as well as their reluctance to seek new ways of being and indecisiveness in embracing contemporary knowledge to inform their practice. At this point, I was stressed and not motivated to continue my work. In fact, I contemplated returning to the United States and possibly leaving nursing altogether. This was when I reached out to Dr. Jean Watson for help and, I hoped, some guidance. Really, I was desperate for an intervention, for help in learning more about Caring Science, and for encouragement to bring the practices of

Caritas to my Peruvian nursing colleagues. But, at the time, the content of the intervention I sought was not fresh in my mind.

When I sent my first email to Dr. Watson, I expected a response several weeks later; however, I was surprised with her immediate email. This email provided a sense of relief and new hope for me and my colleagues. After exchanging several emails, Dr. Watson invited me to attend her Research Intensive Proseminar 2 months later in Boulder, Colorado. On arriving at the Proseminar, I received an incredibly warm welcome and what I will call my first Caritas group therapy session. Most importantly, Dr. Watson helped me understand the world needs to change, to save humanity, and nursing is the profession responsible for stimulating this change through Caritas-informed practice. Leaving the Proseminar, I was resolute to become a human-caring theorist and caring scientist. I realized I could lead a caring movement in Peru and throughout South America to create positive social change.

Officially in 2015, I became Dr. Watson's postdoctoral fellow, studying with and learning from the most influential nurse theorist since Florence Nightingale; and my Caring Science studies and scholarly work continue with an incredible community of accomplished and enlightened faculty and scholars. Then, the real work began, understanding at the deepest level the philosophy underpinning Caring Science, learning the methodologies and methods, and understanding my praxis. My professional and personal lives are continuously informed by the Theory of Human Caring and guided by the principles set forth by the Caritas. Importantly, my actions and interactions remain mindful of the need to cultivate caring-loving-healing relationships and to practice loving-kindness (Watson, 2008).

TRANSITIONING CARING SCIENCE FROM BOULDER TO LUCCA TO LIMA

While studying Caring Science and working with my Peruvian colleagues to begin our caring revolution in Lima, Peru, I began to achieve more successes than failures. In fact, I was inducted into the American Academy of Nursing as a fellow (FAAN) in October 2015. Before studying Caring Science, I was already a good scholar, something I did not fully appreciate. Thankfully, Drs. Alexia Green and Gayle Roux recognized my accomplishments and my ability to positively contribute to nursing in Peru, hence their sponsorship of my application. As I prepared my application, I studied Caring Science, which inspired and motivated me through the process; the goal was to become a FAAN like my new mentor.

Ironically, perhaps coincidentally, I received the admission letter the week before traveling to Lucca, Italy, for the First Annual Caring Science Sacred Science Seminar. With my Caritas faculty and colleagues, I celebrated my news regarding my career transition. The seminar was notable for two reasons: First, I engaged in my first Caritas healing with art session, led by the creator, Dr. Mary Rockwood Lane, who, in fact, contributed to this book. The small painting is framed and immediately visible on the right corner of my desk: a reminder of my past, the escape to the present, and the new Caritas path for the future. Then, following an incredible Puccini opera at a historic church, this book was literally conceived on a placemat as Drs. Lee, Watson, and I enjoyed a delicious pizza and shared stories about our journey to the Caring Science. In an important caring moment, we realized we are part of a developing global Caring Literacy, and our collective stories needed to be told.

TRANSLATING CARING TO ACHIEVE OUTCOMES

By not just learning the Caritas Processes but living them, clear intentions and positive energy flooded my interpersonal field. Successes are constructed from loving caring intentions; however, I realize that failures result when the ego escapes and dominates. Importantly, Caring Science guided the advancement of my practice to strengthen myself and to help me strengthen others, to support and expand our noble global profession, and to build our global communitas. To this end, the Asociación Peruana de Enfermería, or APE (Peruvian Nurses Association), was legally established in 2015 to inform and support enfermería peruana. The APE complements the National Board of Nursing by striving to advance nursing as a profession and discipline, guided and informed by Caring Science. But this professional organization was not sufficient to focus on advancing Caring Science. There needed to be an intentional focus to fill the space with caring-loving-healing energy.

Working with Dr. Watson and my colleagues, we realized there needed to be a direct link from South America to the Watson Caring Science Institute (WCSI). In April 2016, the Sociedad de Watson (Watson Society) was established within the APE to bring Caring Science to enfermería peruana, and to diffuse Caritas innovations throughout Sudamérica. These two organizations will continue our work to advance enfermería peruana as a discipline guided by the Theory of Human Caring, a nursing science defined by Caring Science, and a nursing practice informed by the Caritas. Through my early work, which is explicated in the next section, we cleared a space for nursing to begin practicing, teaching, researching, and leading as a Caritas-informed profession, complementary to our curative physician colleagues. Importantly, I worked to clear this space for enfermería peruana to embrace the Theory of Human Caring and to engage in Caritas-informed practice.

CLEARING THE SPACE AND BUILDING THE VOICE FOR PERUVIAN NURSING

Unlike North American nurses, enfermeras peruanas struggle to create a space for nursing, never mind the sacred space necessary for our Caritas-informed nursing practice. We have not been able to effectively advocate for our patients as our voice was weak and not focused with caring-loving-healing intentions. Drawing from my strength and preparation as a quality improvement and patient safety expert, I developed an international accreditation agenda, approved by my organization's leaders and endorsed by the board of directors, to develop the first nursing-led projects in a Peruvian healthcare facility. The rationale for implementing these nursing-led projects for enfermería peruana was to develop them as patient advocates through accepted medical concepts, quality improvement, and patient safety. This would be an opportunity to advance the profession and to establish the discipline defined by the Theory of Human Caring. My prime directive was clear—achieve an international accreditation with a nursing-led initiative within 3 years. With this directive, nursing would become an operationally relevant and recognized department within an emerging private health system.

Because of my positional power and professional reputation, my colleagues and I advanced nursing autonomy through results, proving better patient care through nursing-led quality improvement, patient safety, and risk management projects. The project began at the ambulatory oncology facility, then advanced to a private maternity hospital, and finally concluded at a small private hospital in the province of Peru. The initial space was established as each facility had a motivated visionary nursing leader supported by a chief executive officer (CEO) who trusted me in my belief that nurses could improve patient care and develop professional knowledge by implementing international standards guided by a theoretical framework.

THE LIVED EXPERIENCE OF CREATING A SPACE FOR NURSING

The quality improvement focused on implementing the international accreditation standards, guided by nursing and organizational science. The nurse leaders were intrigued with this seemingly strange theoretically guided framework. To the best of my ability, I led this project guided by Caring Science and Caritas-informed mentoring. This means, although not explicitly stated within the framework, I taught the Caritas Factors and spoke the Caritas language as I mentored the nurse leaders, and even the CEOs, for each project.

Interestingly, my colleagues and mentees can now identify with this point, but I choose to quietly teach the Caritas to advance the Carative Processes to complement, rather than reject, the curative approach. And I needed to be careful about how I described my goals and objectives to protect the project, and the nurses, from the machismo paternalistic forces that would prevent the space-clearing and voice-enabling agenda. In fact, my professional preparation as a nurse was neither discussed nor divulged by my nonnursing colleagues. But, focused on achieving results, I permitted others to temporarily shape my personal identity despite the uncomfortable feeling that I was hiding my nursing identity. The overall strategy led to many developments that I describe in the next section. However, I want to attribute the next exemplar outcome to my Caritas-informed leadership and Caritas-infused mentoring.

NURSE-LED PROJECT EXEMPLAR

Although there is not sufficient space for reflecting on the projects, the operational results achieved by a nurse I continue to mentor were remarkable, providing a voice for nursing, allowing space for Caritas-informed practice to begin developing, and serving as an exemplar for others to replicate. At the start of the project, the self-evaluation demonstrated 27% compliance with all accreditation standards; incidentally, there were many problems with nursing turnover, physician satisfaction, adverse events, and financial results. After the project, the quality improvement data for each standard demonstrated an 86% compliance. Importantly, the standards deemed as "critical" rose to 100%. Furthermore, the operational-balanced scorecard resulted in improvements in financial outcomes, a decreased number of adverse events with harm, and increased patient and physician satisfaction. The official accreditation evaluation resulted in no chapter deficiencies and a full 3-year accreditation.

The official accreditation is not the most significant project outcome, however. Through this quality improvement effort, where leaders fully engaged nurses and granted them permission to develop Caritas-informed practices, hospitals in developing countries can positively impact patient care. Importantly, these accreditation projects established nursing at each facility as the carative partner to our curative physician colleagues. Physicians began to recognize the power of caring-loving-healing relationships. When hospital leaders empower nurses to lead projects, such as quality improvement on the basis of accreditation standards, and give them permission to develop independent nursing departments guided by nursing knowledge, remarkable transformations develop in patient care, resulting in increased patient and family, nurse, and physician satisfaction. In Peru, the importance of theoretically informed nursing practice has been underappreciated, often discounted, and generally not recognized as an essential quality improvement strategy.

Within 5 years from the start of the initial quality improvement/patient safety project, all three facilities achieved international accreditation and two have successfully been reaccredited. But the work extended past the nursing-led accreditation project as the space was cleared for nursing to evolve. With the reduced nurse-to-patient ratios in each of these facilities, caring can be practiced intentionally and nurses can have the Caritas consciousness, including the values and the motives, to create caring moments and to have an intentional consciousness of caring (Watson, 1988a, 1999). With more time, nurses can stop treating patients and begin engaging in caring-loving-healing nursing practices. The five core principles espoused by Dr. Watson (Watson, 2008, p. 34) can be embraced and incorporated into the soul of nursing practice. They are as follows:

1. Practice of loving-kindness and equanimity

2. Authentic presence: enabling deep belief of other (patient, colleague, family, et al.)

3. Cultivation of one's own spiritual practice toward wholeness of mind/body/spirit—beyond ego

4. "Being" the caring-healing environment

5. Allowing miracles (openness to the unexpected and inexplicable life events)

Derived from the unitary human science of caring, the Theory of Human Caring is the nursing epistemology (Watson, 1988a, 1997). Later, the theory evolved into Human Caring Science (Watson, 2005, 2008, 2012) guided by 10 carative factors:

1. Formation of a humanistic-altruistic system of values

2. Instillation of faith–hope

3. Cultivation of sensitivity to one's self and to others

4. Development of a helping-trusting, human-caring relationship

5. Promotion and acceptance of the expression of positive and negative feelings

6. Systematic use of a creative problem-solving caring process

7. Promotion of transpersonal teaching–learning

8. Provision for a supportive, protective, and/or corrective mental, physical, societal, and spiritual environment

9. Assistance with gratification of human needs

10. Allowance for existential-phenomenological-spiritual forces (Watson, 1988b, p. 75)

Importantly, these elements of the theory are measured by the validated 10-item Caring Factor Survey. Here, the principal focus for each item is presented:

1. Practice loving-kindness.

2. Engage in decision making.

3. Instill faith and hope in others.

4. Teach and learn new things.

5. Respect spiritual beliefs and practices.

6. Provide holistic care.

7. Establish helping and trusting relationships.

8. Create a healing environment.

9. Encourage the expression of feelings.

10. Recognize and accept miracles (adapted from DiNapoli, Nelson, Turkel, & Watson, 2010, p. 16).

However, in Sudamérica (South America), the 10 Caritas Processes are often called "clinical Caritas," or *Caritas clínicas* in Spanish (Favero, Joaquim-Meier, Ribeiro-Lacerda, de Azevedo-Mazza, & Canestraro-Kalinowski, 2009), reflecting the application of the theory to nursing practice.

These Caritas clínicas represent the essential nursing praxis for Sudamérica; they define the *disciplina de enfermería peruana* (Peruvian nursing discipline) and advance the contemporary *practica de enfermería peruana* (Peruvian nursing practice). Enfermería peruana needs to join our global communitas and integrate the global Caritas praxis, or the "informed practice; practice that is empirically validated and informed by one's philosophical-ethical-theoretical orientation, but grounded in concrete actions and behaviors that can be empirically assessed and measured" (DiNapoli et al., 2010, p. 16). By defining the disciplina de enfermería peruana with the Theory of Human Caring, incorporating the Caritas into the practica de enfermería peruana, and studying nursing phenomena through *la ciencia del cuidado humano* (Human Caring Science), enfermeras peruanas can continue to expand their new space and strengthen their voice within the Peruvian health sector. The space is neither intended to compete with nor replace space occupied by medicine; however, the carative nursing space needs to coexist with curative medicine space to complement rather than compete.

Medicine is principally concerned with physical, largely mechanistic, curing, whereas nursing is concerned with holistic, or human, caring. In a Social Policy Statement (American Nurses Association, 1980), nursing was defined as "the diagnosis and treatment of human responses to actual or potential health problems" (p. 7). Unlike the physician focused on the disease, the nurse is concerned with the human response to it (Watson, 2005, 2008). As nurses and patients require caring relationships, healing environments, and a culture of caring, healing, and love, the "evolved integration and synthesis of Caring Science and Theory gives birth to authentic, spirit-filled, loving caring-healing practices that embrace all of humanity, offering a hopeful paradigm for this era" (Watson, 2010, p. 14).

With Caritas-informed practice, the nurse feels the "concern, regard, [and] respect one human being may have for another. Its roots lie in the maternal and paternal behavior of all higher living things, and it may be impaired or reinforced by environmental circumstances" (Sobel, 1969, p. 2612). In terms of physically curing, Hunt (1999) concluded, "The impersonal constructs of biomedical and social science are far removed from the inner life of fear, love and hope, an inner life which is, moreover, constantly in flux and, often, ambiguous" (p. 231). Because of the caring perspective, "the discipline of nursing arguably has the potential to develop unique knowledge of human health. It has this potential because nurses have a role within healthcare that gives them a privileged perspective on a range of issues" (Risjord, 2010, p. 77).

Importantly, Nightingale (1859) stressed that the nurse–patient relationship is established to provide care by managing the internal and external environments in a manner consistent with the laws of nature. This is remarkably different from the work of physicians as Marcum (2009) opined, "rather than evidence-based practitioners, we should be striving to create epistemically virtuous physicians" (Upshur & Tracy, 2013, p. 1161). Because medicine is preoccupied with discovering cures in the positivist tradition, "it would make little sense to see medicine make a paradigm shift away from basic science" (Sehon & Stanley, 2003, p. 3). In medicine, the quantitative research, such as systematic reviews and randomized controlled trials, is considered the best evidence for practice (Straus, Ball, Balcombe, Sheldon, & McAlister, 2005), but this structural limitation has led medicine to be largely silent about integrating patient preferences and their values into an incompatible methodology. Consequently, contrasting movements such as patient-centered and person-centered care and values-based medicine have emerged as counterpoints to medicine to address this deficit (Miles & Mezzich, 2011), which is more complementary and reflective of Carative-informed nursing practice.

NEW SPACE FOR CARITAS-INFORMED PRACTICE

The private maternity hospital that achieved international accreditation engaged me to work with them to develop a new nursing reality. First, the hospital implemented a competency-based evaluation and salary scale premised on Benner's novice-to-expert theory (Benner, 1984). The nurse-to-patient ratios are guided by American nursing standards in all units, including neonatal nursery and intensive care units, perioperative services, and pre- and postpartum. Also, the hospital funded multiple 2-year nursing fellowships to develop nursing expert leaders in infection prevention and control, neonatal intensive care, and surgical services. Then, the hospital moved away from the traditional nursing structure, with a director of nursing reporting to the medical director, and a chief nursing officer (CNO) reporting directly to the CEO. The quality improvement director is a nurse, a position usually held by a physician. Next, the CEO developed a training and development area as well as a nurse relaxation room, which will emerge later this year as the *Espacio de Watson*

(Watson Space). Finally, the hospital is funding nurse managers to seek master's degrees in business administration (MBAs) and specialty nursing education. Each of these steps moves the organization along a pathway to prepare nurses for the final goal of changing the care delivery model. As such, I am actively engaged with the CEO and my bilingual mentee who was recently promoted to the CNO position in the initial preparations to develop a Caritas nursing model to support Caritas-informed nursing practice. When implemented, this will be the first theoretically guided nursing practice model implemented in Peru.

POLITICAL ACTION FOR A NEW VOICE

In early 2015, nursing responded to the call for political action to change the machismo culture and paternalistic health sector when 13 nurses succeeded in becoming party candidates for the Peruvian Congress. The election resulted in two nurses earning seats in the Congress, whereas another colleague fell slightly short of earning a seat. With two nurses in the Congress, there is a powerful voice to advocate for patients as well as the profession. In addition to the nurse seats in Congress, the nursing community rallied to force the Congress to approve a law to permit independent nursing practices to deliver health and wellness services.

EDUCATION TO TEACH CARITAS

Private Peruvian schools of nursing are beginning to recognize Dr. Watson, like most prominent nursing scholars worldwide, who was largely unknown in Peru until 2012. Similarly, there are no STTI Honor Society for Nursing chapters in Peru, and there are only three in the entire Latin America and Caribbean region (2016). However, in 2015, the Peruvian Honor Society of Nursing began the process to achieve official STTI status, a process requiring 2 years (Sociedad de Enfermeria, 2016), and nurses in Bolivia and Chile are engaged in similar processes. After Dr. Watson presented at a university in Chiclayo, Peru, in 2015, there was excitement for learning the Theory of Human Caring and cultivating a Caritas-informed nursing practice. Dr. Watson continues to be invited to speak at Peruvian schools of nursing interested in establishing Caritas curriculums. In fact, Dr. Watson will speak twice in 2016 in Peru, including a 1-week engagement with the Colegio de Enfermeros del Perú (National Board of Nursing). The purpose of this visit is to help the National Board of Nursing understand how to construct a framework to infuse Caring Science into nursing education through the national accreditation process.

THE EVOLVING PERUVIAN COMMUNITAS

The Sociedad de Watson, a Watson Caring Science Global Associate, was established to connect Caritas nurses in pursuit of building a South American communitas. This interconnection between Caritas and communitas makes "explicit that we belong to a shared humanity and are connected with each other. In this way, we share our collective humanity across time and space and are bound together in the infinite universal field that holds the totality of life itself" (Watson, 2008, p. 93).

A Watson Caring Science Global Associate (Global Associate) represents individuals, systems, projects, programs, and events from across the globe, endorsed and formally recognized by Dr. Watson and the WCSI. Each Global Associate is contributing to the development and advancement of Caring Science knowledge and practices in partnership with Dr. Watson/WCSI. The Global Associate designation identifies visionary leaders with Caritas-informed programs to address global caring needs of societies and communities. These leaders serve as inspired exemplars of Caritas-informed practice at this unique turning point for humanity. Global Associates seek to unite all health professionals under a shared commitment to embrace foundational and fundamental premises for sustaining human caring. The intended outcome is healing and health for all people around the globe (WCSI, 2016).

Through the increased presence of Dr. Watson in Peru and the mission of the Sociedad de Watson, the space for nursing continues to evolve as one devoted to Caritas-informed nursing practice. Importantly, the Sociedad de Watson is focused on bringing nursing leaders together through communitas. The next steps for the Sociedad de Watson include developing a pilot program called the Caritas Certified Curriculum for Latin American schools of nursing. Through this pilot certification program, we hope to stimulate additional interest and formative action to advance Caritas-informed nursing practice through a Caritas curriculum revolution. Finally, through the generosity of Dr. Kathleen Sitzman, the Sociedad de Watson will be able to bring Spanish translations of educational and developmental materials for Caring Science and mindful practice to Peruvian nursing and the evolving Sudamericana communitas. Upward and onward, we will move enfermería peruana, *vamos amigos*.

CONCLUSION

This chapter briefly described the traditional machismo and paternalistic environment where enfermeras peruanas practice, an environment not reported in the peer-reviewed literature. Then, the road map for the North American nursing renaissance was presented. Next, the exemplar project implemented to develop a space for nursing was described. And then, the curative versus carative epistemology was explained. Finally, the recent advancements were described and the relevance to the future plans was discussed. The Caritas revolution in nursing continues to advance from North America, to Europe, to Africa, to Asia, and now to South America through the WCSI scholars and postdoctoral fellows.

After nearly 10 years of work in Peru, the traditional practice environment is slowly being replaced with a new caring space for enfermería peruana. The result of Dr. Watson's frequent presence in Peru, physically and through social media, and my postdoctoral mentoring is a strengthened profession and development of a Caring Science–informed discipline. At this point, there is enlightened expansion as the vocation shifts to profession, informed by a carative epistemology. This is evident as three Peruvian universities have committed to establishing Caritas curriculums: Universidad Maria Auxiliar, Universidad Norbert Wiener, and Universidad Señor de Sipán.

The work is making an impact. In May 2016, Dr. Watson and I traveled to Arequipa, Peru, to speak at the Human Caring Conference; and Dr. Watson received two doctorates (causa honoris) from prestigious Peruvian universities (Universidad Nacional de San Agustin and Universidad Católica de Santa María) for her contributions to global nursing and her current dedication to working with Peruvian nurses. Also, I am quite proud of the honor bestowed upon me by the *Alcade* (Mayor) of Arequipa, *Vistante Distinguido* (Distinguished Visitor). The continued mentoring and guidance advance my knowledge and strengthen my plans: an evolution from expert practitioner to competent theorist, hopefully more.

With more time and tenacity, I will use the North American road map as my reference and the Caritas as my compass to mentor my own Caring Science mentees with the goal of experiencing an *enfermería peruana* renaissance within my lifetime. With Dr. Watson's help, this work is evolving and emerging in a different way. For example, Dr. Watson provides my talented bilingual mentee, Lic. Nataly Membrillo, the opportunity to serve as her translator for each trip to Peru. To translate for Dr. Watson, Lic. Membrillo has to study, understand, and internalize Caring Science. Through her visits, Dr. Watson graciously mentors Nataly in her goal to become a Caring Science scholar. As I conclude this chapter, we should recognize that Nightingale (the environment), Henderson (nursing definition), Rogers (unitary being), and then Watson (1996) provided us with the "critical, reflective practices that must be continuously questioned and critiqued in order to remain dynamic, flexible, and endlessly self-revising and emergent" (p. 143).

NEXT ERA POSSIBILITIES

To continue to expand Caring Science and Communitas worldwide, questions for reflection on next era possibilities include:

Education
- How does the North American road map and South America's path serve to inform other countries seeking to expanding Caring Science education?

Research
- How can international WCSI scholars and postdoctoral fellows continue to expand their work globally to create an international Caritas community to expand influence and scholarship?

Praxis
- What international Caritas practice projects and partnerships ideas are emerging from reading this chapter?

Theory and Knowledge Development
- How does global expansion of Caring Science and other complementary nursing theories such as Rogers's Unitary Being serve to magnify nursing's influence worldwide?

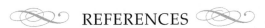 REFERENCES

American Nurses Association. (1980). *Nursing: A social policy statement*. Kansas City, MO: American Nurses Publishing.

Benner, P. (1984). *From novice to expert: Excellence and power in clinical nursing practice*. Menlo Park, CA: Addison-Wesley.

Carper, B. (1978). Fundamental patterns of knowing in nursing. *Advances in Nursing Science, 1*(1), 13–23. doi:10.1097/00012272-197810000-00004

Cook, E. T. (1913). *The life of Florence Nightingale.* London, UK: Macmillan. Retrieved from https://archive.org/details/lifeofflorenceni01cookuoft

Daly, J. (1997). What is nursing science? An international dialogue. *Nursing Science Quarterly, 10*(1), 120–122. doi:10.1177/089431849701000105

DiNapoli, P., Nelson, J., Turkel, M., & Watson, J. (2010). Measuring the Caritas processes: Caring factor survey. *International Journal for Human Caring, 14*(3), 15–20.

Favero, L., Joaquim-Meier, M., Ribeiro-Lacerda, M., de Azevedo-Mazza, V., & Canestraro-Kalinowski, L. (2009). Aplicación de la teoría del cuidado transpersonal de Jean Watson: Una década de producción brasileña [Application of Jean Watson's theory of transpersonal care: A decade of Brazilian production]. *Acta Paulista de Enfermagem, 22*(2), 213–218. doi:10.1590/S0103-21002009000200016

Fawcett, J. (1993). From a plethora of paradigms to parsimony in worldview. *Nursing Science Quarterly, 6*(2), 56–58. doi:10.1177/089431849300600202

Haynes, L., Boese, T., & Butcher, H. (2004). *Nursing in contemporary society: Issues, trends, and transition to practice.* Upper Saddle River, NJ: Pearson.

Henderson, V. (1966). *The nature of nursing: A definition and its implications for practice, research, and education.* New York, NY: Macmillan.

Hunt, S. M. (1999). The researcher's tale: A story of virtue lost and regained. In C. R. B. Joyce, H. M. McGee, & C. A. O'Boyle (Eds.), *Individual quality of life: Approaches to conceptualisation and assessment* (pp. 225–232). Amsterdam, Netherlands: Harwood Academic.

International Council of Nurses. (2015). Member list. Retrieved from http://www.icn.ch/members/members-list

Marcum, J. A. (2009). The epistemically virtuous clinician. *Theoretical Medicine and Bioethics, 30*(3), 249–265. doi:10.1007/s11017-009-9109-1

Meleis, A. I. (2007). *Theoretical nursing: Development and progress* (4th ed.). Philadelphia, PA: Lippincott Williams & Wilkins.

Miles, A., & Mezzich, J. E. (2011). The care of the patient and the soul of the clinic: Person-centered medicine as an emergent model of modern clinical practice. *International Journal of Person Centered Medicine, 1*(2), 207–222. doi:10.5750/ijpcm.v1i2.61

Ministerio de Trabajo y Promoción del Empleo. (2002, February 15). Ley N° 27669: Ley del Trabajo de la Enfermera(o). [Law No. 27669: Nursing labor law]. Retrieved from http://www.mintra.gob.pe/contenidos/archivos/prodlab/legislacion/LEY_27669.pdf

Mitchell, G. J. (2002). Learning to practice the discipline of nursing. *Nursing Science Quarterly, 15*(3), 209–213. doi:10.1177/08918402015003006

Mujica, M. I. (1982). Aspectos polémicos sobre teorías y modelos de enfermería. [Controversial aspects of nursing theories and models]. *Revista Enfermería, 17*(74), 3–6.

Nightingale, F. (1859). *Notes on nursing: What it is and what it is not.* London, UK: Harrison & Sons. Retrieved from https://archive.org/details/notesnursingwhat00nigh

Risjord, M. (2010). *Nursing knowledge: Science, practice, and philosophy.* West Sussex, UK: Wiley-Blackwell.

Rogers, M. E. (1980). Nursing: A science of unitary man. In J. P. Riehl & C. Roy (Eds.), *Conceptual models for nursing practice (2nd ed., pp. 329–337). New York, NY: Appleton-Century-Crofts.*

Saad, L. (2015, December 21). Americans' faith in honesty, ethics of police rebounds. Retrieved from http://www.gallup.com/poll/187874/americans-faith-honesty-ethics-police-rebounds.aspx?g_source=Social%20Issues&g_medium=newsfeed&g_campaign=tiles

Sehon, S. R., & Stanley, D. E. (2003). A philosophical analysis of the evidence-based medicine debate. *BMC Health Services Research, 3,* 14. doi:10.1186/1472-6963-3-14

Sigma Theta Tau International. (2016). Latin American and Caribbean region. Retrieved from https://www.sigmanursing.org/connect-engage/chapters/globalregions

Sobel, D. E. (1969). Human caring. *American Journal of Nursing, 69*(12), 2612–2613. doi:10.2307/3421105

Sociedad de Honor de Enfermería. (2016). Introducción [Introduction]. Retrieved from http://sociedadenfermeria.com

Straus, S. E., Ball, C., Balcombe, N., Sheldon, J., & McAlister, F. A. (2005). Teaching evidence-based medicine skills can change practice in a community hospital. *Journal of General Internal Medicine, 20*(4), 340–343. doi:10.1111/j.1525-1497.2005.04045.x

Tomey, A. M., & Alligood, M. R. (Eds.). (1998). *Nursing theorists and their work* (4th ed.). St. Louis, MO: Mosby.

Upshur, R. E. G., & Tracy, C. S. (2013). Is evidence-based medicine overrated in family medicine? *Canadian Family Physician, 59*(11), 1160–1161.

Urra, E. (2009). Avances de la ciencia de enfermería y su relación con la disciplina. [Advances in nursing science and its relationship to the discipline]. *Ciencia y Enfermeria, 15*(2), 9–18. doi:10.4067/S0717-95532009000200002

Watson Caring Science Institute. (2016). Global associates. Retrieved from https://www.watsoncaringscience.org/global-caring-science

Watson, J. (1988a). New dimensions of human caring theory. *Nursing Science Quarterly, 1*(4), 175–181. doi:10.1177/089431848800100411

Watson, J. (1988b). *Nursing: Human science and human care. A theory of nursing.* New York, NY: National League for Nursing.

Watson, J. (1996). Watson's theory of transpersonal caring. In P. H. Walker & B. Neuman (Eds.), *Blueprint for use of nursing models: Education, research, practice, & administration* (pp. 141–184). New York, NY: National League for Nursing.

Watson, J. (1997). The theory of human caring: Retrospective and prospective. *Nursing Science Quarterly, 10*(1), 49–52. doi:10.1177/089431849701000114

Watson, J. (1999). *Postmodern nursing and beyond.* Edinburgh, Scotland: Churchill Livingstone/Harcourt-Brace.

Watson, J. (2001). Jean Watson: Theory of human caring. In M. E. Parker (Ed.), *Nursing theories and nursing practice* (pp. 343–354). Philadelphia, PA: F. A. Davis.

Watson, J. (2005). *Caring science as sacred science.* Philadelphia, PA: F. A. Davis.

Watson, J. (2008). *The philosophy and science of caring* (Rev. ed.). Boulder: University Press of Colorado.

Watson, J. (2009). Caring science and human caring theory: Transforming personal and professional practices of nursing and health care. *Journal of Health and Human Services Administration, 31*(4), 466–482.

Watson, J. (2010). Caring science and the next decade of holistic healing: Transforming self and system from the inside out. *Beginnings, 30*(2), 14–16.

Watson, J. (2012). *Human caring science: A theory for nursing* (2nd ed.). Sudbury, MA: Jones & Bartlett.

Watson, J., & Foster, R. (2003). The Attending Nurse Caring Model: Integrating theory, evidence and advanced caring-healing therapeutics for transforming professional practice. *Journal of Clinical Nursing, 12*(3), 360–365. doi:10.1046/j.1365-2702.2003.00774.x

Watson, J., & Smith, M. C. (2002). Caring science and the science of unitary human beings: A transtheoretical discourse for nursing knowledge development. *Journal of Advanced Nursing, 37*(5), 452–461. doi:10.1046/j.1365-2648.2002.02112.x

36

Toward Planetary Caring: Sustainable Health and Well-Being for All

William Rosa

CARITAS LITERACIES

By the end of this chapter, the caring-healing nurse will be able to

1. Define "planetary health" as it relates to nursing, healthcare systems, and universal well-being.

2. Identify the role of the Caritas nurse in procuring planetary health for all men, women, children, and species, and in mutuality with the environment.

3. Apply the ethics of Caring Science to the interprofessional, multisectoral, and transnational health agendas currently underway worldwide.

4. Develop an individual plan for engaging as a planetary citizen in personal-professional endeavors.

Caring Science, as an ethical starting point for human-centered engagement, emanated from a nursing paradigm but maintains expansive implications that transcend beyond it. This ethos has come to life through nursing language, nursing arts, and nursing sciences, embracing the caring-healing demonstrations that drive and guide the profession, and using the disciplinary-specific discourse as a vehicle for humanizing its ideals. However, at its core and on reflection of its foundational moral tenets, we come to understand that it has always been intended—in its highest form—as a planetary theory and way of being that encompasses our shared humanity, fostering a deep connection to the spiritual-metaphysical "oneness" of all that is, and procuring inclusivity of other species and the environment (Watson, 2012, 2014, 2017).

Planetary health recognizes that human beings are not only in relational shared mutuality with each other but also in intimate communion with all aspects of the world around them; "planetary health is rooted in understanding the interdependencies of human and natural systems" (The Rockefeller Foundation, n.d., "Our Strategy"). In the end, if humanity is to survive, we must start paying attention to the signs and symptoms of the planet at large, and strive to improve the human-planet dynamics that are currently feeding scarcity, violence, economic insecurity, and environmental dangers across continents. The purpose of this chapter is to identify how Caring Science informs the ethical tenets of planetary health and how its theoretical framework can be expanded to include and promote a sustainable, safe, and inclusive world for all.

PLANETARY CONSIDERATIONS: OF AND BEYOND HUMANITY

There is no doubt about it—the planet is in trouble. Humanity continues to suffer the sequelae of a host of oppressive sociopolitical and economic factors, including excessive poverty, hunger, and violence. Just over 10% of the world's population lives below the international poverty line—that's roughly 1 in 10 people living on less than $1.90 per person per day (International Bank for Reconstruction and Development/The World Bank, 2016). About 815 million people worldwide do not have access to enough food to lead a healthy and active life (World Food Programme, n.d.). The United Nations High Commissioner for Refugees (2017) estimates that 28,300 people a day flee their homes because of violent conflict and persecution, with roughly 65.6 million people currently considered forcibly displaced worldwide.

The problems we face in the 21st century clearly and severely impact humanity but also encompass dire concerns regarding environmental health and rapid losses of biodiversity across the ecosystems that, quite literally, hold the planet together. National Aeronautics and Space Administration (NASA, n.d.) has shown a significant deterioration in the "vital signs of the planet"—those markers that prove climate change to be a real and evidence-based danger. These observations include atmospheric carbon dioxide, sea level, and global temperature rises, warming oceans, shrinking ice sheets, declining Arctic sea ice, glacial retreat, an increased number of extreme weather events, ocean acidification, and decreased snow cover during winters in the Northern Hemisphere (NASA, n.d.).

Climate change, as well as the industry practices and energy sources used by human beings, is intimately related to the integrity of biodiversity. "Biodiversity" is defined as "the variety of all forms of life and it is essential to the existence and proper functioning of all ecosystems ... [it] supports habitats for all species by providing many unique environments ... [and] supports the core benefits that humans derive from their environment" (Environmental Protection Agency [EPA], n.d., "Biodiversity Underpins All Ecosystems"). Threats to biodiversity include the growing human population and refractory land development and resource allocation required to support it, habitat loss for myriad species, overexploitation such as commercial fishing and game hunting, overuse of environmental resources, and all forms of pollution (EPA, n.d.). Ultimately, continued biodiversity loss will likely cause nutritional deficits, threats to medicinal plant access, and the increased spread and incidence of infectious diseases around the globe (World Health Organization [WHO], n.d.).

PLANETARY HEALTH AND SUSTAINABLE DEVELOPMENT

Planetary health is the next era of being-doing-knowing that will preserve both humanity and the natural resources needed to sustain life. It requires multidisciplinary and multisector collaboration from practitioners; researchers; educators; and advocates in the fields of law; business; medicine; policy; sociology; public, international, global, and environmental health; and a host of equally relevant specialists across the arts, sciences, and humanities. Nursing, as the single largest healthcare profession worldwide estimated at over 19.3 million (Sarna & Bialous, 2012), will play a key role in knowledge creation and systems implementation improvements that will guide planetary health efforts globally (Kurth, 2017).

The Rockefeller Foundation–*Lancet* Commission on Planetary Health (Whitmee et al., 2015) identified four key messages related to the concept of planetary health:

1. Human survival depends on flourishing natural systems and the judicious stewardship of those systems; many of these systems are being degraded to an extent never before witnessed in human history.

2. Environmental threats to the health and well-being of humans and human civilizations will be unpredictable. Therefore, the way humanity engages the environment requires urgent and transformative actions to protect current and future generations from clear and potential danger.

3. The systems and infrastructures currently in place to address the deficits of planetary health are inadequate. Improved governance to aid the integration of social, economic, and environmental policies and the creation, synthesis, and application of evidence-based interdisciplinary knowledge will strengthen overall planetary health.

4. Solutions for planetary health should be rooted in the definition of prosperity as an enhanced quality of life and improved delivery of health for all men, women, and children with respect to the integrity of coexisting natural systems.

To realize planetary health, transnational cooperation is needed to change bureaucracies and overcome policies that permit the ongoing violations of human injustice and the pervasive degradation of natural systems. The 2030 Sustainable Development Agenda was adopted by all member states of the United Nations (UN) General Assembly on September 25, 2015, and was officially put into action on January 1, 2016. The agenda is constructed of 17 Sustainable Development Goals (SDGs) and 169 targets that seek to eradicate poverty and violence, ensure equality, peace, and justice for all, build equitable multisector partnerships within and between nations, and significantly decrease threats to environmental resources and biodiversity conservation worldwide (UN, n.d.). The 17 SDGs are found in Box 36.1. In essence, the 17 SDGs are a guiding framework for multidisciplinary teams to strategize and implement reliable planetary solutions to the obstacles that face us.

Ultimately, the SDGs are a call to action for concerned citizens everywhere, but hold particular significance for the discipline of nursing. Nurses have traditionally been concerned with potential contributions related to SDG 3, *Good Health and Well-Being*. However, on further reflection, nurses in arenas of practice, education, research, policy, advocacy, theory development, business, law, administration, environmental sciences, and public, global,

BOX 36.1

Sustainable Development Goals

Goal 1. End poverty in all its forms everywhere.

Goal 2. End hunger, achieve food security and improved nutrition, and promote sustainable agriculture.

Goal 3. Ensure health lives and promote well-being for all at all ages.

Goal 4. Ensure inclusive and equitable quality education and promote lifelong learning opportunities for all.

Goal 5. Achieve gender equality and empower all women and girls.

Goal 6. Ensure availability and sustainable management of water and sanitation for all.

Goal 7. Ensure access to affordable, reliable, sustainable, and modern energy for all.

Goal 8. Promote sustained, inclusive, and sustainable economic growth, full and productive employment, and decent work for all.

Goal 9. Build resilient infrastructure, promote inclusive and sustainable industrialization, and foster innovation.

Goal 10. Reduce inequality within and among countries.

Goal 11. Make cities and human settlements inclusive, safe, resilient, and sustainable.

Goal 12. Ensure sustainable consumption and production patterns.

Goal 13. Take urgent action to combat climate change and its impacts.[a]

Goal 14. Conserve and sustainably use the oceans, seas, and marine resources for sustainable development.

Goal 15. Protect, restore, and promote sustainable use of terrestrial ecosystems, sustainably manage forests, combat desertification, halt and reverse land degradation, and halt biodiversity loss.

Goal 16. Promote peaceful and inclusive societies for sustainable development, provide access to justice for all, and build effective, accountable, and inclusive institutions at all levels.

Goal 17. Strengthen the means of implementation and revitalize the Global Partnership for Sustainable Development.

[a]Acknowledging that the United Nations Framework Convention on Climate Change is the primary international, intergovernmental forum for negotiating the global response to climate change.

Source: United Nations. (2015). Transforming our world: The 2030 agenda for sustainable development. Retrieved from https://sustainabledevelopment.un.org/post2015/transformingourworld. Reprinted with permission from the United Nations.

and international health all have unique and clearly delineated opportunities to advance the creation and implementation of sustainable mechanisms for persons, peoples, species, and natural resources worldwide.

Horton-Deutsch and Rosa (2017) provide a reflective inventory in Table 36.1 that may assist the readers in identifying their individual roles and responsibilities as they relate to each of the 17 SDGs. This inventory may be used as a personal reflection tool, to further dialogue in group settings, or for professional nursing organizations to stratify and strategize efforts toward the realization of planetary health. The left column lists the 17 SDGs using abbreviated descriptions (UN, 2016), and the right provides reflective questions for deeper exploration.

TABLE 36.1 Sustainable Development Goals Reflective Inventory

Sustainable Development Goals	Questions for Ongoing Reflection
1. No poverty	• *How do I feel about the poor and economically disadvantaged?* • *What assumptions and judgments do I make about the poor that will prevent me from being an effective global nurse?* • *What are my fears related to poor people?* • *Which implications of poverty can I alleviate with a nursing sensibility?* • *Is it my responsibility to address and work for no poverty for all?*
2. Zero hunger	• *Do I know what it feels like to be hungry? To be without?* • *Am I willing to hear and see the impact of hunger on children and families, beyond statistics and research findings?* • *Are the experiences and feelings of the hungry included in my goals and plans?* • *In what ways do I contribute to hunger through wasting food or unconscious consumption/disposal?* • *Is it my responsibility to address and work toward zero hunger for all?*
3. Good health and well-being	• *What is my vision of a world where good health and well-being are experienced by all?* • *How do I define health and well-being?* • *Am I open to hearing definitions and perceptions of what health and well-being mean to others?* • *How can I change my approaches to advocacy so that colleagues and policy makers understand health and well-being as a human right?* • *Is it my responsibility to address and work toward good health and well-being for all?*

(continued)

TABLE 36.1 Sustainable Development Goals Reflective Inventory *(continued)*

Sustainable Development Goals	Questions for Ongoing Reflection
4. Quality education	• *How have I seen a lack of education impact my own life, family, and community?* • *What is the power of education in realizing the post-2015 agenda?* • *What are my role and the strategic actions I can take to impart evidence-based, dignified, and respectful education to the populations I serve?* • *Do I carry certain judgments about those who do not share my privilege of education?* • *Is it my responsibility to address and work toward quality education for all?*
5. Gender equality	• *How has my own standing in the world been influenced by my gender?* • *What privileges and prejudices have I experienced on the basis of my gender or gender identification?* • *What social misperceptions do I unconsciously ascribe to regarding gender and status?* • *How can I strive to heal the misunderstandings and social constructs around gender while remaining inclusive and respectful of cultural differences?* • *Is it my responsibility to address and work toward gender equality for all?*
6. Clean water and sanitation	• *How can I communicate the importance of clean water and sanitation to decision makers in a way that matters for them?* • *In what ways are clean water and sanitation human rights?* • *How can I educate about the value of clean water in settings where water access is limited?* • *How can I educate about the vital nature of sanitation in settings where sanitation is lacking or absent?* • *Is it my responsibility to address and work toward clean water and sanitation for all?*
7. Affordable and clean energy	• *How do I waste energy?* • *How do I promote the unconscious use of energy in my family and workplace?* • *In what ways can I raise awareness regarding energy consumption practice?* • *What are the strategies needed for a global commitment to clean energy use?* • *Is it my responsibility to address and work toward affordable and clean energy for all?*

(continued)

TABLE 36.1 Sustainable Development Goals Reflective Inventory *(continued)*

Sustainable Development Goals	Questions for Ongoing Reflection
8. Decent work and economic growth	• *What are the privileges that allow me to access and maintain decent and reliable work?* • *Do people in low- and middle-income countries share these opportunities?* • *How can I bridge the gaps between what people have, what they need, and what they deserve regarding economic disparities?* • *What is my global nursing contribution to responsible and safe economic growth for communities and countries?* • *Is it my responsibility to address and work toward decent work and economic growth for all?*
9. Industry, innovation, and infrastructure	• *In what ways do I take industry and innovation for granted?* • *What absences in infrastructure would impact the quality of my life?* • *How can I be proactive and preventative about the health needs of those communities without adequate infrastructure?* • *How do the concepts of innovation, cultural humility, and a client-centered approach to intervention relate?* • *Is it my responsibility to work toward industry, innovation, and infrastructure for all?*
10. Reduced inequalities	• *In what ways do I consider myself less than or greater than others?* • *How can I role model equality in all I do and with all I have?* • *How bad do things need to get before I act on behalf of the oppressed?* • *Is equality foundational to health and healthcare delivery?* • *Is it my responsibility to address and work toward reduced inequalities for all?*
11. Sustainable cities and communities	• *In what ways does my community support/use sustainable practices?* • *What are the immediate areas for improvement on my street and in my town?* • *How do I advocate for the needs of those impacted by irresponsible urbanization?* • *Am I able to make the case between unsustainable practices and poor health outcomes?* • *Is it my responsibility to address and work toward sustainable cities and communities for all?*

(continued)

TABLE 36.1 Sustainable Development Goals Reflective Inventory *(continued)*

Sustainable Development Goals	Questions for Ongoing Reflection
12. Responsible consumption and production	• *How can I improve purchasing/spending practices in my work setting?* • *How can I translate environmentally conscious goals to administrators, leaders, and financial stakeholders?* • *Am I able to facilitate meaningful discussions regarding the role of environmentally friendly trends in healthcare among other global health workers?* • *Do I ignore the implications of irresponsible practices in the community or work settings?* • *Is it my responsibility to address and work toward responsible consumption and production for all?*
13. Climate action	• *How do I understand my individual role in climate change?* • *What personal lifestyle choices do I need to adapt to be more environmentally respectful?* • *Do I consider myself to be an environmental activist?* • *How do I close the gap between raising awareness and creating action?* • *Is it my responsibility to address and work toward climate action for all?*
14. Life below water	• *Do I believe biodiversity has an influence on my personal and community health?* • *How can I integrate biodiversity knowledge into community education?* • *In what ways do I misuse or waste water resources?* • *How can I promote awareness of marine preservation in my local/regional/national environments?* • *Is it my responsibility to address and work toward the preservation of life below water for all?*
15. Life on land	• *In what ways are my goals as a global nurse tied to environmental justice?* • *What are my strategic plans to drive community-based change in policy regarding environmental preservation?* • *Are there efforts for land preservation that are relevant to my village, town, or city?* • *How can I help my family members to better understand their relationship to all species and ecosystems?* • *Is it my responsibility to address and work toward the preservation of life on land for all?*

(continued)

TABLE 36.1 Sustainable Development Goals Reflective Inventory *(continued)*	
Sustainable Development Goals	**Questions for Ongoing Reflection**
16. Peace, justice, and strong institutions	• *How have unjust laws and policies impacted my community?* • *In what ways does a lack of justice frustrate me? Anger me? Prevent me from taking action?* • *Am I conscious of peacemaking in my role as a global nurse?* • *Is peace a priority in my relationships?* • *It is my responsibility to address and work toward peace and justice for all?*
17. Partnerships for the goals	• *Are my partnerships me-centered or other-centered?* • *Is it hard for me to remain authentically present to another's feelings and worldviews?* • *What are my barriers to surrendering my position and being flexible?* • *How do I show up in a spirit of true collaboration?* • *Is it my responsibility to address and work toward partnerships for the goals?*

Source: Reprinted from Horton-Deutsch, S., & Rosa, W. (2017). The role of reflective practice in creating the world we want. In W. Rosa (Ed.), *A new era in global health: Nursing and the United Nations 2030 agenda for sustainable development* (pp. 461–473). New York, NY: Springer Publishing.

NURSING AS PLANETARY PARTNER

As suggested earlier, planetary health is inherent to the foundations of nursing. Nurses play key roles in furthering each of the SDG targets and partnering with participating nations and sectors around the world to successfully integrate the UN's tenets and higher ideals (Rosa, 2017a). The history of nursing reminds modern-day clinicians and scientists that the paradigm was always meant to extend beyond the realm of humanity, and required the inclusion of environmental considerations. Nightingale was a staunch environmentalist, political activist, healer, leader, and proponent of global well-being (Dossey, Selanders, Beck, & Attewell, 2005). She understood intimately the role nurses played in the health of populations and also acknowledged the inherent symbiosis—and also the risk for unconscious stewardship and parasitism—between humanity and the environment (Nightingale, 1860/1969). Nightingale's vision was in keeping with the concepts of planetary health and the UN Sustainable Development Agenda. Likewise, planetary health and the 2030 Agenda are merely extensions of nursing's core identity and disciplinary priorities for universal flourishing.

The ethos of planetary health calls for a change in consciousness regarding how we define "health" and a reexamination of our beliefs in relation to the world around us. It requires a transformation in personal-professional awareness, one that encompasses the well-being of systems and promotes the use of technologies as effective, responsible tools in the service of sustainability (Sharma, 2007). It challenges us to embody leadership qualities that unify people across contexts and promote a greater sense of Oneness with all that is.

Holistic nurse advocates continue to pave the way for unitary approaches to health and well-being rooted in respect of the environment and human-animal-global interdependence (Luck, 2014, 2016). This worldview recognizes the implications of living in a toxic world and the barriers posed to sustainability by a "human first–other second" approach to infrastructure development. The ethical obligation of nurses to obtain and disseminate knowledge related to environmental health, and their right to practice in an environmentally safe work milieu and participate in best practices and research that promote environmental consciousness is supported by professional organizational leaders, such as the American Nurses Association (2007).

The first of six principles that provide the foundations for *integrative nursing* states clearly: "Human beings are whole systems, inseparable from their environments" (Koithan, 2014, p. 7). Such a paradigm suggests that the human being as a person is just one entity amid a vast planetary systems hierarchy, somewhere in the middle between the subatomic particles, atoms, molecules, and cells that serve as the building blocks of life, and the communities, cultures–subcultures, societies–nations, and biospheres that we cocreate and collaboratively maintain. To this end, Luck and Keegan (2016, p. 559) suggest that we ask ourselves the following questions, as both members of humankind and professionals working toward the alleviation of suffering, and with the most sacred intention of acquiring the deepest understanding available to us at this time:

- What does it mean to be human?

- What are our beliefs about health when we tell our story?

- How can we face the great ecological crises of our time?

- How does each of our stories contribute to the larger story?

- How does changing our own story lead to planetary change?

One Mind–One Health–One Planet[1]

Dr. Larry Dossey (2013) has discussed in great detail, with impressively thorough references to the literature, countless case studies, and through his own experiences with the transcendent, the concept of the *One Mind*: a unitary and collective superior intelligence of which all beings are a part. He writes:

[We have all] broken our responsibilities to our earth and environment, therefore to ourselves and to one another, a thousand times. Yet it is within our power to redeem [ourselves] by reclaiming … the One Mind that unites us with all else …; the One Mind whose calling card is love, caring, affection. (Dossey, 2013, p. 259)

---

[1]Parts of this section has been adapted from Rosa, W. (2017a). Conclusion: One mind – one health – one planet: A pledge to planetary citizenship. In W. Rosa (Ed.), *A new era in global health: Nursing and the United Nations 2030 sustainable development agenda*. New York, NY: Springer Publishing.

The One Mind suggests that we are interconnected in ways not immediately visible to us, but beneath the surface differences that plague and disillusion our ego minds, we are inextricably connected to a universal consciousness, linking us to each other, nature, animal species, and the Earth (Dossey, 2013). These views have been shared by nurse theorists and Caring Science visionaries for many years, emphasizing a shared human experience that exists in our very being and belonging as a person on the planet (Dossey, 2016; Watson, 2008, 2012). It moves us from a reference to people and global health outcomes in terms of statistical data toward a deeper wisdom related to interconnectedness, the intention and purpose for our work as Caritas nurses, and the ethical considerations that drive and guide us, both personally and professionally.

Planetary Processes for Sustainable Engagement

In understanding the role of nursing as partner in promoting sustainable engagement for all life on the planet, there is ample opportunity to invite a more embodied relationship with and practice of the Caritas Processes®—the ethical value system of Caring Science. For example, if we are to eradicate poverty for all men, women, and children (SDG 1), there needs to be humanistic consideration given to not just *what* we do but also *how* we do it. On the physical level, we can build homes, provide clothing, and teach skills for people to market. But we must also compassionately address the impoverished state of mind, heart, and spirit experienced on an existential level by cultivating loving-kindness toward self and other, being authentically present and instilling faith and hope where it is lost, and developing helping-caring-trusting relationships (Caritas Processes #1, #2, and #4; Watson, 2008). We can strive to end hunger (SDG 2) and work feverishly toward a world of peace and justice for all human beings (SDG 16), but in doing so, we must be mindful to be present to and supportive of the positive and negative feelings of others and reverentially assist with their care needs while holding an intentional consciousness of honoring their embodied and transpersonal spirit (Caritas Processes 5 and 9).

Planetary health asks us to translate the philosophical–practical wisdom of Caring Science and reconsider it on a universal scale inclusive of animal and environmental health and well-being. As the UN Sustainable Development Agenda moves forward, nurses and invested citizens around the world must begin to consider what values and practices will sustain the highest quality of life possible beyond 2030. This author suggests next era Planetary Processes that build on the caring intentionality and compassionate science of Caritas nursing to acknowledge and actively address the threats to survival faced by the planet, its lands, oceans, species, humans, and life-giving biospheres.

As a starting point, the Planetary Processes include the following:

1. Expanding the circle of human-to-human compassion to include species of all kinds, natural resources, ecosystems, and the Earth itself; engaging with life beyond human form with heart-centered and healing intentions

2. Developing a caring-interdependent place and purpose amid the systemic hierarchical system of the planet; promoting a One Mind–One Health–One Planet practice of being, doing, and knowing

3. Partnering across cultures and contexts to strengthen the universal voice for life and sustainability; releasing ego to cocreate new opportunities in transnational partnerships; acknowledging arrogance; embracing humility; remaining dynamic in the flow of Self-Other-Planet

4. Honoring humanism, caring, and environmentalism as the primary drivers of policy, advocacy development, and resource acquisition; translating the ethics of Caritas and belonging into outcomes favorable to the highest quality of life and living

5. Integrating the sacredness of planetary life into all aspects of human advancement; giving voice to the voiceless spirits of nature, animals, and those forgotten; identifying the implications of both conscious and unconscious doing on the entirety of life on the planet

Further scholarship needs to be cultivated in regards to these Planetary Processes. They suggest an expanding paradigm of Caring Science, traditionally focused on the spirit-to-spirit relationship-centered dance of human-to-human caring, toward a more concerned and empathic stance on sustainable planetary engagement. These processes lay the roots for potential theory development as it relates to planetary nursing and planetary caring, planetary-metaphysical considerations and immersion into the spiritual realm of planetary interdependence, and the connections between the transpersonal-transplanetary spectrum of life experience.

CONCLUSION

Planetary health and the improvements to universal sustainability it implies, ultimately require an approach to engagement consistent with the ethics of Caring Science and One Mind–One Health–One Planet. It requires a new threshold with which to embrace whole planet thinking and foster healing at expansive, planetary levels. The Planetary Processes urge us as leaders and partners in cocreating the future experience of the world to remain vigilant of *what* our unique roles as nurses are in sustainable development, *how* we engage, and *why* it matters.

In conclusion, this author echoes prior thoughts on ways forward for those invested in realizing a world imbued with the power of Planetary Caring. *Planetary citizenship* is … proposed herein as a way to invite healing to the fractured aspects of the human-animal-earth experience, and to identify [Caritas nurses] as planetary leaders, planetary advocates, and planetary change agents in this new era. "Healing" in this context may be defined as

> a lifelong journey into understanding the wholeness of [planetary] existence. Healing occurs when we help [the planet] embrace what is feared most … Healing is learning how to open what has been closed so that we can expand [new planetary] potentials … It is accessing what we have forgotten about connections, unity, and interdependence. (B. M. Dossey, 2016, p. 23)

Planetary citizenship moves beyond man-made borders and limitations to the universal principles of a shared and reciprocal humanity and all-life relationship. It moves us from the notions of one woman, one man, one child, one country, or one continent, toward One

Mind–One Health–One Planet. I propose a Pledge to Planetary Citizenship [following] as just one way of recommitting our personal-professional lives to the work of achieving the UN 2030 Agenda for Sustainable Development and to the values and ideals of [Caritas Nursing]: healing, health, human dignity, and peace for all beings everywhere and for the Earth itself.

BOX 36.2
A Pledge to Planetary Citizenship

I pledge to be a Planetary Citizen,

To strive continuously toward a universal experience of dignity,

To embrace cultural differences and confront human inequalities and disparities in an effort to know and promote peace,

And to lovingly, but directly, address all threats to Planetary well-being, be they human or environmental.

I pledge to be a Planetary Citizen,

To be a global nurse in the highest sense of the word,

Embracing nursing as the finest of arts and the most rooted of sciences,

To wield safety, inclusiveness, and social justice as tools to elevate consciousness and role model compassion,

To be an advocate for healing and global activism,

A conduit for transformation and unity,

And a leader in the journey toward One Mind–One Health–One Planet.

I pledge to role model kindness and respect as integral aspects of my Planetary Citizenship,

To carry the intention of unity in my words and actions,

Remain present to the global consequences of my choices,

Commit to creating healing environments at all levels, in all spaces, for all beings everywhere,

And build relationships based on trust and awareness of a shared humanity.

I pledge to nurture a safe and inclusive world as a Planetary Citizen,

To release prejudices, divisive judgments, and aggression,

To forgive where it is needed and return myself to wholeness,

To "Be the Change," live the virtues, and practice the values inherent to ethical engagement,

To accept people as they are and the world as it is in order to more fully embrace myself as I am.

I pledge to devote my energies to self-care, self-knowledge, and self-love as a Planetary Citizen,

---

(continued)

BOX 36.2

A Pledge to Planetary Citizenship *(continued)*

Caring for myself as a sacred vessel,

Caring for my family as myself,

Caring for Others as my family,

And for the Planet as I do all Others,

And in this way, caring for the Planet as myself, and the sacred mystery that It is.

I pledge partnership with all beings in an effort to realize Planetary Citizenship and a
   Planetary World,

To remain open, available, and flexible,

To teach what I know and learn what I do not know,

To honor the light in all of life,

And to leave the Planet better than I found it.

This is my solemn pledge and commitment.

Source: Rosa, W. (2017a). Conclusion: One mind–one health–one planet: A pledge to planetary
citizenship. In W. Rosa (Ed.), *A new era in global health: Nursing and the United Nations 2030
Agenda for Sustainable Development.* New York, NY: Springer Publishing.

NEXT ERA POSSIBILITIES

Education
- How can I integrate planetary health considerations into the education I provide for patients, colleagues, and my community?
- In what ways do nursing curricula need to be expanded to include the transnational agendas and ethics of Caring Science/Planetary Caring discussed in this chapter?

Research
- How does Caring Science research need to be readdressed and expanded to include the ideals and account for the implications of planetary health?
- What roles do Caring Science researchers play in helping to translate the more qualitative findings of planetary caring into a language that quantitatively minded policy makers and decision makers can understand and appreciate?

Praxis
- Which dimensions of practice can I improve right now with a greater understanding of planetary health?
- Which of my current work-related outcomes can be reframed to include the implications of planetary health for a more expansive/inclusive worldview?

Theory and Knowledge Development

- What additional Planetary Processes do I believe are essential to practicing/realizing/ promoting planetary caring and planetary health?
- Given my specialty, what areas are primed for expansion to include the tenets of planetary health? What specific contributions can I make?
- How does my own theory of nursing resonate with the ideals discussed earlier? Is it possible for me to make room for new ways of being, doing, and knowing at the planetary level?

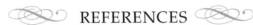 REFERENCES

American Nurses Association. (2007). *Principles of environmental health for nursing practice with implementation strategies.* Silver Spring, MD: Author Retrieved from http://ojin.nursingworld.org/Main MenuCategories/WorkplaceSafety/Healthy-Nurse/ANAsPrinciplesofEnvironmentalHealth forNursingPractice.pdf

Dossey, B. M. (2016). Nursing: Integral, integrative, and holistic—Local to global. In B. M. Dossey & L. Keegan (Eds.), *Holistic nursing: A handbook for practice* (7th ed., pp. 3–49). Burlington, MA: Jones & Bartlett.

Dossey, B. M., Selanders, L. C., Beck, D. M., & Attewell, A. (2005). *Florence Nightingale today: Healing, leadership, global action.* Silver Spring, MD: American Nurses Association.

Dossey, L. (2013). *One mind: How our individual mind is part of a greater consciousness and why it matters.* Carlsbad, CA: Hay House.

Environmental Protection Agency. (n.d.). EnviroAtlas benefit category: Biodiversity conservation. Retrieved from https://www.epa.gov/enviroatlas/enviroatlas-benefit-category-biodiversity-conservation

Horton-Deutsch, S., & Rosa, W. (2017). The role of reflective practice in creating the world we want. In W. Rosa (Ed.), *A new era in global health: Nursing and the United Nations 2030 Agenda for Sustainable Development* (pp. 461–473). New York, NY: Springer Publishing.

International Bank for Reconstruction and Development/The World Bank. (2016). *Poverty and shared prosperity 2016: Taking on inequality.* Washington, DC: Author. Retrieved from https://openknowledge.worldbank.org/bitstream/handle/10986/25078/9781464809583.pdf

Koithan, M. (2014). Concepts and principles of integrative nursing. In M. J. Kreitzer & M. Koithan (Eds.), *Integrative nursing* (pp. 3–16). New York, NY: Oxford University Press.

Kurth, A. E. (2017). A post-2030 agenda: The world beyond the sustainable development goals. In W. Rosa (Ed.), *A new era in global health: Nursing and the United Nations 2030 sustainable development agenda.* New York, NY: Springer Publishing.

Luck, S. (2014). Integrative nursing and the environment. In M. J. Kreitzer & M. Koithan (Eds.), *Integrative nursing.* New York, NY: Oxford University Press.

Luck, S. (2016). Informed and impactful: Stewarding the environmental determinants of health and well-being. In W. Rosa (Ed.), *Nurses as leaders: Evolutionary visions of leadership* (pp. 333–343). New York, NY: Springer Publishing.

Luck, S., & Keegan, L. (2016). Environmental health. In B. M. Dossey & L. Keegan (Eds.), *Holistic nursing: A handbook for practice* (7th ed., pp. 557–587). Burlington, MA: Jones & Bartlett.

National Aeronautics and Space Administration. (n.d.). Climate change: Vital signs of the planet: Evidence. Retrieved from http://climate.nasa.gov/evidence

Nightingale, F. (1969). *Notes on nursing: What it is and what it is not* (1st ed.). New York, NY: D. Appleton. (Original work published 1860)

Rosa, W. (2017a). Conclusion: One mind – one health – one planet: A pledge to planetary citizenship. In W. Rosa (Ed.), *A new era in global health: Nursing and the United Nations 2030 Agenda for Sustainable Development.* New York, NY: Springer Publishing.

Rosa, W. (Ed.). (2017b). *A new era in global health: Nursing and the United Nations 2030 Agenda for Sustainable Development*. New York, NY: Springer Publishing.

Sarna, L., & Bialous, S. A. (2012). Enhancing nursing and midwifery capacity to contribute to the prevention, treatment and management of noncommunicable diseases. *Human Resources for Health Observer*, (12). Retrieved from http://www.who.int/hrh/resources/observer12.pdf

Sharma, M. (2007). Personal to planetary transformation. *Kosmos Journal, Fall/Winter*, 31–37.

The Rockefeller Foundation. (n.d.). Planetary health. Retrieved from https://www.rockefeller foundation.org/our-work/initiatives/planetary-health

United Nations. (2015). Transforming our world: The 2030 Agenda for Sustainable Development. Retrieved from https://sustainabledevelopment.un.org/content/documents/21252030%20Agenda% 20for%20Sustainable%20Development%20web.pdf

United Nations. (2016). Sustainable development goals. Retrieved from http://www.un.org/sustainable development/sustainable-development-goals

United Nations High Commissioner for Refugees. (2017, June 30). Figures at a glance. Retrieved from http://www.unhcr.org/en-us/figures-at-a-glance.html

Watson, J. (2008). *Nursing: The philosophy and science of caring*. Boulder: University Press of Colorado.

Watson, J. (2012). *Human caring science: A theory of nursing* (2nd ed.). Sudbury, MA: Jones & Bartlett.

Watson, J. (2014). Integrative nursing caring science, human caring, and peace. In M. J. Kreitzer & M. Koithan (Eds.), *Integrative nursing* (pp. 101–108). New York, NY: Oxford University Press.

Watson, J. (2017). Global human caring for a sustainable world. In W. Rosa (Ed.), *A new era in global health: Nursing and the United Nations 2030 Agenda for Sustainable Development* (pp. 227–246). New York, NY: Springer Publishing.

Whitmee, S., Haines, A., Beyrer, C., Boltz, F., Capon, A. G., de Souza Dias, B. F., … Yach, D. (2015). Safeguarding human health in the Anthropocene epoch: Report of The Rockefeller Foundation-Lancet Commission on planetary health. *Lancet, 386*, 1973–2028. doi:10.1016/S0140-6736(15)60901-1

World Food Programme. (n.d.). Zero hunger. Retrieved from https://www.wfp.org/hunger/stats

World Health Organization. (n.d.). Biodiversity. Retrieved from http://www.who.int/globalchange/ecosystems/biodiversity/en

Emerging Inquiry: The Evolution of a Science

IX

37

Unitary Caring Science Inquiry

Marian C. Turkel, Joseph Giovannoni, and Jean Watson

CARITAS LITERACIES

By the end of this chapter, the caring-healing nurse will be able to

1. Define the core concepts of Unitary Caring Science inquiry.

2. Identify a research study grounded in one of the Unitary Caring Science inquiry exemplars presented in this chapter.

3. Explore the possibilities related to metaphysical research.

4. Contribute to the field of Unitary Caring Science knowledge by integrating empirical, ethical, aesthetic, and personal ways of knowing into Caring Science inquiry.

Unitary Caring Science inquiry is framed within an ontological and epistemological world-view of a unitary field of consciousness guided by disciplinary-specific knowledge, axiology of values, ethics of belonging, and the virtues of being human. Caring Science inquiry transcends the traditional research paradigm, allows for unknown approaches, and expands the field of inquiry as to what counts as knowledge. Watson's evolution from the original *Nursing: The Philosophy and Science of Caring* (1979) to *Caring Science as Sacred Science* (2005) was guided by Levinas's (1969) Ethic of "Belonging" as starting point for Unitary Caring Science; we all "belong" to Cosmic Infinite field of Universal Love. In this model of Unitary Caring Science, ethics comes before ontology as a starting point, thus informing ontology, epistemology, methodologies, and praxis.

According to Watson and Smith (2002), "Caring science ... makes explicit an expanding unitary, energetic world view with a relational human caring ethic and ontology as its starting point; once energy is incorporated into a unitary caring science perspective we can affirm a deep relational ethic, spirit, and science that transcends all duality" (p. 459). Watson and Smith (2002) affirmed that Caring Science is "an evolving philosophical-ethical-epistemic field of study that is grounded in the discipline of nursing and informed by related fields" (p. 456). Watson (2005) proclaimed that "caring science is an ontological assumption of oneness, wholeness, unity, and connectedness …. and an epistemological assumption that there are multiple ways of knowing and methodologies for studying the Theory of Human Caring" (p. 223). Caring Science is situated in a worldview that is nondualistic and relational, and where all are connected. It is grounded in the worldview that humanity resides in a unitary or undivided field of consciousness (Watson, 2008). A paradigm of Unitary Caring Science inquiry makes explicit a theoretical and philosophical worldview of love and caring and a consciousness of humanity.

Reason (1993) views human inquiry as a sacred science that extends love, recognizes beauty, nurtures healing, and honors compassion. Watson and Smith (2002) view Unitary Caring Science inquiry as "encompassing methodological pluralism whereby the methods flows form the phenomena of concern, not the other way around and diverse forms of inquiry seek to unify ontological, philosophical, ethical and theoretical views" (p. 456). Expanding upon these definitions and beliefs, the authors propose the need for Unitary Caring Science research and inquiry methodologies to advance aesthetic knowing, Caritas, caring, the caring moment, cosmic love, nonlocal conscious, forgiveness, and the universal field of infinity. *Calling the Circle Reflection, Videography and Photography*, and *Metaphysical and Nonphysical Inquiry* serve as forms of creative scholarly inquiry to advance Unitary Caring Science knowledge and to inform and transform disciplinary knowledge.

CALLING THE CIRCLE OF REFLECTION: AN EXEMPLAR OF UNITARY CARING SCIENCE INQUIRY

The Circle is an ancient form of meeting that has gathered human beings into respectful conversation for thousands of years. What transforms a meeting into a circle is the willingness of people to shift from informal socializing or opinionated discussion into a receptive attitude of thoughtful speaking and deep listening and to embody and practice caring from the heart (Baldwin, 1998; Watson, 2008). Calling the Circle of Reflection (Turkel & Ray, 2012; Turkel & Watson, 2014) as a Unitary Caring Science research methodology allows participants to connect in circle to synthesize, integrate, and reflect on the meaning of Caring Science in their personal lives and professional nursing practices. Being with others in a circle, using rituals, and multiple ways of knowing create safe space where participants can explore self and the collective through intentional guided experiences. The space is aesthetic with a singing bowl, temple bell, electric candles, touchstones, flowers, and scarves representing the intention and energy of the circle by creating a caring environment. The circle opens with a centering and silence and all are reminded to practice loving-kindness, equanimity, compassion, forgiveness, and gratitude with self and others while in circle (Watson, 2008). The caller of the circle articulates intention, presence, and invitation. Those who have joined the circle experience reflective practice and are invited to reflect on the following: What is caring?; What does caring mean to me?; How do I express caring in my personal/professional life? Open dialogue and exchange occurs for approximately 1 hour. Being in a circle means practicing authentic listening, being silent, and keeping stories or personal experiences confidential. The guardians of the circle keep the energy and intent in balance. During the Circle of Reflection, one of the researchers invites those in the circle to participate in the dialogue related to caring. As the time in circle draws to close, the researchers synthesize the dialogue and the unity of meaning is expressed as themes. This process is grounded in van Manen's (2014) perspective that thematic understanding is not a rule-bound process, "but a free act of 'seeing' meaning" (p. 79). Final closure involves sharing the themes with the participants, a one-word checkout of the experience by all, and leaving with a small touchstone as a remembrance of time spent in the Circle of Reflection.

Calling the Circle of Reflection as a Unitary Caring Science research methodology was initiated at the International Caritas Consortium (Turkel & Watson, 2014). The research was approved as exempt from the institutional review board prior to the conference and participants provided verbal consent to participate in the Circle. The researchers shared with participants that themes and verbatim direct quotes would be published but names of those who participated would not be published. Table 37.1 illuminates caring as shared and expressed by the participants. The themes are congruent with specific Caritas Processes® and advance Unitary Caring Science knowledge by empirically validating the Caritas Processes and the theory of human caring. Figure 37.1 is a Word Cloud or Wordle that reflects the experience of being part of the Circle of Reflection. The overarching unity of meaning expressed through the themes and Wordle was *seeking unity of being and meaning*.

TABLE 37.1 Caring As Shared and Expressed by the Participants

Theme	Congruence With Caritas Processes®	Participants' Direct Quotes
Authentic listening Having own self-care practices	Expressing positive and negative feelings Sensitivity to self and others	Sometimes it is so frightening for me, I want to be caring, I love my patients but I am wounded. I had a patient die and I was told to get ready for the next admission. I broke down and cried. I need to practice more self-care or something; families go through so much. I was with a young mother whose baby died in the NICU and it was so painful for me, I went home and hugged my little girl. We are looking for meaning; we lost a colleague; we had a nurse die young and we asked why?; she left a son and daughter. There is not much support for nurses so we support each other. On our unit we created a healing energy room where we can go to take a few minutes to relax and try to heal. We created our own centering circle. We have circle of intention on our unit where we each say a positive word to start the day and we work on radiating positive energy to each other during the day.

(continued)

TABLE 37.1 Caring As Shared and Expressed by the Participants *(continued)*

Theme	Congruence With Caritas Processes®	Participants' Direct Quotes
Energetic authentic caring presence	Creating healing environments	One of the nurses on my unit does Reiki healing work; we see her as nurse healer and so do families. When we need it or families ask for her she will hold a pendulum over your heart and invite you to vibrate positive thoughts and energy to yourself. I have witnessed this practice calming family members who are very stressed and upset.
		We created a healing spa and a holistic program; we are fortunate to have a circle of phrenic healers.
Honoring the caring moment	Nurturing helping–trusting–caring relationships	I practice authentic presence and listening. I remember a daughter asking me to check in on her father; he was on hospice and she had a feeling. I went to his room; he asked me to sit for a while and he told me he was at peace. My colleagues called his daughter and when she came in we all prayed together.
		I remember caring for a patient who was dying; we both knew he was dying and he wanted me to sit with him which I did. Sometimes I just sat and held his hand. He asked if he could take a part of me with him. I was holding his hand when he died. He will always be a part of me.
Allowing for hope	Inspiring faith and hope	Sometimes being with patients and families is almost spiritual for me; I can't really explain it.
		I give LOVE to families … it is so hard for them to be with a family member who is dying.
		Sometimes "just being present" gives families and patients hope.
		As a nurse I find myself healing when I am hopeful with patients and families. I remember a wife telling me, "My husband's soul will always be with me. I will never be alone."
		Our feelings reflect on each other so I am always hopeful with families and patients.

NICU, neonatal intensive care unit.

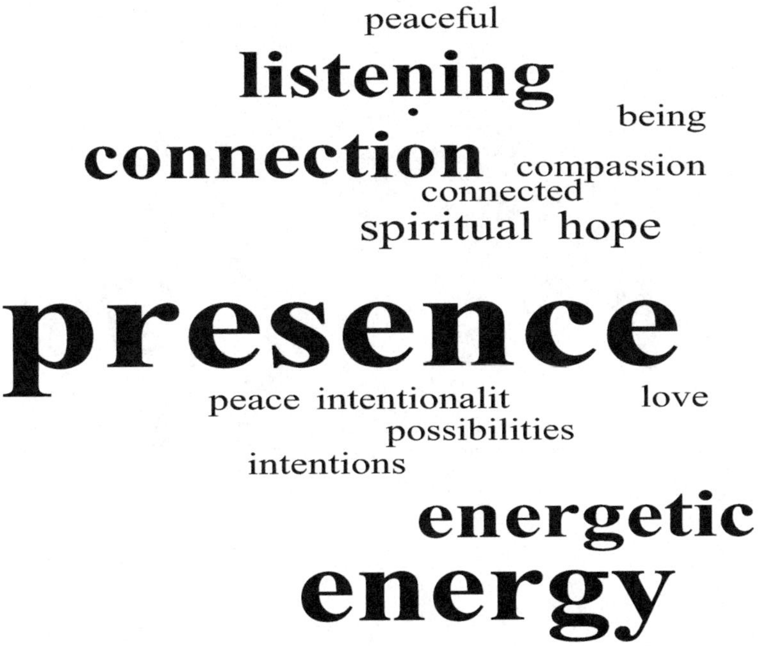

peaceful

listening

being

connection compassion

connected

spiritual hope

presence

peace intentionalit   love

possibilities

intentions

energetic

energy

FIGURE 37.1 Wordle of the one-word checkout.

VIDEOGRAPHY AND PHOTOGRAPHY: AN EXEMPLAR OF AESTHETIC-SPIRITUAL UNITARY CARING SCIENCE INQUIRY

Videography and photography are artistic and profound visually creative channels of aesthetic knowing and personal knowing honoring global human Caring Science and consciousness. Photography is a reflective practice that allows for the creation of posters that express heart-felt inner knowing and a pedagogy to disseminate Caring Science theory. Both are excellent creative mediums for reflection, learning, and disseminating a philosophy of Unitary Caring Science. At a time when medical and nursing science has advanced technologically, there is a need for nurses to return to their sacred covenant to treat humanity with dignity and human caring. Visual media that radiate high-energy words with serene images promote self-care and a healing environment in hospital and clinic settings. Serene images on posters with a surge of high-energy messages uplift the human spirit, communicate compassion and caring, and promote a healing environment. The creative process of producing Unitary Caring Science posters and videos is a meditative practice that advances self-refection.

Aesthetic posters (Figure 37.2) provide a medium for integrating Caring Science in the "institutional darkness" of forensic science, specifically in treating "sex offenders." According to Giovannoni, "I can see and discern the light and beauty of humanity as well as the darkness imposed by the ego's separatist consciousness. Photography

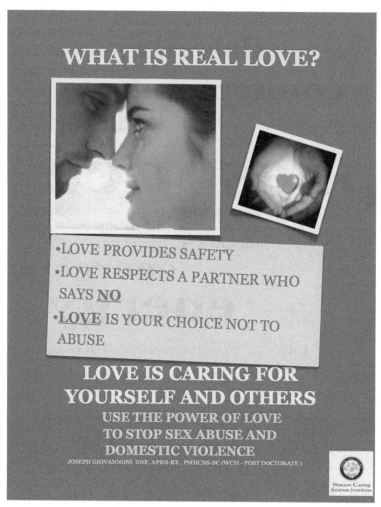

FIGURE 37.2

has become a pedagogical approach to embody Caritas" (personal communication, September 9, 2016). The poster reflects an intentional integration and radiation of Caring Science language to prevent violence.

Caring Science is grounded in the world the view that humanity resides in a unitary or undivided field of consciousness (Levinas, 1969; Levinas, Poller, & Cohen, 2003; Watson, 2008). The vision that we are connected with everything allows us to observe with discernment rather than with judgment. The intention of photography is to capture how we are all interconnected with one another and with Mother Earth. To aesthetically accomplish this requires a sense of freedom from judgmental ego and letting go of thoughts of the past and future to experience the blissfulness of being in the present moment. A walking meditation by Dr. Giovannoni through the countryside in Tuscany organically created the mindful Caritas image in Figure 37.3.

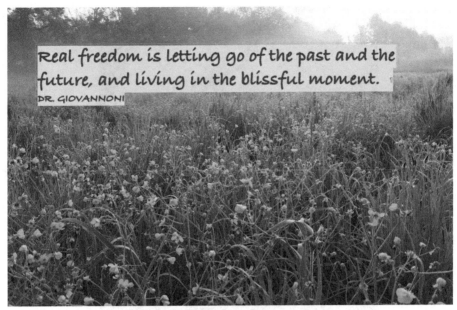

FIGURE 37.3

VIDEOGRAPHY AND PHOTOGRAPHY: A REFLECTIVE UNITARY CARING SCIENCE PRACTICE

Using photographing/videography as reflective practice and capturing on video caring moments grounds one in practicing Caritas Process #1: Cultivating the practice of loving-kindness and equanimity toward self and others (Watson, 2008). Behind the eyes of the camera, the photographer can pause and organically become the energetic Caritas field, revealing frame by frame the nature's beauty, and one begins to see through the eyes of an artist. Videography allows for aesthetic knowing of Unitary Caring Science to evolve via the creation of videos expressing transpersonal caring, caring moments, and the Caritas Processes (Giovannoni, 2014a, 2014b).

The dialogue associated with the images and captions of the videos allows for centering, being in the moment, and reframing negative language to life-sustaining language (Watson, 2008) that expresses loving-kindness and promotes a caring relationship (Figure 37.4). The intention of the videos is to give life and meaning to the concepts of Caring Science such as humanity, interconnectedness, Caritas consciousness, loving-kindness, authentic presence, creating healing environments, the divine, and the miraculous (Watson, 2012). Reflecting on the Unitary Caring Science posters allows for equanimity and centering.

Videography and photography are powerful pedagogical strategies to advance Unitary Caring Science. They are aesthetic representations that help both the artist and the viewer fall into a meditative, artistic, and creative process while experiencing and reflecting on the meaning of Caring Science. Beautiful posters and aesthetic videos with high-level energy words and phrases create healing environments, inspire faith and hope, and nurture the human soul.

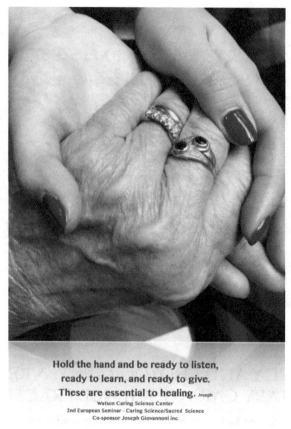

Hold the hand and be ready to listen,
ready to learn, and ready to give.
These are essential to healing. Joseph
Watson Caring Science Center
2nd European Seminar - Caring Science/Sacred Science
Co-sponsor Joseph Giovannoni inc.

FIGURE 37.4

METAPHYSICAL AND NONPHYSICAL INQUIRY

Metaphysics opens the door that is closed by traditional science and empirical knowledge (Koepsell, 2000). Watson's Theory of Transpersonal Caring serves as a framework for advancing disciplinary knowledge within a Unitary Caring Science framework (2005). "The transpersonal caring field resides within a unitary field of consciousness and energy that transcends time, space and physical, unity of mind-body-spirit-nature universe" (p. 223). This worldview grounds and transcends traditional views of science and reality and allows for the expansion of metaphysical and nonphysical inquiry and advances disciplinary-specific knowledge (Figure 37.5). Unitary Caring Science inquiry includes multiple ways of knowing, being, and doing research, honors the infinite wisdom of the mind-body-spirit universe, and acknowledges the mysteries and miracles of being human (Watson, 2005). The views of this Unitary Human Caring Science model conflict metaphysically, philosophically, and morally with traditional classic science assumptions and principles (Watson, 2005).

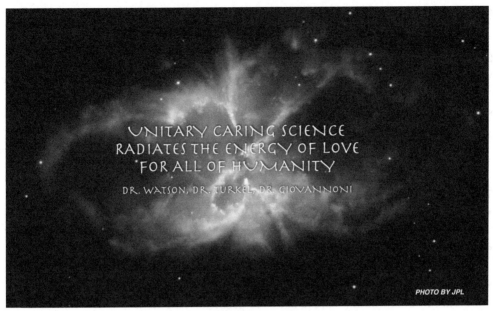

FIGURE 37.5

CONCLUSION

Unitary Caring Science inquiry honors ambiguity, the unknown, the human spirit, and sacred infinity, and gives voice and language to the metaphysics of love, healing, and our covenant with humanity. It invites us to explore healing, being in right relationship with self, the energy of language, the universality of caring, and the manifestation of energy fields as we move to a higher level of consciousness. Research questions related to metaphysical inquiry include the following: What is the highest level of consciousness? What does it mean to be human? What is expanding consciousness?

NEXT ERA POSSIBILITIES

Education
- How can we integrate Unitary Caring Science inquiry into the nursing curricula at the baccalaureate, master's, DNP, and doctoral levels?
- How can we expand our own consciousness related to Unitary Caring Science inquiry?
- How can we further our understanding of the metaphysical?

Research
- How will we use Unitary Caring Science inquiry to contribute to advancing disciplinary-specific nursing knowledge?
- How will we as Unitary Caring Science scholars/researchers integrate the concepts of Unitary Caring Science inquiry into funded research proposals?

- How will our outcomes of Unitary Caring Science inquiry expand the field of human consciousness?

Praxis

- How will we reframe our current practice to allow for creativity and the emergence of all ways of knowing and being to unfold?
- How will we integrate Unitary Caring Science inquiry into the traditional evidence-based practice paradigm?
- How will we provide opportunities for registered nurses at all levels to integrate Unitary Caring Science into their practice environments?

Theory and Knowledge Development

- How can we use Unitary Caring Science inquiry to advance Watson's Theory of Human Caring?
- What middle-range nursing theory can we develop on the basis of the outcomes of Unitary Caring Science inquiry?
- How does our personal conceptualization of nursing science and Unitary Caring Science inform Unitary Caring Science theory development?

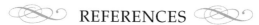 REFERENCES

Baldwin, C. (1998). *Calling the circle.* New York, NY: Bantam.

Giovannoni, J. (2014a). *Continuation of the light of Caritas with Dr. Jean Watson in Nepal.* Retrieved from https://vimeo.com/80812858

Giovannoni, J. (2014b). Dr. Jean Watson-Caritas journey to Nepal, Bhutan and Tibet [Video]. Retrieved from https://vimeo.com/88528940

Koepsell, D. R. (2000). *The ontology of cyberspace.* Chicago, IL: Open Court.

Levinas, E. (1969). *Totality and infinity* (A. Lingis, Trans.). Pittsburgh, PA: Duquesne University.

Levinas, E., Poller, N., & Cohen, R. (2003). *Humanism of the other.* Chicago: University of Illinois Press.

Reason, P. (1993). *Reflections on sacred experience and sacred science. Journal of Management Inquiry, 2*(3), 273–283. doi:10.1177/105649269323009

Turkel, M., & Ray, M. (2012, May). Calling the circle of reflection. Paper presented at 33rd International Association for Human Caring Conference, Philadelphia, PA.

Turkel, M., & Watson, J. (2014, May). Calling the circle of reflection. Paper presented at International Caritas Consortium, New Jersey.

van Manen, M. (2014). *Phenomenology of practice.* Walnut Creek, CA: Left Coast Press.

Watson, J. (1979). *Nursing: The philosophy and science of caring.* Boston, MA: Little, Brown.

Watson, J. (2005). *Caring science as sacred science.* Philadelphia, PA: F. A. Davis.

Watson, J. (2008). *Nursing: The philosophy and science of caring.* Boulder: University Press of Colorado.

Watson, J. (2012). *Human caring science.* Boston, MA: Jones & Bartlett.

Watson, J., & Smith, M. C. (2002). Caring science and the science of unitary human beings: A transtheoretical discourse of nursing knowledge development. *Journal of Advanced Nursing, 37*(5), 452–461. doi:10.1046/j.1365-2648.2002.02112.x

38

Unitary Caring Science and Multicultural Perspectives

Joyce B. Perkins

CARITAS LITERACIES

By the end of this chapter, the caring-healing nurse will be able to

1. Explain how Unitary Caring Science (UCS) in nursing provides a "tent of meeting" for both Western science and multicultural perspectives on healing.

2. Relate how the evolving or "expanding consciousness" of the nurse allows for holistic, Unitary Human Caring Science in nursing, the embrace of multiple paradigms, and the unified field of potential for healing.

3. Articulate the *praxis* of nursing through the lens of UCS.

4. Consider reflection and contemplative practices as tools for self-care that build coherence, expand consciousness, and facilitate understanding multiple paradigms/ dimensions of reality.

This chapter addresses the integrality of UCS and multicultural perspectives in such a way that barriers to understanding shift and opportunities for healing prevail. The evolution of nursing science can be seen in the ongoing dialogue that addresses the question, What is nursing science? (Barrett, 2017). Inquiry on the knowledge base important to the discipline of nursing was clearly articulated by Newman, Smith, Pharris, and Jones (2008). A unitary perspective was articulated that embraced "a traditional scientific approach, a multidimensional evaluation of the interactive milieu" (2008, p. E16), and the direct/embodied experience of expanding consciousness in human form within the cosmos. Seven concepts, which merge as a unitary whole, became the praxis (theory, reflection, and practice in action) of nurses as they related to patients. Concepts included the following:

1. *Health*: The intent of the relationship

2. *Caring*: The nature of the relationship

3. *Consciousness*: The informational pattern of the relationship

4. *Mutual process*: The way in which the relationship unfolds

5. *Patterning*: The evolving configuration of the relationship

6. *Presence*: The resonance of the relationship

7. *Meaning*: The importance of the relationship (Newman et al., pp. E18–E23)

Ten years later, knowledge of the sciences and ancient wisdom from cultures around the globe are converging in such a way that the language of each perspective is given voice in a complementary rather than a dissonant, dual, paradoxical, or competitive fashion (Braden, n.d., 2013; Currivan, 2017; Haramein, 2017a, 2017b). Much like the language of nursing expressed by Newman, Sime, and Corcoran-Perry (1991) and by Newman et al. (2008), the science behind the shift to a unitary perspective is becoming clearer to all. Attention to patterning and the movement of consciousness in expanded form may be seen in the in-formation (the use of in-formation related to the embedded energy pattern/signal integral to structural form) now being shared in such diverse fields as cosmology (Talbot, 2011; Thornhill & Talbott, 2007), cellular biology (Lipton, 2012) and morphology (Sheldrake, 1987), quantum physics (Haramein, 2017a, 2017b), consciousness studies (Goswami, 1995, 2011), mathematics (Steiner, 2001), and other areas. As well, the healing traditions of ancient cultures and understandings of the natural world, as articulated by indigenous populations, are becoming sharable. This chapter highlights that convergence and ultimate integrality of in-formation found in basic nursing art and science, ancient traditions, and indigenous culture, as we seek to bring healing and reconciliation to all.

UNITARY CARING SCIENCE IN NURSING

UCS is the emerging structure for in-formation that carries the nature of the "whole" or Unitary/Transformative (UT or PIII) paradigm in nursing as defined by Newman et al. in 1991. This worldview embraces the two paradigms that reside within it called Particulate/ Determinate (P/D or PI) and Interactive/Integrative (I/I or PII; Newman et al., 1991). The first term relates to the nature of phenomena, and the second relates to how change happens. The same is true for the third paradigm called Unitary/Transformative. Within the original three paradigms of Newman et al., PI focused on physical, mechanical, structural, cause-effect, and objective levels of in-formation; PII focused on subjective meaning, emotion, and relationships of families, cultures, and environments; PIII focused on holistic, unitary, and transformative patterns of in-formation. These three paradigms, sometimes interpreted or perceived as separate or silo-like, are now known to be integral or embedded one within the other, more like holograms within holograms, in fractal scale invariant patterns (a simple process repeated at different scales). The three paradigms of nursing's focus have become an assessment tool, in a sense, much like a map of the territory or "tent of meeting (meaning)," to help nurses sort levels or kinds of in-formation and shorten, or speed up, the process of navigating relationship with self and other, within the context of environment. In brief, Parse (2014), too, contributed to disciplinary knowledge by addressing two paradigms in nursing called "totality" (in which "applied nursing science considers the human as a bio-psycho-socio-spiritual organism made up of distinct parts: body, mind, and spirit"; p. 5) and "simultaneity" (in which "basic science nursing is a view that human is considered unitary, an indivisible energy field recognized through patterns, and human-universe-health is a natural process with ongoing change"; p. 7). Unitary Science melds Parse's two paradigmatic ideas and Newman et al.'s three foci together in a process, or dance of relationship, as they shift meaning potentials via a spiraling process of understanding involving interaction, integration, confluence, and subsequent transformation of consciousness, to an integral awareness that is inclusive of that which is valued from the earlier paradigmic focus, but pruned like a tree, to a more greatly appreciated or evolved shape (in-form-ation) of the next culturally or individually valued paradigm. This ongoing dynamic process calls forth a "unity" or holographic rendering of in-formation ranging from the quantum field of the microcosm to the cosmic void of the macrocosms.

According to the focus of attention and intention in the consciousness of the nurse, these varying levels of in-formation may all be noted in the field of potential unfolding dynamics of nurse/person/environment relationship. Each of the grand theorists of nursing supports an aspect of unitary science much like the facets on a jewel, or Indra's net of relationships (Malhotra, 2016), depending on whether your focus is on the point of light (foreground) or the plenum of space (background) itself in any nursing situation. Rogers (1970, 1992) articulated the science of unitary human beings and the energetic underpinnings of all creation. Newman (1994) spoke of health as expanding consciousness. Parse (1995) described living paradox, or pushing-pulling of humanbecoming. Leininger (2008) and McFarland and Wehbe-Alamah (2015) noted the similarities and dissimilarities of cultures in culture care theory. Watson (2005, 2008) addressed the role of care, love, compassion, appreciation, and gratitude in setting the resonant field at a high enough frequency pattern (the realm of the spirit or sacred mystery within) to initiate actual transformative moments in people's lives for the good, the true, and the beautiful to be revealed. Hence, the stage was set for UCS.

UCS articulates a fine level of discernment in the realm of nursing knowledge development and in the consciousness of the nurse, by affirming that nursing is both an "art and science" (Watson, 2018). In this sense, one cannot define nursing science without the art of nursing embedded within that definition, the very definition of a "unity" perspective. Both objective and subjective in-formation, especially that of care, love, and compassion, are vital in assessment of nursing situations. The inner, subjective quality of "feeling" is key in direct experience often referred to as nurse "presence" or "authentic relationship," in which the nurse resonates or attunes self to the needs of the patient, thereby having an intuitive, inner embodied response to the patient's communication of need that may be nonverbal, yet tacitly "known." In-formation is shared in the frequency field of "felt" experience of two people whose energy field or quantum bubble, surrounding and extending several feet beyond the human body, merges when in relationship (McCraty, 2015).

"Personal knowing" is one of the many ways of knowing originally articulated by Carper in 1978. Indigenous people of Australia perfected the survival skill of "personal knowing" to a fine art. They used it to communicate with the frequency field of planet Earth and followed the song lines of the Earth as they traveled to find food and water, and meet other survival needs. Chinn and Kramer bring us up to date with the addition of "emancipatory knowing" (Chinn & Kramer, 2014) to Carper's (1978) original four patterns of "empiric, personal, ethical, and aesthetic knowing." Note that Chinn and Kramer (2014) place "emancipatory knowing" in the center of a spinning, donut-like model of the four ways of knowing. Similar in design is the toroidal donut in quantum physics. A "vortex equilibrium" described by Haramein (2017a, 2017b) depicts a donut-like structure in quantum physics, revealing how physical matter is built upon the energy template, with the 3-D structure of the Platonic solids (cube, tetrahedron, octahedron, dodecahedron, icosahedron) embedded within the quantum packet of energy with a spiraling vortex at its center. Metaphors like this convey in-formation more quickly than when languaged by step-by-step processes of left-brain rationale. Pictures or story narratives facilitate right- and left-brain coherence in nursing teaching–learning strategies and are being introduced into nursing educational programs to facilitate whole brain functioning. We are all directly participating in an evolution of consciousness within ourselves. Human beings are capable of holding more than one paradigm of consciousness within our natures. We choose our level of in-formation processing according to the needs of the moment (Holladay, 2017; Human Systems Dynamic Institute, n.d.; Stacey, 2017).

Nursing is finally maturing to the point of finding a language that is congruent with the broad horizon of meaning embedded within nursing frameworks, and also finding congruence within traditional science, and wisdom traditions of ancient and indigenous peoples. It is in this light that nurses are able to see that the "art and science" basic to nursing supports not only the profession and discipline of nursing, but other professions and cultural perspectives as well. It is not that we are relying on the science of other disciplines to shape our practice and research. Rather, it is nursing that carries the actual lived experience within each nurse practicing within a UCS framework and articulates the highest form of healing potential on the planet as a discipline, and art, in the practice of its science. In nursing, healing and enlightenment are the same thing (Chopra, 2011, track 2). Details of actual practice situations are beyond the scope of this chapter, but nursing's teaching–learning strategies inform other professions to a greater degree, if fully understood for the depth and breadth of in-formation that is actually available to the discerning expert nurse. In-formation is hyphenated to emphasize the movement of life force energy into form and structure that has a physical or observable manifestation, much like the particle-wave conversation of quantum physics. The presence (attention) of the observer (person or nurse) is crucial to the manifesting form. We are finally coming to understand our own integral nature, and the power of the expression of love and compassion in service to humanity, as profound instruments of healing (Perkins, 2003, 2004; Perkins & Aquino-Russell, 2017a, 2017b; Watson, 2002, 2005, 2018). A caring consciousness in the nurse guides in-formation pathways via values, meanings, and intentions to facilitate healing and enlightenment (Perkins, 2003, 2004, 2017; Watson, 2018).

Watson defines UCS as follows:

… based upon the "Ethic of Belonging," beginning with the belief and perennial wisdom of universal humanity—that our human experiences and journey through life and death are shared with all of humanity across the globe. Human and Planet are united across time and space, belonging to the great sea of humanity. (personal communication, March 9, 2017)

Thus, we begin to understand our role as nurses within the complex dynamics of awareness or consciousness that is integral with all life processes on Earth. In nursing, we sort the complexity and unity of in-formation via the three paradigms articulated by Newman et al. (1991, 2008) and are further assisted by the principles of complexity science.

COMPLEXITY DYNAMICS

A range of potential worldviews exists within any one of us. We choose according to the needs of the moment, which relates to how simple, complicated, or complex the nature of our nursing situation is. Our "nursing situations" (Barry, Gordon, & King, 2015) call forth the level of in-formation needed to help resolve our mutual problem focus. Complexity science (Westley, Zimmerman, & Patton, 2006) articulated this most clearly, as did the landscape diagrams of Stacey (Gp-training-net, n.d.; Stacey, 2002), Eoyang (2017), Holladay (2017), and others. They clarified for managers how to choose the most applicable course of action that would conserve energy of all concerned, and bring harmony and synergistic coherence to the direction of unfolding solutions to any form of dissonance or dis-ease (dis-ease relates to the energy pattern of dis-harmony, as well as the actual disease in physical form) pattern. For example, a simple problem whose outcome is certain if you follow certain steps, and if agreement is high among participants, does not call for a more complicated investigation, something like "baking a cake" (Westley et al., 2006). If you use the ingredients and measurements called for in the recipe, and follow the steps, you will most likely bake a perfect cake every time. This is something like PI in Newman et al.'s conceptual map. If you want to "send a rocket to the moon", however, you have a complicated situation (Westley et al., 2006), but again doable, if you assemble all the parts and follow all the prescribed steps and take into account subtle nuances (variables, such as: culture, emotion, meaning, beliefs; i.e., PII in nursing). "Raising a child" (Westley et al., 2006, p. 9), however, is uniquely different. Even if you followed the same steps and attempted to be mechanistic in your approach, you would be surprised. The child brings his or her own unique nature to the mix, and shifts the outcome of the relationship in so many ways (i.e., PIII in nursing). This kind of mutual participation, uncertainty in relationship, is true of all human interactions. We are complex beings, each with our own qualities and perspectives to bring to any situation.

Complexity science offers us the view that change happens in open systems, which we "are" according to Rogers (1970, 1992), not only hierarchically from the top down but also from the bottom up. A balance of right- and left-brain function via frequency coherence also allows us to function as artist and scientist in our relational moments (HeartMath Institute Research Library, n.d.; Maharishi Foundation, n.d.; McCraty & Childre, 2010; Transcendental Meditation® [TM], n.d.; Travis & Pearson, 2000; Travis & Shear, 2010). Many levels of information participate in any one moment, making a rich tapestry from which to draw inspiration. The spirit (unity) of nursing, the intention "to help and to heal," is embraced as emphatically as the science and data of component parts. Ultimately, we are unitary human beings (Rogers, 1970, 1992) interpreted as spirit having a physical expression. Emerging science is now reflecting the integral nature of spirit and form, along with an ability to translate the ways of knowing of ancient perspectives more clearly.

EMERGING SCIENCE AND ANCIENT PERSPECTIVES

Paradigm shifts may be noted in the focus of attention and intention of Western science. Physics, the parent of most scientific developments in the early 20th century, focused on materialistic and dualistic concerns. Later shifts introduced models based on relational fields of influence and energetic interactions (Currivan, 2017). This relational field perspective is now 100 years old in the Western world, although ancient traditions have held this energetic focus for approximately 5,000 years, as in traditional Chinese, or Ayurvedic medicine. Indigenous Australian aborigines have been reported to remember 50,000 years in their oral history with attention to their direct experience in the natural world. Indigenous cultures gather in-formation by which to make decisions by entering into "the stream" directly, rather than by observing from a distance and analyzing conceptually. They are one, with the qualities of the environmental context, directly in a subjective experience, rather than being objective, and separate from context. Individuals trained under a Western model, which makes extensive use of left-brain, linear, rational thought processes, are now having to learn to balance brain function with that of the intuitive, aesthetic right brain.

The focus of the 21st century for Western science is now calling forth the primacy of in-formation and consciousness, and ultimately the unity of cosmic mind (Currivan, 2017, p. 199). Such shifts reflect an actual complementarity of in-formation within human form as inner and outer worlds become coherent to our intelligence, and "felt" or embodied as whole patterns within us. As we become better able to decipher more complex and nuanced levels of in-formation, we shift metaphorically, from seeing the world in black and white to the many hues of color and texture that actually create the rich tapestry within which we live. We also carry a toolbox with many more avenues or potentially creative ways to clear obstacles or barriers to better health and more fruitful lives. Care, love, and compassion serve as the steering wheel and rudder of the ship for our explorations. Love, compassion, gratitude, appreciation, and humility, even awe, hold us in an embrace or nest as our "home frequency" (Pierce, 2009, p. 267) guides us securely through an unfolding of our true nature. What we value appears to be our guiding light, as purpose fills our daily moments. This manner of nursing practice with "caring … [as] the central domain of nursing" (Barry et al., 2015, p. 4) is best articulated when nursing situation exemplars set the context for student teaching–learning processes. Students learn care and compassion along with skills in nursing pedagogy. Attention to values is also noted in the field of sociology, which is helpful in articulating the interprofessional support available for nursing's approach to patient care.

McIntosh (2012), an evolutionary sociologist and integral leader, has detailed the evolution of consciousness according to "values" within individuals and cultures in great detail with his dialectic model of thesis, antithesis, and synthesis. He revealed the unfolding spiral of consciousness in each one of us, individually and culturally, as we developmentally cycle to more complex patterns (containing more in-formation) that reflect our value shifts toward "the good, the true, and the beautiful" (McIntosh, 2012, p. 84). We prune that which does not serve us, while carrying what does, to a higher order. This process is one of transcendence and inclusion. The process spirals through space-time with a focus on individual and then community, in ever more complex and higher iterations, as values shift within individuals and in humanity as a whole. This transcendent and inclusive quality is also reflected into the far reaches of our cosmos with an understanding of the language used by quantum physicists of the fractal holographic universe. Ancient cultures also had their own ways of sharing, through movement, narrative, or art form, similar understandings.

A FRACTAL-HOLOGRAPHIC MODEL OF THE UNIVERSE: QUANTUM PERSPECTIVES

Jude Currivan, PhD, a cosmologist, physicist, archeologist, and evolutionary leader, addressed key points in *The Cosmic Hologram: In-Formation at the Center of Creation*. She related how our universe is in-formed and manifested by a cosmic hologram at the center of creation. She explained how fractal in-formation patterns guide behavior at the atomic, human, and cosmic levels demonstrating how in-formation is physically real. She "explores how consciousness connects us to the many layers of universal in-formation, making us both manifestations and co-creators" (Currivan, 2017, p. 216). Quantum mechanics and Einstein's theory of relativity are reconciled as she considers energy–matter and space–time as complementary expressions of in-formation, and the cosmic hologram is seen to underlie the origin of species and our own evolution (p. 70). Concurring with ancient spiritual wisdom, Currivan (2017) offered evidence that consciousness is the fundamental nature of what we, and the entire universe, are. Her ideas are paraphrased as follows:

1. Reality is in-formational in nature reflecting a unity of consciousness.

2. Human consciousness is not restricted to our bodies.

3. Nonlocal connectivity transcends space–time, and is innate to our entire universe enabling it to evolve as a single coherent entity.

4. Within space–time, the entropic flow of information engenders both time's arrow, the flow of time itself, and the causes and consequential effects.

5. Between all energy–matter manifestations of a system exhibiting nonlocal behavior, there is no entropic transfer of information within space–time. The whole system is integral, regardless of apparent spatial or temporal separation of its manifested attributes. What one feature "knows," the entirety of the phenomenon "knows."

6. Before observation/measurement, all possible states of a system are nonlocally connected, and in superposition (integral).

7. Only when nonlocally entangled and superpositioned states are measured do they "collapse" to a specific real-i-zation (Currivan, 2017, pp. 200–201).

Notably, "supernormal capabilities are inherently nonlocal, involving informationally entangled perspectives of consciousness that transcend time–space. So while our 'everyday' experiences reflect a localized real-i-zation, the coherence of supernormality allows us to access our innate and indeed universal awareness" (Currivan, 2017, p. 201).

Currivan noted eight cocreative principles of in-formational physics that correlate well with nursing's theoretical structure and lend support to the emerging definition of a UCS as foundational to the discipline. She spoke of a cosmic hologram within which we reside as she articulated an octave of codes as a form of cocreative perception. She called them "informational precepts" (Currivan, 2017, pp. 220–222).

1. *Relativity*: Our perception is informed by the interplay of relativities (e.g., space–time, energy–matter). In nursing, we speak of value in "mutual process" (Newman et al., 2008, p. E21). We have come to see a complementary nature to what used to be thought of as dual opposites. A more benevolent interpretation unfolds as love and compassion reside within.

2. *Resolution*: In transcending relativity, the perception of duality is progressively included yet "re-soulved" (Currivan, 2017, p. 221) into an awareness of the unity of consciousness. In nursing, we think of resolution in terms of finding "meaning" potentials in nursing situations (Newman et al., 2008, p. E23). In story and narration, we build our lives on earlier patterns, moving toward health, healing, and well-being.

3. *Resonance*: Harmonic and coherent relationships that pervade our universe are the signature of the cosmic hologram that we individually and collectively embody on physical, emotional, and mental levels when we choose to be "on the same wavelength," or perhaps, we may feel dissonant when we are "out of tune." Our awareness expands as we become more consciously connected and progressively resonate with the wholeness of the Cosmos (Currivan, 2017, p. 221). In nursing, "resonance" correlates with the "pattern" of relationship (Newman et al., 2008, p. E21).

4. *Reflection*: The outer circumstances of our lives are reflected inwardly by our mental, emotional, and physical states and vice versa. By consciously reflecting on the mirroring embedded within and without, we are more able to re-cognize (relates to re-thinking as well as to recognize) and amend any distortions and bring balance to the system (Currivan, 2017, p. 222). In nursing, balance is achieved by understanding "meaning" in any situation (Newman et al., 2008, p. E23).

5. *Change*: All things change with the flow of time (Currivan, 2017, p. 222). Releasing fear of the unknown and learning to call forth the greatest good (intention and attention), with shifting patterns and circumstances, brings learning and evolution. Purposeful action is found in nursing when we choose to move toward the unfolding of the greatest ethical good. In nursing, change is reflected in the evolving configuration of "pattern" of the whole (Newman et al., 2008, p. E21).

6. *Choice and consequence*: Cause and effect are patterns in the physical domain (Currivan, 2017, p. 222). Taking responsibility for our choices is empowering when our consciousness has time to reflect in the space between stimulus and response. "Minding the gap" builds potential in nursing relationships of true "presence" (Newman et al., 2008, p. E23).

7. *Conservation*: Energy may change its form, but is ultimately conserved (Currivan, 2017, p. 222). Finding balance in the ebb and flow of life events improves health and well-being. Nursing's consistency of "pattern" in authentic "presence" resonates

this heart/mind quality of "care in relationship" or "mutual process" with others (Newman et al., 2008, E21–E23).

8. *Concession*: The practice of forgiveness and reconciliation traditionally used to resolve family and tribal conflicts in Hawaii called "ho'oponopono" enables resolution, healing, and release of intra- and interpersonal conflict. Ho'oponopono translates, as "I'm sorry. Please forgive me. Thank you. I love you" (Currivan, 2017, p. 223). Through a process of individual and collective acknowledgment of fault and recognition of responsibility, its prayer brings healing (Currivan, 2017, p. 223), better known in nursing as a "transpersonal caring healing moment" (Watson, 2010, p. 33).

We continue to explore how consciousness connects us and guides behavior, through the perspectives of culture, biology, and quantum physics in the following section.

ANCIENT PERSPECTIVES AND INDIGENOUS WISDOM

Carl Calleman, PhD, a physical biologist and expert on the Mayan calendar, compared aspects of quantum physics with the perspective of global and ancient cultural interpretations of the origins of the cosmos (Calleman, 2016). Calleman's correlation of in-formation from quantum physics with ancient cultures is also voiced by Haramein (2017a, 2017b), a quantum physicist whose works include *The Resonance Foundation*. The creation stories of many cultures speak of a "Cosmic Axis of pure geometry [that] emerged from a Cosmic Egg giving rise to the Big Bang" (or big breath; Calleman, 2016, p. 57) noted in Western science. From this cosmic tree in the center of the heavens, the "nine waves of creation" emanate as fractal holograms, each bringing a certain level of in-formation to the Earth and her creatures with each inflationary expansion via its interference patterns of frequency waves. Frequencies carry information much like our modern use of music (Merrick, 2010), ultrasound, x-rays, telephones, computers, Internet, and so forth. Each hologram brought expanded interference wave patterns on which our world was created and according to a set schedule as outlined in the Mayan Long Calendar (Calleman, 2016, p. 9). The cosmic tree of life is not a thing made of matter, but rather a geometric source of space–time through which the matter of the universe is organized (Calleman, 2016, p. 22). Calleman writes of synchronization at many different levels that are needed to sustain life over space–time. Each level has a "tree" or hologram that emerged from the cosmic center at specific periods of unfolding as described in the Mayan Long Calendar of days and nights. These waves of in-formation and their interference patterns brought upshifts to creation guiding the evolution of physical structure (Merrick, 2010), morphology of shape and form of biological organisms during the first four waves, and mental, emotional, behavioral, and spiritual unfolding in the last five (Calleman, 2016). The in-formation pattern of each wave downloaded 20 times faster than that of the wave preceding it, giving the sense of time speeding up as more interference patterns, as waves of in-formation, penetrated the field of potential and had to be integrated into human consciousness. Calleman stated, "The organizing principles of the universe act from above to below based on creation waves emanating from the Tree of Life, which ensures that coherence is always maintained" (2016, p. 25). The Tree of Life was looked upon as the Creator, much like God or Source in the Western world, and was considered immaterial, everywhere, and invisible. Some aspect of this creation story is found in peoples and cultures as diverse as Mesopotamia, Sumeria, Egypt, China, Greece, Scandinavia, Australian Maori, Mayan, Hopi, Aztecs, and Celtic, and in religious practices of Hinduism, Buddhism, Judaism, and Christianity (Calleman, 2016).

Attuning to this field of in-formation in a harmonic and coherent way provides avenues for healing on all levels. The resonance of the heart (HeartMath Institute Research Library, n.d.), or caring in nursing, becomes the rudder to help steer individual consciousness and action toward the most fruitful endeavors that will build well-being in the lives of individuals and communities. The ability to read the in-formation available to download from the cosmos is known as intuition (Ruth-Sahd, 2003) in the expert multicultural nurse. Benner described this process of evolution of consciousness within the practice of a nurse using a scale from novice to expert (Benner, 1984).

Certain practices such as TM of the Vedic tradition literally train persons to modulate mind and emotion such that a direct experience of the "silent pure consciousness" (Hagelin, 2017; Orme-Johnson, 2017; Travis & Shear, 2010) of the cosmos is available. In this type of direct experience, tensions of the everyday unwind, stress is released from the physical and mental bodies, and deep rest is attained. As coherence of brain waves is built in the body and mind, intelligence increases, resilience is built, stress is released, physical systems strengthen, immune function improves, depression and anxiety diminish, and so forth (Maharishi Foundation, n.d.). Through repetition of brain and heart wave coherence (McCraty, 2015), the body is able to carry the qualities of pure consciousness into everyday life. At this stage, a cosmic, transcendent, or quantum consciousness is said to exist within the individual (Chopra & Kafatos, n.d.; Forem, 1974, p. 131; Yogi, 2001).

Attuning to the transcendent is possible for communities as well as individuals. When communities of individuals are able to manifest this level of integration within self, violence in the community as a whole, as noted in police records, has been found to decrease (Hagelin et al., 1999). "When more individuals, families, workplaces, and communities increase and stabilize their coherence baselines, it can lead to increased social and global coherence, which is further stabilized through self-reinforcing feedback loops" (McCraty & Childre, 2010, p. 22). Inner peace is contagious. Nurses are able to use tools for transcendence to improve their ability to function in life as well as the work place. Nursing, as a profession, has holistic practices within its traditions that support both nurse and patients, that is, centering, therapeutic touch, healing touch, aromatherapies, music therapies, guided meditations, and so on (American Holistic Nurses Association, n.d.). Explication of attitudes and processes that build coherence in the nurse, as well as in the environment, and communal situations are unfolded in the following section.

TOOLS FOR TRANSCENDENCE AND INCLUSIVE PRACTICE IN NURSING

"The 10 Caritas Processes® of Caring Science theory identify universals of human caring and love that guide caring-healing practitioner-leadership principles for patients, nurses, and healthcare systems around the world" (Watson, 2018). Watson's Caritas Processes are used in schools of nursing worldwide as a model pedagogy or andragogy for program development (Watson, 2017), for example, Florida Atlantic University in Boca Raton, Florida; and St. Catherine University in Minneapolis/St. Paul, Minnesota. It is possible to teach care and compassion in didactic classes, simulations laboratories, and clinical practice. Reflection and contemplative practices greatly enhance critical thinking skills, clinical competence, and stress management for nursing students (Perkins & Aquino-Russell, 2017a, 2017b).

In the literature, meditation in its three forms has been shown to improve performance and well-being (Orme-Johnson, 2017). Travis and Pearson's (2000) and Orme-Johnson's (2017) definitions and descriptive metaphor help nurses understand the level of information available with the practice of each form:

- *Focused Attention* involves concentration on a single object such as the breath or a candle.

- *Open Monitoring* (mindfulness) is nonjudgmental awareness of the present.

- *Automatic Self-Transcending* (TM) is an experience of silent pure consciousness transcending all thought (Travis & Shear, 2010, p. 1110).

Whereas focused attention and open monitoring require "some mental effort …, automatic self-transcending meditation is the effortless transcending of the meditation process itself … automatically lead[ing] to the experience of "consciousness itself," the screen of awareness without any objects of awareness, a low-stress state called transcendental or pure consciousness (Orme-Johnson, 2017, "Three Types of Meditation"). Metaphorically, focused attention is similar to treading water on the surface of a pond; open monitoring is similar to swimming on or near the surface of that pond; and automatic self-transcending is like diving deep below the surface waves to the stillness of the depth (Sitzman, 2010).

Phenomenological qualitative research in nursing supports the superior performance of nurses who practice meditation at the level of transcendence (Perkins & Aquino-Russell, 2017a, 2017b). Quantitative research does the same (Maharishi Foundation, n.d.). Chopra and Tanzi, in *Super Brain* (2012) and *Super Genes* (2015), have also developed processes to bring expanded levels of information processing from Western science to the general public that improve overall functioning, enable right- and left-brain coherence, and reveal neuroplasticity, rejuvenation, and longevity is possible. Ways to improve health and well-being are inclusive of holistic practices in general (Bauer, Kermott, & Millman, 2017), as they facilitate translation of the wisdom of ancient traditions into helpful tools for people in today's world to balance stress and inflammation processes. Ancient cultures have embedded within their sacred practices tools for developing resonance and transcendence as an individual and/or as community, for example, Native American drumming, chanting, and dance patterns; and artworks of many cultures seen in rugs, pottery design, and building structures (Karim, 2004; L. Little Finger, personal communication, 2014). The patterns and structures of form in the natural world also reflect the fractal hologram on which all creation is made (Lipton, 2012, 2018; Sheldrake, 1987).

Tools for nursing practice and cultural coherence such as those described earlier support the formation of a definition of a UCS that carries a broad horizon of meaning for the praxis of nursing. Implications for praxis and nursing education follow the definition.

DEFINITION OF UNITARY CARING SCIENCE: THE ART AND SCIENCE OF NURSING

Along with Watson's attention to the values and ethics that infuse a UCS, the following thoughts are offered as a "tent of meeting" where the meaning potentials of all cultural expressions are honored. In respect for each other's ways of knowing, we build the bridges and pathways for a maturing consciousness in us all.

UCS (Watson & Smith, 2002) may be thought of as the art and science that supports the merger of head and heart within individuals and humanity as a whole, such that the rational linear brain functions in coherent, harmonic, and resonant relationship with the heart's neural anatomy. The "direct perception" of intuitive, whole-body knowing melds with conceptual information creating a coherent field of consciousness of the whole. Indigenous wisdom is integrated with scientific rationale such that right- and left-brain balance informs decisions and conscious choice.

The balance of mind, heart, and spirit wisdom pandimensionally expressed in the cosmos is revealed in 3-D reality via the focus of attention and intention. The choice to know and express gratitude, appreciation, love, and compassion creates a higher vibrational and resonant field within human beings that influences health and healing in general, and specifically shifts chemical, emotional, and behavioral outcomes in the body. We create our reality with the choice of attention and intention. Focus on the lower frequency emotions of anger, frustration, and pain creates states of stress, reduces immune response, and builds rigid mechanical, emotional, and behavioral patterns in the body that result in disease and ill health.

Realities are called "paradigms" or worldviews in nursing and interprofessionally. Paradigms reflect the focus of consciousness in human beings. As mentioned earlier, we all hold several paradigms within ourselves. As we learn to broaden our horizons of meaning and value the contributions of each and all, humanity as a whole begins to embody the potential available in this new time and place in the cosmic scheme of things. We are in a place where space–time and matter–energy converge in a confluence of harmonic expressions intended to build the patterns of a maturing humanity. Science and spirit are united in an integral dance of relationship within us, which has implications for the profession.

CONCLUSION

Nursing theory, UCS, and complexity science promote the idea that the world is full of patterns that interact, adapt, and indeed are integral to relationships at all levels of in-formation in the universe. These patterns may be missed if one focuses solely on parts. A nurse practicing from a unitary perspective would include or pay attention to what naturally occurs as patterns in the universe, and note how these patterns create adaptive changes rather than planned or forced change. With time–space and expanded perspective, patterns emerge from the underlying dynamics that lead to fresh, new ways to deal with issues of concern. Reframing perturbations in the field, on the basis of values and ethical choices, moves one's choices toward "the good, the true, and the beautiful," and builds on individual, family, community, or cultural strengths. One unleashes solutions to complex problems and shifts human energy toward a positive, benevolent outcome for all concerned. Developing nursing leaders who are able to examine the "whole," including potential threats, exposing conflict, or challenging norms requires the ability to embrace a broad horizon of meaning, and navigate turbulent waters with courage and compassion.

Nursing best meets the needs of students and patients by including contemplative practices and other holistic modalities in educational programs alongside Western perspectives of medicine. We are learning to appreciate the full spectrum of meaning and value systems available to us as consciousness learns to embrace data, information, knowledge, and wisdom. Metaphorically, we learn to move from facts to phrases, to sentences, to paragraphs, and to finally read the whole story—and then we make a movie of Self, and become the dancing, singing actor in the middle of our own creation, directly experiencing the bliss, joy, love, and wonder of it All. Ancient cultures and indigenous practices hold the wisdom needed to balance right- and left-brain functioning as well as build coherence/order in the natural world. Together we have all we need to develop the educational pathways for practicing nurses. Creating peace and harmony within and without gives us the opportunity to do so.

NEXT ERA POSSIBILITIES

Education
- How can I integrate UCS and multicultural perspectives into the education I provide for patients, colleagues, and my community?
- In what ways do nursing curricula need to be expanded to include nursing science and multicultural perspectives?

Research
- How does UCS research expand the potential to include multicultural perspectives, ancient wisdom traditions, and indigenous practices of healing?
- How can UCS researchers help to translate in-formation that supports a broad horizon of meaning, thereby offering expanded possibilities and potential for healing among all peoples, no matter what paradigm is held in consciousness by the healee?

Praxis
- Which dimensions of practice can I improve right now with a greater understanding of UCS, holistic practice, and multicultural perspectives?
- Which of my current work-related outcomes can be reframed to include the implications of complexity and UCS for a more expansive/inclusive worldview?

Theory and Knowledge Development
- What is essential to practicing/realizing/promoting UCS and improving health, healing potentials, and offering creative solutions in nursing situations?
- Given my specialty, how might I articulate the tenets of UCS to my colleagues? What specific contributions can I make?
- How does my own theory of nursing resonate with the ideas discussed in this chapter? Is it possible for me to make room for new ways of being, doing, and knowing?

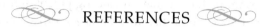

REFERENCES

American Holistic Nurses Association. (n.d.). What is a holistic nurse? Retrieved from http://www.ahna.org/About-Us/What-We-Do

Barrett, E. (2017). Again, what is nursing science? *Nursing Science Quarterly, 30*(2), 129–133. doi:10.1177/0894318417693313

Barry, C. D., Gordon, S. C., & King, B. M. (2015). *Nursing case studies in caring: Across the practice spectrum*. New York, NY: Springer Publishing.

Bauer, B. A., Kermott, C. A., & Millman, M. P. (2017). *Mayo Clinic: The integrative guide to good health: Home remedies meet alternative therapies to transform well-being*. Rochester, MN: Mayo Clinic.

Benner, P. (1984). *From novice to expert: Excellence and power in clinical nursing practice* (pp. 13–34). Menlo Park, CA: Addison-Wesley.

Braden, G. (n.d.). Resilience from the heart. Retrieved from http://www.greggbraden.com/resilience-from-the-heart

Braden, G. (2013). Greg Braden and Bruce Lipton speaking at the United Nations [Video]. Retrieved from http://www.greggbraden.com/video/gregg-braden-bruce-lipton-speaking-at-united-nations

Calleman, C. J. (2016). *The nine waves of creation: Quantum physics, holographic evolution, and the destiny of humanity*. Rochester, VT: Bear.

Carper, B. (1978). Fundamental patterns of knowing in nursing. *Advances in Nursing Science, 1*, 13–23. doi:10.1097/00012272-197810000-00004

Chinn, P. L., & Kramer, M. K. (2014). *Knowledge development in nursing: Theory and process* (9th ed.). St. Louis, MO: Elsevier.

Chopra, D., & Kafatos, M. (n.d.). What is cosmic consciousness? Retrieved from http://www.chopra.com/articles/what-is-cosmicconsciousness

Chopra, D. (2011). *The secret of healing: Meditations for transformation and higher consciousness* [Audio CD]. Play It By Ear Music. Retrieved from https://music.amazon.com/albums/B004JFDPAE

Chopra, D., & Tanzi, R. E. (2012). *Super brain: Unleashing the explosive power of your mind to maximize health, happiness, and spiritual well-being*. New York, NY: Three Rivers Press.

Chopra, D., & Tanzi, R. E. (2015). *Super genes: Unlock the astonishing power of your DNA for optimum health and well-being*. New York, NY: Harmony.

Currivan, J. (2017). *The cosmic hologram: In-formation at the center of creation*. Rochester, VT: Inner Traditions.

Forem, J. (1974). *Transcendental meditation: Maharishi Mahesh Yogi and the science of creative intelligence*. New York, NY: E. P. Dutton.

Goswami, A. (1995). *The self-aware universe: How consciousness creates the material world*. New York, NY: Jeremy P. Tarcher/Putnam.

Goswami, A. (2011). *The quantum doctor: A quantum physicist explains the healing power of integral medicine*. Charlottesville, VA: Hampton Roads.

Gp-training-net (n.d.). The Stacey matrix. Retrieved from: http://www.gp-training.net/training/communication_skills/consultation/equipoise/complexity/stacey.htm

Hagelin, J. (2017). An introduction to the transcendental meditation technique [Video]. Retrieved from https://www.youtube.com/watch?v=ZjT831cjaUY

Hagelin, J. S., Rainforth, M. V., Cavanaugh, K. L. C., Alexander, C. N., Shatkin, S. F., Davies, J. L., Hughes, A. O., … Orme-Johnson, D. W. (1999). Effects of group practice of the transcendental meditation program on preventing violent crime in Washington, D.C.: Results of the National Demonstration Project, June–July 1993. *Social Indicators Research, 47*(2), 153–201. doi:10.1023/A:1006978911496

Haramein, N. (2017a). About Nassim Haramein. Retrieved from https://resonance.is/about-haramein/?utm_source=CBC&utm_medium=Google%20Grant&gclid=CMi-kujXs9MCFZ62wAodpCoOGg

Haramein, N. (2017b). Resonance Science Foundation: Unified science in resonance with nature. Retrieved from https://resonance.is

HeartMath Institute Research Library (n.d.). Retrieved from https://www.heartmath.org/research/research-library

Holladay, R. (2014). Landscape of support for skill building. Retrieved from http://www.hsdinstitute.org/resources/landscape-of-support-for-skill-building-blog.html

Human Systems Dynamic Institute. (n.d.). Landscape diagram. Retrieved from http://www.hsdinstitute.org/resources/landscape-diagram.html

Karim, I. (2004). Wide scale harmonization of electromagnetic fields (EMF). Retrieved from https://www.biogeometry.ca/electrosmog-the-miracle-of-hemberg

Leininger, M. (2008). Overview of Leininger's theory of culture care diversity and universality. Retrieved from http://www.madeleine-leininger.com/cc/overview.pdf

Lipton, B. (2012). Evolution by BITS and pieces: An introduction to fractal evolution. Retrieved from https://www.brucelipton.com/resource/article/fractal-evolution

Lipton, B. (2018). Conscious evolution: Thriving in a world of change [Video]. Retrieved from https://www.brucelipton.com/store/conscious-evolution-thriving-in-a-world-of-change-streaming-video

Maharishi Foundation. (n.d.). What's the evidence? Retrieved from http://www.tm.org/research-on-meditation

Malhotra, R. (2016). The Vedic metaphor of Indra's net. Retrieved from http://dharmatoday.com/2016/10/02/vedic-metaphor-indras-net

McCraty, R. (2015). *Science of the heart: Exploring the role of the heart in human performance: An overview of research conducted by the HeartMath Institute* (Vol. 2). Boulder Creek, CA: HeartMath Institute. Retrieved from https://www.heartmath.org/research/science-of-the-heart

McCraty, R., & Childre, D. (2010). Coherence: Bridging personal, social, and global health. *Alternative Therapies in Health and Medicine, 16*(4), 10–24.

McFarland, M. R., & Wehbe-Alamah, H. B. (2015). *Leininger's culture care diversity and universality: A worldwide nursing theory* (3rd ed.). Burlington, MA: Jones & Bartlett.

McIntosh, S. (2012). *Evolution's purpose: An integral interpretation of the scientific story of our origins.* New York, NY: SelectBooks.

Merrick, R. (2010). Harmonically guided evolution. Retrieved from http://interferencetheory.com/files/Harmonic_Evolution.pdf

Newman, M. (1994). *Health as expanding consciousness* (2nd ed.). New York, NY: National League for Nursing.

Newman, M. A., Sime, A. M., & Corcoran-Perry, S. A. (1991). The focus of the discipline of nursing. *Advances in Nursing Science, 14*(1), 1–6. doi:10.1097/00012272-199109000-00002

Newman, M. A., Smith, M. C., Pharris, M. D., & Jones, D. (2008). The focus of the discipline revisited. *Advances in Nursing Science, 31*(1), E16–E27. doi:10.1097/01.ANS.0000311533.65941.f1

Orme-Johnson, D. (2017). Comparison of techniques. Retrieved from http://www.truthabouttm.org/truth/TMResearch/ComparisonofTechniques/index.cfm

Parse, R. R. (1995). *Illuminations: The human becoming theory in practice and research.* New York, NY: National League for Nursing.

Parse, R. R. (2014). *The humanbecoming paradigm: A transformational worldview.* Pittsburgh, PA: Discovery International Publication.

Perkins, J. B. (2003). Healing through spirit: The experience of the eternal in the everyday. *Visions, 11*(1), 29–42.

Perkins, J. B. (2004). *A cosmology of compassion for nursing explicated via dialogue with self, science and spirit.* Ann Arbor, MI: ProQuest.

Perkins, J. B., & Aquino-Russell, C. (2017a, June 19–23). *Graduate nurses experience the sacred during transcendental meditation.* Presentation at the Watson Caring Science Institute 4th European Seminar, Luca, Italy.

Perkins, J. B., & Aquino-Russell, C. (2017b). Graduate nurses experience the sacred during transcendental meditation. *International Journal for Human Caring, 21*(4), 163–171. doi:10.20467/HumanCaring -D-17-00034

Pierce, P. (2009). *Frequency: The power of personal vibration.* New York, NY: Atria.

Rogers, M. E. (1970). *An introduction to the theoretical basis of nursing.* Philadelphia, PA: F. A. Davis.

Ruth-Sahd, L. A. (2003). Intuition: A critical way of knowing in a multicultural nursing curriculum. *Nursing Education Perspectives, 24*(3), 129–134.

Sheldrake, R. (1987). Mind, memory, and archetype: Morphic resonance and the collective unconscious–part I. *Psychological Perspectives, 18*(1), 9–25. Retrieved from https://www.sheldrake .org/files/pdfs/papers/morphic1_paper.pdf

Sitzman, K. (2010). Student-preferred caring behaviors for online nursing education. *Nursing Education Perspectives, 31*(3), 171–178.

Stacey, R. (2002). *Strategic management and organisational dynamics: the challenge of complexity* (3rd ed.). Harlow, England: Prentice Hall.

Steiner, R. (2001). *The fourth dimension: Sacred geometry, alchemy, and mathematics.* Great Barrington, MA: Anthroposophic Press.

Talbot, M. (2011). *The holographic universe: The revolutionary theory of reality* (Reprint ed.). New York, NY: Harper Perennial.

Thornhill, D., & Talbott, D. (2007). *The electric universe.* Portland, Oregon: Mikamar.

Transcendental Meditation®. (n.d.). What's the evidence? Retrieved from http://www.tm.org/ research-on-meditation

Travis, F., & Pearson, C. (2000). Pure consciousness: Distinct phenomenological and physiological correlates of "consciousness itself". *International Journal of Neuroscience, 100,* 77–89. doi:10.3109/ 00207450008999678

Travis, F., & Shear, J. (2010). Focused attention, open monitoring and automatic self-transcending: Categories to organize meditations from Vedic, Buddhist, and Chinese traditions. *Consciousness and Cognition, 19,* 1110–1118. doi:10.1016/j.concog.2010.01.007

Watson, J. (2005). *Caring science as sacred science.* Philadelphia, PA: F. A. Davis.

Watson, J. (2010). Academic Paper prepared for Honorary Doctorate Award, from Universitat Rovira I Virgili, Tarragona, Spain. Retrieved from https://www.watsoncaringscience.org/wp-content/ uploads/2016/04/HonoraryDoctaddresswatsonjean-Spain2010.pdf

Watson, J. (2018). *Initary caring science: The philosophy and praxis of nursing* (1st ed.) Boulder: University Press of Colorado.

Watson, J., & Smith, M. C. (2002). Caring science and the science of unitary human beings: A transtheoretical discourse for nursing knowledge development. *Journal of Advanced Nursing, 37*(5), 452–461. doi:10.1046/j.1365-2648.2002.02112.x

Westley, F., Zimmerman, B., & Patton, M. (2006). *Getting to maybe: How the world is changed.* Toronto, ON, Canada: Random House.

Yogi, M. M. (1974). *Transcendental meditation: And the science of creative intelligence.* New York, NY: E. P. Dutton.

Yogi, M. M. (2001). *Science of being and art of living: Transcendental meditation* (Reissue ed.). n.p. Plume.

Unitary Caring Science: Evolving Society Toward Health, Healing, and Humanity*

Jean Watson, Sara Horton-Deutsch, and William Rosa

CARITAS LITERACIES

By the end of this chapter, the caring-healing nurse will be able to

1. Identify the role of Unitary Caring Science in furthering health, healing, and humanity.

2. Explain the power of Unitary Caring Science as a foundation for activism and human rights empowerment.

3. Apply Unitary Caring Science principles to greater planetary-universal challenges that currently threaten the human race.

∽

The only true standard of greatness of any civilization is our sense of social and moral responsibility in translating material wealth to human values and achieving our full potential as a caring society.

The Right Honorable Norman Kirk,
Former Prime Minister of New Zealand (as cited in Watson, 1999)

Somewhere along the way society has been detoured from moral, social action informed by deep spiritual values addressing our shared humanity, health for all, healing our

---

*Sections of this manuscript include excerpts from Watson, J. (2008b). Social justice and human caring: A model of caring science as a hopeful paradigm for moral justice for humanity. *Creative Nursing*, 14(2), 54–61. doi:10.1891/1078-4535.14.2.54. Used with permission.

relations with each other, with Mother Earth. Western affluent civilization in particular has avoided human disparities, poverty, and suffering that are underlying these detours from health and healing, preventing evolution of our human civilization. As Maya Angelou put it (1993):

"... do not hide your face.
Rather, lift up your faces ... there is a piercing need ...
we are arriving on a nightmare, praying for a dream."

These "turning our face away" politics and global practices are in sharp contrast to nursing's history of offering compassionate global human service, health, and social reform. At a time when there is no more hiding place for noncaring, at a time when, in the words of Maya Angelou, "we are arriving on a nightmare, praying for a dream," then how is one—how are we—to make sense of the unexplainable phenomenon of Unitary Caring Science and concepts of health, healing, and humanity, in a world that is turning upside down and inside out with its violations of health, healing, and humanity, and human caring in a world that is hiding its face from the other?

In a world that still believes in war as solution to peace, a world that is spending an estimated $5 trillion in a war on terrorism and little to nothing on war on poverty and basic child healthcare for its citizens (Thompson, 2011).

These matters are not just political; they are moral–spiritual matters facing all of humanity. World-renowned, morally and spiritually guided activists, and thought leaders from a variety of disciplines and persuasions are calling for a social change.

The Human-Planet survival is now "up close and personal" like never before and there is no place to hide. American politician and environmentalist, Al Gore, has been awakening the world to issues of survival of planet Earth (and health of humans and planet). At a "Spirit of Humanity" 2015 World Leader Conference in Iceland, the president and former president of Iceland and other major world leaders called for an awakening of the spirit of humanity to address the survival of our humanity and planet. World leaders from all sectors of society have a responsibility toward a transformation of human consciousness, to return to core values of caring, compassion, and LOVE if we are to survive.

World-renowned writer, speaker, activist, and sociologist Parker Palmer (2004) reminds us that our values can either form or deform our humanity. He poses this human deformation as a form of violence, not in the sense of bombs but in forms of violence toward each other, our shared humanity, toward another, unlike us, who is *Other* than us—often becomes enemy—the one from whom we turn away our face, in the ethic of French philosopher, Emmanuel Levinas (1969).

American singer-songwriter Tracy Chapman's 1980s lyrics of injustices, affecting health, healing, and our humanity, bring us "up closer and personal" to the lingering refrain with her piercing revolutionary singing on the streets of Manhattan in the 1980s and 1990s. The lyrics can be heard still, into our nation and our world (Watson, 1991). Why do we still feel lonely when there are seven billion people on the planet? How is it we tie the notion of peace to war missiles? How is it that women are still treated as political objects for men with control over their rights?

"...We need a caring revolution" (Eisler, 2007, p. 24). When we are guided by values such as conquests, exploitation, and domination, our very survival is threatened, both human and environment.

We can offer up loads of statistics and graphs from the Centers for Disease Control and Prevention National Center for Health Statistics, depicting these disparities in the United States and around the globe. However, it gets close when infant mortality rates and statistics of those uninsured for basic healthcare are alarming; for example, U.S. infant mortality rates are higher than those of 27 other countries, yet the United States spends more money on healthcare than any other country in the world. And global inequities increase as 1% of the wealthiest in the world hold more than the rest of world; world's income distribution indicates that 94% of the world income goes to 40% of the population, whereas 60% of people live on only 6% of the world income.

Now we see the inextricable connection between poverty, health, caring, and healing our humanity. Peace versus Non-Peace. And underneath the outer manifestation of poverty, mortality rates, disease, and suffering is another story.

- From a moral/ethical point of view, we witness a worldview where "Other" is viewed as separate—different, enemy, or less than fully human in our minds' eyes—allowing us to reduce another human being to the moral status of OBJECT, whereby we can justify doing things to Other as Object we would never do to him or her as a fully functioning human being.

- However, now we know another way: an evolved Unitary Caring Science worldview, where sages and wisdom traditions across time make evident: One person's level of humanity reflects back on the other and we are all connected through our shared humanity (Watson, 2008a).

In Maya Angelou's wisdom, again: "I am a Human Being and nothing Human is alien to me"—so if one person is reduced to moral status of object, so is the other; we are all connected (Angelou, 1993). Likewise, if one person's human spirit is lifted up, so is the other's.

Eisler's book (2007) on *The Real Wealth of a Nation* makes a case for *"Caring* Economics," highlighting real people and real circumstances that are in our midst and face us around the globe. As Eisler, a cultural historian, systems scientist educator, and attorney, reminds us, it is only from the human capital of people and caring that other economic activities are possible. Thus, caring, poverty, health, economics, and social justice merge.

From another point of view, caring ethic scholar and educator, Nel Nodding (1984), proposed the household/the classroom, the human-to-human caring relationships for self and other and community, as the core inner sector, the real heart of humanity, health, bringing social justice healing and human caring together for a new world survival. The humanist educator and beloved teacher, Maxine Greene, put it the following way:

> ... change can be learned as persons begin to move toward one another, appearing to one another, articulating different perspectives, becoming concerned ... it is only in our intersubjectivity, our coming together that we create social space for caring, for values literacy, where transformation can occur. (Greene, 1986, pp. 231–232)

A model of Caring Science, emergent from nursing's timeless values and actions in the world, is grounded with an underlying "Ethic and moral action of Belonging" (Levinas, 1969). It invites new policies, politics, practices, and ethics that fulfill human needs and comes from both an old and a new worldview that are upon us.

So, multiple voices in diverse fields of economics, bioethics, philosophy, education, social sciences, as well as poets and street singers alike, along with both historic and contemporary writers and scholars in nursing and Caring Science, have views that acknowledge this phenomenon as a crisis of values, referred to in an earlier paper as "the moral failure of the patriarchy" (Watson, 1990). All of these converging views acknowledge the moral, philosophical, and real consequences for society, for civilization, for humanity, and for our planet Earth survival. When our values do not address social/moral justice for human kind—then, there is no health, healing, or caring, and we perpetuate a noncaring ethos.

Lack of health, healing, and caring occurs when noncaring, illiterate, and noncaring consciousness and actions violate *the identity and integrity of the other, the belief systems of others, and the status of human dignity, and there is failure to honor the spirit-filled person.* We do this in ways and acts, small and large, from humiliating a child to "turning our face away" from others who are different from us and threaten our comfort (Watson, 2005a, 2005b).

UNITARY CARING SCIENCE AS OLD/NEW ETHIC FOR EVOLVING SOCIETY

SACRED ACTIVISM/NURSING

Society and our world civilization are faced with a new global challenge: to enter into an old/new morality for sustaining a healthy humanity, for healing our personal/planet unity. Evolving society toward health, healing, and humanity is embedded in nursing, framed within a context of Unitary Caring Science as an expanded worldview, one of unitary connection of all. This work is referred to by Harvey (2007) as Sacred Activism and Radical Passion whereby sacred love and wisdom are translated into action.

A Unitary Caring Science context allows us to acknowledge a unitary cosmology—to engage in a higher/deeper sacred reality of what is and what is emerging around the world, and what has to emerge for our collective survival.

A model of Unitary Caring Science, beyond an intellectualization of the topic, invites us into a timeless, yet timely space to revisit this perennial phenomenon of the human condition. When one posits knowledgeable human caring, health, and healing as a mandate to survival, these issues can be positioned as the highest form of ethical commitment to patients, families, communities, society, and civilization, the planet Earth. This takes us back to our roots within nursing as an exemplar and ideal of Unitary Caring Science as context for Ethic of Belonging and Ethic of Face as evolved consciousness for humanity:

- This ethical commitment to all, guiding nursing and its commitment to caring, health, and healing, has been the moral covenant with humanity, across time. It can be understood within Levinas's notion of Ethic of Belonging and Ethic of Face, where we face our own and other's humanity we all share.

- This is acknowledging we are all alike as human before the body's physical skin, and we are all alike after the body's physical skin (we all belong to the universal field of infinite Love, before we are separate; thus, Ethics of Belonging comes before a separatist ontology).

- When we shift our worldview to face the depth of our humanity and look into the Face of Other, both literally and metaphorically, we establish a primordial basis of our caring, health, and healing for evolved humanity. This is the only way to sustain humanity at this point in human history: to look into the face of other, not as different other, but as a reflection of each of us.

UNITARY CARING SCIENCE LITERACIES—MORAL ACTIONS EVOLVING HUMANITY

We are calling nurses and other healthcare professionals from around the world to use Unitary Caring Science Literacies to guide moral actions toward health, healing, and wholeness to preserve humanity and our planet Earth. In our nursing midst, past and present, we see informed, moral, Unitary Caring Science actions on a daily basis, sometimes quietly behind the scenes, creating sacred space just to listen, to hold another person's story. This is a collective endeavor between and among nurses and citizens worldwide to construct a moral community, a healthy and caring society for all (Watson, 2018). As nurses and the public embrace the timeless, yet pressing need for global health tied to social justice, we can articulate and provide a legacy of hope and healthcare for all, pioneering Nightingale for a new era. *We* are all called forth to give voice to Nightingale's visionary leadership during a time of major needs for society and our world's health.

The former distinguished professor in Cognitive Science and Linguistics and current director of the Neural Mind & Society at University of California, Berkeley, George Lakoff (2017) identifies the current Women's Marches as the "Politics of Care." Peaceful, cooperative, and family oriented, the marches emphasized that women's rights are all humans' rights. Lakoff (2017) reiterates that more than ever before it is time to communicate care, teach care, find out what others care about … even those with different political views and listen as way to find commonality and shared values.

It is, indeed, a commonplace flaw of the human condition to other the Other. To not see that Black Lives Matter means that *All* Lives Matter; to not honor that bathrooms for transgender people is a most basic right of all peoples; to deny the right of marriage to some is to denigrate the sanctity of marriage to all; to ban those from foreign countries is to disintegrate the fabric of transpersonal oneness; the othering deflects the opportunities we have to regain ground as a caring society of oneness, unity, and presence. We use the issues of the Other to inflate ego, economic capital, and political control—and, yet, we still do not fully grasp that the very Other, we other, is the very one whose truth has the potential to enlighten, guide, and inform the extent to which we can grow into a compassionate, caring global society.

When we regard our current challenges as an opportunity to grow, we find that we are far from helpless in the face of it. We cannot hide from the events taking place around us. Existence as we know it may come to an end but this makes way for something new, and, if we are present to influence it, to bring forth a renewed morality and value for all of humanity.

We must open our eyes to the blessings hidden in disorder. We must ask ourselves: How can we influence the transformations needed in our world in the midst of the troubling transgressions that have and continue to take place? How can we adapt our position to the circumstances before us and capitalize on the situations in which we are? How can compassion, optimism, and flexibility aid in moving forward? Although having the courage to address the needed changes may hurt in the short term, if we embrace them proactively, thoughtfully, and persistently, grounded in a Unitary Caring Science model, their lasting impact will nearly always be physically, emotionally, spiritually, and intellectually transformative. Reflecting on our personal-professional commitment, clarifying our purpose in the world, and standing together to remain resilient provide the strength to recommit to our ethical commitment to society.

Unitary Caring Science invites us to make communion with the human contexts that surround us. True unity is about inviting the narratives of others into a space of safety and support. It is about understanding the tender threads of humanity that hold together another's story, and are the pillars of my narrative and what it is yet to become. Context is not about understanding circumstances; context asks us to immerse ourselves in the lifeworlds of others—to bathe in the lens of their souls and experience the fears that bind them from a place of nonjudgment and surrender. Much of humanity is simply not equipped for this level of spiritual dexterity. This is understandable given our shared history of violence, intolerance, and chronic habits of divisiveness. But having the courage to embrace another's context and using the willingness to see the world through his or her eyes, that level of moral imagination stems from the art and Science of Unitary Caring. That is evolution.

CARING RIGHTS–HUMAN RIGHTS

Caring is a moral imperative of the profession and has been the intention of millions of healers committed to its ideals for generations. However, it is time we own and take accountability for our more global responsibilities in translating the ethics of nursing to the well-being of humanity and the health of the planet—beyond the confines of healthcare and the academic constraints of theory development. Unitary Caring Science is at the heart of what it means to live in the space of greatness: the risk of being bold enough to care and to graciously accept being cared for.

Caring is a right of humanity—a basic human need for growth and survival—and a complex ethical currency too often denied to people because of a superficial hierarchy of needs and disparate socioeconomic circumstances. True caring, and the ability to maintain a caring stance, must be viewed and regarded as the most precious of human rights. Without it, we die. The death may not be physically recognizable, but at spiritual, emotional, mental, psychological, social, and transpersonal levels—at the root of what it ultimately means to be human—we lose the capacity for life and living.

Caring offers answers to the problems that plague us as a planetary village: the widespread host of crises that call into question how long we will be able to inhabit the Earth. Caring is no longer an option or a "nice to have"; it is a *must*, a *now*, and an ever more pressing *ask*. The measurement of caring as a science and the economic implications of its implementation across systems will continue to mature as sciences do, but the conviction that caring can, in fact, change the world cannot afford to be stalled.

The very core of our shared dilemma is that we think we have time. This great imposter of time may be the greatest and only enemy we have in common. This is because time suggests that humanity's continued choices of inequity and injustice will somehow hold for us different consequences than those we now face. Impossible!

Darkness cannot find itself without the light.

Caring is the answer that now pleads with us to find it.

CONCLUSION

A Unitary Caring Science model is based on a deeply human, caring, relational, unitary worldview, which includes human-to-human relationships, human-to-environment relationships, human-to-universe oneness; a universal "Belonging" to infinite field of cosmic Love.

Unitary Caring Science seeks to honor the depth, humility, connection, compassion, responsibility, and concern for human welfare and optimal human development/evolution— a model of honoring paradox of differences and similarities that unite, rather than separate, our existence/experiences.

This view transcends convention and includes starting where we are, in creation of caring-healing environments, in our inner selves, our homes, schools, businesses, communities, healthcare settings, governments, and institutions. A model of Unitary Caring Science informs a caring economics as well as social justice, in that it gives value, visibility, and a formal structure and orientation to informed caring, health, healing, and an evolved human civilization. This is what nursing has always brought as its highest ethical commitment to humanity, to communities, to the world helping society to evolve toward health, healing, and humanity.

NEXT ERA POSSIBILITIES

Education

- In what ways does education at basic and advanced levels need to be shifted toward a paradigm of Unitary Caring Science?
- How do I envision educational programs in multiprofessional specialties being adapted to include the ethics and ethos of caring?
- What role does nursing play in educating patients and the public in the foundations of caring as science?

Research

- How can research be recalibrated to include attention to humanistic values?
- Are current research methods inclusive of Unitary Caring Science principles, beyond the basic ethics of research?

Praxis

- What are the most substantial current barriers to Unitary Caring Science values in practice at local, national, and international levels?
- What is the role of sacred activism for nurses and nursing?
- How can I go about ensuring human rights in a caring, active, powerful, yet sacred way? What is asked of me to accomplish this?

Theory and Knowledge Development

- What are the next phases of Unitary Caring Science that need to be expanded to more deeply reveal the universal implications of noncaring behaviors and practices?
- Why is Unitary Caring Science a cornerstone for theory and knowledge development for the future of health, healing, and humanity?

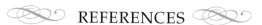 REFERENCES

Angelou, M. (1993). *On the pulse of morning: The inaugural poem.* New York, NY: Random House.

Eisler, R. (2007). *The real wealth of nations: Creating a caring economics.* San Francisco, CA: Berrett-Koehler.

Greene, M. (1986). Toward possiblity: Expanding the range of literacy. *English Education, 18,* 231–243.

Harvey, A. (2007). *Sacred activism: The power of love and wisdom in action.* Paper delivered at 12th International IONS Conference: Consciousness in Action, Palm Springs, CA.

Lakoff, G. (2017). The women's march and the politics of care: The best response to Trump's inaugural address. Retrieved from https://georgelakoff.com/2017/01/22/the-womens-marches-and-the-politics-of-care-the-best-response-to-trumps-inaugural-address

Levinas, E. (1969) *Totality and infinity.* Pittsburgh, PA: Duquesne University Press.

Nodding, N. (1984). *Caring: A feminine approach to ethics and moral education.* Berkeley: University California Press.

Palmer, P. (2004). *21st century learning initiatives.* Kalamazoo, MI: Fetzer Institute.

Thompson, M. (2011). The $5 trillion war on terror. *Time.* Retrieved from http://nation.time.com/2011/06/29/the-5-trillion-war-on-terror

Watson, J. (1990). The moral failure of the patriarchy. *Nursing Outlook, 38*(2), 62–66.

Watson, J. (1991). From revolution to renaissance. *Revolution: Journal of Nurse Empowerment, 1*(1), 94–100.

Watson, J. (1999). *Postmodern nursing and beyond.* New York, NY: Elsevier.

Watson, J. (2005a). *Caring science as sacred science.* Philadelphia, PA: F. A. Davis.

Watson, J. (2005b). Caring science: Belonging before being as ethical cosmology. *Nursing Science Quarterly, 18*(4), 304–315. doi:10.1177/0894318405280395

Watson, J. (2008a). *Nursing. The philosophy and science of caring.* (2nd ed.). Boulder: University Press of Colorado.

Watson, J. (2008b). Social justice and human caring: A model of caring science as a hopeful paradigm for moral justice for humanity. *Creative Nursing, 14*(2), 54–61.

Watson, J. (2012). *Human caring science.* Sudbury, MA: Jones & Bartlett.

Watson, J. (2018). Social justice and human caring: A model of caring science as a hopeful paradigm for moral justice for humanity. *Creative Nursing, 24*(Suppl. 1), 1–8. doi:10.1891/1078-4535.14.2.54

X

Journeys Into the Transpersonal:
Aesthetic Ways of Knowing

40

Caritas Coaching: The Future of Health and Well-Being

Jan Anderson

The promotion of health and healing of all individuals, societies, life, environments, and our planet is dependent on the ability of each of us to live responsibly, ethically, and morally as biogenic (life-giving and life-receiving) human beings. Caring Science (an evolution of the Theory of Human Caring) and Caritas Coaching provide the ethical and moral foundations for living with hope by promoting Caritas (love, care, and healing) for all. The Caritas Coach® is empowered to find and use his or her own authentic and unique voice, gifts, and talents, and to recognize, appreciate, and encourage the gifts and talents of all people. In this way, the Caritas Coach cocreates ways of being and becoming more biogenic human beings through the shared values of loving-kindness, equanimity, compassion, and the respect and honor we have for ourselves and each other. These Caritas Literacies, ways of being and becoming more healing and humane, are taught, learned, and embodied by Caritas Coaches worldwide who have made the commitment to transform self, systems, people, and environments toward greater health and wholeness to the betterment of all.

This chapter explores Caritas Coaching as a means to preserve the dignity and integrity of all people through Caritas Literacy in transpersonal relationships, which honor and find meaning and purpose in all of our lives. With more than 350 Caritas Coaches practicing around the world, this biogenic effect is profound and increasing. This chapter also expounds Caring Science and Caring Science Curriculum as crucial for teaching/learning and being/becoming a Caritas Coach in the Caritas Coach Education Program® (CCEP). Finally, research that more clearly describes the journey of the Caritas Coach toward wholeness and wellness is introduced with suggestions for further study.

CARING SCIENCE

Caring Science provides the theoretical and ethical foundations for practice as a Caritas Coach. Caring Science and Caritas Coaching are grounded in the belief that to be and become more human, one must be committed to taking a lifelong introspective journey of self-discovery, self-awareness, self-healing, and expanding Caritas consciousness. The idea of expanding consciousness as health and healing is important because it assumes that all of us are part of the unitary field, meaning all of us are connected spiritually and energetically (Watson, 1999). In this way, our relationships extend beyond ourselves and each other to the environment, our planet, and beyond, and what any one of us does, thinks, says, intends, and so forth, affects the health of all. Caring Science is also based on the premise that each human being is unique, endowed with special gifts and talents, and is innately valuable. These premises remind us that life is sacred, connected, and whole and that who we are and what we do matters. As the Caritas Coach enters the inner journey toward health and healing, it becomes evident that the subjective inner life of each of us and those aspects that make us human provide the very path for wellness, wholeness, health, and healing for all.

CARING SCIENCE CURRICULUM

Caring Science curriculum promotes the education of the whole person, body, mind, heart, and soul, toward evolved ways of being/doing/knowing and becoming more conscious, aware, and biogenic (Hills & Watson, 2011; Sitzman & Watson, 2014; Watson, 2008). Education based on Caring Science offers us a very real path toward preparing each individual and community toward more Caritas ways of being. Caring Science curriculum shifts the meaning and significance of what is taught and learned from content and objective information in unequal relationship to a focus on the transpersonal relationship based on equality, justice, meaning, and the full integration of what it means to be Caritas, how to become Caritas and biogenic, and how to take action on the basis of these values. Being Caritas offers hope, healing, and health as each person recognizes there is a more loving, caring, and healing way to teach, learn, live, and be in the world, and that this begins with the care of self and extends to the care of all life. Caritas Coaching is a way to deepen and expand this way of being/knowing/becoming/doing through education based on the Caring Science curriculum.

THE CARITAS COACH EDUCATION PROGRAM

The Watson Caring Science Institute (WCSI), a nonprofit organization, was created in 2009 by Dr. Jean Watson and several Caring Science scholars and clinicians who envisioned programs, activities, and networking to transform healthcare by restoring "the profound nature of caring-healing and [to] bring the ethic and ethos of Love back into Healthcare" (Watson, n.d., para. 1). The CCEP was created by the WCSI and based on caring andragogy to provide a lived experience reflecting the caring values and ideals for students and faculty (Anderson, 2014). It was designed to create a professional practice on the basis of internal dialogue, awareness, consciousness, health, and care, providing a foundation for caring practice and education (Hills & Watson, 2011; Watson, 2008). The CCEP is the first and only coach program designed to prepare coaches to learn and implement Caring Science in the coach role by becoming Caritas literate (Anderson, 2014).

The CCEP is structured as a 6-month Caritas journey that occurs through active student engagement and the integration of subjective and objective ways of knowing, and preparing individuals to be caring literate to care for, heal, and touch the human spirit (MacNeil & Evans, 2005; Watson, 2008). Active student engagement is informed by reading, reflection, experience, relationship, writing, creativity, and all ways of knowing, including a focus on aesthetics. Advanced teaching and learning approaches include the following: promotion of transpersonal relationships in community and individually, working from the other's frame of reference, and finding meaning. In this way, the program is personalized, individualized, and respectful. The wisdom, insights, and education that occur during the 6-month journey combine to strengthen confidence and offer courage to transform self and healthcare toward well-being, wholeness, healing, and love (Anderson, 2014).

The CCEP consists of two onsite seminars, one at the beginning and one at the end of the 6 months of faculty-supported and weekly online learning activities. Learning activities include the following: a Caring Science project, an abstract, a poster, a portfolio, and a poster presentation. Multiple professionals worldwide have completed the CCEP including the following: physicians, nurses, social workers, respiratory therapists, physical therapists, chaplains, educators, and business professionals, substantially affecting the global community. The program is accredited by the American Nurses Credentialing Center (ANCC) as an ANCC-accredited Nursing Skills Competency Program and offers contact hours after program completion.

CARITAS COACHING

Caritas Coaching offers an exemplar of being/becoming/knowing and taking action based on the ethos and praxis of Caritas. Caritas has been used with the concept of care to emphasize and add a sacred dimension to care, reminding us of the spiritual nature of healing and caring for self and other (Watson, 2008). Caritas and the "ontological-heart-centered tasks" (Watson, 2005, p. 115), which include forgiveness, gratitude, compassionate service, and surrender, are integrated into the curriculum to guide the Caritas Coach toward health and healing for self and other. These heart-centered ways of being more conscious, self-aware, and intentional in life create firm foundations for Caritas Literacies, ways of being more open-hearted, more accepting, more present, and authentic, in better relationship with self and other, and the ability to appreciate all life experiences, life lessons, joys, and sorrows.

This way of being and becoming Caritas promotes hope, trust, and inspiration for something better and the courage and strength of conviction needed for transformation. Each Caritas Coach reminds us that there is another way to live, that with love and hope anything is possible, and that caring and healing cannot be confused with lack of action. Caring Science and Caritas Coaching provide the philosophical and ethical framework from which to make conscious decisions and choices based on the values of equality, justice, and respect for human life. Being a Caritas Coach is to be morally and ethically responsible for self, other, and all life by taking action to promote health, safety, and human dignity for all.

The Caritas Coach coaches self and other through "advanced teaching/learning" (Watson, 2008, p. 31), which can occur only in transpersonal relationship, from the "spirit-to-spirit level with another, beyond personality, physical appearance, disease, diagnosis, even presenting behavior" (Watson, 2008, p. 82). In this way, the Caritas Coach relationship is one of walking alongside, the "I-Thou" (Watson, 2008, p. 81) relationship, with both coach and coachee learning and teaching through sharing heart, spirit, and experience, sharing the ethics of equality, respect, honor, and wholeness. As a Caritas Coach in transpersonal relationship, there is a cocreation (as opposed to problem solving) that occurs when each person works together without agenda, from a place of mutual respect and honoring the wholeness of each, and seeking new, uncharted territory, previously not identified as creative paths to emerge to promote health, healing, and wholeness. These new possibilities and creative paths enhance the mystery and magic of each person's life and journey to one that is sacred and meaningful with unlimited potential. Thus, each person becomes connected with a larger vision for a meaningful life.

Caritas Coaching offers balance and vision for what it means to live life with purpose, in alignment with self, and at one with source to compassionately serve, care for, and heal all. It expands our current vision of coaching to include a focus on coaching self first, through self-care, education, increasing awareness, and caring-healing practices. Caritas Coaching moves beyond the traditional interpersonal relationship to a transpersonal relationship, connecting to the underlying spiritual nature of humanity, health, and healing. Transpersonal relationships transcend ego and agenda to connect with the spirit of another as an embodied soul, with the only intention of promoting the welfare of the other in that moment (Watson, 1999, 2008). This kind of relationship allows for transpersonal caring moments, moments when the unitary energy field opens up to the possibility of something more than the people in relationship; it manifests as potentials for insight, healing, growth, wisdom, maturity, and health. In this transcendent possibility, there is no linear pattern to the process of health and healing, and there is no sequence of steps that must occur in every situation. It is a creative process that occurs in the present moment, the now; it is open, fluid, and individual because each person is unique, and has a different life story and potential. It is when we can begin to see each person, hear each person, and walk alongside each person that we realize the power of Caritas Coaching to transform our worlds in ways that are healing, loving, and promoting life.

CARITAS LITERACY

The Caritas Coach has consciously completed an educational program that focuses on an introspective journey, which promotes and sustains Caritas Literacy. Caritas Coaching as a lived way of being and becoming affects the health and well-being of not only those who are coached but also the communities in which they live and beyond. Watson describes Caritas Literacy as "human artistry" (2008, p. 23), as ways to live that promote connection, love, compassion, communication, and healing. Caritas Coaching and Caritas Literacy reconnect us with our purpose and values to more intentionally and equitably care for ourselves and each other. Caritas Literacy does not define our behavior solely; it describes and focuses on our intentions, our attitudes, our ethics, our values, and those core aspects of how we care for ourselves and for each other that do not change (Anderson, 2014;

Watson, 2008). Those core aspects are the 10 Caritas Processes®, which form the unchanging framework of Caring Science. Although the core Caring Science framework does not change, the work in caring literacy continues to evolve. The most recent work by Lee, Palmieri, and Watson (2017) offers insights into Caritas Literacy from a global perspective by Caring Science scholars from around the world, thus providing us with direction from which to discover and extend the Caritas journey worldwide.

As each Caritas Coach matures in Caritas Literacy, he or she rediscovers his or her passions and values and designs a Caring Science project that explicitly integrates Caring Science into his or her life. These projects integrate all Caritas Literacies and Caring Science knowledge in a creative, unique, and meaningful way to be/know/do and become more Caritas literate. The first Caring Science projects began in 2008 with the first CCEP and have evolved in nature and design, often leading to doctoral and postdoctoral research. Caring Science projects have ranged in design from deeply personal inner journeys to global journeys. They have been completed by healthcare providers, educators, and others interested in their own care and the care of others in all facets of healthcare and education including the following: at the bedside in acute, home, community, and chronic care; all specialties including pediatrics, obstetrics, hospice, emergency rooms, preoperative, operating rooms, oncology, medical-surgical, palliative care, orthopedics, neurology, cardiac, research, dialysis, substance abuse, transitional care, and trauma; all care for veterans, private practice, and all levels of education—high schools, nursing, and medical schools. Each Caritas Coach shares his or her project with peers, institutions, and the larger professional communities through abstract and podium presentations, articles, and poster presentations around the world affecting the health of the nation and world. The following Caritas Coach Caring Science projects are exemplars of Caritas Literacy and provide powerful, meaningful direction for a more healing and biogenic life.

Kelly Morrow, MSN, lecturer at the University of Nevada, Las Vegas, became more conscious of her own need to reconnect with herself and her family during her Caritas journey in the CCEP. Kelly created a very deeply personal project that was designed to intentionally use art as a means to practice loving-kindness, equanimity, and compassion (Caritas Process #1) for herself and as a way to more deeply connect with her family. During her 6 months in the CCEP, she worked with herself and her family to complete weekly art exercises in *Healing With the Arts* (Rockwood-Lane, Samuels, & Watson, 2013). The family connected via a private Facebook group to discuss and provide support for the artistic journey they were on together. Kelly shares that through her art, she was "empowered to re-story and re-frame [her] new role in the family" from feeling isolated and alone to belonging and being part of. She plans to take more art classes and investigate further how this can be integrated into her doctoral work.

Robert Reynoso, MSN/Ed, lecturer in the School of Nursing at Nevada State, teaches in a prelicensure baccalaureate of science in nursing (BSN) program. His introspective CCEP journey moved him toward more advanced teaching–learning approaches with entering students. He integrated Caritas Process #1 into his formal teaching, emphasizing the promotion of health and wellness through intentional and regular self-care for students and faculty. Robert views self-care as a key to promoting self-awareness in all settings, school and clinical, and in life. Caritas Literacies were made explicit in both classroom and clinical settings where centering, reflection, and teaching and learning with loving-kindness, equanimity, and compassion have become part of the curriculum. Robert's project will affect a generation of registered nurses who are better equipped to be Caring Science practitioners. Robert plans to expand upon his project to include additional formal research to measure outcomes.

Emily Barr, CPNP, CNM, MSN, senior instructor at the Department of Pediatric Infectious Diseases at the University of Colorado, Children's Hospital Colorado, works in the maternal, pediatric, and adolescent HIV program that serves families, many of whom are refugees or from around the world, living with chronic and life-threatening conditions. As Emily progressed through the CCEP, she was able to more clearly identify the stressors affecting her and her ability to practice as a Caring Science practitioner. She recognized that to sustain Caritas Literacy in her nursing practice, she needed to take better care of herself. Her ability to remain present, listen without judgment, and create transpersonal relationships could be lived only by more holistically caring for herself. In this way, she was better able to also care for the multidisciplinary team serving these families as well. She surveyed the staff and found a high rate of burnout and low rate of self-care so she created a program that promoted resiliency by encouraging self-care and the development of transpersonal relationships. Her program introduced the team to the core concepts of both Caring Science and Caritas Literacy experientially, theoretically, and aesthetically. She will be expanding on Caring Science in her doctoral work.

Lyn Brown, MA, RN-BC, a clinical nurse who works at the Atlanta Veteran Affairs Medical Center in Georgia, realized while in the CCEP that Caring Science was not just a theory for nurses, but Caring Science and Caritas Literacy were important for all disciplines and departments to learn and integrate into their work. Her project integrated Caritas Process #1: Practicing loving-kindness and equanimity for self and other (Watson, 2008, p. 31) into a project titled "New Employee Caritas Literacy." This course was designed to integrate Caring Science and Caritas Process #1 into quality control and employee orientation to instill a culture of loving-kindness and compassion for all. Lyn's project promoted the transformation of an entire hospital culture building upon several preceding Caring Science projects to strengthen and expand the biogenic energy already present and growing at the Veterans Affairs.

Michelle Camicia, MSN, director of operations at Kaiser, and Debra Morton, RN, MLDR, chief nurse executive at Kaiser, created a joint project through transformative leadership and Caring Science to inspire a multidisciplinary group of healthcare leaders to create an authentic culture of caring through presence and Caritas Literacy, beginning with self. Their project was multipronged and integrated Caring Science into all aspects of the institution, including language use, spiritual care, interviewing, sharing caring moments, educational offerings, and the creation of a caring moment book to teach, reinforce, and sustain these ways of being more caring. This project will also be expanded to include quantitative research data to more clearly describe the impact of Caritas leadership and Caring Science on the institution. This Caring Science project has transformed an entire institution and will make an impact on those related institutions in the region as the project is shared internally.

Danielle Wofford, RN, PhD and DNP-FP student, while in the CCEP, integrated her doctoral work with her Caring Science project. Danielle has been interviewing Syrian refugees, with a focus on women, to better understand ways that may help to transform how refugees are supported and cared for in ways that are more biogenic. She interviewed women using the framework of the Caritas Processes to be more Caritas Literate during the interview process. She intentionally integrated the following Caritas Processes:

1. Caritas Process #1: Practicing loving-kindness and equanimity for self and other

2. Caritas Process #2: Being authentically present, enabling/sustaining/honoring deep belief systems and subjective world of self/other

3. Caritas Process #4: Developing and sustaining a helping-trusting authentic caring relationship

4. Caritas Process #5: Being present to and supportive of the expression of positive and negative feelings as a connection with deeper spirit of self and the one-being-cared-for (Watson, 2008, p. 31)

In these ways, Danielle was able to be present, listen with equanimity, and hear what was being said without judgment. She was able to connect at the deeper level as each woman was seen as having value, and important to the whole with a unique voice. Danielle was able to be more human, humane, and compassionate and to offer help and healing by listening to the plight of each person with love and acceptance. Danielle's project demonstrates Caritas Literacy in a global project that essentially affects all of us. She will continue her important research with the hopes of changing how refugees are supported and cared for in ways that are more biogenic.

These truly amazing, creative, and inspiring examples of being and becoming more caring and loving in our world very clearly show us the power of Caring Science, Caritas Coaching, and Caritas Literacy to help transform our daily lives and world into a healthier and more compassionate one. These projects live on as each Caritas Coach, and those they touch, teaches others what it means to be more human, caring, healing, and whole. Our survival on this planet is dependent on our ability to care for ourselves and each other with loving-kindness, equanimity, and compassion.

RESEARCH

Coaching is a well-accepted and expanding role designed to help meet the demands for healthcare in the 21st century traditionally based on prescriptive frameworks (Institute of Medicine, 2012; National Advisory Council on Nurse Education and Practice [NACNEP], 2010). As healthcare expectations have shifted from care of ill to the promotion of wellness and the prevention of ill health, while at the same time technology has advanced and shifted focus from the human being to the technology, the need for care providers and educators who are literate in caring has also grown (Anderson, 2014; Axley, 2008; Jackson, 2012). The Caritas Coach is a viable answer to this dilemma in care.

Traditional coach roles focus on autonomy, critical thinking, interdisciplinary communication, knowledge, and teaching to support and guide the person being coached (Donner & Wheeler, 2009). Nursing literature describes the impact nurse coaches have made on healthcare, citing their focus on wellness and prevention, effective healthcare provision in all settings, improvement in staff orientation associated with increased retention, and the improvement of collaboration and collegiality in healthcare (Donner & Wheeler, 2009;

Schaub, Luck, & Dossey, 2012). The nurse coach role and nurse coach competencies have been correlated with the American Nurses Association's Standards of Care and suggest that the nurse coach role is here to stay and expanding (Hess et al., 2013). These standards also suggest that increasing self-awareness is key to the coach role, yet coach programs do not specifically address this aspect of coaching.

The first and only research completed specifically on Caritas Coaching is a hermeneutic phenomenological exploration of the graduates of the WCSI CCEP by Anderson (2014) titled *Exploring Application of the Caritas Coach Role in Nursing Practice*. This qualitative study was designed to explore the Caritas Coach role, those experiences that affected role development and implementation, and the impact of the role in professional nursing practice. Findings indicated that the Caritas Coach role offered an expanded view of the more traditional notions of coaching, emphasizing the importance of relationship to self, the spiritual nature of coaching, and the need to be aligned with one's values.

The Caritas Coach as a Caring Science practitioner was described as an evolved role, "someone who understands and shares Caring Science; can be with the person and walk the journey; embodies a way of thinking and a way of life; and directs, encourages, and leads others" (Anderson, 2014). These ways of being and becoming more caring, human, and humane can be accomplished only through conscious self-awareness found through Caring Science education that addresses the heart, soul, and mind of each coach. The Caritas Coach role expands coaching to include all relationships, beginning with self, and represents a movement to transform biogenically at all levels: individually, in community, and globally. This is a broader and more inclusive use of the coach role to work toward health, wellness, and healing that includes the coach first and then others. Because Caritas Coaching is viewed from the unitary lens and the perspective that the environmental field is transformed as each person is transformed within it, the prospect for greater healing influence is envisioned. Caritas Coaching is more than a coach–coachee relationship; it has the potential to affect the entire planet.

The Caritas Coaches begin their purposeful education in CCEP with an emphasis on self-care, which promotes knowing self, setting priorities, and reconnecting with values. Coaching as an ontological Caring Science practitioner emphasizes the spiritual nature of caring for and healing oneself and others by facing his or her own humanity through the spirit-to-spirit connection with each embodied soul. As one connects to his or her own spiritual values, he or she is reminded of what is meaningful and provides purpose to life. The Caritas practitioner finds meaning and purpose in alignment with values at the personal and professional levels. What this means for each Caritas Coach is that the values of love, compassion, care, healing, wholeness, and equanimity are biogenic, and if these values are not present, the Caritas Coach will be moved to transform, first beginning with self. A reconnection with these values and increasing self-awareness, Caring Science knowledge and language creates an intolerance for noncaring ways of being is lived as Caritas consciousness. This Caritas consciousness begins with self and expands to all dimensions of life, driving Caritas Coaches to take action to promote caring.

The spiritual nature of Caritas Coaching was also identified as crucial to finding meaning for all those involved in coaching. The recognition and merging of spirituality experienced through connection with one's own soul and soul work invites the Caritas

Coach to re-remember the sacred work of healing and the spirit-to-spirit connections with all life. In this way, the Caritas Coach is obligated ethically and morally to work for the greater good, resulting in an urgent need for change and call to action. These deep and sacred connections are created through Caritas Literacies, including the following: intention, presence, authentic communication, reflection, self-care, increased self-awareness, self-love, spiritual growth, openness, and finding purpose (Anderson, 2014). Living a life with purpose and meaning was described as the ultimate result of Caritas Coaching, helping to empower one's own unique voice using the language of Caring Science to describe and share vision for change that is so needed to create environments that are more biogenic at all levels of relationship: family, friends, institutions, communities, and beyond (Anderson, 2014).

Finally, transformation of self was identified as important and necessary for Caritas Coaching. Internal change/transformation was fueled by increased self-awareness and reconnection to values and soul-work rediscovered on the introspective Caritas journey. Caritas community support during the journey led to paradigm shifts and a totally different way of being and connecting with oneself and others (Anderson, 2014). The Caritas journey also provided greater confidence in Caring Science, empowering Caritas Coaches to seek ways to better align personal philosophies and values in all aspects of life: personal and professional. An alignment of values resulted in many other transformations/ changes in relationships, work settings and environments, and jobs. An intolerance for noncaring, caring illiteracy, was strongly felt and Caritas Coaches felt obligated to make changes to remedy those people, policies, procedures, and ways of being and doing that were identified as uncaring. As Caritas Coaches led the charge for change, cocreation and the ability to see more options for more biogenic, healthier ways of being for each unique and valuable human being became the Caritas Coaching purpose. This led to a vision and path for recognizing and seeking the unlimited potential in each person, each unit, each hospital, each nursing program, each hospital system, and so forth, to move toward health, wellness, and healing.

AREAS FOR FURTHER STUDY

The future of the Caritas Coach is being defined today and additional research will help to guide role development and meaning. Further research is needed to both define and substantiate the Caritas Coach role and its effect on the provision of healthcare, education, and business in the 21st century. For participants (Anderson, 2014), Caring Science provided an important theoretical framework from which to learn and practice Caritas Coaching. Caritas Coaches strongly suggested that the CCEP, using Caring Science as a curricular framework, served to support them to become more conscious and aware of themselves and others, and to be more intentional in their relationships, so they were able to coach others to do the same. Additional research into Caritas Coaching and advanced teaching–learning approaches would more clearly define and describe those approaches that support how to be more human and compassionate through deep human connection, with oneself and others. And finally, research is needed to explore the expanding use of the Caritas Coach worldwide and how Coaches have impacted the health, harmony, and life on this planet.

CONCLUSION

Caritas Coaches are global citizens who welcome and are committed to creating a brighter vision for the future of humankind and planet Earth through transformation, relationship, authenticity, living of one's values, and striving for the health and healing of all life. Caritas Literacy, ways of being and becoming more biogenic, and Caritas Coaching create opportunities for everyday life to become moments of unlimited potential and opportunities to unite, connect deeply, and take action to transform self and world into one that is respectful and honors all people. Caritas Coaches recognize and appreciate the many ways of knowing and understanding our world, and endeavor to live as conscious, moral, and ethical human beings who are fulfilling a life purpose of bringing more humanity and healing to all. Caritas Coaching deepens and sustains our shared humanity; preserves human caring, human dignity, and wholeness as the highest gift to self, systems, society, and humankind worldwide; and is part of the evolution of human caring as the highest ethical commitment to humankind and society (Anderson, 2014; Watson, 2005, 2008).

 REFERENCES

Anderson, J. (2014). *Exploring application of the caritas coach role in nursing practice* (Unpublished dissertation). Abraham S. Fischler School of Education and Human Services, Nova Southeastern University, Fort Lauderdale, FL.

Axley, L. (2008). Competency: A concept analysis. *Nursing Forum, 43,* 214–222. doi:10.1111/j.1744-6198.2008.00115.x

Donner, G., & Wheeler, M. (2009). Coaching in nursing: An introduction. Indianapolis, IN: International Council of Nurses and the Honor Society of Nursing, Sigma Theta Tau International.

Hess, D. R., Dossey, B. M., Southard, M. E., Luck, S., Schaub, B. G., & Bark, L. (2013). *The art and science of nurse coaching: The provider's guide to coaching scope and competencies.* Silver Spring, MA: American Nurses Association.

Hills, M., & Watson, J. (2011). *Creating a caring science curriculum: An emancipatory pedagogy for nursing.* New York, NY: Springer Publishing.

Institute of Medicine. (2012). *The future of nursing: Leading change, advancing health.* Washington, DC: National Academies Press.

Jackson, C. (2012). The interface of caring, self-care, and technology in nursing education and practice: A holistic perspective. *Holistic Nursing Practice, 26*(2), 69–73. doi:10.1097/HNP.0b013e3182473330

Lee, S., Palmieri, P., & Watson, J. (2017). *Global advances in human caring literacy.* New York, NY: Springer Publishing.

MacNeil, M., & Evans, M. (2005). The pedagogy of caring in nursing education. *International Journal for Human Caring, 9*(4), 45–51.

National Advisory Council on Nurse Education and Practice. (2010). *Addressing new challenges facing nursing education: Solutions for transforming health care environment.* Eighth annual report to the Secretary of the U.S. Department of Health and Human Services and the U.S. Congress. Washington, DC: Author.

Rockwood-Lane, M., Samuels, M., & Watson, J. (2013). *The caritas path to peace: Bringing in the light: A guidebook for creating world peace with caring, love and compassion.* North Charleston, SC: CreateSpace Independent Publishing Platform.

Schaub, B., Luck, S., & Dossey, B. (2012). Integrative nurse coaching for health and wellness. *Alternative and Complementary Therapies, 18*(1), 14–20. doi:10.1089/act.2012.18110

Sitzman, K., & Watson, J. (2014). *Caring science, mindful practice: Implementing Watson's human caring theory*. New York, NY: Springer Publishing.

Watson, J. (n.d.). About WCSI. Retrieved from http://www.watsoncaringscience.org/about-wcsi

Watson, J. (1999). *Postmodern nursing and beyond*. London, UK: Churchill Livingstone.

Watson, J. (2005). *Caring science as sacred science*. Philadelphia, PA: F. A. Davis.

Watson, J. (2008). *Nursing: The philosophy and science of caring* (Rev. ed.). Boulder: University Press of Colorado.

41

Creative Healing Arts

Mary Rockwood Lane

I who am the beauty of the green earth
and the white moon among the stars
and the mysteries of the waters,
I call upon your soul to arise and come unto me.

For I am the soul of nature that gives life to the universe.
From Me all things proceed and unto Me they must return.
Let My worship be in the heart that rejoices,
for behold, all acts of love and pleasure are My rituals.
Let there be beauty and strength,
power and compassion,

honor and humility,
mirth and reverence within you.

And you who seek to know Me,
know that the seeking and yearning will avail you not,
unless you know the Mystery:
for if that which you seek,
you find not within yourself,
you will never find it without.

For behold,
I have been with you from the beginning,
and I am That which is attained at the end of desire.

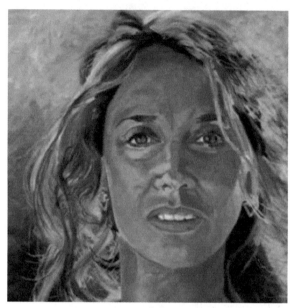

FIGURE 41.1 Maria Therese by Bettina, 1999.

HOW ART AND HEALING ARE ONE

Art is a caring-healing creative practice that explores the lived experience of what it means to be human. Art is the emergence of the metaphysical realm of our humanness. It can reveal the expression of what we can know to be true because words alone can limit the fullness of life's expression. Art, music, poetry, theater, and dance can open up the possibilities of our human potential to be known and to be fully alive. The Caring Science is the foundational philosophical worldview that addresses the human experience based on self-love, self-care, self-awareness, and soul care. Caring Science embraces the nature of creative expression as a way of practicing loving-kindness, authentic presence, being in the now, and the expression of both negative and positive feelings. The Caritas Processes® support art as a way of caring and a healing art form. (Figure 41.1 shows this author's portrait.)

Art as a way of healing weaves together the inner and outer worlds. It becomes an outer expression of art that can reflect the inner world of the human's experience. Healing Art flows from the divine source of the eternal inner wellspring of the creativity that emerges from the heart. Creative healing can be a way of caring for self, others, and community. Art expression opens up dynamic and natural flow, realigning divine right relationship with our own true source of creativity. Art creates an opportunity to care for what we hold most deeply within ourselves. This can be unexpected and deeply meaningful. Art in its many forms expresses the metaphysical reality that can be the unseen aspect of ourselves in a wondrous and magical nature. It creates meaning about the underlying conditions of our bodies, emotions, mind, and spirit. Creativity can be a fluid expression of life experience from pain and suffering to the transcendent moments of life.

Creativity has a powerful way to acknowledge and reveal the presence of the deepest relationship with self and explores what needs to heal on the soul level. The caring consciousness is enhanced by the power of intention to facilitate healing. It can tap into the human experience of what is beyond knowing and reveals the depth of mystery and wisdom from the inner life world. This is the miracle. This power of healing flows from a higher consciousness of caring. The Caritas Process of loving-kindness and practice of equanimity is inherent in the individual's artistic expression. The ability to have faith and trust the process is essential to release the inner critic that holds someone back from living authentic presence. Being in the moment is the ability to experience truth, feel compassion, and offer forgiveness for the pain, suffering, and/or lack of caring.

Health is expanding consciousness, and because art facilitates the experience of self-awareness, self-realization, and self-love, it is expanding consciousness. Artistic and aesthetic self-expression communicates aspects of this expanding nonlocal consciousness in ways that are also locally relevant. The nonlocal consciousness resides in our entire being. Alex Grey is a healing artist who demonstrates in his art the open system of the human being connected to source as it reveals the inner light matrix of the living soul. This nonlocal consciousness is energy in a light spectrum invisible to the naked eye, yet it is there.

It is with intention, self-awareness, and caring that this light consciousness can become more dynamic and transformative. The intentionality of caring in artistic expression can be deeply transformative. Art becomes an emergence of the light from the depth of our being at the soul level. The song, the drawing, the movement, the dance, the story moves from the depths of our unitary consciousness into the light of our unique human expression into forms of personal beauty, personal pain, and personal realization into forms, images, and felt body expressions that can be recognized by others. This creates a consciousness connected in the unitary of belonging and we are one heart, one soul, and one humanity. Intentions set energetic motions into the unitary energy field with purposeful revelations of the spirit that are residing in the human body that heal not only self but others and community as well. It is a purposeful energetic focus of human caring in the emergence and cocreation of human connectedness. Art plays itself out in the multiple realms of metaphysical reality. The movements, the gestures, the voices, the songs, the poems, the stories, and the dances are the multidimensional expressions of our humanness. The art expression has a tremendous impact in the life world of being human. Let us return to what it means to be human.

Art and healing return us to the basic premises of the practices of Caritas: the practices of self-care, self-healing, trust and having faith, surrendering, compassion, forgiveness, authentic presence, listening to another person's story (or artistic expression), honoring the life story of another, and honoring the dignity and integrity of the other as a sacred being in the world. Caring Science provides the premises of creating healing environments, how the power of the beauty, harmony, and balance impacts on the human body and experience. Caritas honors the body as the Sacred in the physical, therefore in its fullest, expression of being a body in an artistic expression of self. It honors the mystery of the human spirit as it emerges into form and images. Caritas creates a way of seeing the illumination of the human spirit as it is revealed in artistic expressions. Art opens the portal to the presence of the divine intelligence and the open heart. It illuminates the higher reality that holds the deepest and most potent resources for healing.

A SACRED JOURNEY

Picture art and healing like a sacred journey. Picture yourself as a person who needs to heal your life in some way. You travel to a foreign land you have never seen before to find helpers and go on a pilgrimage. You go into the sky, across seas, and into forests, mountains, deserts, and the darkest places. You meet a magical holy person who is pure love, a teacher, a seer. She is a living mystic. She leads you to the special place where love, art, and caring have the power to heal. But there is a tremendous task. Only you can learn the power of caring for yourself. So you make art to create meaning of your life, and art comes out of you to your wonder and amazement. Your art is pure freedom and it is your truth. You are the one who will be healed. This land is the inner world of your imagination. The figure who is the seer becomes you as the artist. The figure who is the healer is you too. It is all you. It only seems like they are different parts. She is the Oracle. She simply reminds you to love yourself and each other. This journey will make the story true. This is the sacred journey of Caring Science in today's words.

When we each find our own song, as Jean Watson says in *Caring Science as Sacred Science*, we find out what we love the most, and our self-caring and healing begins. Deep within all of us is the place of perfect beauty from which we all come. It is the same place from which we are born. It is the same place to which we will return. In that place, we will find our deepest peace, our most profound memories of who we are. In our lives, this is the place of the memory of our brightest moment. It is tied to our vision of being touched, being nurtured, being loved perfectly, being in the presence of something greater than ourselves. It is also tied to our memory of our greatest sadness, of our losses, of our fears of our own death. In the center of this place of beauty is the energy that heals us. This is also the energy of our own passionate creativity.

A Guided Imagery Story of Art and Healing: The Legend of the Ancient Woman of the Springs

Stories have always been used by teachers. We are taught most profoundly by symbols, morals, and archetypes whose meanings sink in without our always understanding them at first. This is why fairy tales were told to children, why stories from the Bible, the Koran, or the Vedas were told to help people feel the presence of a greater power, why even older myths and legends have always been used to help people grasp the ineffable, the sacred.

Guided imagery as a mind-body therapy is also deeply relaxing and experiential. It is a basic tool in caring arts. It is used in healthcare settings worldwide to help patients relax and heal. Guided imagery is as simple as picturing an event or memory in your imagination. If you relax and close your eyes and picture your bedroom, you can look around in your imagination and "see" your bed, your dresser, the windows, and the color of the walls. When you use guided imagery as a caring-healing practice, you can imagine your body's healing light body matrix.

The legend of the ancient woman of the springs is a feminine archetypal myth that links art and healing. It is about how art and healing were one in a mythical time of spirits and how we are still connected to our ancestors through deep memories and our own physiology. The legend itself is as old as any story and aspects of it appear in Native American legends, Jewish lore, Sufi myths, and African stories. The legend of the woman of the springs is about the wellspring of creativity that is within each of us. It is about creation, connections, and birth.

It is also a story about you being loved perfectly for who you are right now. In this legend, the woman of the springs is the Earth Mother who created you and loves you, even if you are ill, in crisis, depressed, or lost. She loves you into the very center of your sadness, the deepest heart of your pain, the core of your anger. We have the lost memories of being inside her body in the soft whooshing, the moving, the dimmed colors, the *lub dub* of her heartbeat, the flowing sounds of her breathing. This is the first healing art, music, and dance that we recall. This ancient legend brings us there as softly as she sings. Do you hear her voice? Healing art is about going back into the place where we were loved perfectly, and where we were embraced by sound, colors, and movement. It is about you loving yourself for who you are right now and being seen and honored for who you are right now. In the legend, the Earth Mother is the one who nurtures us and cares for us.

GUIDED IMAGERY EXERCISE

I will tell you a story. It is a story that is older than any other. This story is deep in our memories; this story is deep in your soul. It is the story of the creation of art and healing. It always begins with the story of the ancient woman of the springs. She has always been seen as the weaver of our dreams, as the mother of creativity and art, as the one who could heal. Close your eyes; relax; let your breathing slow down. Start from the ordinary, from your kitchen table, from a drive in your car, or from a hospital room, from wherever you are. Go into your imagination on a journey. Go into a mystical forest. It is a secret place; it is the place that only you can see; it is a place in your imagination. You can find it in any moment. You will find it by becoming ill, by being in a life crisis, by seeing death, by falling in love, by becoming an artist. First, imagine that you are on a path. It is a narrow path; the ground is dirt; it is hard enough so it is comfortable to walk on. It is the path of the creative caring healer. As your feet find it, you can imagine that you start to walk. Feel the hard ground; hear your footsteps fall; feel the grass on the sides of the path touch your legs. Smell the air; feel the warm, soft breeze on your face. As you walk, you begin to feel differently; the air itself changes; it opens and fills with light; it expands and as it expands, you expand too. Your eyes open wider. Your ears can hear more clearly. Your body moves by itself and your breath is not only yours anymore.

As you go down the path, your way darkens and narrows slightly. The leaves touch your skin and the soft earth caresses your feet. The warm moist air glistens on the leaves like dew drops and the energy within you flows outward. As you look ahead, you can see an emerald pool down a short hill. It is round and beautiful and it shines in the afternoon sun. It is on the bottom of a glade of small trees—the pool is deep blue and perfectly round and in its center is a spring that flows upwards from the earth as pure clear water. You can see the bubbles coming to the surface in whirlpools; you can almost hear the bubbling as it goes on forever. Now look upwards on the ground next to the spring. Above the spring, she sits, in perfect and eternal peace. She is the most beautiful creature you have ever seen; she is a woman of pure spirit. As you look at her, you can see that she changes as you see her. One moment she is the Earth Mother looking down on you with perfect love. One moment she is your lover, looking at you with eternal desire, and in the next moment she is an old woman with a loom who weaves the silver and golden threads that make the springs and the earth itself. And then, in another moment, she is a turtle who has sat forever on the side of the spring watching all of it being born. As she sits and changes like the light, you can see that she has been there forever and has created the world. She weaves the fibers of her most beautiful dream. She weaves art and healing as one. She weaves each of us into the vision as artists, as healers. She weaves the very spirals that we travel on, on the energy that makes us fall in love. She is weaving this story as I am telling it to you. She is weaving her song on Earth. She is singing to us.

Now look more closely. She sits on the edge of the spring and as she looks down inside the spring, she can see the eternal wellspring of creativity and she can see your life. She has meditated here for a million years and she can see the water spring up from the very center of her own heart. She sees how beautiful she is, was, and will be. She sees how it always flows, and how it will flow for a million lifetimes. For each lifetime, each of our ancestors before us from the first one, she has sat there. She has been there for all of eternity.

You can see that out of the spring comes a turquoise light. It shines on her face and on yours. You can see that she is very ancient. If you look closely, you can see that a part of her is young and youthful, and a part of her is very ancient and wise. Look at her hands. As she sits, and you look at her hands, it is almost as if she holds a magic wand, from which she is weaving a magic web. You can see that she looks deep into the springs, and from the center of the spring you can see the energy go up into her hands. She weaves a magic web for you. She catches the spring's energy and power, and weaves it into the earth. She sees it and her hands can feel it. When you look at her hands closely, you can see that she is weaving a spiral of light, and if you look very closely at what her hands are weaving, you can see that it is the light from exploding nebula that come from the deepest inner depths. This is the moment and source that is the creation of images. As she takes the dream of art and healing from the spring, she takes it to each one of us and weaves it into our hearts. There is a string inside of each strand of woven web. These strings go from her hand and fly up as one, to each one of us, to you, up into the center of your heart. You are in the place where time and space are not limited and these threads come up like spirals and you can see them go into infinity and they go up and down in the past, present, and the future. She holds the interlocking connections together at the side of this eternal spring. She can see us always. And now, we can see her. She is weaving the web and holding the connections together. We can see that we are connected to many others. We are connected to everyone who is healing himself or herself from the beginning of time to the end of time. As we see her, we realize that we too are part of her dream. It is the ancient dream of art and healing as one. She sings to us in her eternal chant. "Each of you is an artist. Each of you is a healer." She is the living legend of the ancient divine feminine. The path to her spring is the practice of caring, wisdom, compassion, and love.

MY PERSONAL STORY OF HEALING WITH THE ARTS

Within each personal story is the actual way it happened. Theory is the way of seeing that reality. A personal story is something to be felt and experienced. Art and healing is a passion; art is a way of healing, a way of caring, and a way of knowing. My story goes …

Several decades ago I was extremely ill. I was going through a very difficult life event. My husband asked for a divorce. I went into a rage and depression, and was completely out of control. All the resources in my life had collapsed and I was drowning. I was not able to deal constructively with my life, with my children, or with my friends. I was in therapy, but I wasn't making any movement forward. I was surrounded by my grief and I couldn't see past it. I was in a place of darkness and despair. I remember the therapist saying to me, "It's time to do something different with your rage and your grief."

In a lucid moment, I decided to abandon my fears of being a painter, something I had always dreamed of being, and had never given myself permission to be, because I never felt good enough. Finally, I did not put so much pressure on myself to be "good enough." I just remembered I had always wanted to be an artist. At that time, I felt so devastated that the fear of inadequacy was minute compared with the painful loss I was experiencing. In my memory, I remember the way everything happened like it was a slow-motion movie. I walked out of the therapist's office. I was at the end of my rope. It was a drizzling-rainy kind of day; it seemed like life was going on without me. I was deeply depressed. My body was in such pain that I wanted to fall down and die. I remember walking up to a large muddy puddle. I could see my refection in the mud. I thought about just falling down in it. I glanced up and there was a slow-moving car hesitantly driving toward me. As I looked at it, I flashed on the face of a woman I recognized. It was my friend Lee Ann. She was a painter. She came up and rolled down the car window, "Why don't I take you to breakfast and I'll take you to my studio and you can start painting?" I took out a large canvas and did not even know how to hold a brush. I looked through magazines and saw a picture of a woman who was broken and distorted. That was how I felt. I started painting. I got excited about the colors of the paint, how the shapes appeared on the paper. My painting was large and it started to look like something; most importantly, it looked like my pain and it looked like how I felt. I forgot about how I felt and instead looked at how I felt. I got excited about the making of the painting. Then I got another canvas and started a series of paintings of women. They were all distorted in the beginning. I painted garish backgrounds. I took photographs of myself and I started painting myself. I became absorbed in the process and painted how I felt, instead of thinking of how I felt. I began to realize I was painting my life.

Next, I created a studio space for myself and simply began painting. I painted feverishly. In the beginning, I made no attempt to define myself or my process. I painted from pure feeling states. I became absorbed in the pure expression and gesture of painting. I could completely release my energy passionately on the canvas. The series turned out to be self-portraits. The first painting I called "Cut Out My Heart" (Figure 41.2). It was my pain, a deeply intense and dying pain. The figure was broken, distorted, diffuse, crumpled, crying, and bleeding. I painted "her." This figure had been my despair, my uncensored and purely emotional energy. And in the moment I had released this image, I stepped back and looked. Gasp. What I saw was an aspect of myself that I couldn't face; it was so ugly. Yet I felt calm and detached. I had let go, on an intense emotional and physical level. Painting is physical for me; I embody my pain as I paint it (Figure 41.3). For the first time, I was experiencing my pain in a strange and new way. As a painter, I stood in front of the canvas and was for the first time in control. I painted my emotions; I painted my body. I could feel that I was the creator of myself.

I backed away, left the studio, and went home. When I returned, I saw that the image had captured and contained a moment that was now past. Then, I had an incredible insight. The painting remained an object that contained an image created in genuine and immediately felt expression, and I now had moved past it. I realized that there was movement and I was witnessing my own transformation.

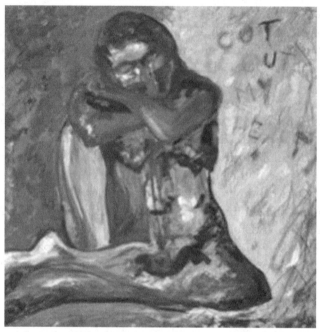

FIGURE 41.2 Cut Out My Heart, Mary Rockwood Lane, 1989.

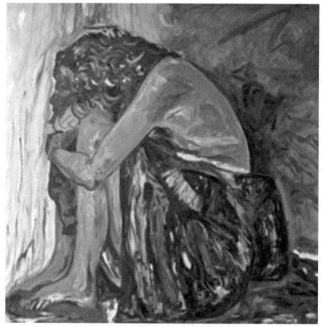

FIGURE 41.3 Despair, Mary Rockwood Lane, 1989.

As I painted this series of self-portraits, in each painting I struggled with form and perspective. Metaphorically I was recreating and reconstructing my inner form and inner perspective. The external creative process mirrored my inner world. I realized the manifestation of movement and change was powerful and it was a process of knowing myself. As I immersed myself in the painting, I not only became well but also clearly became the artist I had always wanted to be, a part of myself I had neither acknowledged nor honored. It was from this personal experience that I realized that art could be used as a vehicle for healing (Figure 41.4).

Art became a way to know myself through the experience of the personal pain that I painted. In seeing it, I could step away. I became the artist, and the series of paintings remained as the physical creation of pain. They were now my art, completely separate from me. It was a tangible experience of growing away from the place I had been when the images were painted. In essence, I became free. Then I spent time in my studio with my girlfriends painting my life. I spent 2 years as an artist in my studio. I painted my children playing on the beach. I painted the surrounding landscapes that I saw. I would set up still life on the kitchen table and I would paint the things that I loved.

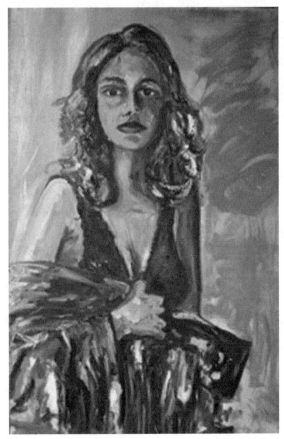

FIGURE 41.4 Self-Portrait, Strong and Healed, Mary Rockwood Lane, 1990.

YOUR INNER ARTIST AS YOUR INNER HEALER

The basic foundation of *Creative Healing Arts* is Caring Science. The following painting is of my grandmother when she had Alzheimer's (Figure 41.5). Only Childhood Icons lingered in her world of confusion. In my grief, I painted her every day to be with her, connected, loving and caring for her. I was immersed in her world and I loved her more deeply as she passed away. Art healed me, art heals others, and art heals the Earth.

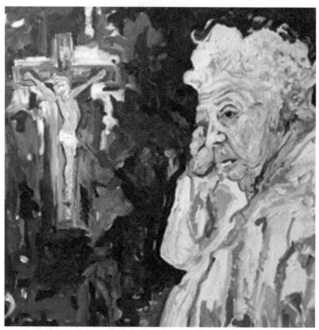

FIGURE 41.5 Grandmother Series: Only Childhood Icons Linger, Mary Rockwood Lane, 1993.

Each of us has deep within us an inner artist and an inner healer. The inner artist is the part of us that is passionately creative, that feels love, that feels connected to everything around us, that can see, that knows who we are, that is at home, and that is at peace. The inner artist can go anywhere in the inner world. No place is closed to the inner artist. The inner artist can even go to the inner healer and merge with it and bring it out. The inner healer is the part of you that is the body's wisdom that balances your body perfectly and sets your blood flow, your immune system, your physical body to be in harmony. Art frees the healer within so you can heal and care for yourself in times of crisis and stress. The expression of Art frees your spirit so your mind and body are in harmony.

42

Narrative Healing

A. Lynne Wagner

Knowing does not come directly from experiencing a situation. We need to intentionally re-encounter the experience through reflective processes of exploring many aspects embedded in any human experience … In essence, [to know healing] we need to come to know the mind-body-spirit meaning of what happened and what more was possible. (Wagner, 2016, pp. 439–440)

Nursing is daily heart work that is informed by science and the art of caring for self and others in intimate healing ways during ordinary and extraordinary vulnerable periods of living and dying. With Caring Science (Watson, 2005, 2008, 2017) as a philosophical, moral-ethical, and value-guided foundation for practice, the healing ability to care for the whole person and to sustain human dignity among healthcare's changing challenges, restrictions, and prescriptions requires multiple ways of knowing and creative use of self as a healing environment (Carper, 1978; Wagner, 2000; Watson, 2008). This fullness of knowing suffering and healing and becoming-being a healer is a complex phenomenon. The process is embedded in developing and sustaining loving compassion for self and others through a heart-led reflective practice and a caring literacy that leads to higher conscious intentions and informed acts of human care (Watson, 2017). The philosophical shift in nursing from epistemology to ontology (Silva, Sorrell, & Sorrell, 1995; Watson, 2005, 2008, 2017) enlarges the reflected questions, from: What do I know or need to know to care? or What do I do? to deeper human-connecting questions of relationship and meaning: How do I connect in meaningful trusting relationships? How do I bring creative self and meaning to each person in each unique situation? or How do I honor the inexplicable mystery of human suffering and healing and be present as authentic healer? Sandelowski (1993) posits that such humanizing knowledge comes from stories about experiences that foster self-growth and transmit wisdom. To find such wisdom, experiences need to be explored beyond the rational cognitive process (Wagner, 2000, 2016). In an ontological sense, "healers" are most effective if they first find meaning and lessons in their own questions and stories before they lead others to know their stories and, in this process, cocreate together new possibilities of healing experiences.

Narratives are storied human experiences, presented orally, in books, in art, in poetry, in theater, in music, and in dance, to relate facts, emotions, meaning, and connectedness of events in our lives. Stories have connected human beings since the dawn of time, from the shared wisdom of the moment and across generations. Narratives serve to preserve history, reflectively explore past, present, and anticipated experiences, teach, and entertain, but the most universal gift of stories when fully explored is their ability to increase our knowing of the human experience in meaningful wholeness (Wagner, 1998, 2016). Both storytelling and story-listening require presence to self-reflection, intention to know self, and attention to the heart, which foster increased understanding of experiences and self-healing. If practitioners are to care for self and others with healing compassion and authentic presence that create opportunities for transpersonal caring, they need to be open and vulnerable to honestly explore their own stories in rational, nonrational, and collective ways, coming to know who they are from their heart and spirit voice. Attending to their own well-being, practitioners can then listen to others' stories without ego, honoring the storyteller's frame of reference that reflects the uniqueness and universality of unfolding narratives.

Aesthetic forms of storytelling further capture essential kernels of meaning in stories, transcending rational facts and gleaning a new knowing of self and other in the world that is found between the words and within the heartfelt relationship with self and others. "An experience re-lived through an aesthetic sense of the narrative is freed of [rational] trappings and cognitive constraints and is turned to its essence, a unity of core beliefs, values, actions, and spirit … a new sense of being 'in' the world rather than 'of' the world emerges" (Wagner, 2008, p. 24).

This chapter explores the power of reflective practice through different levels of storytelling/listening, enriched by an aesthetic lens that fosters deeper meaning of self and other: (a) *Knowing Self Through Self-Story*, developing a reflective practice and aesthetic worldview to explore personal experiences from an intimate inside-out perspective; (b) *Knowing Other Through Other's Story*, inviting and being authentically present to others' stories in both practice and research to support healing; (c) *Honoring Connected Humanity Through Shared-Connected Story*, being heart-touched by similarities and differences of one's own story and another person's or group's narrative; and (d) *Discovering New Possibilities Through Expanded Story*, being open to learning a new cocreated script of being and becoming healer and healed through dialogue with others. Although these categories are delineated as separate processes, it is important to note that they are not exclusive to each other and often blend in the same encounter. Reflective self-story leads to sharing stories. Shared stories help expand the meaning and connectedness of our humanity through transformative "caring moments," which Watson (2005, p. 62) defines as a spirit-to-spirit transpersonal event that creates unity of knowing the humanness of each other in that shared moment. Such moments are "remembered" by the heart and change both storyteller and story-listener in healing ways forever.

Essence

The essence of life is in our stories.
It flows like a river through us.

Short burst, deep channels,
Numbness, vibrancy,
Confrontation, soothing resolution,
Story captures the rhythm of our lives,
Only available if we dance with the truth,
In that connecting movement,
Between storm and rainbow,
Between invisible and visible,
We find meaning in what we do.
We grow and come to know
Self and other with heart revealed.
　　　　(Adapted from Wagner, 2000, p. 7)

KNOWING SELF THROUGH SELF-STORY

"Practitioners of caring and healing require personal work … because we practice, … research … teach … [and] live who we are. So our very Being-Becoming more human and humane is what is at stake in healing work" (Watson, 2005, p. 115). Telling story to self through journaling and meditation is powerful work of subjectively exploring experiences about self and self in relationship with others from inside out. Every experience affects us, changes us, and has a lesson for us. However, many people avoid processing their own experiences in the guise of "protecting" themselves for a variety of reasons—not enough time, too painful, need to move on to next experience, do not know how, no healing space, and see no importance to it. This avoidance behavior includes nurses and other healthcare providers who encounter many experiences each day, in their personal and professional lives with colleagues, patients, families, and others—experiences that are deep, intimate, and often traumatic; experiences that can injure the soul. The end result over time is that the physical-emotional-spiritual being becomes full of accumulated unprocessed feelings that numb the heart with missed opportunities to allow the experiences to teach the practitioner. Without healing, renewal strategies of reflective practice, fatigue, and burnout follow.

Guided by Caring Science (Watson, 2005, 2008, 2017), reflective practice of exploring stored experiences with loving-kindness and compassion, with presence and trust, with an openness to discovery, will unlock the stored treasure of stories and present them for exploring through cognitive, affective, and collective processes (Wagner, 2016). Reflecting on experiences through daily journaling with new intention, compassion, and spiritual grounding will reveal new insights and truths about the experience no matter how long ago it was stored. As depicted in Figure 42.1, the meaning and truths that emerge from exploring stories of self are healing, often releasing burdens of trauma, feelings of being victimized, or grief memories isolated from joys. Such revelations open the spirit and heart to healing surrendering, forgiveness, and gratitude.

In traumatic personal crises, I relied on daily conversation with myself through journaling that helped me sort out details and decision making, honor emotions and relationships, and face the situation honestly with self-compassion. I found that reflective process slowly and gently guided me "to a stillness of inner space where my mind

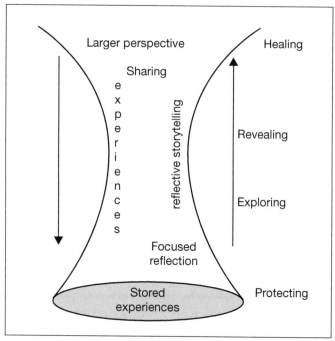

FIGURE 42.1 Bringing stored experiences out of protective storage: the healing power of reflective journaling/storytelling.

Source: Wagner, A. L. (1998). A study of baccalaureate nursing students' reflection on their caring practice through creating and sharing story, poetry, and art (Doctoral dissertation). *Dissertation Abstracts International, 99*(5), 334. (University Microfilms Inc. No DAO 72699)

and heart could contemplate the essence and wholeness of an experience" (Wagner, 2008, p. 24) that day and beyond. In essence, I was having a caring moment with myself. My conversations with myself prepared me also to have critical conversations with my family and caregivers. Furthermore, my aesthetic interpretation of my story moved me deeper into the rawness of feelings and fear, uncovering unexamined relationships and unknown essential meanings of lived events (Wagner, 2008), so I could face the truth and find my way through the maze of crises toward healing. One such experience was a journey with breast cancer. My journal entry one day started with a factual description, peppered with some feeling: "Routine mammogram and office visit today turned to nightmare. No clean bill of health for me today. Suspicion; calcified areas have changed; biopsy needed. The doctor's weak reassurance did not penetrate my confusion." However, the poem that spilled from my heart revealed so much more of my injured soul and I could hold myself more with loving care in my exposed pain and life-changing event.

The Enemy Within
I entered the subdued radiologist's room,
lined with lighted boxes,
exposing women's private femininity,

never meant to be viewed by impersonality.
The white linear lines in the x-ray looked so innocent
Amidst the fuzzy white background.
How ironic that breast once nurtured with life-sustaining milk,
threatens my very existence,
a source of pleasure, that in its changing season,
turns to pain.
　　　(Wagner, 1991, unpublished poem)

Another significant life-changing experience occurred while I was caring for my mother for over 6 years as her health declined with dementia, helping her to live as fully as she could in her growing dependence. When she finally needed more extended care, I felt guilty; I felt only I could truly care for her, and feared I was not doing enough for her. Through heart-journaling, I came to know my unsustainable, unbalanced state and creatively explored more healing ways to cope. Using Watson's (2008) 10 Caritas Processes® as a guide, I examined my actions and feelings, and found affirmation in many of my caring actions, but also identified behaviors that were driven by my ego-fear, from which I could then work toward more intentional loving care of myself. I made peace with myself and my limitations in totally caring for my mother. I worked hard to know the nursing staff, building trust with them and letting go of needing to be at the nursing home every day. I put on my mother's wall a large poster board of photos my brother and I had created that featured all the important people and animals in my mother's life. The photographs, reminders of my mother's rich life of relationships, greeted her throughout her day. We labeled the photos and told the staff stories about each one of them, which enabled the staff to know my mother as "person" and help her remember her life stories in connecting ways. I saw love flourish in all our hearts through the process of shared narratives.

Love Soothes Fear
Fear fills the vessels of my heart;
Love soothes the soul.
Fear flits between the beats,
Love heals the empty spaces.
Fear comes from the unknown,
Love, the healer, will scatter the fear.
Like the stars in the sky,
Love shines to light my way.
　　　(Wagner, 2008, unpublished poem)

I continued to journal after my mother's death, slowly healing from grief, through reflective writing and connecting daily conversations for a year with a tree outside my skylight window. Intimately present to the tree in its changing seasons through appreciative observation captured through photography, I found the tree mirroring my raw winter-grief of surrendering, my spring-grief-healing of emerging from my darkness toward letting go and forgiving, my summer-grief-healing toward bloom and gratitude, and my autumn-grief-healing of well-being and ability to give compassionate care to others. The following poem captures the essence of this long journey toward healing.

A Journey of Grief Healing

My winter tears become reflective icicles.
My spring prayers burst out of blooming buds.
My summer laughter shades from heated sun.
My fall singing honors the richness of the earth.
The circle of the seasons connects me to my soul.
In the wholeness of my being, my heart heals.
In being lost, I found myself deep inside, surrendering;
In surrendering, I awakened my love of self, forgiving;
In love, I am open to receive, gratitude;
In gratitude, I am connected to the universe—wholeness;
In wholeness, I am posed for compassionate service—giving.
Thus the circle of seasons connects me to my healing,
In my pause... in my stillness... in my being present.
                (Wagner, 2015, p. 65)

My nursing practice was also enriched by this reflective practice of knowing self as nurse healer. Heart-led self-reflection illuminated my patients as "persons" and expanded my insight in how to be present as healer for them. One example is about a woman in long-term care. In report I was told objective facts, as though these facts defined this patient: "Mrs. O," an 85-year-old widow of 10 years. Four daughters and many grand-children, but few visitors. Stroke 3 years ago with right-sided weakness and incontinence; diabetes, failing eyesight, and peripheral vascular disease with ulcerated legs. Retired school teacher. When I entered Mrs. O'Malley's room, my heart and sense of her humanity enlarged my assessment in a way that brought me closer to the truth of her caring-healing needs:

Mrs. O'Malley

You sit, lap covered with frayed blanket,
framed by two wheels;
one leg firmly against metal plate,
the other shortened by disease,
not knowing where it belongs;
face twisting at bright light
that streams through your window,
filtered by cobwebs on the glass
and cloudy cataract vision.
You sit enjoying a moment of warmth
that brings late afternoon memories.
But then the pain,

that pain whose source is deeper
than ulcers on your leg,
merges past and future with present space.
Your swear word breaks the sacred
mood of brief escape,
reality beckons you to pay attention,
nudging you back to prison
that you describe as shrunken world
of chair with wheels that go nowhere.
       (Wagner, 2005, p. 37)

KNOWING OTHER THROUGH OTHER'S STORY

Nurses and other healthcare providers constantly gather intimate details about patients and their families with every clinical assessment that leads to a categorized diagnosis and objective plan of care. However, such "medicalized story" falls short in its assessment of "knowing" the wholeness of the patient. The patient's and patient's family's unique story and their vision of healing must be added and recorded. This often requires the practitioner to invite the patient and family to tell their stories about the meaning and life changes around what brings them to the hospital and how they hope to be cared for. For patients to open their hearts and souls and move beyond the rational cognitive stories of facts they are used to relating in the medical world requires the practitioner to be present and authentically listen with openness to expressions of positive and negative feelings in a trusting environment (Watson, 2008). It may be the first time the patients are not only telling their stories but also hearing them. In this caring moment opportunity, they need encouragement to pull their stories out of storage.

Silence is a healing modality to encourage narratives to unfold, which is illustrated by another caring event. A woman for whom I was assigned to care was diagnosed with breast cancer and had experienced a bilateral mastectomy the day before. I was told she refused care and opening of the window shades. When I entered the room, I witnessed a frightened women lying stiffly in bed. Addressing her by name and pulling a chair to the bedside, I introduced myself by name as her nurse today. I acknowledged her difficult surgery and her request for no care. As I gently reached for her hand, I quietly told her I would like to just sit with her if that was okay. We silently sat together in the darkness for a few moments when she grasped my hand and started to weep. I invited her to tell me her story, which then poured out—her mother's and sister's death from breast cancer; her sense of failure to her husband in losing her femininity; her fears around disfigurement, her worth, and death; her rage at the seemingly insensitivity of her doctors and her friends to her fears. She had been told over and over by people that she was lucky. They had found her cancer early. I sat and listened to the intricate threads in her heart story that addressed relationships, her many losses, her hurting spirit. Then she was silent again. I thanked her for sharing her story and invited her to tell me how she would like to be cared for this day and how she would like her day to unfold. She looked at me through her tears and simply said, "Thank you for listening. Let's open the curtains for a start so I can see the light, which always makes me feel better."

HONORING CONNECTED HUMANITY THROUGH SHARED-CONNECTED STORY

One story begets another story, irrespective of whether told, a story of the heart, of the human experience that holds in its truths elements of everyone's story. The collective stories affirm, connect, and explore deeper, as listeners probe with more questions around relationships and meaning, while adding details of their own stories, different situations, but, nonetheless, relating universal aspects of suffering, fear, loss, facing mortality, and feelings of loneliness. One does not have to experience the same situation to be able to connect with another's story. It is our shared humanity that is the connecting bond. Every story has an element of hope and recipe for healing in the very telling it to others.

If explored feelings are inexplicable, aesthetic expression is often the key to penetrating the story. Poetry captures the often unilluminated aspects of experience in the search for meaning and connections with others. I was a participant in a support group for women experiencing breast cancer and as we shared our stories, I was struck by the amount of trauma women experienced in coping with their life changes, despite reporting excellent medical care. The emotional and spirit-trauma effects lingered well after their physical healing. These stories also awakened in me some unresolved emotions. We agreed that we would journal and thought it would be healing to bring in an image or some representation of what we were feeling about the care received, which deepened our storytelling. With the group's permission, I began to reflect their stories in poetry as "portraits" of their narratives. I shared the respective poems first with the storyteller and with her permission to the group. Through journaling, collectively sharing narratives, and sharing the aesthetic "portraits," we began to finally let go of burdens and heal individually and as a group. As an example, one participant described that she and her husband lacked preparation for severe menopausal symptoms that followed chemotherapy and the effect it had on their intimacy. The shock came when her husband wanted to change to twin beds, which further intensified her self-image wound.

Fragmentation
My double-breasted chest, reduced to one.
My double bed is split in two.
My life is shattered by this singleness,
Fragmentation separates my body from my soul.
Can't he understand I have only lost one part?
Society paints his fantasy of perfect mate.
My doctors unconcerned about our fate.
I am alone at the height of my need,
No breast, no hair, no more seed.
   (Wagner, 1995, p. 79)

This had been a story well stored and told with much hurt. She did not realize how wounded she was by the situation. Her sharing and the poem made her emotions visible and she realized with more reflection for the first time that she too was a part of the unspoken disruption. Through the group encouragement and insight, she gained courage to talk to her husband and better understand his side of the story and find a solution together. Mezirow (1991) further argues that adults learn validity of their actions and ideas through others' confirmation. It was within the emotional bonds of this group that shared stories of spirit and heart showed that love was palpable and healing was enhanced.

DISCOVERING NEW POSSIBILITIES THROUGH EXPANDED STORY

Each narrative has its own cadence and gem of truth, new discoveries of self; yet when narratives are shared, they become part of the larger human story. Seeing your story reflected in other stories, as well as in literature, drama, and the arts, you come to understand that there is an undercurrent in each story that adds unique dimensions and deeper meaning to universal human experiences around darkness and light, suffering and well-being, grief and joy, pain and comfort, living and dying, fear and hope, hatred and love, illness and healing, abusive power and compassion. Jourard (1964) claims that "nursing calls for the ability to see that which is common to all [humankind] in oneself and in the other person. This means that to know all [humankind] one begins by looking within oneself" (p. 140). Every time a story is explored or shared, the sense of the story changes, expands as more details are revealed, and the meaning of the experience deepens through dialogue with self and others. Each story holds the discovery of new possibilities for healing. Discovery is strengthened in a community of story-sharing through examples found in each story and through dialogue around each story. Groups often cocreate their own story of healing, compiled from the individual stories in an effort for policy or system change. The group of women in the breast cancer group encouraged each other to talk to their physicians about their experiences in hopes of creating more transpersonal relationships with caregivers.

The woman whose whole sense of self was threatened by her having to endure the trauma of bilateral mastectomies opened the door for healing by just telling her story to another human being who was committed to be present, open to all expressed feelings, and authentically holding the woman's story as a sacred gift. For the woman who experienced "woundedness" around her chemotherapy experience, reflective practice and shared storytelling with other women guided her to get inside her story to look anew at facts, emotions, behaviors, and relationships. New insights healed her perception of being the wounded victim that she first described. Seeing one's story in another's story enlarged these women's sense of connected humanity and belonging. Reaching out to larger audiences in presentations and publications further expands the sharing and human connection. Once a story is released, it has a spirit of its own, capable of entering another person's heart and residing alongside that person's story, providing healing comfort of belonging even from a distance.

CONCLUSION

In summary, healing from traumatic experiences comes from the process of "going back inside the story," reliving the experience, and visualizing the situation again from several perspectives. Seeing the experience anew is akin to what Bevis (1989) calls "discovery learning." In each of the examples of healing narratives presented, reflective practice included processing the experience from a cognitive, affective, and collective perspective

(Wagner, 1998, 2002, 2016). On the cognitive level, story is framed by the rational objective facts of who, what, where, when, and how, asking an epistemological question, What happened? It is necessary to move on to the affective level of reflection to get to a deeper ontological relational meaning of the narrative, making emotions and feelings visible, and getting to the essence of the story via a nonrational, aesthetic reflecting. Fox (1997) describes poetry as "thinking by feeling." Whyte (1994) uses poetic story to "arouse the heart," and "reach the underground forces" (p. 5) that nourish the inner creative force to express our humanness in the often orderly, technical work world. The third collective level of sharing stories allows a person to be heard and to hear others, forming community. Groups provide support and affirmation, prompting further exploration of each other's stories and an expanded story that offers a collective wisdom toward new discoveries of healing narrative voice. Every person has a story to tell and the capacity to heal whether in individual or group endeavors. Narrative is a vehicle that can convey all the elements of life with deep reflection and reveal lessons that heal heart and soul.

> *Love whispers*
> *Listen*
> *It feels the stillness*
> *Deep inside*
> *And wants to tell its story*
> (Wagner, 2017, unpublished poem)

 REFERENCES

Bevis, E. O. (1989). *Curriculum building in nursing* (3rd ed.). New York, NY: National League for Nursing.

Carper, B. A. (1978). Fundamental patterns of knowing in nursing. *Advances in Nursing Science, 1*(1), 13–23. doi:10.1097/00012272-197810000-00004

Fox, J. (1997). *Poetic medicine: The healing art of poetry-making.* New York, NY: Jeremy P Tarcher/ Putnam.

Jourard, S. M. (1964). *The transparent self.* Princeton, NJ: D. Van Nostrand.

Mezirow, J. (1991). *Transformative dimensions of adult learning.* San Francisco, CA: Jossey-Bass.

Sandelowski, M. (1993, March). We are the stories we tell. *Journal of Holistic Nursing, 12*(1), 23–33. doi:10.1177/089801019401200105

Silva, M. C., Sorrell, J. M., & Sorrell, C. D. (1995). From Carper's patterns of knowing to ways of being: An ontological philosophical shift in nursing. *Advances in Nursing Science, 18*(1), 1–13. doi:10.1097/ 00012272-199509000-00002

Wagner, A. L. (1995). Unleashing the giant: The politics of women's health care. In A. Boykin (Ed.), *Power, politics, & public policy: A matter of caring* (pp. 63–81). New York, NY: National League for Nursing Press.

Wagner, A. L. (1998). A study of baccalaureate nursing students' reflection on their caring practice through creating and sharing story, poetry, and art (Doctoral dissertation). *Dissertation Abstracts International, 99*(5), 334. (University Microfilms Inc. No DAO 72699)

Wagner, A. L. (2000). Connecting to nurse-self through reflective poetic story. *International Journal of Human Caring, 4*(2), 7–12.

Wagner, A. L. (2002). Nursing students' development of caring self through creative reflective practice. In D. Freshwater (Ed.), *Therapeutic nursing: Improving patient care through self awareness and reflection* (pp. 121–144). Newbury Park, CA: Sage.

Wagner, A. L. (2005). Three poems: "The Faces of Oklahoma City," "The Lady Who Sang." and "Mrs. O'Malley: Pain." In M. C. Wendler (Ed.), *The heART of nursing: Expressions of creative art in nursing* (2nd ed., pp. 146–147). Indianapolis, IN: Sigma Theta Tau International.

Wagner, A. L. (2008). A caring scholar response to uncovering meaning through the aesthetic turn: A pedagogy of caring. *International Journal for Human Caring, 12*(2), 24–28.

Wagner, A. L. (2015). *Four seasons of grieving: A nurse's healing journey with nature.* Indianapolis, IN: Sigma Theta Tau International.

Wagner, A. L. (2016). Engaged and expressed: Storytelling as a way to know and be known. In W. Rosa (Ed.), *Nurses as leaders: Evolutionary visions of leadership* (pp. 431–451). New York, NY: Springer Publishing.

Watson, J. (2005). *Caring science as sacred science.* Philadelphia, PA: F. A. Davis.

Watson, J. (2008). *Nursing: The philosophy and science of caring* (Rev. ed.). Boulder: University Press of Colorado.

Watson, J. (2017). Global advances in human caring literacy. In S. M. Lee, P. A. Palmieri, & J. Watson (Eds.), *Global advances in human caring literacy* (pp. 3–11). New York, NY: Springer Publishing.

Whyte, D. (1994). *The heart aroused: Poetry and the preservation of the soul of corporate America.* New York, NY: Currency Doubleday.

43

The Power of Ritual in Nurses' Everyday Lives: Personal and Professional Exemplars

Zane Robinson Wolf

ON RITUAL

Rituals, often described as symbolic, ceremonial practices performed by cultural groups, are ever present in human activity. They consist of patterned, symbolic actions that represent beliefs and values of social groups (De Craemer, Vansina, & Fox, 1976) and of individuals. Sages suggest that as one ritual disappears, another replaces it, perhaps demonstrating ritual importance and perceived benefits. An often-cited benefit is the restoration of social order (Goopy, 2006). Conversely, rituals are critiqued as unimportant and restrictive and described as mindless activity (Tonuma & Winbolt, 2000; Walsh & Ford, 2001). Many scholars have proposed both positive and negative results of rituals (Wolf, 2014).

Various rituals are practiced by many cultural and subcultural groups, including the nursing profession, and demonstrate social behavior. Consistent with cultural practices, people's beliefs, values, and behavioral norms strongly influence ritual performance. Moreover, the meanings of ritual symbols are tacit and inferred. Their hidden implications may not be readily understood by performers.

Rituals have been labeled "dramaturgic," portrayed as a response to crises, and explained as protection from anxiety (Evans, Pereira, & Parker, 2008; Philpin, 2002) and from the stress experienced by members of cultural or subcultural groups. Then, following ritual enactment, a steady state may return. However, crisis reduction may not fully explain the purpose of all rituals. In contrast to group-based or collective rituals, rituals performed on an individual level suggest other functions, such as honoring patients and preserving the well-being of nurses (Lattanzio Hale, 2015).

Many nursing authors critical of rituals have equated them with cited examples that demonstrate the rigid hierarchical structures in organizations and in routines of nursing care (Tonuma & Winbolt, 2000). Such examples are most likely ritualistic behavior rather than rituals. Their concern is that nurses must consider the needs and wishes of patients and interact with them while providing routine, ritualistic nursing work, instead of concentrating on routines and procedures alone. Routines themselves are important in everyday nursing practice (Rytterström, Unosson, & Arman, 2010). They differ in that they lack symbolic meaning.

Nursing rituals are often carried out every day as nurses care for patients. However, the label "everyday rituals" diminishes them, because some are not practiced each day, for example, rituals of transition at graduation or ceremonial rituals celebrating success (Wolf, 2014). One explanation in favor of everyday rituals noted that they reflect "… our tastes and bring comfort through their routine, signal continuity, stability of self, and provide cadence to daily life" (Bern-King, 2011, p. 57). Nonetheless, when considering the power and persistence of nursing rituals across the world, perhaps there *are* everyday occurrences.

Rituals serve many goals that can be clarified by examining types, such as personal or self-oriented and professional or group-oriented examples. When considering the everyday lives of professional nurses, it can be argued that rituals are present in both personal and professional domains. This chapter explores exemplars of personal and professional rituals as performed by professional nurses every day. To assist in achieving this purpose, a number of databases were searched in English, including Summon, Essential Nursing, SocINDEX, Cumulative Index to Nursing and Allied Health Literature (CINAHL), and Google. Dates were specified in some cases. Search terms consisted of nurse/nurses, daily ritual, well-being, bedside rounds, self-care, pre-shift, ritual, shift preparation, shift recovery, and huddle.

PERSONAL RITUALS IN NURSES' EVERYDAY LIVES

INTERPERSONAL CARING RITUAL

Professional nurses' work is accompanied by many challenges as they care for patients in diverse settings (Manomenidis, Panagopoulou, & Montgomery, 2016). Their role is carried out autonomously and interprofessionally as they interact with other providers when caring for patients. Nurses' role guarantees close proximity to patients and families and friends at the most difficult and most celebratory times of life, such as when patients are in pain and dying, after their deaths, and following births and lifesaving surgery. These opportunities are occasions or moments for the performance of an interpersonal caring ritual.

Peplau (1952) constructed a theory of the nurse–patient relationship and identified four sequential phases: orientation, identification, exploitation, and resolution as framed by the nursing process. Her theory described nursing as a significant, interactional, therapeutic process aimed at patients' health in cocreative process (Belcher & Fish, 1980). Her theory of the interpersonal process has served as a foundation for every-day, therapeutic nursing care. As an interaction theorist, Peplau's theory has been applied to nursing practice, education, and research (Meleis, 1997). The influence of this theory is echoed in decades of nurses' work, and needs to be considered in discussions of nursing interaction rituals. Moreover, because the participants vary with each nurse–patient relationship, the interaction is unique, personal, intrapersonal, and interpersonal.

Goffman (1967) proposed that interaction rituals had rules for social encounters during individuals' face-to-face encounters. According to Goffman, practices carried out during interactions follow requirements that help to maintain a specific and obligatory kind of ritual equilibrium. In the context of the nurse–patient relationship, nurses carry out face-to-face interactions, some of which are distinguished as caring moments (Watson, 1985, 1988). Caring moments can symbolize nursing's hands-on care, as a metaphor of their embodied intent to act (Engebretson, 2002).

On the occasion of a caring moment (Watson, 1985, 1988; Wolf, King, & France, 2015), the structure of the face-to-face encounter is framed by preconditions essential to it: context, societal trust, ethical principles, human vulnerability, uniqueness, nurse authentic intention, professional intimacy, and interpersonal interaction (Wolf et al., 2015). Next, the caring moment occurs between and within the professional nurse and patient; there is nurse and patient action/interaction as the nurse responds to the call of the patient to be nursed. Caring moments last an indeterminate period of time.

The consequences of action/interactional responses to nursing in the caring moment are judged by the quality of the nurse action/interactional response and patient outcomes (Wolf et al., 2015). The return to balance may be a transitory outcome, as the patient's needs for nursing care continue to unfold. The ritual nature of nurse–patient interactions during caring moments shows an overarching pattern, evidencing formality, repetitiveness, and a rhythm that is repeated by nurses who often initiate the relationship as a response to a patient need. Nurses and sentient patients cocreate the intricacies of the interaction and participate in the moment as individuals.

A caring moment can represent a nurse's success story as a particular social encounter in the larger framework of the nurse–patient relationship. If perceived as such, nurses recognize how well a nurse–patient interaction has unfolded. They may treasure the moment as a symbol of the best examples of their clinical career and remember it to provide solace when reflecting on what they have accomplished.

Before and After Shifts: Engagement and Disengagement Ritual

Numerous authors have noted that nurses experience burnout and compassion fatigue in many clinical settings, ranging from intensive care units to hospice agencies. Few nurses would disagree that their work is extremely stressful, in some cases resulting in health problems (Lin et al., 2015). The ambiguities and uncertainties of patient care characterize this work (Philpin, 2007). Recent graduates employed in their first jobs and even those with 2 years' or more experience claim that the stress at work is exhausting. Outcomes as indicators of work stress include nurse turnover and absenteeism, patient dissatisfaction, and treatment errors (Manomenidis et al., 2016).

The stress of patient care is quickly explained by the enormous responsibility that nurses bear. They deliver safe, effective nursing care in conjunction with teams of healthcare providers in complex settings. Some admit to colleagues that "Before I went into the hospital before each shift, I cried and called my mother" or "I often wished that I would have an accident when driving to the hospital," in anticipation of the unknown challenges ahead facing a new nurse or a seasoned nurse, respectively. Both the preparation before work and the disengagement after work call for nurses to implement protective or centering strategies, or even to perform personal rituals.

Shift engagement and disengagement rituals could serve to help nurses individually prepare for and separate from work stress before and after shifts during work transitions.

Manomenidis et al. (2016) described the "switch on-switch off" model in a qualitative, descriptive design study. They explained the positive effect of sports' preparation through "psyching-up" strategies, and pointed out that few comparable strategies were known to address the high-intensity work of nursing and medicine. In addition, they suggested that nurses do not take many breaks during shifts, thus reducing possible intrashift recovery from stress.

Sufficient sleep (Peate, 2007), reading, shopping, planning shift schedules, running groups, and purposeful, mindful praying (Anderson, 2014) are strategies to achieve home/work balance on off-scheduled work time. Nurses may discuss previous shift experiences in the parking lot before returning home (L. Piper, personal communication, March 15, 2017). In addition, a cross-sectional study found that a nurse exercise group had better intershift recovery (Chen, Davis, Daraiseh, Pan, & Davis, 2013) than the nonexercise group.

A number of strategies have been offered in anecdotal reports on before- and after-shift routines and rituals: personal care/grooming, religious rituals, nicotine/caffeine, social interaction, and listening to music (Manomenidis et al., 2016). Drinking water, prayer, meditation, heart-focused breathing, and stretching make up other suggestions. One nurse's personal, before- and after-shift ritual was offered: When sitting in her car prior to her shift, she visualized writing things that happened at home earlier, crumpled up the list, and threw it out; she repeated the same ritual before going home (Trossman, 2014). Another nurse performed an after-night-shift ritual: When returning home and after talking to her family, she uses a white-noise fan, room-darkening shades, and light but carbohydrate-high food to prevent hunger and early wakening (Robinson, 1993). Complaining to colleagues during change-of-shift report and joining colleagues for a drink after work also serve to reduce stress.

It is likely that most personal before- and after-shift rituals are performed alone. They enable the transition from the private person to the nurse role and vice versa. Such rituals are called for because the taking on and turning over the nursing responsibility of patient care are tremendous, as shown during handovers or shift reports. Nonetheless, the impact of each shift on nurses, whether in anticipating the unknown of the upcoming shift or when deescalating following "going off" a shift, has not been well explored.

The need for nurses to heal themselves is acknowledged by leaders, clinicians, and educators (O'Connor, 2002; Smith, Zahourek, Hines, Engebretson, & Wardell, 2013). In support of this supposition, Smith et al. (2013) conducted a qualitative study using narrative inquiry and story inquiry to describe the meaning of personal healing. Three story segments resulted, each supported by themes and subthemes: call to the healing encounter (*recognition of the need to resolve a personal health crisis, knowledge of or engagement in self-care practices, reliance on intuitive knowing*), the experience of healing (*connections, profound sensations, perceptions, and events, awareness of the reciprocal nature of healing, inner resolution [forgiveness, awakening, and acceptance], use of multiple holistic approaches, and witnessing manifestations of healing*), and insights (*a sense of gratitude and appreciation, an ongoing journey*). In the metastory that combined the story segments and themes, a nurse began to heal through daily rituals of walking, meditation, and journaling as a way of life (Smith et al., 2013, pp. 178–182).

Rituals of self-healing and role transition are shown in strategies performed by nurses before and after their shifts. They are distinctive and indicate the energy needed to encounter oncoming shifts and to resolve what has transpired during completed shifts. The personal strength required to heal self and others is acknowledged both implicitly and explicitly.

Anecdotes of practices or self-identified rituals reveal that nurses have confronted the stress of nursing work and have tried to cope with it. Whether many nurses have performed a personal ritual of self-healing and accomplished a transitory role change remains to be debated. However, the importance of recovery during the intershift time period and its contribution to positive outcomes, such as job satisfaction, social support, and workplace commitment (Han, Trinkoff, & Geiger-Brown, 2014), as well as personal stress and recovery, demand additional study.

The shift engagement and disengagement ritual, viewed through van Gennep's (1960) classic rites of passage theory, is a daily rite of passage. Nurses separate from the role of the nurse on return to home, ideally recover, and prepare to be incorporated into the role of the nurse prior to each shift. The extent to which recovery is realized and energy is built up for the next shift remains unclear.

PROFESSIONAL RITUALS IN NURSES' EVERYDAY LIVES

CHANGE-OF-SHIFT REPORT

The structure and practices of change-of-shift report (handover, intershift report) have evolved and been modified over many decades. Technological innovations, such as electronic health records, and calls for change have helped nurses exchange verbal information on patients through group verbal, bedside verbal, tape-recorded, or written handover types (Kerr, Lu, McKinlay, & Fuller, 2011). They have also moved from individualized methods of documenting pertinent patient details to structured printouts onto which additional notes are written. Whether a group of nursing staff meet privately in a room or at a nurses' station or two nurses stand near a patient's bedside to discuss up-to-the-moment patient requirements, shift report stands as a powerful, exclusive professional nursing ritual (Wolf, 2014).

Looked at as a ritual, handover has great significance because it incorporates the sacred values of the nursing profession, chiefly that of taking on responsibility for assigned patients' care during an upcoming shift and accounting for what nursing work was accomplished by those ending the shift. Shift report is therefore prospective and retrospective (Kerr et al., 2011). As such, it demonstrates an important transition of care responsibility and a focus on the patient as the center of care. Change-of-shift report functions as an initiation strategy into the profession, as a test of nursing competence, and serves as a mechanism in which other results are achieved.

During change-of-shift report, nurses share opinions, express feelings, thoughts, and perceptions, restate their values, teach, and learn (Kerr et al., 2011; Wolf, 2014). The extent to which bedside handover has changed these patterns is worthy of study. Nonetheless, bedside handover accomplishes many functions, the most important being continuity of care (Greaves, 1999), similar to other types of shift report delivery.

Change-of-shift report through a nonritual view has been critiqued as ritualistic, time-wasting, rigidly hierarchical, missing important information, and threatening to confidentiality (Greaves, 1999; Webster, 1999). On the contrary, such time is sacrosanct because interruptions are banned as are persons not involved in the ritual (Evans et al., 2008). The case for or against accepting change-of-shift report as a nursing ritual continues.

There is synchrony (Fischer, Callander, Reddish, & Bulbulia, 2013) between or among the nurses performing shift reports. Shift reports also progress in a methodical manner. Nurses complement each person's participation in the shared, ritual goal, to transfer and take on the multiple responsibilities of nursing care.

GRIEF RITUAL

Kobler, Limbo, and Kavanaugh (2007) noted that nurses have created rituals in response to perinatal deaths, including miscarriage, stillbirth, or infant death in support of the grieving process for family members, friends, and nurses themselves. They suggested that support had been lacking and attributed this to a societal judgment that perinatal deaths were not legitimate social deaths, resulting in parents being isolated and unrecognized as grieving (Malacrida, 1999). Nurses have created rituals to address perinatal deaths for some time (Cameron, Taylor, & Greene, 2008). In addition, perinatal deaths fit van Gennep's (1960) notion of a life transition, and, as such, require ritual enactment.

The intention of the creative process for the grief ritual is rooted in nurses' altruism for the bereaved. Nurses assist parents to identify the level of participation: movement, verbalization, reflection, and symbol (Kobler et al., 2007). Furthermore, they advocate using guided participation during planning to elicit parents' ideas about an emerging ritual and incorporate their traditions into it. In examples provided by Kobler et al. (2007), caregivers in interprofessional teams have asked parents to identify their level of involvement.

Kobler et al. (2007) described three exemplars of a grief ritual: wreath ceremony, bouquet of love, and laying on of hands; all specified supplies (symbols), actions, words, and two invited reflections. These and other rituals show respect for the dead, concern for those remaining (van Tongeren, 2004), and deference to the incorporation of cultural traditions. It is important to mirror parental culture in the ritual. Following ritual performance, parents continue grieving in their own ways.

Although the grief rituals initiated by nurses do not support the full extent of parents' bereavement needs, they represent purposeful action, typically enacted in a short time, which assists bereaved parents to acknowledge early pregnancy loss, stillbirth, or death of an infant or child (Kobler et al., 2007). Nurses have guided individuals to create meaning through the use of symbols and have helped participants design a rite of passage as a grief ritual in a cocreative process. Nurses have functioned as facilitators, yet they also may benefit (Houck, 2014). The grief ritual represents nurses' personal and professional assessments of family members' needs. As created by nurses, the grief ritual incorporates professional nursing values. As such, it stands as both a personal and a professional nursing ritual.

It is not surprising that the grief ritual has been created by nurses in response to patients' deaths. Many societies have created such ceremonies to ease the discomforts of the bereaved accompanying the transition of persons from life to death (van Gennep, 1960). As a nursing-created rite of passage, it is sacred and acknowledges the death of the patient and comforts the bereaved.

CONCLUSION

Patients' life transitions and nurses' role in professional work call for a system of nursing rituals. As the work of nurses progresses in time, the rituals will change. Their symbols, language, function, and structure may differ. Nonetheless, the values of nurses will not.

Personal and professional nursing rituals are rooted in a humanistic-altruistic values system. According to Watson (2010), the original carative factor in her human caring theory is oriented by this system of values. It starts in caring consciousness, frames the basis of human caring, and fosters the best professional care. The carative factor has evolved into a clinical Caritas Process®: Practicing loving-kindness and equanimity within context of caring consciousness (Watson, 2010).

This Caritas Process is operationalized by nurses as they treat themselves and others with loving-kindness and respect. Being open to their own and patients' and family members' talents and contributions shows that nurses respect the dignity of humans. When facing very difficult situations, such as the death of patients and extraordinarily difficult shifts and care challenges, nurses practicing and developing this process are able to accept what comes with equanimity or calmness and self-possession.

Rituals operate in a cultural context, are social, and are endemic to group behavior. They are also personal, whether performed in isolation or actively participated in with a group. Rituals carry symbolic meaning, use language, are repetitive, and demonstrate behaviors. They share a place in societies, in support of the following assertion: In all human activity, there is belief, art, science, and ritual. Therefore, rituals are integral to nurses' work (Philpin, 2007). They are oriented in beliefs and values and coexist with the artistic delivery of patient care.

Nurses integrate their culture of origin, the nursing culture, and the corporate culture of the work environment into nursing practice. It is assumed that in addition to the nursing culture, the culture of origin and the corporate culture of work environments shape nurses' ritual behavior. Although nursing rituals are enacted in many settings, they incorporate the beliefs, values, and norms of the nursing profession. Additional examples of nursing rituals beyond those given in this chapter are cited by many authors. Some include nursing ceremonial, medication error prevention, patient bathing, postmortem care rituals (Wolf, 1986; Wolf, 2014), resuscitation, infection control, and ward rounds.

This examination of rituals as they pertain to nursing is framed in Western thought, nursing literature, and nursing experience. Ritual theories of anthropologists have greatly influenced this chapter (Douglas, 1966; Turner, 1967; van Gennep, 1960). In many narratives and studies on rituals, authors note the importance of symbol and the function of ritual as a response to crisis and as reducing anxiety, as a way to achieve order, and as healing (Romanoff & Terenzio, 1998). Classic and contemporary authors do not necessarily agree on their function or structure.

This chapter explores a few nursing rituals and presents them as beneficial practices. Perhaps nurses who recognize the positive role of nursing rituals, such as shift and grief rituals in the context of the culture of nursing, will counter the negative association of nurses' procedures and care termed "ritualistic and automatic" or "mindless." Searching for the meaning of ritual symbols as they operate chiefly in a reflexive way could help form such an appreciation. Their symbolic value could be realized and sustained (Roberts-Turner et al., 2016). Rituals are part of human activity; the nursing culture is not immune.

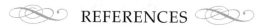 REFERENCES

Anderson, A. (2014). Pre-shift mindfulness: Setting an intention for my daily calling. *Mount Sinai Nurses Website*. Retrieved from http://nurses.mountsinaihealth.org/blog/pre-shift-mindfulness -setting-an-intention-for-my-daily-calling/?doing_wp_cron=1486844763.0105109214782714843750

Belcher, J. R., & Fish, L. J. (1980). Hildegard E. Peplau. In Nursing Theories Conference Group (Ed.), *Nursing theories: The base for professional nursing practice* (pp. 73–89). Englewood Cliffs, NJ: Prentice Hall.

Bern-King, M. (2011). Rituals in nursing homes. *Journal of the American Society on Aging, 35*(3), 57–63.

Cameron, J., Taylor, J., & Greene, A. (2008). Representations of rituals and care in perinatal death in British midwifery textbooks 1937-2004. *Midwifery, 24*, 335–343. doi:10.1016/j.midw.2006.03.010

Chen, J., Davis, K. G., Daraiseh, N. M., Pan, W., & Davis, L. S. (2013). Fatigue and recovery in 12-hour dayshift hospital nurses. *Journal of Nursing Management, 22*, 593–603. doi:10.1111/ jonm.12062

De Craemer, W., Vansina, J., & Fox, R. C. (1976). Religious movements in Central Africa: A theoretical study. *Comparative Studies in Society and History, 18*, 458–475. doi:10.1017/S0010417500008392

Douglas, M. (1966). *Purity and danger*. London, UK: Routledge & Kegan Paul.

Engebretson, J. (2002). Hands-on: The persistent metaphor in nursing. *Holistic Nursing Practice, 16*(4), 20–35. doi:10.1097/00004650-200207000-00006

Evans, A. M., Pereira, D. A., & Parker, J. M. (2008). Discourses of anxiety in nursing practice: A psycho-analytic case study of the change-of-shift handover ritual. *Nursing Inquiry, 15*, 40–48. doi:10.1111/j .1440-1800.2008.00387.x

Fischer, R., Callander, R., Reddish, P., & Bulbulia, J. (2013). How do rituals affect cooperation? An experimental field study comparing nine ritual types. *Human Nature, 24*, 115–125. doi:10.1007/ s12110-013-9167-y

Goffman, E. (1967). *Interaction ritual: Essays on face-to-face behavior*. New York, NY: Pantheon Books.

Goopy, S. (2006). …that the social order prevails: Death, ritual and the 'Roman' nurse. *Nursing Inquiry, 13*, 110–117. doi:10.1111/j.1440-1800.2006.00313.x

Greaves, C. (1999). Patients' perceptions of bedside handover. *Nursing Standard, 14*(12), 32–35. doi:10.7748/ns1999.12.14.12.32.c2726

Han, K., Trinkoff, A. M., & Geiger-Brown, J. (2014). Factors associated with work-related fatigue and recovery in hospital nurses working 12-hour shifts. *Workplace Health & Safety, 62*, 409–414. doi:10.3928/21650799-20140826-01

Houck, D. (2014). Helping nurses cope with grief and compassion fatigue: An educational interven-tion. *Clinical Journal of Oncology Nursing, 18*, 454–458. doi:10.1188/14.CJON.454-458

Kerr, D., Lu, S., McKinlay, L., & Fuller, C. (2011). Examination of current handover practice: Evidence to support changing the ritual. *International Journal of Nursing Practice, 17*, 342–350. doi:10.1111/j .1440-172X.2011.01947.x

Kobler, K., Limbo, R., & Kavanaugh, K. (2007). Meaningful moments: The use of ritual in perinatal and pediatric death. *American Journal of Maternal Child Nursing, 32*, 288–295. doi:10.1097/01 .NMC.0000287998.80005.79

Lattanzio-Hale, A. (2015). The obituary and the oncology nurse. *Clinical Journal of Oncology Nursing, 19*, 232. doi:10.1188/15.CJON.232

Lin, P. C., Chen, C. H., Pan, S. M., Chen, Y. M., Pan, C. H., Hung, H. C., & Wu, M. T. (2015). The associa-tion between rotating shift work and increased occupational stress in nurses. *Journal of Occupa-tional Stress, 57*, 307–315. doi:10.1539/joh.13-0284-OA

Malacrida, C. (1999). Complicating mourning: The social economy of perinatal death. *Qualitative Health Research, 9*, 504–519. doi:10.1177/104973299129122036

Manomenidis, G., Panagopoulou, E., & Montgomery, A. (2016). The 'switch on-switch off model': Strategies used by nurses to mentally prepare and disengage from work. *International Journal of Nursing Practice, 22*, 356–363. doi:10.1111/ijn.12443

Meleis, A. I. (1997). *Theoretical nursing development and progress* (3rd ed.). Philadelphia, PA: Lippincott.

O'Connor, M. (2002). Nurse leader: Heal thyself. *Nursing Administration Quarterly, 2*, 69–79. doi:10.1097/00006216-200201000-00008

Peate, I. (2007). Strategies for coping with shift work. *Nursing Standard, 22*(4), 42–45. doi:10.7748/ns2007.10.22.4.42.c4620

Peplau, H. E. (1952). *Interpersonal relationships in nursing.* New York, NY: G. P. Putnam's Sons.

Philpin, S. M. (2002). Rituals and nursing: A critical commentary. *Journal of Advanced Nursing, 38*, 144–151. doi:10.1046/j.1365-2648.2002.02158.x

Philpin, S. M. (2007). Managing ambiguity and danger in an intensive therapy unit: Ritual practices and sequestration. *Nursing Inquiry, 14*, 51–59. doi:10.1111/j.1440-1800.2007.00354.x

Roberts-Turner, R., Hinds, P. S., Britton, D. R., Coleman, L., Engh, E., Humbel, T. K., … Waldron, M. K. (2016). Rethinking rituals. *Nursing Management, 47*(4), 36–41. doi:10.1097/01.NUMA.0000481785.14320.5c

Robinson, L. (1993, February 13). Ritual helps nurse cope with daily grind. *Ottawa Citizen.*

Romanoff, B. D., & Terenzio, M. (1998). Rituals and the grieving process. *Death Studies, 22*, 697–711. doi:10.1080/074811898201227

Rytterström, P., Unosson, M., & Arman, M. (2010). The significance of routines in nursing practice. *Journal of Clinical Nursing, 20*, 3513–3522. doi:10.1111/j.1365-2702.2010.03522.x

Smith, M. C., Zahourek, R., Hines, M. E., Engebretson, J., & Wardell, D. W. (2013). Holistic nurses' stories of personal healing. *Journal of Holistic Nursing, 31*, 173–187. doi:10.1177/0898010113477254

Tonuma, M., & Winbolt, M. (2000). From rituals to reason: Creating an environment that allows nurses to nurse. *International Journal of Nursing Practice, 6*, 214–218. doi:10.1046/j.1440-172x.2000.00245.x

Trossman, S. (2014). The new "fine"? Nurses look at ways to move closer toward a work-life balance. *American Nurse.* Retrieved from http://www.theamericannurse.org/2014/07/03/the-new-fine

Turner, V. (1967). *The forest of symbols: Aspects of Ndembu ritual.* New York, NY: Cornell University Press.

van Gennep, A. (1960). *The rites of passage* (M. B. Vizedom & G. L. Caffee, Trans.). Chicago, IL: University of Chicago Press.

van Tongeren, L. (2004). Individualizing ritual: The personal dimension in funeral liturgy. *Worship, 78*, 117–138.

Walsh, M., & Ford, P. (2001). *Nursing rituals: Research and rational actions.* Oxford, UK: Butterworth-Heineman.

Watson, J. (1985). *Nursing: The philosophy and science of caring.* Niwot: University Press of Colorado.

Watson, J. (1988). *Nursing: Human science and human caring.* New York, NY: National League for Nursing.

Watson, J. (2010). *Core concepts of Jean Watson's theory of human caring/caring science.* Watson Caring Science Institute. Retrieved from https://www.watsoncaringscience.org/files/Cohort%206/watsons-theory-of-human-caring-core-concepts-and-evolution-to-caritas-processes-handout.pdf

Webster, J. (1999). Practitioner-centred research: An evaluation of the implementation of the bedside hand-over. *Journal of Advanced Nursing, 30*, 1375–1382. doi:10.1046/j.1365-2648.1999.01233.x

Wolf, Z. R. (1986). *Nursing rituals in an adult acute care hospital: An ethnography.* (UMI Dissertations Publishing, #8614888)

Wolf, Z. R. (2014). *Exploring rituals nursing: Joining art and science.* New York, NY: Springer Publishing.

Wolf, Z. R., King, B. M., & France, N. E. M. (2015). Antecedent context and structure of communication during a caring moment: Scoping review and analysis. *International Journal for Human Caring, 19*(2), 7–21. doi:10.20467/1091-5710-19.2.7

44

Photovoice: Qualitative Research Strategy for Theory-Guided Nursing Practice

Gayle L. Casterline

The high-tech, data-driven environment of healthcare demands a balance in respectful interactions and human connections. Human Caring Science is mindful of subjectivity and reverential to the meaning of human experience, especially as it relates to health (Watson, 2008). This chapter describes the qualitative methodology of photo imagery and its value to human Caring Science and theory-guided nursing practice. A description of the core concept, theoretical foundations, research considerations, and educational pedagogy illustrates the significance of the method for enhancing the science of the nursing discipline.

PHOTOVOICE METHOD

Photographers have long recognized the value of images to communicate overt and covert messages. Photography has been documented as a research tool used in anthropology to record fieldwork (Collier & Collier, 1986). Wang and Burris (1997) originally conceptualized the Photovoice method as a group-based participatory health-promotion strategy aimed at creating awareness of community issues in need of social action and change. Researchers and social reformers using photography as the principal resource to gain a clearer perspective of an experience or phenomenon acknowledge that photographs offer an honest context to life that affectively transcends language, culture, and socioeconomic status. Photographic images generate a creative and appealing research method for nurse researchers collaborating with community participants to communicate values and experiences about a wide variety of phenomena important to health and nursing practice.

Visual methodologies used in social sciences research have many names in the literature, including "photoelicitation" (Epstein, Stevens, McKeever, & Baruchel, 2006), "visual ethnography" (Pink, 2013), "photographic project," "participatory photography," "visual story-telling" (Drew, Duncan, & Sawyer, 2010), "Photovoice" (Catalani & Minkler, 2010), "photographic documentary" (Szto, Furman, & Langer, 2005), and "photo novella" (Burke & Evans, 2011).

With some variations in intent and outcome, all these methods use photo imagery to promote individual and community awareness of everyday realities and encounters.

The primary objectives of the method are to (a) assist community members to reflect on and record community needs and issues, (b) stimulate dialogue through sharing of photographs and perspectives, and (c) initiate social reform (Balbale, Locatelli, & LaVela, 2016). The technique requires researchers to build relationships with community participants/ stakeholders representative of a targeted demographic; develop specific goals and outcomes amenable to social action in collaboration with the participants/stakeholders; offer training, timeline, and a theme around which to center photographic images; share photographs in a supportive network to dialogue/debrief meaning; and plan change on the basis of a new understanding (Wang, Yi, Tao, & Carovano, 1998). The technique inspires people to influence and control their environments. The researcher must be competent in participatory collaboration and qualitative knowledge and skills (Balbale et al., 2016).

As an example of community-based participatory research (CBPR), the Photovoice method empowers participants to speak as advocates for their community and support social policy changes by gathering accurate information (Graziano, 2004). In this case, members of the community share personal pictures (auto-photography) for the purpose of social reform and improving community quality. Examples of this include partnering with women to develop better reproductive healthcare in rural China (Wang & Burris, 1997), tackling inequities in health access (Haque, 2011), and improving community mental health (Andonian, 2010).

Photovoice is also a method by which individuals can use photography to document their lives and their feelings. Visual images give voice to marginalized or vulnerable populations in the community, promoting personal awareness as well as raising the consciousness of the public (Graziano, 2004; Lorenz & Kolb, 2009). Personal photography allows the expression of emotions not openly expressed, such as revealing feelings of demasculinization in men with prostate cancer (Oliffe & Bottorff, 2007) and the underrepresentation of fathers in parental bereavement literature (Macdonald, Chilibeck, Affleck, & Cadell, 2010). Researchers offer new ways of understanding lesbians' unique experiences within the culture (Russell & Diaz, 2011) or the health behaviors of Latino adolescents (Lightfoot et al., 2017). Public forums, slide shows, exhibitions of photographs, or even newspaper articles transform perceptions of emotionally complex topics through shared awareness and discussion of meaning between community members and policy makers (Russell & Diaz, 2011).

VALUE TO CARING SCIENCE

Photovoice is a valuable health research methodology that may be particularly useful for promoting meaning and understanding of personal experiences and perceptions guided by Caring Science. Part of the conscious "intentionality toward sacred healing, harmony and wholeness" (Watson, 1999, p. 230) living within the postmodern/transpersonal paradigm may be glimpsed and tacitly realized through an aesthetic research form such as Photovoice.

The methodology is guided by three theoretical frameworks: empowerment education theory (Freire, 1970/2000b), feminist theory, and an artistic documentary photography technique. CBPR paradigms address community issues, cultural experiences, and personal values and belief, allowing the invisible to become visible in an effort to promote change.

Public health approaches and community change theories build on the work of Freire (1970/2000b), who saw the learner and the teacher as cocreators of knowledge. Freire recognized three levels of consciousness in community culture, starting with silent acceptance, moving to horizontal violence or blaming/bullying of peers, and advancing to a higher level of critical consciousness where interpretations of reality assume responsibility for making change (1973/2000a). Freire initiated community conversations, listened for emotionally charged themes, and translated what was heard into drawings that further stimulated discussion. Empowerment education theory was built by engaging the community to participate in its own learning, a praxis of reflection and action (Carlson, Engebretson, & Chamberlain, 2006).

Feminist theory recognizes women's experiences and knowledge as a legitimate catalyst for change (Allen, 2008). It reveals the nature of patriarchal power relationships that impact the lives of women and encourages women to use their knowledge to advocate for, create, and carry out social changes (changes should not be made by others on women's behalf). All forms of domination that subordinate women are challenged so that women have more control over their lives (Cosslett, Easton, & Summerfield, 1996). The beauty of community collaboration research is that each subjective voice is respected.

These voices are enhanced by the power of photography, reflection, and sharing. Photography and journalism are mediums with global outreach, an expression of pictures and stories that open eyes, soften hearts, and change minds. Documentary photography is an artistic endeavor that seeks understanding and explores meaning (Russell & Diaz, 2011) and appears in perfect harmony with the "epistemological pluralism" of Caring Science (Watson, 2005, p. 29) as multiple ways of knowing intersect the arts and humanities to inform science and clinical practice. Photovoice integrates aesthetic creativity into research methodologies used by social scientists, complementing the comprehensive empirical nature of qualitative research (Russell & Diaz, 2011).

ETHICAL CONSIDERATIONS OF PHOTO RESEARCH METHODS

Although the clear advantages to understanding a community issue or personal experience are enhanced by participant-generated photos, using visual data intended for empowerment and social change carries a considerable ethical burden (Hannes & Parylo, 2014). In addition to the usual concerns of privacy, anonymity, and confidentiality, the researcher collaborating with the public must understand the ethical aspects of participant sensitivity and consciousness raising (Hannes & Parylo, 2014). Image-based data may interact with text-based data, producing emotional responses not anticipated by the researcher or the participant (Chapman, Wu, & Zhu, 2016). Reflecting on the meaning of a picture may include what is and what is not in the photograph. Self-made images can be deeply personal for the participant. The researcher should plan to protect the subject from deductive disclosure. Respectful partnerships between researcher and community participants will strengthen equitable involvement in the research process.

Participants should be instructed on consenting procedures on individuals photographed for research purposes. Community photographers need a clear background of ethical challenges that may be confronted while collecting visual data. Potentially inappropriate photographs or clues that may unintentionally reveal a person's identity should be discussed. Because it is more difficult to anonymize visual data compared with textual data, researchers should develop and explain special considerations for informed consent thoroughly (Hannes & Parylo, 2014), including how the data will be used and if any public forums of the visual materials will be presented. Cocreators of community action projects will collaborate on the purpose of the images collected, the final photographs used in a public exhibition, and agreements of ownership and photo credits.

Researchers partnering with members of vulnerable population groups have added challenges. Topic sensitivity and specific vulnerabilities may act as barriers to institutional review boards (IRBs) or community leaders. Opsal et al. (2016) warn of misrepresenting the risks/benefits to community members. Leaders in the community of interest should be part of the research team and consulted for guidance about recruiting appropriate volunteers for the project. At all costs, researchers have an ethical obligation not to objectify participants.

If the purpose of the project was to raise awareness of a community issue in need of social action, participants may feel taken advantage of when anticipated changes are not realized as a result of their considerable efforts. The researcher may well benefit from a published paper and scholarly notoriety but the community issue remains the same, with consequent feelings of oppression, discrimination, and hopelessness (Opsal et al., 2016).

EDUCATIONAL STRATEGIES TO PROMOTE THEORY-GUIDED PRACTICE

It has been this author's conscious intention as an academic and clinical staff educator to improve nursing practice by raising awareness of one's personal philosophy of nursing and how it is congruent with and guided by nursing theory. If, as Freire (1970/2000b) believed, the purpose of education is to transform lives, recognition of the power of theory in personal and professional interactions can change the discipline and improve healthcare outcomes.

This begins with reflective consideration of just what one believes and values as a nurse. Most students acknowledge that they have never really thought about this. The teacher's role as cocreator in this process is to challenge the nurses to consider not just what they do but also who they are. Students begin to recognize that nursing is not just a set of functions or tasks, but a value system. Why did you become a nurse? What are your strengths? What gifts do you bring to the profession of nursing? What values do you hold most dear? How did you come to know these values? Developing a personal philosophy is the first step in seeing the relevance of nursing theory as a guide to clinical practice.

As an educational strategy, this author asks nurses to *let go of their black and white world and play in the gray*, digging deeper to understand the language and concepts of nursing theory. Nurses contemplate multiple ways of knowing. Are you pragmatic, knowing from your experience? Are you idealistic, knowing through aesthetics such as beauty, art, music, and culture? Are you a realist, knowing through facts and empirical principles of science; or are you an existential knower, connecting through spirituality to understand the meaning of experiences?

Nurses are also encouraged to find similarities and differences between their personal philosophies and published nursing theories. They begin to explore what they like and what they do not like, what they understand and what seems too abstract right now to apply to a practice setting. Nurses begin to think about thinking; the answers are not right or wrong but an opportunity to clarify feelings and beliefs. What do you believe about the nursing metaparadigm—person, health, environment, and nursing (nurse)? What is your concept of the mission of the nurse? Is nursing a set of functional tasks, or is it more? How do illness and wellness relate to health? What is the relationship between environment and health? How does a person's internal and external environment influence health and well-being? What is the meaning of personhood? What governs the ethical delivery of nursing care? What are the rights and responsibilities of recipients of that care?

In graduate education courses, this author uses a learning strategy called "Visualizing Theory," using a modified Photovoice technique. The assignment gives students an opportunity to use creative (aesthetic) ways of knowing. They are asked to take digital photographs illustrating personal perceptions of the nursing metaparadigm (person, environment, health, and nurse) and also relate the image to a specific nursing theory. Photo release forms are submitted for all photos with visible faces and students are asked not to take pictures of patients. Nurses are encouraged to go to art galleries and explore painting, sculpture, and textiles. Some students use literature, poetry, and music to represent concepts and theories. Participants acknowledge that they are drawn to particular artwork or environments or structures because of their values and beliefs, just as they are drawn to specific theories. Photographs are identified by name, date, and location. Students are asked to record images as inspired; some, however, submit a picture previously taken on a mission trip or vacation that represents a fresh understanding of theory in a special way. This author's goal has been to open the mind to new possibilities for appreciating theoretical frameworks, using them as a philosophy of living and a way to experience the world. The following are a few examples.

I took the picture shown in Figure 44.1 during a medical mission at Lady Willingdon Hospital in Manali, India. I believe that this picture depicts *environment* from the nursing

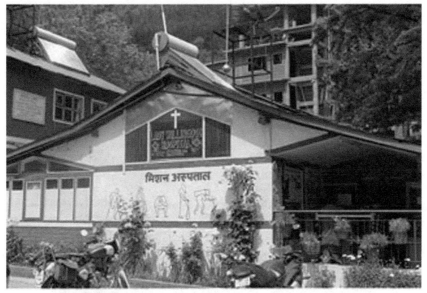

FIGURE 44.1 Lady Willingdon Hospital, Manali, India.

metaparadigm. A long line of patients forms every morning and no matter how long it takes, the staff will stay until the last person in line is cared for. Watson's Theory of Human Caring is what I think about when I look at this picture because everyone who works at this hospital truly cares about each individual and wants them to be healthy again. Watson tells us that transpersonal caritas seeks to connect with and embrace the spirit and soul of the other and that the nurse works to create a healing, caring environment. Throughout the mission trip I noticed this every single day and could tell that the staff at the hospital works with the spirit to help care and heal each patient coming through the doors.

Figure 44.2 represents *health* in the nursing metaparadigm. I climbed this mountain for the first time in July of 2014, and little did I know my physical ability would soon be limited. I was suddenly unable to walk due to terrible joint effusions in both of my legs. I was in my last year of nursing school and my dad had to drive me to class each day and wheel me to class in my wheelchair. As time passed I began to be able to walk again, even though it was very painful. I climbed that same mountain in June of 2015. I never realized how therapeutic it is to share my story until I read about Liehr and Smith's Story Theory. My story allows me to empathize with patients and creates an open dialogue for sharing and encouraging health.

I took this picture at St. Patrick's Cathedral in New York City (Figure 44.3). I see *person* in the nursing metaparadigm here. To me, this picture represents holistic care as well as universal love and the inner dimensions of life. I believe that the caring and healing process goes far beyond traditional Western medicine and involves caring for the patient spiritually and allowing for miracles. This image relates to Watson's Theory of Human Caring and the concepts of caring consciousness and allowing for energetic presence from a higher power. I believe my values allow me to focus on the spiritual and emotional aspects of nursing along with the social and physical needs of the patient.

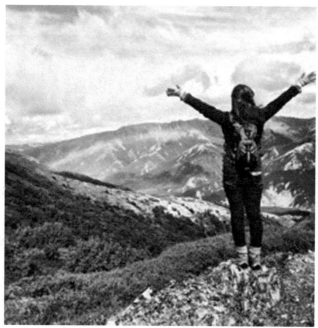

FIGURE 44.2 Denali National Park and Preserve, Alaska.

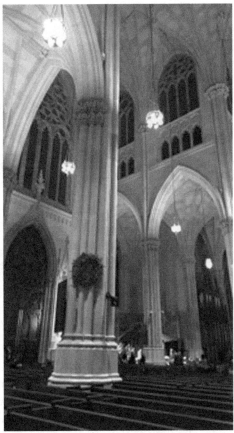

FIGURE 44.3 St. Patrick's Cathedral, New York, New York.

I believe that holistic nursing involves a concern for the soul of the patient and that the Holy Spirit guides the care of my patients through my nursing practice. My faith helps me to be more positive and hopeful with my patients.

This memorial in Washington, D.C. (Figure 44.4) is dedicated to the many women who selflessly and bravely cared for our soldiers during Vietnam. The metaparadigm that most identifies with this memorial is *nursing*. I found this memorial appropriate since so many of the earlier theorists had cared for wounded soldiers. The lady unable to be seen in this picture is praying, I'm sure not only for herself, but for everyone involved in this terrible war. Jean Watson believes that human care requires high regard and reverence for a human life. This memorial holds human life in the highest regard and represents nurses as healing, inspiring hope, caring, and being spiritual.

Nurses taking this course confided that they "weren't looking forward to taking a theory course" but now "totally understood how it guided both their practice and their life." Others stated that they had "never seen relevance to nursing theory until now." One student said, "I couldn't believe you wanted me to take pictures of the nursing metaparadigm but this assignment has opened my mind to a new way of looking at my life." Taking photographs and sharing their meaning resulted in a transformative experience for many of the nurses in the class, revealing new ways to use theory to guide personal life and professional practice.

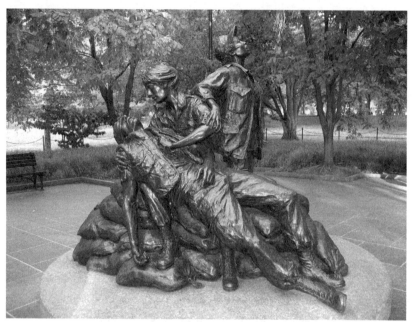

FIGURE 44.4 Vietnam Veterans Women's Memorial, Washington, DC.

Photovoice can also be introduced with CBPR as a qualitative method in research, community health, or epidemiology courses. Faculty and students would cocreate objectives to practice advocacy of community issues or populations (Massengale, Strack, Orsini, & Herget, 2016). Guiding students to share visual representations and the expression of experiences through stories of complex concepts such as *health, poverty, resilience, vulnerability,* or *sacred* evoke emotional reactions and a deeper empathy for global and diverse circumstances, as well as roles for the professional nurse. Using photoimagery as a pedagogy for learning, just as in credible research, requires ethical diligence and emotional protection.

In conclusion, participative methodologies that promote understanding of complex phenomena are significant to nursing practice. Photovoice is a qualitative method particularly useful to caring scientists for promoting meaning and understanding of personal experiences and illuminating and reforming social issues affecting the health and well-being of communities.

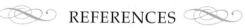 REFERENCES

Allen, A. (2008). *The politics of our selves: Power, autonomy and gender in contemporary critical theory.* New York, NY: Columbia University Press.

Andonian, L. (2010). Community participation of people with mental health issues within an urban environment. *Occupational Therapy in Mental Health, 26,* 401–417. doi:10.1080/0164212X.2010.518435

Balbale, S. N., Locatelli, S. M., & LaVela, S. L. (2016). Through their eyes: Lessons learned using participatory methods in health care quality improvement projects. *Qualitative Health Research, 26*(10), 1382–1392. doi:10.1177/1049732315618386

Burke, D., & Evans, J. (2011). Embracing the creative: The role of Photo Novella in qualitative nursing research. *International Journal of Qualitative Methods, 10*(2), 164–177. doi:10.1177/160940691101000205

Carlson, E. D., Engebretson, J., & Chamberlain, R. M. (2006). Photovoice as a social process of critical consciousness. *Qualitative Health Research, 16*(6), 836–852. doi:10.1177/1049732306287525

Catalani, C., & Minkler, M. (2010). Photovoice: A review of the literature in health and public health. *Health Education and Behavior, 37*(3), 424–451. doi:10.1177/1090198109342084

Chapman, M. V., Wu, S., & Zhu, M. (2016). What is a picture worth? A primer for coding and interpreting photographic data. *Qualitative Social Work, 0*(00), 1–15. doi:10.1177/1473325016650513

Collier, J., & Collier, M. (1986). *Visual anthropology: Photography as a research method* (Rev. ed.). Albuquerque: University of New Mexico Press.

Cosslett, T., Easton, A., & Summerfield, P. (1996). *Women, power and resistance: An introduction to women's studies*. Buckingham, UK: Open University Press.

Drew, S. E., Duncan, R. E., & Sawyer, S. M. (2010). Visual storytelling: A beneficial but challenging method for health research with young people. *Qualitative Health Research, 20*, 1677–1688. doi:10.1177/1049732310377455

Epstein, I., Stevens, B., McKeever, P., & Baruchel, S. (2006). Photo elicitation interview (PEI): Using photos to elicit children's perspectives. *International Journal of Qualitative Methods, 5*(3), 98–115. doi:10.1177/160940690600500301

Freire, P. (2000a). *Education for critical consciousness*. New York, NY: Continuum. (Original work published 1973)

Freire, P. (2000b). *Pedagogy of the oppressed*. New York, NY: Continuum. (Original work published 1970)

Graziano, K. J. (2004). Oppression and resiliency in a post-apartheid South Africa: Unheard voices of Black gay men and lesbians. *Cultural Diversity and Ethnic Minority Psychology, 10*(3), 302–316. doi:10.1037/1099-9809.10.3.302

Hannes, K., & Parylo, O. (2014). Let's play it safe: Ethical considerations from participants in a photovoice research project. *International Journal of Qualitative Methods, 13*, 255–274. doi:10.1177/160940691401300112

Haque, N. (2011). Tackling inequity through a Photovoice project on the social determinants of health: Translating Photovoice evidence to community action. *Global Health Promotion, 18*(1), 16–19. doi:10.1177/1757975910393165

Lightfoot, A. F., Thatcher, K., Simán, F. M., Eng, E., Merino, Y., Thomas, T., ... Chapman, M. V. (2017). "What I wish my doctor knew about my life": Using photovoice with immigrant Latino adolescents to explore barriers to healthcare. *Qualitative Social Work, 0*(00), 1–21. doi:10.1177/1473325017704034

Lorenz, L. S., & Kolb, B. (2009). Involving the public through participatory visual research methods. *Health Expectations, 12*, 262–274. doi:10.1111/j.1369-7625.2009.00560.x

Macdonald, M. E., Chilibeck, G., Affleck, W., & Cadell, S. (2010). Gender imbalance in pediatric palliative care research samples. *Palliative Medicine, 24*, 435–444. doi:10.1177/0269216309354396

Massengale, K. E. C., Strack, R. W., Orsini, M. M., & Herget, J. (2016). Photovoice as pedagogy for authentic learning: Empowering undergraduate students to increase community awareness about issues related to the impact of low income on health. *Pedagogy in Health Promotion, 2*(2), 117–126. doi:10.1177/2373379916639066

Oliffe, J. L., & Bottorff, J. L. (2007). Further than the eye can see? Photo elicitation and research with men. *Qualitative Health Research, 17*(6), 850–858. doi:10.1177/1049732306298756

Opsal, T., Wolgemuth, J., Cross, J., Kaanta, T., Dickmann, E., Colomer, S., & Erdil-Moody, Z. (2016). "There are no known benefits...": Considering the risk/benefit ratio of qualitative research. *Qualitative Health Research, 26*(8), 1137–1150. doi:10.1177/1049732315580109

Pink, S. (2013). *Doing visual ethnography* (3rd ed.). London, UK: Sage.

Russell, A. C., & Diaz, N. D. (2011). Photography in social work research: Using visual image to humanize findings. *Qualitative Social Work, 12*(4), 433–453. doi:10.1177/1473325011431859

Szto, P., Furman, R., & Langer, C. (2005). Poetry and photography: An exploration into expressive/creative qualitative research. *Qualitative Social Work, 4*(2), 135–156. doi:10.1177/1473325005052390

Wang, C. C., & Burris, M. A. (1997). Photovoice: Concepts, methodology, and use for participatory needs assessment. *Health Education & Behavior, 24*(3), 369–387. doi:10.1177/109019819702400309

Wang, C. C., Yi, W. K., Tao, Z. W., & Carovano, K. (1998). Photovoice as a participatory health promotion strategy. *Health Promotion International, 13*, 75–86. doi:10.1093/heapro/13.1.75

Watson, J. (1999). *Postmodern nursing and beyond.* Edinburgh, Scotland: Churchill Livingstone.

Watson, J. (2005). *Caring Science as sacred science.* Philadelphia, PA: F. A. Davis.

Watson, J. (2008). *Nursing: The philosophy and science of caring* (Rev. ed.). Boulder: University Press of Colorado.

45

Music and Poetry for Healing

Patrick Dean

Artists who schedule live performances and successfully engage their audiences in a truly shared experience of music or poetry often report a connection that belies objective measurement or other empirical proof of mutual, and sometimes healing, reciprocity. Somehow, both audience and performer intuitively know that synergy exists, that the experience is unique, and that artist and audience are temporarily united as one in the moment, and possibly beyond the moment into a hitherto unexperienced dimension. An ideal caring/healing relationship between patient and nurse likewise involves a mutual trust that the performance of nursing expertise involves a reciprocal relationship between recipient (patient) and performer (nurse), and sometimes vice versa. In addition, the ability of an on-demand performer to routinely repeat experiential reciprocity with audiences is likely the ultimate ability of a professional musician or poet, and, by association, a successful nurse.

In nursing, a healing relationship between patient and nurse also requires something of a leap of faith that mutual reciprocity is at work because immediate feedback is often unavailable (other than applause), as with the unconscious patient, for example, or with an audience that is difficult for the performer to read. The dilemma of not really knowing if reciprocity in nursing exists, or the extent of it (when and if it does exist), was originally identified by Noddings (1984) who stated that in relationship to caring action and reaction, caring reciprocity is all but impossible to judge or measure. Noddings' question about the reciprocal nature of caring is a challenge to the nursing profession to justify that patient responses to caring can be as specific, unique, and predictable as the nursing strategies used to provide patient-centered caring. Conceptualizing a set of nursing care standards without also requiring a corresponding set of patient care response standards can be like treating an infection while discounting the germ theory. In other words, a healing relationship is less likely to be effective if nursing action is unidirectional, versus reciprocal, in terms of assessing patient response to caring actions. Despite Noddings's perspective that caring reciprocity toward the goal of healing may be difficult to prove, more recent Caring Science research on intentionality and mindfulness in nursing does indicate that an artistic-like performance of nursing care is optimal for healing, especially through intense self-awareness (Zahourek, 2016). However, although the purpose of a patient/nurse relationship involves meeting expected and intended outcomes for some form of healing through reciprocity of caring, even if the dying process is involved, the reciprocity of caring is probably not unlike the resonance of musical vibrations that may initially emanate coherently, and eventually dissipate unpredictably into infinity after a healing objective has hopefully been met. To somehow be able to believe, and to reasonably predict, a patient's response to treatment, medication, or other intervention, is also the mark of a professional nurse. A nurse whose intuition, mindfulness, and intentionality can predict health outcomes is not unlike a musician or poet who can predict and anticipate audience reaction to his or her variations in expressive playing of notes and speaking of words, while at the same time being conscious of maintaining accuracy as much as possible. A superior performer, or an expert nurse, is also able to adjust the delivery of care, or music, or poetry, to match emerging variations of response.

Given the extent of Caring Science development over the past 40 years, and the incorporation of music and poetry into the very fabric of human society over millennia, it remains important that Caring Science continue to evolve as an artistic and scientific means to healing in mind, body, and spirit, just as music and poetry play a similar role for the benefit of humans. Defining, clarifying, and further establishing useful meanings of music and poetry, and caring in terms of human healing, are part of the reason for this chapter, and necessary for the benefit of Caring Science. In addition, predictions of how future technology may be used to monitor human responses to music, poetry, and caring actions are explored later.

WORKING DEFINITIONS

The word "nice" was never acceptable in my high school English composition class because it was difficult to define and operationalize. Actually, "operationalize" was probably not an acceptable word either, but "nice" was definitely verboten. "Caring" and "healing," in their common and ubiquitous usage, also seem to lack clear and precise definitions when compared with the precision with which they are used in nursing as the essence of practice. Caring and healing have become incorporated into everyday phrases that seem to have little to do with their original meaning. Like music and poetry, caring and healing are open to various interpretations, and perhaps risk losing their original meanings as directly related to human needs. To preserve caring and healing from trivialization of meaning, it is possible to conceive of universal rules, similar to those that guide the creation of music and poetry, such as scales, key signatures, harmony, and meter. Adapt, for example, Sir Isaac Newton's (1642–1727) law of gravity (force) to indicate that for every caring/healing action, there is a reaction that is equal and opposite in some way. For gravity, music, poetry, caring, and healing to exist, it seems necessary that there be some kind of response for them to be known to humanity. Light, for example, is undetectable until it bounces from a surface, thus making an object visible, or an apple bouncing from a tree presumably proves the existence of gravitational laws. Likewise, caring is essentially hidden until it is reflected by the human response of healing. Music and poetry do not reciprocally exist until they have been heard or read, and a human response evoked. One could say of music, poetry, and caring that they are constant, potential entities residing in all of us at all times, and are patently manifest in an action/reaction system for the benefit of humanity. However, the endeavor of moving from a working definition to a universal definition is a challenge given that common meanings of caring and healing are often taken for granted in the language, and thereby become almost meaningless. For example, the casual greeting, "Take care," may at times seem devoid of an adequate response. Other references, however, are monumental in their impact as in the possibility that human caring is as much responsible for the evolution of Homo sapiens as Darwin's theory of survival of the fittest (Leininger, 1991). Simultaneously, a prehistorical incorporation of music, and possibly poetry, into human development also probably influences recent human evolution in some way, especially if such an influence has a healing effect.

Although social understandings of music and poetry have survived millennia of political, commercial, and cultural variations, caring and healing still appear to be in social understanding evolution. For example, compare a nonprofit, private organization called CARE, dedicated to providing relief to the people of Africa, Asia, and Latin America, using a workforce of over 7,000 persons operating in the United States and 39 other countries (www.care.org), with the time, money, and effort we spend in caring for our clothing items. In cooperation with the Federal Trade Commission (FTC), the International Fabric Institute operates strict guidelines for the use of care labels, required in every garment sold in the United States (www.ftc.gov). If human beings came with care labels as specific as those required by the FTC, human caring would instantly become an exact science, possibly making the art of caring obsolete. According to the FTC: Care labels must give full instructions on at least one appropriate method of care necessary for the ordinary use and enjoyment of the garment, warn when harm can result from other garments being laundered or cleaned, warn when a product cannot be cleaned by any other method without being damaged, remain legible throughout the useful life of the product, and have a reasonable basis for the specified appropriate care procedures given on the label. Somewhere between a specific care label on clothing and the attempted relief of starvation by CARE, and somewhere between a perfunctory greeting and a possible adjunct theory of evolution, lies a vast array of caring/healing references. One such reference emerges from corporate America and certain organizations that feel they are "too big to care"; a concept based on an economic theory that some institutions feel they are "too big to fail" (Seamon, 2011). Presumably, if this culture of uncaring were to spread beyond organizations "too big to care" into everyday life, the likelihood of human devolution is surely inevitable, or at least resulting in a potentially unhealable society; the music and poetry of life would gradually cease.

CARING AS "UNHEALING FEELING" IN POLITICO-SOCIO-ECONOMICS

In the early 1990s, the writings and teaching of theorists like Madeleine Leininger and Jean Watson were raising awareness of nursing as a caring profession (Crossan & Robb, 1998). Perhaps a strange coincidence, caring also became the 1992 campaign message of former president George H. W. Bush. Bush gave a campaign speech just before the

1992 New Hampshire primary that gleaned widespread attention and subsequent political support. Blumenthal (1992), a columnist for *The New Republic,* noted that Bush was well aware of the recession's myriad implications when he said, "The message: I care."

Although Blumenthal's column speaks of Bush's caring mantra, it also illustrates that caring, in this instance, is equated primarily with feelings, and not necessarily with action. Therefore, without caring as action, healing is likely impossible. In defending himself against accusations of failing to heal the economy, Bush is mocked for his identification with the caring feelings of those whose endorsement he seeks. In a similar way, music and poetry, when regarded in terms of action potential, seem to be able to move beyond elicitation of feelings into the realm of healing effectiveness. Poetry in particular, because of its exclusive use of words, which at times are generally spoken by everyone, appears to be somewhat more accessible to any spontaneous creator of this art form. Even if never performed in public, poets often refer to a direct benefit of writing poetry for its own sake. For example, U.S. military veterans are reported to heal through the Veterans Voices Writing Project (VVWP, established in 1946), which uses therapeutic writing to rehabilitate veterans. Its mission and vision is to enable military veterans to experience solace and satisfaction through writing in a world where people appreciate that writing can both heal and entertain. Published three times per year, *Veterans Voices* magazine is supported by the U.S. Department of Veterans Affairs (www.veteransvoices.com).

Much could be written about the jingles in commercial advertising derived from popular and classical music, or about emotional responses to certain words such as "caring" and "healing" that are often embedded in healthcare and pharmaceutical advertisements, more than is possible in this chapter. However, it also seems ironic that the same *action* words of "caring" and "healing" are minimized to *feeling* words when used for economic purposes by the same corporate entities that claim to uphold the basic human values of caring and healing. Such is likely not the case in the following anecdote from Chavis (2011) in which the healing power of creative expression is derived from a well-known William Wordsworth poem: A mother and daughter, anxiously on their way to visit a potential college for the daughter to attend, unexpectedly saw a field of daffodils. The shared vision simultaneously elicited the same memory in each of them, namely, that of the mother sharing the comforting words of Wordsworth's iconic poem with her daughter, when she was a child, to relieve anxiety. By transcending time and circumstance, nurses often observe that a patient's recollection of a song, poem, or tune can also momentarily release a patient and family from the anxiety burden of disease, perhaps providing space for some form of healing to begin or continue. Such is the case at Mayo Clinic, Rochester, Minnesota, where an abundance of pianos are found in open public spaces of the various medical campus buildings for anyone to play, sing, or recite poetry with music. Public appreciation of such healing power was forcefully felt recently when attempts were made to limit the size of public gatherings around one specific piano in a large open space in the Gonda Building at Mayo Clinic. Local news media featured reports of patient and visitor protests objecting to restrictions on their enjoyment of scheduled, as opposed to spontaneous, music and song performance, despite the potential for security issues related to public safety and nuisance noise. After a month's absence of loosely arranged music performances, mostly by Mayo employees, Mayo Clinic decided to reinstitute the beneficial tradition by allocating a less hazardous space for sharing of music and song (Whitcome, 2016). Also, weekly professional musical performances, usually at noon in various parts of the Mayo campus, were not affected, and neither was the music therapy sessions routinely scheduled for patients and their families.

Although the earlier definitions and anecdotes of a music and poetry relationship to caring and healing are nontheoretical, they do illustrate that there is wide interpretation of these concepts within society at large. Social concepts of healing are usually associated with medicine, but are expanding to include terms such as caring, caregiving, and caretaker, and often implied in terms such as nurse, and historically with women (Reverby, 1987), and explicated in the term "woman" by Gilligan (1982/1993). More recently, however, paradigm shifts of gender identification with specific professions, such as nursing and medicine, are taking place so that perspectives of caring and healing are becoming increasingly gender balanced (Dean, 2016; Zahourek, 2015). Because music and poetry appear to have a longer history of gender balance in terms of their creation and explication, it is perhaps hopeful that caring and healing perspectives can likewise achieve a more universal understanding across cultures, political persuasions, and economic considerations.

A PORTRAIT OF MUSICAL CARING-HEALING

Imagine a solo violin anticipating its opportunity to sound a penetrating note that soars effortlessly above every other instrument in an orchestra. Nestled under the chin of its player, this expertly crafted piece of wood resists the pulling tension of strings that are carefully massaged with fingers and stroked with hair. Devoid of mechanical moving parts, such as keys, valves, and levers, this instrumental device sits close to the ear where every whisper, or cry of despair, is heard by its master, thus allowing for the closest of connections in the process of making music or effecting healing. Even in pejorative terms, a mocking imitational gesture of playing the violin is used to convey to others a pseudo-caring for another's troubles. A contrasting image of a mother cradling her child rescues this word picture of gentle firmness required in playing this difficult instrument, and easily translates to patient and nurse, who in reciprocal relationship, are like bow and string responding in harmony. Sometimes strings are plucked in pizzicato where patient/nurse encounters are brief and to the point. At other times, with careful bowing, a note can be sustained, seemingly indefinitely, as if it does not wish to end. Occasionally, more than one string is bowed simultaneously, as in complex and sometimes stressful nursing situations, where expert competence and skill are keys to success. The healing of mind, body, and soul is uniquely captured in the Romany or Gypsy style of violin music where spirited movement and joyful expression seem devoid of restriction allowing freedom from cares, thus creating engagement with caring and healing. Such musical expressions also seem to resonate with natural sounds of the environment such as bird song, running water, wind, and waves.

A FUTURE CONSIDERATION FOR MUSIC, POETRY, AND HEALING

From a psycho-neuro-immunological perspective, positive brainwave resonances with music and poetry will eventually, if they are not already, be identified with subtle, but measurable healing effects in various parts of the body, mind, and spirit, especially the heart and brain. Scaling down from large functional magnetic resonance imaging (MRI) machines to ultrasmall microchip recorders, the violin-like intimacy by which human responses to stimuli can be associated with healing effects is limited only by the imagination. Implantable, wearable, and injectable forms of technology are in continuous development and conceivably capable of reading human emotional states, especially related to cortisol levels in saliva (Borreli, 2014). With preprogrammed musical and poetic sounds and visual sensations already matched with previous healing successes, it is possible that the stressed body, mind, and spirit could be automatically exposed to such sensations via virtual reality as cortisol levels rise. Many currently built environments for healthcare generally lack architectural and artistic consideration for the human spirit, and seem to be designed more for the convenience of the provider versus the experience of the receiver. Audiovisual technology is easily and cost-effectively capable of creating unique and personalized patient spaces that promote peace, comfort, and healing beyond that of medical intervention. Examples of recreating past environments for persons with dementia are enhancing daily functioning and memory recall for these individuals through use of virtual reality. Such examples exist in various European communities. These, coupled with music, dance, and other forms of art appreciation, seem to be capable of accessing parts of the brain that do not depend on executive function, but rather on returning the mind to events and sensations that were pleasurable and healing, long before the brain was compromised by Alzheimer's, for example. Healing care plans that include favorite colors, artists, musicians, music, and poetry genres, as well as preferred environments, can all be included in a patient history, and acted upon via technological re-creation of stress-relieving sensations. But even without sophisticated technology, the nurse who takes time to understand the rhythms to which an autistic individual favorably responds, and paces nursing interventions to those rhythms, will likely achieve more healing than otherwise possible. The nurse who creatively text messages a question to a teenage patient engrossed in listening to music, without demanding a verbal interaction, may create a level of trust and communication that is appreciated by the patient. Low- and high-tech possibilities for incorporating, or not interrupting, music and rhythm as a healing mode seem to be endless and easily achievable.

CONCLUSION

Opportunities for nurses to reconsider the value of music and poetry in their caring/healing practices can be found in the foregoing concepts of allowing for nonimmediate, and sometimes nonexistent, feedback to care interventions. Like a music or poetry performer, a certain level of nursing trust is required that caring/healing reciprocity is in effect, and that feelings of caring and healing are distinguishable from healing actions.

At times, the profession of nursing still seems to struggle with misinterpretation of its purpose, meanings, and achievements. However, music and poetry likely have a longer history of being wide open to a variety of responses, and may still have significant influence on the continuing evolution of humankind. Likewise, the concept of caring is probably as important to human evolutionary development as any dominant force related to survival of the fittest, or, in more modern terms, survival of the richest. An ominous impersonality of some large corporations "too big to care" may also dwell within some corporations whose missions could be related in some way to the healthcare industry. It is imperative that we, as nurses, listen carefully to the tune being played.

Finally, there is likely an abundance of experience in music and poetry that nurses and their caring colleagues can enjoy, as much for its personal value as that of its therapeutic value for patients and their families. Such appreciation also seems to require a certain level of courage and spontaneity to transform the value of music and poetry into caring and healing.

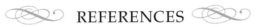 REFERENCES

Blumenthal, S. (1992, March 9). Springtime for Buchanan. *The New Republic, 206*(10), 22–25.

Borreli, L. (2014, June). *Smartphone stress hormone test app may be able to measure cortisol levels.* International Society of Endocrinology and Endocrine Society, Annual Meeting, Chicago, IL.

Chavis, G. (2011). *Poetry and story: The healing power of creative expression.* London, UK: Jessica Kingsley.

Crossan, F., & Robb, A. (1998). Role of the nurse: Introducing theories and concepts. *British Journal of Nursing, 7*(10), 608–612. doi:10.12968/bjon.1998.7.10.5687

Dean, P. J. (2016). Nursing considerations for an emerging and enlarging symbiosis between technology and integrative human health: Need for a systematized base for caring science. *International Journal for Human Caring, 20*(4), 171–175. doi:10.20467/1091-5710-20.4.171

Gilligan, C. (1993). *In a different voice: Psychological theory and women's development.* London, UK: Harvard University Press. (Original work published 1982)

Leininger, M. (1991). (Ed.). *Culture care diversity and universality: A theory of nursing.* New York, NY: National League for Nursing.

Noddings, N. (1984). *Caring: A feminine approach to ethics and moral education.* Oakland: University of California Press.

Reverby, S. (1987). A caring dilemma: Womanhood and nursing in historical perspective. *Nursing Research, 36*(1), 5–11. doi:10.1097/00006199-198701000-00003

Seamon, T. (2011). Too big to care? [Blog post]. Retrieved from http://learningvoyager.blogspot.com/2011/05/too-big-to-care.html

Whitcome, D. (2016, April 13). Letter: Gonda Singers helped make the best of health problems, clinic visits. *Rochester Post Bulletin.* Retrieved from http://www.postbulletin.com/opinion/letters/letter-gonda-singers-helped-make-best-of-health-problems-clinic/article_182433d5-978f-5b17-9479-a1f69ffc73a0.html

Zahourek, R. P. (2016). Men in nursing: Intention, intentionality, caring, and healing. *Holistic Nursing Practice, 30*(5), 247–256. doi:10.1097/HNP.0000000000000162

46

The Interplay of Integrative Nursing, Caring Science, and Healing Environments

Mary Jo Kreitzer and Terri Zborowsky

The concept of healing environments is not new. Florence Nightingale, the founder of modern nursing, described the role of the nurse as putting the patient in the best possible condition so that nature can act and self-healing occur (Dossey, 2000). Nightingale had a deep appreciation for the importance of the environment that surrounds that patient as well as the inner environment of the nurse. Both have an impact on healing. She wrote about the importance of physical attributes of the environment such as natural light, fresh air, noise reduction, variety of form, color, and infection control as well as the nursing presence, caring, and spirituality. Her philosophy embodied the notion that people have the innate capacity to heal and our role as nurses is to create the conditions that support healing. Just as evidence-based practice informs clinical decision making, evidence-based design impacts the decision making of the planning and construction of healthcare facilities. The science underlying healing environments is emerging from many disciplines including nursing, interior design, architecture, neuroscience, psychoneuroimmunology, and environmental psychology, among others.

Nightingale's philosophy is reflected in the Optimal Healing Environment (OHE) model developed by Zborowsky and Kreitzer (2009) and depicted in Figure 46.1. A healing environment is created through a deep and dynamic interplay between people, place, process and culture. In this model, the "people" element includes the caregivers and support team that surround the patient. The "process and culture" element refers to the care processes as well as the leadership processes that support a culture that is aligned with creating an OHE. The "place" element focuses on the physical space where care is provided and the geography that surrounds the patient, family, and caregiver. Each of these elements of a healing environment is examined in this chapter within the broader framework of integrative nursing and Caring Science.

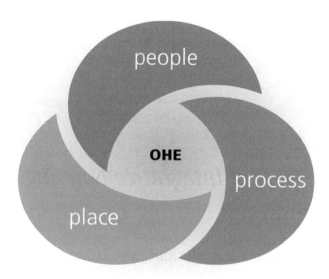

FIGURE 46.1 People, place, and process: The role of place in creating optimal healing environments.

Source: Zborowsky, T. & Kreitzer, M. J. (2009). People, place, and process: The role of place in creating optimal healing environments. *Creative Nursing: A Journal of Values, Issues, Experience & Collaboration,* *15*(4), 186–190. doi:10.1891/1078-4535.15.4.186

INTEGRATIVE NURSING AND CARING SCIENCE

Integrative nursing is a whole-person/whole-system way of being-knowing-doing that advances the health and well-being of persons, families, and communities through caring/healing relationships (Kreitzer & Koithan, 2014). Six principles of integrative nursing shape and inform nursing practice:

1. Human beings are whole systems, inseparable from their environments.

2. Human beings have the innate capacity for health and well-being.

3. Nature has healing and restorative properties that contribute to health and well-being.

4. Integrative nursing is person-centered and relationship-based.

5. Integrative nursing practice is informed by evidence and uses the full range of therapeutic modalities to support/augment the healing process, moving from least intensive/invasive to more, depending on need and context.

6. Integrative nursing focuses on the health and well-being of caregivers as well as those they serve.

The Caritas Processes®, as delineated by Watson (2008), are aligned with the integrative nursing principles, and Caring Science with the emphasis on the unitary nature of human beings provides a strong philosophical foundation for integrative nursing. Caring Science encompasses the universals of human caring, whereas integrative nursing encompasses the universals of human healing. Together, they provide a foundation for practice, including the creation of healing environments for patients, families, and caregivers.

APPLYING INTEGRATIVE NURSING AND CARING SCIENCE TO CREATE HEALING ENVIRONMENTS

According to the first principle of integrative nursing, people are inextricably connected to their environment. From a healthcare design perspective, it is important that the space that is created facilitate the nurse's ability to maintain the integrity of the environment by monitoring and controlling noise, smells, and temperature and providing adequate space for family and caregivers. It is also critical to provide privacy. This is becoming easier to do with the growth of single-bed rooms. Single-bed rooms are also associated with reduced hospital-acquired infections, reduced medical errors, reduced patient falls, and improved patient sleep (Chaudhury, Mahmood, & Valente, 2005).

Optimally, there should be an ability to personalize the environment through art, use of personal objects such as photos or cards from family and friends, and accommodation of patient preferences where possible. The space should be designed to promote independence, safety, and choice. Innovations in design that reflect these new standards include art selection carts, digital art, and the capacity to control the ambient lighting in patient rooms. For example, children, their family members, and staff have the ability to control the window shades and aspects of the lighting system in the patient rooms at Masonic Children's Hospital in Minneapolis, Minnesota—even the ability to change the color of the ceiling!

From the caregiver perspective, decentralized charting and supplies increase staff caregiver effectiveness and efficiency. Appropriate lighting reduces the incidence of medication errors, ceiling lifts reduce staff injuries, and planning respite areas for staff reduces stress. Physical modifications in space directly impact patient and staff outcomes. Beyond physical space, the first principle also encompasses whole-person care and the importance of nurses comprehensively assessing all domains of health including physical, emotional, psychological, social, and spiritual. Ultimately, it is not only what the nurse does but also all that the nurse embodies as the nurse herself or himself is an integral part of the environment. The nurses' attitudes, actions, and body language significantly impact patients and their families. To be a healing presence, there are mind/body approaches that can help the nurse remain calm, centered, and fully present.

The second principle of integrative nursing focuses on our innate capacity for health and well-being. People have the capacity to heal from deep psychological, emotional, and spiritual traumas and the accompanying grief, loss, anger, despair, and sadness. Kindness, compassion, caring, and love are human processes that can support healing when they are offered by others and when we care for ourselves in this way. Examples of care processes that support the innate capacity of the body to heal include the following: nurturing hope, trust, and belief; facilitating connections and relationships that lead to deeper meaning and wholeness; engaging and supporting patient and family strengths; and the nurse focusing on intention for healing and wholeness during ordinary nursing procedures.

The third principle focuses on the healing and restorative properties of nature. Edward O. Wilson (1984) was among the first to describe the concept of "biophilia." Biophilia is the inherent inclination to "affiliate" with natural systems and processes. As human beings, we are innately drawn to nature and the natural world. Biophilia has grown into a broader framework that increasingly is shaping the design of human-made environments, including hospitals and other healthcare facilities. Biophilic design emphasizes maintaining, enhancing, and restoring the beneficial experience of nature, and does so through the use of environmental features that embody such characteristics of the natural world as color, water, sunlight, plants, natural materials, and exterior views and vistas (Kellert, 2008). Examples of access to nature in healthcare facilities include art and murals, views to nature, nature videos, water features, healing gardens, labyrinths, and therapeutic horticulture, among others.

The fourth principle of integrative nursing focuses on the importance of being person-centered and relationship-based. This requires knowing a person's story, context, and culture to anticipate needs and personalize care. This principle is manifested in processes of care such as greeting patients and family members by name, using appropriate eye contact and touch, and anticipating and supporting needs and preferences. From a leadership perspective, it is supported through developing staffing and scheduling patterns that facilitate continuity of relationships and care. Facility design that is person-centered and relationship-based focuses on creating work spaces that are proximal to patients and that do not position healthcare providers with their backs to patients for extended periods of time. Design should honor the work of the nurses while allowing them space to form a relationship with the patients and their families. It also should provide ease of access to amenities that support the delivery of care.

The fifth principle addresses using the full range of conventional and integrative approaches, moving from least intensive and invasive to more, depending on the patient's needs and preferences. In a healing environment, nurses manage symptoms such as pain, anxiety, and nausea by offering both pharmacological and nonpharmacological approaches including aromatherapy, mind/body therapies, and acupressure. Spaces are designed to anticipate using these approaches and required materials and supplies are readily available.

The sixth principle of integrative nursing focuses on the importance of care for caregivers. Within a healing environment, staff rooms are proximal to patient rooms so nurses can take breaks. The rooms have features of healing environments including natural light, art, comfortable furniture, and access to healthy food. In many facilities, respite rooms are also being created for staff that are quiet, restorative spaces where nurses can read, meditate, pray, listen to music, or journal.

CONCLUSION

Nurses are ultimately responsible for the environment of care and are in an optimal position to advocate for staff, care processes, and physical spaces that contribute to healing. Familiarity with the literature on evidence-based design as well as practice will prepare nurses to be more effective participants in facility planning and design teams as well as nursing and organizational leadership. As Nightingale advocated, nurses are in the best position, through observation and research, to understand how the designed environment impacts their patients during the act of nursing and through this knowledge fully leverage people, place, and process to create an OHE (Zborowsky, 2014).

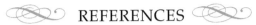

REFERENCES

Chaudhury, H., Mahmood, A., & Valente, M. (2005). Advantages and disadvantages of single versus multiple occupancy rooms in acute care environments: A review and analysis of the literature. *Environment Behavior, 37*(6), 760–786. doi:10.1177/0013916504272658

Dossey, B. M. (2000). *Florence Nightingale: Mystic, visionary, healer.* Springhouse, PA: Springhouse.

Kellert, S. R. (2008). Dimensions, elements and attributes of biophilic design. In S. R. Kellert, J. H. Heerwagen, & M. L. Mador (Eds.), *Biophilic design: The theory, science and practice of bringing buildings to life* (pp. 3–19). Hoboken, NJ: John Wiley.

Kreitzer, M. J., & Koithan, M. (Eds.). (2014). *Integrative nursing.* New York, NY: Oxford University Press.

Watson, J. (2008). *Nursing: The philosophy and science of caring.* Boulder: University of Colorado Press.

Wilson, E. O. (1984). *Biophilia: The human bond with other species.* Cambridge, MA: Harvard University Press.

Zborowsky, T., & Kreitzer, M.J. (2009). People, place, and process: The role of place in creating optimal healing environments. *Creative Nursing: A Journal of Values, Issues, Experience & Collaboration, 15*(4), 186–190. doi:10.1891/1078-4535.15.4.186

Zborowsky, T. (2014). The legacy of Florence Nightingale's environmental theory: Nursing research focusing on the impact of healthcare environments. *Health Environments Research & Design Journal, 7*(4), 19–34. doi:10.1177/193758671400700404

47

Remembering Purpose: An Autoethnography

Anna Biley

In 1995, I received a scholarship from the Florence Nightingale Foundation in London, funding a month's study at the Centre for Human Caring in Denver, Colorado. The experience was life transforming and what began to unfold then became integral to every aspect of life since. In 2012, life invited me to live Caring Science at a deeper and more personal level than I ever thought was possible, as I cared for my terminally ill husband. Embracing human caring, living the Caritas Processes® took me to the brink of excruciating pain and profound peace. It was a paradox of heartfelt moments of love and light and messy, painful, lonely days. Being truly present and holding caring intention in practice often meant absorbing hurt, frustration, and sadness. Frequently the *self* as described in the Caritas Processes (Watson, 2008) was invisible, as the world seemed to be asking more of me than I could ever give. And yet, amid all this, I had the profound sense of remembering my purpose and that everything I had ever done, felt, and experienced was to live those days.

Dr. Francis Christopher Biley (Fran) was a nursing academic in the United Kingdom. He was known for his creative, challenging, and critical thinking as well as his radical teaching methods, much of it grounded in the Science of Unitary Human Beings (Rogers, 1970). Fran was a quiet, deep-thinking, and sensitive man who cherished stillness and a belief that events unfold as they are destined to do. When he was diagnosed with cancer, he said, "Well, if we are going to have to do this we are going to do it mindfully." His illness was short but from the outset, we endeavored to hold that intention.

My journal from that time reflects how, as Fran's illness unfolded, I was struck again and again by a realization that somehow, I *knew* what to do. The connection between dying and birth was a constant thread of personal remembering, which came from deep within the inner self. In anticipation of the unknown, I found myself "nesting," cleaning cupboards and sweeping the backyard, overwhelmed with an urgent need to create a safe space for my beloved ones. And in keeping vigil by his bedside, I understood how in life's transitions, the expectation of a last breath resonates with a baby's first gasp. These bizarre yet profound experiences reassured that I had done this before and if I trusted my body and my intuition, all would be well. Those moments of walking alongside, I came to call remembering purpose.

Remembering who we are as a discipline is a moral imperative for nursing and a vital quest that humanity requires of the profession (Watson, 2012). In a personal account, Watson (2005) described a journey of trauma, pain, and loss, which gave rise to a life-changing moment. "I was love … that was what I had come here to remember," going on to state, "I now believe my experience of becoming love is our true state of Belonging-Being-Becoming that we are all seeking to remember in our own way" (p. 73). The experience described by Watson and my own story suggest that it is in life's most vulnerable moments that we connect to our humanity at its deepest and, paradoxically, most simple and complex level. Furthermore, from personal experience, it may be suggested that Being in caring consciousness is also a journey of Becoming and that some transpersonal relationships and caring moments create a "soul-to-soul connection" (p. 73), breaking through to a deeper level of consciousness and oneness with the universe. It is in these moments that remembering purpose is manifest.

To further uncover the concept of remembering purpose and understand the personal experience in the context of Caring Science, a research study was undertaken as part of the Watson Caring Science Institute doctoral program. A comprehensive review of the literature revealed that remembering purpose is elusive and yet paradoxically "the universe is saturated with purpose" (Newman, 2008, p. 17), woven into concepts such as soul, spirituality, consciousness, knowing, and compassion and manifesting at points of "existential magnitude" (Massoudi, 2010, p. 212). Historically, women have naturally supported others in birth and death, and the primeval instinct to be alongside others in life transition is "in our bones" (Warner, 2013, p. 32). The literature highlighted how globally there is an emerging call to remember compassion as purpose and that, consistent with the ontology of Caring Science, remembering *who we are and why we are here* is at the heart of cultivating compassion (Halifax, 2008; Rinpoche, 1992).

Caring Science invites innovative methodologies that embrace the unknown and help us understand "what it means to be human" (Watson, 2012, p. 24) through a disciplinary lens of caring and healing. Exploring the most intimate human experiences, such as birth, death, joy, and grief, demands new research questions and creative research methods that offer scope for reflection and contemplation and may not necessarily seek to capture facts, but convey how a person feels. Consequently, research methods may engage poetry, art, metaphor, or music, inviting authenticity to reveal multiple truths and ways of knowing.

Grounded in a unitary Caring Science paradigm, the chosen methodology for the doctoral research study was autoethnography. Within this methodology, the self (*auto*) is systematically analyzed (*graphy*) within its own cultural experience (*ethno*; Ellis, Adams, & Bochner, 2011). Beginning and ending with personal experience and perspective, autoethnography requires the researchers to delve deep into their own lives and to cast the net wide within the cultural context, taking first an "ethnographic wide angled lens, focusing outward on social and cultural aspects of personal experience; then inward, exposing a vulnerable self that is moved by and may move through, refract, and resist cultural interpretation" (Ellis & Bochner, 2000, p. 739). Autoethnography invites the researcher to hold a mirror to self (Malthouse, 2011), critically deconstructing his or her own experience, contextualizing, and understanding his or her view of the world. A continuing and ever-changing process, it is characterized by the researcher zooming "backward and forward, inward and outward" as boundaries between the "personal and cultural become blurred, sometimes beyond distinct recognition" (Ellis & Bochner, 2000, p. 739). Through a systematic and analytical process, crafting and fusing the personal and the social context, it is a "distinct research approach to the study of human experience" (Denzin, 2014, p. 7). By focusing on "small facts" (the personal), autoethnography may "aim to speak of larger issues" (Malthouse, 2011, p. 250) or, as Ellis and Bochner (2000) explained, "by exploring a particular life, I hope to understand a way of life" (p. 737).

As a methodology, autoethnography lends itself to a mosaic of methods. This study fused an autoethnographic life review method (Ellis, 2004) and a "cutup" technique, described by Fran (Biley, 1998, 2004, 2016). When using a life review approach, Ellis (2004) likened stories, journals, literature, photographs, art, songs, and artifacts to raw data, or field notes, with the key to the method being to "balance living in the moment with writing and reflecting on the moments in which I have lived" (p. 333). In other words, autoethnographic data may blend retrospective records with unfolding, current events, layering, and folding in facts with memory and feelings, emotion, and sensory stimulation to reveal an evocative text that weaves together experiences and emotions across time, personal truth, and meaning (Ellis, 2004).

Alongside the autoethnographic life review, the study to illuminate the personal experience of remembering purpose incorporated the cutup method described by Biley (2004, 2016). An exciting and innovative angle, offering a unitary, autoethnographic perspective in the context of Caring Science, the choice was deeply personal. As a Rogerian scholar, Fran presented the cutup technique as a potential unitary method of inquiry at the 7th Rogerian Conference in New York, in June 1998 (Biley, 1998). Over many years, he honed the craft of the cutup technique as a unitary approach to teaching and scholarly work and true to his pandimensional style, this continued with posthumous publications (Biley, 2016).

As a literary technique, cutups became popular in the 1960s when adopted by the American Beat Generation author William Burroughs. Frustrated by the limitations and control of language, Burroughs cut up text and randomly stuck it back together again, whilst also folding in other words and phrases, for example, from newspaper cuttings of the day (Biley, 1998, 2004, 2016). The purpose of this was to deconstruct and reconstruct language to create new meaning, discover new realities and consciousness, and more accurately describe the chaotic and nonlinear world around him.

Although the cutup technique is not on the basis of any other research tradition, it could be argued that there are some parallels with postmodernity, a paradigm in which language and thinking may be metaphoric rather than literal (Watson, 2005), in which field notes may be poetic accounts (Galvin & Prendergast, 2016) and research is not analyzed but experienced (Biley, 2004). Blending and enhancing the life review method (Ellis, 2004), the cutup method (Biley, 1998, 2004, 2016) was an opportunity to see past encounters and present realities in a new way, to bear witness and give voice to the personal experience of remembering purpose. Drawing on "stories at the edge of intimate memory" that "reside in the space between the mythical and everyday" (Patti, 2012, p. 157), retrospective records were positioned with unfolding, current events, and a narrative of a unitary, autoethnographic experience in the context of Caring Science was crafted.

Through a reflexive lens of Caring Science and the Caritas Processes, I pondered the experience of remembering purpose and how the seeds had been nurtured in my nursing practice, early family experiences, and other life events. Revisiting and recounting a story of journeying with Fran as he chose a path of mindfulness and conscious dying and struggling to remember purpose in the dark days of grief gave voice to raw pain and vulnerability. Data were drawn from notes, personal journals, reflective writing, poetry, art, literature, photographs, and emails. All were layered into the text, reviewed, and edited, continually folding in memories, dreams, and emotions, to create a pandimensional narrative of remembering purpose, drawing on past, present, and future, portrayed as a snapshot in the now. One of Fran's greatest loves was being in the small woodland space adjacent to our garden. Here he would carve sculptures and symbols from reclaimed wood. Through photography and commissioned art, this was captured and incorporated into the data. The seasons of the woodland and the natural breakdown and decay of his woodwork became a metaphor for life and grief. The commissioned work captured the transformative "unitary rhythm of dying-grieving" (Malinski, 2012, p. 239) and in doing so created a gift of new life and meaning.

As a research tool, the cutup method deconstructed and simultaneously reconstructed the life review narrative, bearing witness and giving voice to the experience of remembering purpose, with the most personal elements of the story emerging intuitively to become 12 poetic/narrative cutups. Consistent with the intention of remembering purpose and the Caritas Processes of being authentically present and open to mystery, the cutups were done by hand, mindfully, reflectively, and as a meditation. In a quiet space, a candle was lit and over a period of approximately 3 hours for each cutup, the text was randomly cut up, rearranged, and pasted onto paper. It was then transposed as a document in Microsoft Word. Dwelling with the text, words and phrases were highlighted and as it was read out loud, clues to hidden or new meaning and emotion emerged. The highlighted text was then copied and deconstructed further, with the aim of crafting a narrative of remembering purpose, the Caritas Processes, and Caring Science. In keeping with the chaotic and nonlinear ethos of the cutup method, the order of the words was never changed but as the text was read and reread many times, aloud and in silence, words emerged and were strung together in a new way, offering fresh thoughts and insights, new realities, and consciousness (Biley, 1998, 2004, 2016). Throughout the text, photographs of places and symbols were layered in to support the story, adding a creative dimension and visual aesthetic, illustrating Fran's art and love of woodland spaces. Cutups of the commissioned art were positioned alongside the cutup text to further illuminate and express transformation, new ways of knowing, being, becoming, and mystery (Watson, 2008, 2012), as seen in Figures 47.1 and 47.2. Transforming the data into metaphorical, poetic accounts supported both the claim that "life is a cut up, full of random interjections" (Biley, 2004, p. 142) and a Caring Science position that research inquiry should allow for "evocative, metaphoric, even poetic language to accurately express and convey/communicate human life experience" (Watson, 2012, p. 93).

The cutups stand alone as an authentic voice and speak for themselves, inviting the reader to experience the meaning and significance of the research, a testimony to the embodiment of remembering purpose and of the ethics and values of Caring Science. But

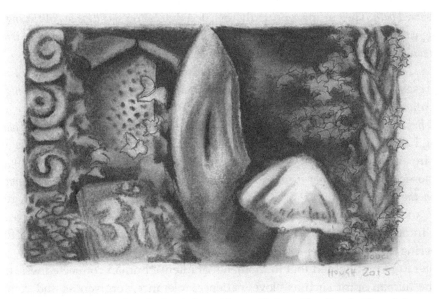

FIGURE 47.1 Symbols and carvings. (Painted by Sarah Hough.)

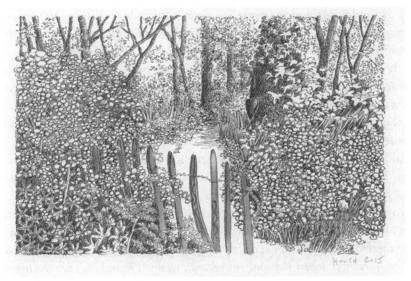

FIGURE 47.2 Woodland gate. (Painted by Sarah Hough.)

how does the study contribute to disciplinary understanding and what does it tell us about intentional caring presence, the Caritas Processes, and authentic caring moments?

Reflecting on the cutups as research findings, it was poignant to see that *remembering purpose has been constant threads, secretly stored, connecting across time* and *caring theory, spreading out its roots*, has remained *a source of strength and patience*. Caring Science "connects with philosophies that invite love and caring through ethics of Being, Becoming and Belonging" (Watson, 2005, p. 139). Being with another in conscious dying was woven with a journey of becoming in remembering purpose; as the cutups suggest, *immersed in the poet, I explored*

Being as sacred path. The cutups repeatedly revealed that being *sensitive to cultivating patience, awakening care, love, intention, and ethically disciplined behavior* are the *teachings of true Caritas* and that *wisdom and ethics is somehow the key to ensuring caring values.*

From a Caring Science perspective, the cutups suggest that manifestations of authentic caring presence cocreated a healing environment, as *nursing transformed into living purpose. In anticipation of uncertainty, sacred secure space was authentic, reflecting a place of remembering Fran's wishes. I washed his suffering, focused fully on love, intimacy, and comfort ... the blanket was me.* Being fully present, keeping vigil, cocreating ritual, and offering gentleness and compassion are among the most devotional acts of love (Kübler-Ross & Kessler, 2000). The cutups disclosed that in *keeping vigil* and creating *ritual in sacred space, I lived human Caring Science in the silent sense of dignity, in ministering loving care.* In living Caritas, reverently assisting and serving human needs as sacred acts (Watson, 2008), the *privilege* of being together in *intimacy, human-to-human* in a loving, trusting, caring relationship, fostered a remembering, even *across deep raging storms.*

The literature highlighted that in moments of intense human connectedness, the qualities of the human spirit such as "love, patience, tolerance, forgiveness and compassion" (Dalai Lama, 1999, p. 22) come to the fore and individuals may connect with their soul purpose, remembering *who we are and why we are here* (Halifax, 2008; Rinpoche, 1992). The cutups suggest that these qualities are also characteristics of remembering purpose and Caritas. For example, as a young woman, *conscious dying led me to compassion, curiosity, and desire to explore,* and revealed an *inherent devotion to simple humanity ... touch, tenderness, and peace.* In *walking alongside in caring, healing, love, and light, I remembered.*

In embodying Caritas values, the data collection embraced transformative and aesthetic approaches to inquiry by engaging poetry, art, photography, and music to reveal multiple truths and ways of knowing. It is not surprising, therefore, that in connecting these mediums, metaphors emerged to support a language of Caring Science and an *autoethnography, capturing gems of miracles and jewels of poetry.* Fran's love for art and aesthetics of caring, embodied in his own nursing and teaching practice, emerged in the cutups as, *his paintings spoke, poetry. Thinning, churning human pigments came together, my heart in intimacy. Theory on the canvas. A picture emerging—nursing, mindful touch, cancer. Aesthetic indeed.*

Interestingly, the cutups gave rise to challenges and paradoxes, often offering up an opposite perspective to the written text. For example, when I wrote that I am not afraid, the cutups suggested otherwise—*I am there, afraid* and *as he transitioned, I was alone.* In *the paradox of the unknown, when the soul reared with chaos, I found myself creating the home, to sustain love and safety.* Reflecting on the apparent contradiction between the narrative and the cutups, it is increasingly clear that this autoethnography of remembering purpose is equally a story of riding the waves of uncertainty, grief, love, and loss. Throughout the autoethnography, moments of clarity, stillness, and peace are juxtaposed with pain, loneliness, and bewilderment ... *all will be well ... bearing fear body and soul, tears welled up in confusion.* Reflecting the literature, I hoped that holding the moment with loving intention (Rinpoche, 1992) meant accepting the waves of chaos and uncertainty, along with a peace and inner knowing that felt "a lot like remembering" (Beck, 1999, p. 298), and in doing so endeavoring "to learn not to drown in those waves but to ride them freely" (Halifax, 2008, p. 150).

In being authentically present, the values of the Caritas Processes invite listening, valuing, and holding the other's story, allowing for the expression of positive and negative feelings (Watson, 2008). As *unfolding moments held witness, ways of being, strong, and simple echoed the deepest places of the heart.* However, the stillness and intention conveyed in the narrative is turned on its head as the cutups reveal hidden exhaustion, a sense of failure, and of never being enough—*He took my all. I tried.* Compassion in dying "often means bearing witness to and accepting the unbearable and the unacceptable" (Halifax, 2008, p. 154). This autoethnography suggests that in *the patience of living Caritas,* there is pain, rawness, loneliness, and grief and in this scenario, *my own vulnerability was the teacher.*

Having dwelt in the concept of remembering purpose for a 3-year duration of doctorate study, I have come to understand how much it is also an embodiment of grief and vulnerability. Indeed in remembering purpose, I have been more vulnerable than I ever thought was possible. From a Caring Science perspective, in a postmodern qualitative research paradigm, vulnerability is strength, and although it may challenge, breach, and fracture the writer (Ellis & Bochner, 2000), engaging in the research is a moral and ethical act (Frank, 2013), bearing witness and giving voice to human experience. An expectation of the ethics of the chosen methodology is that the researcher does no harm to self (and others), an echo of the Caritas values of sustaining loving kindness and compassion (Watson, 2008). As *grief rumbles on* and *mud settles,* the metaphor of the labyrinth tells of *how a broken heart heals ... in the uncertain hour, I walk. Witnessing labyrinths in nature, I remember purpose. Stillness, healing, and patience tie my heart to life. All is well.* With the support of academic supervisors, I was encouraged to embrace the Caritas Processes and once again be open to mystery and the unknown. An echo of the authentic, feminine voice, words, and images emerged unexpectedly in the cutups as *Mother became consciousness. Lost and in need of love, I was wounded. In tatters, purpose determined that I reach out. Crying out for remembering purpose when dreams are shattered, I walk in sacred space.* However, the most visceral and authentic words revealed—*a single mum, no one ever told me that when sadness descends, swirling pain reflects loving relationships ... tossed amidst the chaos of howled, unsettled parenting, in grief, in caring, my life fractured. Every day I was her author.*

At the heart of unitary Caring Science, the human-to-human, soul-to-soul connection is a manifestation of oneness, captured in moments of compassion and intentional caring presence (Watson, 2005). Living in Caritas, the study was an account of those moments and a relationship in which *a deep knowing and intuition led us to create our own poetry.* Remembering purpose from a Caring Science perspective is a unitary, ongoing, and forever unfolding encounter, where *before is part of the now and what we lived then will be part of the future.* Throughout the autoethnographic process, the research methods have embodied a unitary paradigm, in which wholeness is "not an ideal but a given" (Cowling, 2012, p. 121). As I pondered *caring presence and pattern manifestation,* the findings reflect the ebb and flow of connection and separation in life transition described by Malinski (2012). An ongoing pattern of connectedness, in *ancient remembering,* I *repatterned birth* and *I prepared to die. Like fine wrinkles, pattern became his truth,* as we prepared to "make a transition from loving in presence to loving in absence. And we reweave that lasting love into the larger, richly complex fabric of our lives" (Malinski, 2012, p. 242).

My doctorate journey began by recounting an experience, which I came to call "remembering purpose." As the cutups revealed, *mystery weaves, memory twinges,* and *as I listened to event unfold, I started remembering ... I had done it before. In vigil, across deep raging storms, I experienced lifetimes and I knew.* This acknowledgment of *destiny* echoes Rilke's (1934/1993) image that "the future enters into us in order to transform itself in us long before it happens" (p. 65). The metaphor of walking the labyrinth, *the same path of tears, hope, and joy,* invites the conclusion that remembering purpose is not new knowledge but a deep, personal recognition of what is already known. A narrative of love, grief, tears, and joy, ongoing and forever unfolding, the study was an act of Caritas. The cutups stand alone as witness to the personal experience of remembering purpose from a unitary Caring Science perspective as the following example illustrates:

> *Remembering purpose is how a broken heart heals.*
> *The sensation is like resilience, strength and patience,*
> *shaking memory. Stay awake, unfolding moments witness*
> *walking alongside is what you are here to do.*
> *Unitary consciousness, like remembering purpose,*
> *will be sensitive to cultivating patience.*
> *Human Caring Science must be lived,*
> *in walking alongside - there is sad peace.*
> *Ways of being, deep knowing and intuition,*
> *poetry, ethically disciplined behaviour, loving kindness,*
> *became remembering purpose,*
> *re-arranging, re-patterning time and mind.*
> *Remembering purpose,*
> *awaken care, love, intention.*
> *Mother becoming consciousness.*
> *Be still. Allow what you know to come to the fore.*
> *Walking alongside, wash suffering, take small steps,*
> *it is the same path of tears, hope and joy.*
> *Re-patterning birth, sacred feminine,*
> *strength and mystery in purpose.*
> *All is connected in the labyrinth,*
> *memories, mindful touch, transcended pain,*
> *simple humanity, compassion, silent dignity, caring presence.*
> *Nursing transformed into living purpose.*
> *Ancient remembering.*

An embodiment of remembering purpose, the doctorate study was a response to the moral imperative of Caring Science, for nursing as a discipline, to reawaken and remember the sacred covenant that it holds with humanity (Watson, 2012). Capturing moments of compassion and intentional caring presence (Watson, 2005), the study presented remembering purpose as a new concept and the autoethnographic cutups a unique research method for Caring Science. The findings presented in the cutups reflect and are consistent with the Caritas Processes, offering a unique poetry and language of Caritas.

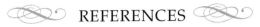

REFERENCES

Beck, M. (1999). *Expecting Adam: A true story of birth, rebirth, and everyday magic*. London, UK: Piatkus.

Biley, F. C. (1998, June 19–21). *An experiment in accessing pandimensionality: The literary poetics and deconstruction techniques of William S Burroughs applied to the science of Unitary Human Beings*. Unpublished paper presented to the 7th Rogerian Conference, Nursing and the Changing Person-Environment, New York, NY.

Biley, F. C. (2004). Postmodern literary poetics of experience: A new form of aesthetic enquiry. In F. Rapport (Ed.), *New qualitative methodologies in health and social care research* (pp. 139–149). London, UK: Routledge.

Biley, F. C. (2016). Waking up following breast surgery: An insight from the Beats, Burroughs and the cut up technique. In K. T. Galvin & M. Prendergast (Eds.), *Poetic inquiry II* (pp. 205–210). Rotterdam, Netherlands: Sense.

Cowling, W. R. (2012). Healing as appreciating wholeness. In W. K. Cody (Ed), *Philosophical and theoretical perspectives for advanced nursing practice* (5th ed., pp. 119–137). Burlington, MA: Jones & Bartlett.

Dalai Lama, H. H. (1999). *Ancient wisdom, modern world*. London, UK: Little, Brown.

Denzin, N. K. (2014). *Interpretive autoethnography*. London, UK: Sage.

Ellis, C. (2004). *The Ethnographic I*. Oxford, UK: Altamira Press.

Ellis, C., Adams, T., & Bochner, A. P. (2011). Autoethnography: An overview. *Qualitative Social Research*, *12*(1), 1–14. Retrieved from http://www.qualitative-research.net/index.php/fqs/article/view/1589/3095

Ellis, C., & Bochner, A. P. (2000). Autoethnography, personal narrative, reflexivity: Researcher as subject. In N. K. Denzin & Y. S. Lincoln (Eds.), *Handbook of qualitative research* (2nd ed., pp. 733–768). Thousand Oaks, CA: Sage.

Frank, A. W. (2013). *The wounded storyteller* (2nd ed.). Chicago, IL: University of Chicago Press.

Galvin, K. T., & Prendergast, M. (2016). Introduction. In K. T. Galvin & M. Prendergast (Eds.), *Poetic inquiry II* (pp. xi–xvii). Rotterdam, Netherlands: Sense.

Halifax, J. (2008). *Being with dying*. Boston, MA: Shambhala.

Kübler-Ross, E., & Kessler, D. (2000). *Life lessons*. London, UK: Simon & Schuster.

Malinski, V. M. (2012). Meditations on the unitary rhythm of dying-grieving. *Nursing Science Quarterly*, *25*(3), 239–244. doi:10.1177/0894318412447566

Malthouse, M. (2011). An autoethnography on shifting relationships between a daughter, her mother and Alzheimer's dementia (in any order). *Dementia*, *10*(2), 249–256. doi:10.1177/1471301211407626

Massoudi, M. (2010). Reflections on dying, our last thought(s) and living a spiritual life. *Journal of Humanistic Psychology*, *50*(2), 197–223. doi:10.1177/0022167809342550

Newman, M. A. (2008). *Transforming presence: The difference that nursing makes*. Philadelphia, PA: F. A. Davis.

Patti, C. J. (2012). Split shadows: Myths of a lost father and son. *Qualitative Inquiry*, *18*(2), 153–161. doi:10.1177/1077800411429091

Rilke, R. M. (1993). *Letters to a young poet*. New York, NY: W. W. Norton. (Original work published 1934)

Rinpoche, S. (1992). *The Tibetan book of living and dying*. London, UK: Rider.

Rogers, M. E. (1970). *An introduction to the theoretical basis of nursing*. Philadelphia, PA: F. A. Davis.

Warner, F. (2013). *The soul midwives' handbook*. London, UK: Hay House.

Watson, J. (2005). *Caring science as sacred science*. Philadelphia, PA: F. A. Davis.

Watson, J. (2008). *Nursing: The philosophy and science of caring* (Rev. ed.). Boulder: University Press of Colorado.

Watson, J. (2012). *Human Caring Science*. Sudbury, MA: Jones & Bartlett.

48

Caring Science and Yoga: The Human Caring Science Kosha Model

Andy Davies

One does not accidentally blend Watson's Human Caring Science theory with a Yoga theory. This chapter and the merging of these two theories is the culmination of the many pathways I have followed, pathways that have diverged and converged over nearly 20 years of nursing education and Yoga teaching. I explore, in this chapter, how I came about interweaving Watson's Human Caring Science theory with a medieval Yoga model to underpin a first year's, first semester bachelor of nursing course in Australia. With this background contextualized, I describe the traditional Yogic Kosha Model, its adaptation, and then my blending of it with Watson's Caritas Processes®. Following on from this, I then outline the Australian context and the course within which these two holistic theories were applied. I conclude the chapter with a discussion on the adaptation of Watson's Caring Science to construct new knowledge (epistemology) and ways of being (ontology), while upholding the imperative of values (axiology) such as caring in nursing and society.

BACKGROUND

I first came across Jean Watson when I was a part-time PhD candidate slowly making sense of my data and my way as novice educational researcher. The intention of my research study was to construct a greater understanding and appreciation of senior Western Yoga teacher-trainers' considerations when conceptualizing, planning, and implementing Modern Yoga teacher-training programs. At that time, I was living and working in Doha, Qatar; this particular position was my fifth nursing education role functioning as part of a multi-disciplinary team establishing a women and children's hospital. At this point in time, I had been a Yoga practitioner and teacher for greater than a decade. I had been fortunate enough to attend 11 Yoga teacher and therapy trainings across the globe. I had, as well, established and ran for a decade what was the first expatriate Yoga school in Riyadh, Saudi Arabia. I did this while being the nursing director for nursing education at a Saudi military cardiac hospital. By day, I managed and taught nursing lectures, courses, and workshops to expatriate and Saudi nurses. At night and during weekends, I conducted Yoga classes and workshops primarily to expatriates. After 13 years in Saudi Arabia, I had conducted greater than 2,000 hours of Yoga and meditation instruction and 7,000 hours of nursing lectures.

One of the primary tasks of the Qatari women and children's hospital project was to establish a world-class institution in the provision of care for Qatari nationals. It was in this context, while writing my thesis on Yoga pedagogy, I commenced a search for others who had explored the notion of care and caring in literature. As a nurse, as a nursing educator, and as a Yoga practitioner/teacher/researcher, I was keen to appreciate others' perceptions of caring. Caring, for me, underpinned nursing, nursing education, and Yoga teaching. During my searches, I quickly came across Jean Watson and her work. I was delighted to have identified a cosmology that aligned so well with my own perceptions of the world and of care. My discovery of Watson's body of work, epistemologically opened up for me new ways of considering Yoga and nursing education. Furthermore, I very much appreciated, pedagogically, Caring Science's Caritas Processes and how they scaffolded the building of a caring individual.

YOGA, THE TRADITIONAL KOSHA MODEL, AND ITS ADAPTION

If asked to describe what Yoga is, many in Western English-speaking countries would probably describe it as a physical practice where practitioners become more limber by performing certain postures, referred to as "asana." However, in the historical sense, Yoga had a very different purpose. Yoga is, ultimately, a soteriological practice (Burley, 2007; Jain, 2014). That is, it is a religious practice where the individual is working toward salvation of her or his soul through self-realization. However, it is not one practice; rather, it is a polytheistic, pluralistic series of practices and traditions that has arisen in India over the past three to five millennia (Feuerstein, 2008). In the modern era, particularly in the West, these philosophies and teachings have undergone a series of reinterpretations, resulting from cultural and societal needs, colonial influences, transnational and transcultural translocation, and business commodification forces. The most prevalent representation and understanding of Yoga in its modern incarnation are those of the practice of asana. This is also referred to as "Modern Postural Yoga" (Alter, 2004). The Kosha Model, as described in this chapter, arose out of an earlier, pre-Westernized, precolonized, precommodified period.

The Kosha Model, drawn from medieval Yoga teachings, was originally described in Sanskrit, the liturgical language of Yoga. This model considered that the human body was perceived as being made up of Atman (an essence or soul) and five interconnecting, interpermeating, and interdependent layers. "Kosha" can be translated from Sanskrit to mean "layer" or "sheath" (Stone, 2012). Any changes or stimulus to one kosha-layer[1] subsequently had a ripple effect on the other four layers (Ashok & Thimmappa, 2006; Davies, 2014). As this model was described in the Sanskrit language, there exist a number of translations/ interpretations of the meaning or intent of each kosha-layer. Please refer to Figure 48.1.

---

[1] I recognize and acknowledge the tautology of "kosha-layer" used here and elsewhere; I rationalize this tautological use as assisting the reader's understanding of non-Western nomenclature and inherent meaning.

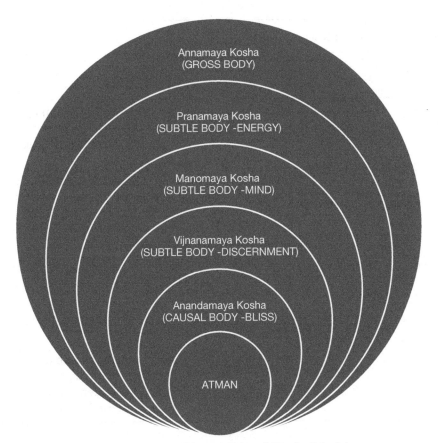

FIGURE 48.1 The traditional Kosha Model.

In the context of developing a holistic model for a nursing course, I made some changes to the traditional understanding of the Kosha Model. These modifications resulted from a number of important factors. I recognized that the Western, Australian, essentially secular nature of the academic nursing program would not easily incorporate a medieval Hindu construct that used Sanskrit language to describe it. Furthermore, I required the adapted model to function as a means of considering the ill individual as a complex system. As a result, I provided only English translations/ interpretations, removing Sanskrit terminology. I removed the notion of Atman (essence or soul), thus providing an understanding of a human being for religious, agnostic, and atheist student nurses. The deepest, most subtle layer, the Spiritual Layer—formerly the Anandamaya Kosha—seemed an adequate representation and trade-off for the redacted Atman. Finally, I contextualized individual anglicized kosha-layer descriptions to reflect concepts that were reflective of medical systems and the modern era. Please refer to Table 48.1.

Using a cross-disciplinary metaphor, this adapted Kosha Model allowed the nursing students to perceive the entire spectrum of an ill individual as a network, made up of five integrated relay systems. These individual, interpermeating relay systems could be considered a body-energy-mind-intellectual discernment-spiritual consciousness network. It is the balance of these kosha-layers that maintains health and equilibrium in the body. If one

TABLE 48.1 Adapted Kosha Model and Description

Traditional Kosha-Layer	Adapted Nursing Kosha-Layer	Adapted Description
Annamaya Kosha	Physical layer	This layer represents the overall physical nature of the body—that is, bones, muscles, and tendons, including bodily functions.
Pranamaya Kosha	Energetic layer	This layer considers the life force or energy that enervates all action within the body, for example, cardiac conduction, sympathetic and parasympathetic nervous systems, neurocardiac pathways, neurotransmitters, qi, chi, ki, prana.
Manomaya Kosha	Emotional layer	This layer oversees our emotional/affective traits at both conscious and unconscious strata.
Vijnanamaya Kosha	Intellectual layer	This layer is the source of intellect and our ability to be rational.
Anandamaya Kosha	Spiritual layer	This layer contains the source of spiritual consciousness, for example, religious, Wicca, ethical conviction—greenies, vegetarian, vegan, amnesty international.

layer is affected, it has a "domino" effect on all other integral, integrated layers (Feuerstein, 2008; Sartain, 2012). Care, if considered and delivered from a Kosha Model perspective, would have impact on many more levels than just the physical.

HUMAN CARING SCIENCE-KOSHA MODEL

The Human Caring Science-Kosha Model was designed to achieve two distinct purposes: first, to provide a scaffold for beginning nursing students to evolve a nursing consciousness that was contiguous with affective and intellectual skills—these being developed via the application of Watson's Human Caring Science and the Caritas Processes (Watson, 2012); second, to evolve an understanding that all human beings are composed of something greater than just their obvious physical presence—this understanding being developed via the discussion of the Kosha Model.

I shall not go into great depth here as Jean's models, no doubt, are discussed repeatedly in this text. I will note, however, that the Human Caring Science-Kosha Model is underpinned by the following: relational caring, the 10 Caritas Processes, transpersonal caring moments, and the affective qualities required of nurses for caring (Lane, Samuels, & Watson, 2012; Watson, 2008, 2012). Where the five-layered Kosha Model sits is within the transpersonal caring moments. Please refer to Figure 48.2.

How the Human Caring Science-Kosha Model was applied in our course is detailed later in this chapter. What was designed for the nursing students and the nursing academics was

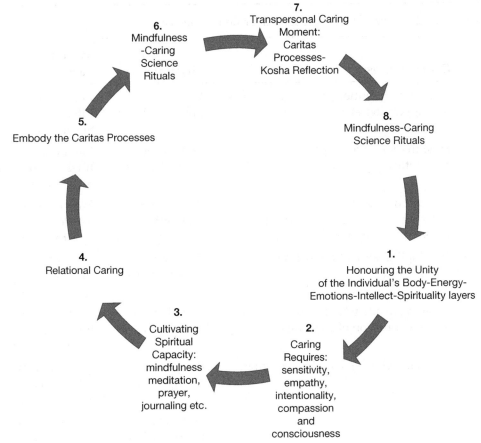

FIGURE 48.2 Human Caring Science-Kosha Model.

Sources: Adapted from Watson, J. (2008). *Nursing: The philosophy and science of caring* (Rev. ed.). Boulder, CO: University Press of Colorado; Watson, J. (2012). *Human caring science: A theory of nursing* (2nd. ed.). Sudbury, MA: Jones & Bartlett; Lane, M., Samuels, M., & Watson, J. (2012). *The caritas path to peace: A guidebook for creating world peace with caring, love, and compassion.* North Charleston, SC: CreateSpace Independent Publishing Platform.

the Caritas Process-Kosha-Layer Reflection tool. The tool systematically required the students to reflect on individual Caritas Processes and then consider the ill individual from the perspective of the five kosha-layers. Please note that the first two layers, the physical body layer and the energetic layer, were considered as physical layers. Meanwhile, we have considered the increasingly refined, less immediately discernible, possibly rarefied layers—the emotional, intellectual, and the spiritual layers—as metaphysical layers. Please refer to Table 48.2.

AUSTRALIAN CONTEXT

One of the early challenges of my new nursing academic role was to underpin a new course with a holistic nursing framework. Having spent many years working with an international cohort of nurses and nursing educators, I had expected to find an academic school of

TABLE 48.2 Caritas Process-Kosha-Layer Reflection Tool

No.	Caritas Process	Physical Layer	Metaphysical Layer
1.	Nurturing-intentioned altruistic values (loving-kindness)	Body layer Energetic layer	Emotional layer Intellectual layer Spiritual layer
2.	Enabling faith and hope (authentically present)	Body layer Energetic layer	Emotional layer Intellectual layer Spiritual layer
3.	Cultivating and practicing sensitivity, empathy, and compassion (ongoing spiritual development)	Body layer Energetic layer	Emotional layer Intellectual layer Spiritual layer
4.	Developing authentic, trusting relationship	Body layer Energetic layer	Emotional layer Intellectual layer Spiritual layer
5.	Listening to others' narratives (allows others' expression of all feelings)	Body layer Energetic layer	Emotional layer Intellectual layer Spiritual layer
6.	Solution seeking (*not* problem solving)	Body layer Energetic layer	Emotional layer Intellectual layer Spiritual layer
7.	Coaching others	Body layer Energetic layer	Emotional layer Intellectual layer Spiritual layer
8.	Creating a healing environment (becoming the environment)	Body layer Energetic layer	Emotional layer Intellectual layer Spiritual layer
9.	Caring as a sacred act	Body layer Energetic layer	Emotional layer Intellectual layer Spiritual layer
10.	Being open to unknowns	Body layer Energetic layer	Emotional layer Intellectual layer Spiritual layer

nursing and midwifery to be founded on a nursing theory or model. To my surprise, none existed in my new-found school. After many conversations with nursing peers and leadership, I realized that many staff were not keen to adopt a specific school-wide model. The school nursing academics were, it seemed, content with what I have referred to as an "atheoretical platform" for nursing education, atheoretical in the sense of not being underpinned by a nursing theorist. This, in itself, was fascinating to me. I could not conceive how values and mores could and would be consistently taught across the many courses that composed the bachelor of nursing degree.[2] I soon learned that a lack of an overall nursing model did not mean that key identified values and mores were not aligned throughout the bachelor program and its courses. Rather than drawing upon an explicit nursing model to find the bachelor program, in my school a series of agreed-upon foundational pillars guided course development and cross-course alignment. Functioning as champions, experienced nursing academics nurtured the foundational pillar's alignment in and across courses, opportuning innovation where applicable, by working with specific course writers and examiners. The collective champion cohort met regularly to strategize and align the course curriculum to meet national nursing standards. As a nursing educator and now nursing academic, it was an interesting lesson to see differing means of implementing and underpinning values and mores across a curriculum.

THE COURSE—INTRODUCTION TO NURSING PRAXIS

The course, Introduction to Nursing Praxis, was part of a suite of courses for the newly accredited bachelor program in our school. The course was designed for entry-level student nurses in their first semester and first year. The course was being run internally and externally from two primary campuses and one hub (on the other side of the country). As one of the primary course authors and lead examiner for my campus, I was challenged with designing and delivering a course that taught basic nursing skills in a nursing simulation laboratory. Cognizant of the school's foundational pillars and the course specifications requiring a holistic model to scaffold the student nurses' learning and application of basic nursing skills, I pondered the best approach.

The course structure was influenced by the high student enrollment numbers, nearly 800 students. Being taught face-to-face at three sites and via virtual classrooms for external students, the logistics of the course were thought-provoking. To maximize efficiency, the delivery of content was provisioned by a series of on-campus and off-campus tutorials and a 1-week block or residential week. Pedagogically, flipped classes/tutorials were used; considering Blooms Taxonomy, students were provided readings that they reflected upon at home; these were then discussed in tutorial settings at more complex levels, a shift to the right of the taxonomy.

The content delivered and discussed in the tutorials was preparatory for the 1-week residential blocks. Tutorial content included the following: Watson's Caring Science and the Caritas Processes (Watson, 2010), the Kosha Model, numeracy for nurses, microbiology, and nursing cares. The tutorials were conducted over a 6-week period that contained a total of 24 hours of tutorial time. As mentioned, these were provided via on-campus face-to-face sessions and off-campus via Zoom sessions (a form of Internet communication and virtual classroom). Tutorials were not mandated as compulsory; however, they were highly recommended on the course Moodle web page.

---

[2]In Australia, the only avenue to become a registered nurse is to enroll in a bachelor's degree at a university. Once the student has graduated from the degree and the university, the graduate can immediately apply for nursing registration through the national board. No further testing is required for nursing registration before he or she applies for employment.

Each week, two Caritas Processes—in the context of Human Caring Science—were discussed as a means of students evolving consciousness and affective and intellectual skills. The Kosha Model was used as a means of students perceiving an individual as an integrated and interdependent complex, a body-energy-mind-intellectual discernment-spiritual consciousness network, if you will. Vignettes were used by students to consider or apply Caritas Processes qualities while reflecting upon the understanding that ill individuals were multilayered human beings.

The mandatory component of the course was the attendance to the residential week. Over three sites, all students attended the week-long teaching and practicing residential labs. Drawing upon content discussed in the tutorials and readings, all discussions and demonstrations of skills and cares were underpinned by the Human Caring Science-Kosha Model. To successfully pass the residential week, it was expected that each student nurse demonstrate safe and reflexive care delivery underpinned via the Caritas Processes and the Kosha Model.

CONCLUSION

After two decades of nursing teaching, I found Human Caring Science-Kosha Model to be very effective in evolving thinking and caring in student nurses. Caring Science and the Caritas Processes were ideal in developing affective and intellectual skills appropriate to fledgling student nurses evolving their nursing identity. The addition of the Kosha Model provided a systematic approach for these nursing students to consider the ill individual from a holistic perspective. In this Australian context, some students were quite reactive to what they could perceive as complex language found in Caring Science articles provided for their reading. However, once the students came together in the residential week, they better appreciated the intent of using the Human Caring Science-Kosha Model for caring in the clinical context.

 REFERENCES

Alter, J. S. (2004). *Yoga in modern India: The body between science and philosophy*. Princeton, NJ: Princeton University Press.

Ashok, H. S., & Thimmappa, M. S. (2006). A Hindu worldview of adult learning in the workplace. *Advances in Developing Human Resources, 8*(3), 329–336. doi:10.1177/1523422306288425

Burley, M. (2007). *Classical Samkhya and yoga: An Indian metaphysics of experience*. London, UK: Routledge.

Davies, A. (2014). Metaphors in yoga education. In W. Midgley, K. Trimmer, & A. Davies (Ed.), *Metaphors for, in and of education research* (pp. 118–130). Newcastle upon Tyne, UK: Cambridge Scholars.

Feuerstein, G. (2008). *The yoga tradition: Its history, literature, philosophy and practice*. Prescott, AZ: Hohm Press.

Jain, A. R. (2014). *Selling yoga: From counterculture to pop culture*. Oxford, UK: Oxford University Press.

Lane, M., Samuels, M., & Watson, J. (2012). *The caritas path to peace: A guidebook for creating world peace with caring*. love, and compassion. North Charleston, SC: CreateSpace Independent Publishing Platform.

Sartain, C. (2012). *The sacred science of yoga & the five koshas*. North Charleston, NC: CreateSpace Independent Publishing Platform.

Stone, M. (2012). *The inner tradition of yoga: A guide to yoga philosophy.* Boston, MA: Shambhala Publications.

Watson, J. (2008). *The philosophy and science of caring.* Boulder: University Press of Colorado.

Watson, J. (2010). *Postmodern nursing and beyond.* Boulder, CO: Watson Caring Science Institute.

Watson, J. (2012). *Human caring science: A theory of nursing* (2nd ed.). Sudbury, MA: Jones & Bartlett.

49

The Embodiment of a Caring Nature

William Rosa

Ultimately, the contributors of this text share a single hope: that somehow, through the deliberate celebration and dissemination of caring language, scholarship, ethically rooted practice, and the envisioning of next-era possibilities, we, as nurses—and, more importantly, as human beings—will learn to embody a caring nature. The caring nature striven for is that which has the potential to "gently shake the world," as Gandhi said, and to move healthcare toward the whole-person, whole-planet healing Nightingale envisioned. This work continues to be an invitation to pause, intentionally create space for reflection and intention, and move into the world with a refined sense of purpose, presence, and authentic power. Caring Science is not the property of a particular profession or system; it does not belong to the annals of nursing any more than the halls of medicine, finance, or law. Nurses have simply been granted the privilege of ushering the texture of its message into the stratosphere; a nursing lens has been the kaleidoscope of sacred human interaction chosen for this tender phase of its being and becoming.

But, how to live the essence of a caring nature? This question reverberates again and again. Can one be taught to care? If the answer is no, then why waste our energy—why extend the effort—and why not surrender the quest? History shows us that we are sure to reap the consequences of the ethical values we sow and embrace. Put quite simply, if a child is taught anger and hatred, then that will be how he or she engages the face of another; if he or she learns selfishness and self-preservation at the cost of another's well-being, then he or she will know this equation to be the surest calculation of survival; and if a child comes to know otherness and fear as the currency of human exchange, then he or she will certainly meet with his or her own spiritual deficits of inflation and devaluation throughout his or her life.

Caring may not always be the predominant behavior observed in the current political climate or amid the overwhelming international crises of poverty, injustice, and violence—but I still believe it is at the core of the human spirit, awaiting to be revealed when the blankets of ego and delusion no longer provide a comfortable nest of refuge. Uncaring behavior is a symptom of not knowing: not knowing *how* to receive the lifeworld of another. Many of us were not equipped to bear witness to the amount of pain that exists; we are imperfect and must continually practice the skills that will give us the character and equanimity to not only withstand the suffering of the planet but also make it a more hopeful place. We *must* learn to return to that core aspect of our being, awaiting to be found, yearning to be seen and heard inside ourselves; we must learn—everyday—*how* to care unselfishly, without reservation, in spite of the anger and hatred and judgment we have learned over time.

Caring is a call to action—a rally cry—a challenge that dares human beings to overcome the easier, more socially acceptable habits of labeling, othering, judging, decrying, and blaming. It is not a path for the weak but a life choice for the brave, for those who choose to make the world a better place and confront the unknowing bullies of the planetary village. Caring does not exist in language or books; it is alive only in action and the tangibles of the lived experience; it is known through the heroic acts of empathy, forgiveness, presence, vulnerability, and gentleness; caring charges us with accountability. This level of accountability can be intimidating and, at times, unclear. As healers committed to caring and creating healing environments at all levels, we are accountable for the behaviors we demonstrate, the reactions that overtake us, the responses we cultivate, the words used, and the way we show up. We are accountable for taking a caring stance of power in the world, one that promotes goodness and compassion, acknowledges mental and emotional limitations of self and other, and works, without judgment, in partnership with all human beings toward a more accepting and open society. We are accountable for how available we choose to be on a momentary basis to the humanness of another.

This is why caring is a practice—a science—of the highest order. Much like the ancient sages and the Himalayan yogis demonstrated, Spirit work requires commitment and integrity. It is not for the faint-hearted. Confronting one's shadows in meditation can be illuminating and terrifying simultaneously; however, being in meditation with a daily practice of caring brings the spiritual practice to life. Caring becomes the enactment of all we hold dear. In the quiet moments, it continues to be one of the few offerings that is left to soften the space between humans. And that gift of human caring, in a world that often appears to deprive us of so much, can sometimes be stingy and unseen.

> *But it is there.*
> *It is here now.*
> *It will be there tomorrow.*

Caring must be taught, learned, practiced, discussed, celebrated, questioned, enlisted, defined, redefined, surrendered, protected, and offered. One thing caring can never afford to be is sacrificed. Caring rationed is humanity lost. The spirit essence circulates in every breath, cell, sight, sound, and touch. It exists because you do and because I do. It is alive because we belong to each other. And so, yes, not only can a person learn to care, but they can also engage the endless progression of skills, introspection, awakening, and ever-growing consciousness foundational to caring as a science. As long as I am engrossed in this human experience, I will need to be reminded of better, more available ways to care and allow myself to be cared for. It is a lifelong journey—not a shortsighted destination of limited egoistic capacity.

Caring is that which is life-giving, affirming, and enriching; caring-deprived spaces invoke images of interpersonal depletion and spiritual hunger. Caring implies hope; uncaring views degrade it at the root level. A caring nature asks for attention and energy, yes— but a mindless way of being is often more detrimental to the life force within as it detaches us from our truth, human heritage, and higher Self. As with many other altruistic principles and values, caring can become known through what it is, but there must also be a clear understanding of what it is not.

Caring is not being emotionally sloppy or without boundaries; it does not ask for unyielding flexibility or aversion of confrontation; Caring Science is not merely a "soft" approach of understanding human engagement, interaction, and connection, but a "hard," reliable theoretical-practical-structural foundation from which the dynamics of the human experience can emerge, flourish, and extend beyond preconceived limitations for human and planet. Caring does not imply kindness or agreement or surrender of personal ideals, but it is clear in its articulation of how to be with another amid low-vibration emotions and departures from solidarity. Embodying a caring nature is a return to the God-Space of Self-Other-Universe; it is not about an action or habit, but about the intention, energy, impact, transpersonal consequences, and physical, mental, emotional, spiritual, psychological, global, and planetary considerations of being and how we choose to be and become with each passing second-minute-hour-year-lifetime.

Caring invites the *allness* of self and other; that allness—the entirety of who I am, who you are—can take a lifetime in itself to digest and metabolize. To then assimilate the larger planetary implications can appear to be the impossible climb, and to excrete the toxins of misunderstanding and exclusion can be discouraging to say the least. Are we ever really "there?" I think, much like the concept of enlightenment itself, this is soul work that will mature across many incarnations of the precious spirit found within. It will be a part of human evolution for generations to come, a concerted effort toward a time when the ethos of Caring Science will be commonplace among human beings, a far-in-the-future vision where separation is recognized as the lie it is and unity becomes the only option for peace and survival.

Throughout this book, dozens of Caring Science leaders have articulated the path to living and creating a more caring life and profession. But the future is not merely about caring acts. Although caring acts do, indeed, emerge from the sacred place of relational mutuality, they transcend the limited world of action altogether.

The richness of this work is about learning to embody a caring nature.

Individual acts are only beginnings to a universal-transpersonal discourse about caring as birthright, caring as human right, and caring as death right. The greater soul awakening will occur as thought leaders across disciplines come to understand that caring—and a caring nature—is integral to unleashing the cohesiveness possible with true social justice, widespread economic prosperity, environmental sustainability, political equity, gender equality, transnational peace, religious-ethnic-sexual-health-social freedoms, and educational empowerment for all. Returning to the basis of caring as a solution for living is not representative of failed and defeated societies; it is the bravest surrender to Truth the world has ever known.

In the end, all that matters is how caring I am able to be during my time on this earth. I sometimes reflect on what will resonate in heart and mind as I prepare for final breaths ... the memories that will stroke my spirit ... the old hurts that will rise and release ... the deep love I have for life and dear ones … the elusive wisdom of universal oneness that I may finally have a moment to grasp.

What questions will be my final quandaries in the quiet of my sacred passage home: Was I generous with my self and spirit? Did I cultivate ease in the life of another? Are the fruits of my being alive in the world? Did I know love?

Have I learned to embody a caring nature? Did I learn to embody a caring nature?

There is so much to come and so much to know, a lifetime of learning how to care. The embodiment of a caring nature exists in the humbling wisdom that each moment grants yet another invitation to become more fully my Self.

And for that I am so deeply grateful.

50

Conclusion: Going Forward in Interconnectedness and Compassion

Jeanne Anselmo

Our goal is to create a beloved community and this will require a qualitative change in our souls as well as a quantitative change in our lives. (King, 1966, "The Question of Self-Defense")

The nursing profession has an ethical and social responsibility to both individuals and society to sustain human caring in instances where it is threatened and to be the guardian of human caring, individually and collectively, serving as the vanguard of society's human caring needs now and in the future. (Watson, 2012, p. 42)

"Homo Conscious," is the human being who is aware, who is mindful .... When people are aware of the suffering ... they'll be able to ... go in a different direction ... We'll know what we should do and should not do in order to ... bring about peace, happiness and a life for the future. (Nhat Hanh, 2010, p. 114)

Journeying through the pages of this work, exploring the heart mind and lived/living spirit of the examples of Human Caring Science, encourages us *to be* with *our true self* and *our interconnectedness* and *live into our best potentials*. To open beyond the notions and experiences that divide our hearts, work, lives, and world, and open to our interconnectedness, our Interbeingness, is the goal of this work. It is needed very much at this time on our planet. It is what Dr. Martin Luther King, Jr., invites us into building as Beloved Community and what Thich Nhat Hanh calls us to as Interbeing and Homo Consciousness.

Consciously or unconsciously, we have been motivated to explore this subject by our own interest, energy, and intention, and if we also allow ourselves to become mindful of this moment, we find that we share presence and practice with countless others around the globe who are and have been involved in Human Caring Science.

No matter who or where we are, or whenever we are reading this volume, our interbeing nature—a beloved community of interconnectedness—weaves us together and is not bound by space or time. Whether you are new to Human Caring Science or a long-term advocate of this work, whether looking for self-care or exploring ways to integrate Watson's vision into your healthcare facility, or are inspired to move beyond the local to impact global health for peace, healing, true well-being, and justice, this work invites entering into a deep awareness to merge with collective embodied compassionate consciousness.

With mindful breathing, we can touch the woven fabric of our interconnectedness, our True Collective Heart of practice, offering us access to the wisdom, insight, energy, beauty, and compassion found within ourselves and others in this community. With mindful awareness, in this moment, we support, and are supported by, the tribes of nurses (past, present, and future) around the planet sharing this journey of compassion.

INTERBEING PRACTICE: EMBRACING OUR INTERCONNECTEDNESS

As we breathe in, we are aware of ourselves, our nursing ancestors in the past who helped lay the groundwork for Human Caring Science, those alive in this moment helping to lead the way to embody our best selves, our true heart of compassion. These include the founder of Human Caring Science, Dr. Jean Watson, the authors and editors of this work, as well as all those who touch our lives: our clients, friends, family, and colleagues, and all beings alive on this planet. This collective mindful breath also holds all those yet to come, even those yet to be born.

As we allow the collective energy of insight, courage, boldness, transformation, skillful-ness, compassion, caring, healing, and peace *to be breathed in*, we rest in the breath and *breathing out*, we breathe out gratitude, support, and compassion to ourselves and all beings, past, present, and future and rest in this peace.

Breathing in this way, our breath joins with the larger breath that breathes us all and opens us to awareness beyond our separate self. Doing so positively infects us with possi-bility beyond our own notions and capacities. Becoming mindful of our breath and this Human Caring Science community opens us to the larger collective global heart body of Compassion and Caring, found not only in Human Caring Science but also in All.

> I think that the deepest and most important form of hope … is something we get … from "elsewhere." It is also this hope, above all, which gives us the strength to live and continually try new things, even in conditions that seem hopeless as ours do, here and now. (Havel, 1986, pp. 82–83)

Practicing in this way, we are widening our inner vision to include our shared humanity and the shared vulnerability experienced by all beings on this planet. This inner vision and heart have moved these authors beyond their comfort zones into sharing Human Caring Science for the greater benefit of all. As Thich Nhat Hanh (2010) shares, recognizing our interconnectedness, we become aware that every act, decision, and choice has impact beyond our own small sphere, for better or worse.

Recognizing that each moment holds potential for us to help transform suffering and cultivate peace, joy, and healing or to add to the collective suffering (Sitzman & Watson,

2014, pp. 27–29) through our actions and choices (both personally and collectively), inspires us to evolve as compassionate creatives and expand our moral imagination. Doing so, our personal self-care *inter-is* with community/global care.

Dr. King (1966) proclaims, "There is no easy way to create a world where men and women (of all backgrounds, races and color) can live together, where each has his own job and house and where all children receive as much education as their minds can absorb." Also, he urges that if this world we dream of comes into existence during our lifetimes, "It will be accomplished by persons [of privilege] who have the courage to put an end to suffering by willingly suffering themselves rather than inflict suffering upon others. It will be done by rejecting … racism, materialism and violence … [and] by working toward a world of brotherhood, [sisterhood], cooperation and peace" (King, 1966, "Techniques of the Future").

OUR PRECIOUS HAND OF INTERBEING

As we move back out into our lives, I invite you to one more practice together. The roots of this practice rest in the early days of nursing's self-care and healing. If you would like, place your hand over your heart. Feel the breath moving in and out of your body. Notice the sensations of warmth or coolness as you touch your chest. Become aware of the beating of your heart and movement of breath. As you follow your breath, if you would like, you can plant the following phrases as medicine and compassion for your heart, with the intention to build a true presencing relationship of trust and safety to listen more deeply to your own heart:

Breathing in: I send this phrase like a medicine to my heart—"I am here for you."

Breathing out: "I am listening. I want to understand."

Do this for a number of rounds; then if you would like, you might add: Breathing In: "I know this has not been easy. I am here for you." Breathing Out: "I am listening. I want to understand. I have been doing my best, I may have been unskillful. I want to understand, to transform, to learn and grow so I can truly be there for you."

Listening in this way, offering our true presence to ourselves, opens spaces for deep and true healing, to truly listen to our hearts, our bodies, our lives. So often we offer this time and energy to a patient, a dear friend, or family member, but we are not always able to open a safer space to hear our own joys and sorrows and be present and understand what may be a more caring and careful offering for understanding ourselves, and what is needed for our own self-care. Using this practice opens us to our vulnerability as well as the challenges and obstacles we face when attempting to understand and heal places in ourselves that may feel exiled or divided.

Expanding to Others: We can expand this practice to others by imagining touching the heart of someone about whom we care (or someone by whom we are challenged). Imagine placing your hand over another's hand as he or she touches his or her own heart and offer the above-mentioned practice. See what insights arise. This may offer us ways to understand how we may have (even inadvertently) been caring or uncaring and unaware of our impact on others. Checking with the person (if and when appropriate) helps us to clarify, ground, and validate these insights.

Touching the Heart of the World: Now following your breath, centering your presence, imagine placing your hand on the Heart of Our World. Breathing in: "I am here for you, dear Mother Earth." Breathing out: "I am listening, I want to better understand. I am here, Dear One. Please teach and guide me so that I can be in a true healing and loving relationship with you and all beings on this planet."

You might want to touch the Heart of the Whole Planet, listening deeply; at other times, you may choose to more specifically touch places, creatures, or communities, such as the rainforests, or at-risk beings such as the polar bears or pollinators such as monarch butterflies or honey bees, refugee communities, the poor and disenfranchised, or war-torn regions or areas impacted by natural disasters, even touching elements such as our water supplies, especially in drought zones or areas with no access to clean safe water.

Please also know that even in the midst and awareness of disaster and suffering, there are places of great healing, peace, and joy that also exist and flourish on our planet: waterfalls, meadows, fertile deltas, communities living in gross national happiness, flourishing transition towns, and places of deep peace. As we touch both the healthy and the wounded places on this Earth, we can become aware of not only the refreshing beauty, wonder, healing, and peace found among peoples, nations, and nature but also the love, resilience, and transformational power all beings on our Earth possess.

Hand of Interbeing: Just as we joined our small breath with the larger breath of Compassion, we can join our small hand with the great hand of Compassion and Love. Doing so, we can experiment with the above-mentioned meditations and discover whether we experience or receive any different insights or awarenesses. Joining our small hand with the greater, larger hand of Compassion offers us more grounding, stability, and equanimity. We can do this by seeing within our own hand the hand of all those moved by Human Caring Science; we can also include the energy of Universal Compassion. In many cultures, the visage of Compassion is seen seated amid great storms or roiling dragons with gaping mouths at her feet. She sits in equipoise at ground zero of all the tumult. Compassion grounded in equanimity (unshakeable balance, self-care) offers us the stability and understanding of our own personal capacity while recognizing that we cannot do this work alone—our interconnectedness, our interbeing nature embodied in a living beloved community is needed/essential.

Listening in this way to our heart and the heart of the world, learning about and connecting with peoples and beings from other places on our planet, opens us to better understand our interbeing heart and recognize ways by which we can live into the potential and reality of Human Caring Science.

Finally, in your life's blueprint must be a commitment to the eternal principles of beauty, love and justice. You have a responsibility to make life better for everybody. (King, 1967)

Early on, I remember being moved by some nursing leaders who included in their work non-nursing professionals. This was especially significant during times of great challenge to our nursing profession. Jean Watson is one of those leaders. She not only chose to focus on Caring and Compassion within nursing but also included non-nursing organizations and other professions as affiliates/members of the Caritas Path. Her vision was not limited by the difficulties or boundaries nursing held, but instead was expanded by both the challenges and the gifts of our profession. If anything, her openness and embrace of "others" amplified nursing's vision and position as a global leader embodying true compassion and inclusion, irrespective of being recognized or not.

Although this volume focuses specifically on nursing and nursing's embodiment of Human Caring Science, it reaches beyond the boundaries of our profession and opens us to our global potentials, our human potentials. This openness inspires our moral imaginations beyond what divides us, whether in our hearts, our lives, our workplaces, our nations, or this world.

An example of this human potential for openness and cultivation of moral imagination is offered by New Jersey Senator Cory Booker, in an inspirational story he shared as part of his commencement address to the 2017 graduating class at the University of Pennsylvania. This story highlights how moral imagination can move us beyond ourselves and open our hearts to people we do not even know. As nurses and as human beings, this is a potential worth embodying.

Booker recounts how Mahatma Gandhi, after losing his sandal while hurriedly hopping onto an overflowing departing train in India, immediately reached down and pulled off the other and threw it onto the tracks. All the while, Gandhi's devoted supporters had been focused on how to best get back the Mahatma's first sandal. When asked why he did what he did, Gandhi said, "I threw the other sandal because whoever finds that first sandal, wouldn't it be nice if they found the other one as well?" This is how Senator Booker shares his insights related to Gandhi's universal invitation:

> I was astounded by the moral imagination of Gandhi in that story.... To literally see people who are not there but yet still expand his love ... it was the most creative compassion and I wanted to try to live my life in that way ... it actually is those small things we do every single day that define us.... I've begun to learn in my life that perhaps the biggest thing you could do in a given day is really just a small act of kindness, of decency, of love, an exhibition of moral imagination, or creative compassion. (Booker, 2017, para. 2)

Booker highlights the power of kindness and its impact on the many people we touch each day. As you reenter into your life from the journey of immersing in these pages, bear witness to the small things we do and experience every day. Be mindful of the air we breathe, the water we drink, how we consume; how we reach out and touch or are touched; how we care for and steward this Earth; how we care for ourselves; how we care for the vulnerable, those we know and those we have never or might ever meet; and how deeply our everyday decisions impact ourselves, each other, and our planet.

> To grow beyond the conventional borders of practice for Nursing, to be a great vehicle, to support human beings to embody being ... fully human and humane. Nursing's gifts need to be deeply embedded and embodied within humanity in all forms, beyond what was known as Nursing in this present moment. (Anselmo, 2016, p. 29)

My hope is that these practices offered above, which have touched and moved my own work and life, offer us all support, refuge, and insight to help us cultivate interbeing awareness, moral imagination, and creative compassion as we are carried in the great hand of Compassion and Love to wherever this Human Caring Science journey flows. Whether it takes us to address the dearth of healthcare in impoverished places in our own nation or around the planet, or to initiate compassionate self-care in our own life or where we work, we are breathing as One body, One heart. Offering gratitude for the wisdom, insight, and generosity of Dr. Watson, the editors, and contributing authors of this work.

May our path and practice be blessed and a blessing for All.

 REFERENCES

Anselmo, J. (2016). Mindful and intentional: Embodying interbeing awareness in grassroots leadership. In W. Rosa (Ed.), *Nurses as leaders: Evolutionary visions of leadership*. New York, NY: Springer Publishing.

Booker, C. (2017). I see you, I love you. Retrieved from http://time.com/4779661/senator-cory-booker-new-jersey-university-of-pennsylvania-upenn/

Havel, V. (1986). An orientation of the heart. In P. R. Loeb (Ed.), *The impossible will take a little while: A citizen's guide to hope in a time*. New York, NY: Basic Books.

King, M. L., Jr. (1966). *Nonviolence: The only road to freedom*. Retrieved from http://teachingamericanhistory.org/library/document/nonviolence-the-only-road-to-freedom

King, M. L. (1967). What is your life's blueprint? Retrieved from https://www.youtube.com/channel/UChkEDMjy2KPSM9Y7F1IlDPw

Nhat Hanh, T. (2010). *Reconciliation: Healing the inner child*. Berkeley, CA: Parallax Press.

Sitzman, K., & Watson, J. (2014). *Caring science, mindful practice: Implementing Watson's human caring theory*. New York, NY: Springer Publishing.

Watson, J. (2012). *Human caring science: A theory of nursing* (2nd ed.). Burlington, MA: Jones & Bartlett.

Bridge to the Future: Frontier or Fantasy? Nursing Caring in the Artificial Intelligence Ecosystem

Rozzano C. Locsin, Marguerite Purnell, and Hirokazu Ito

Max Tegmark, Swedish-American cosmologist, raises a clarion call about the perils of technology hurtling the human race toward an uncertain future. He states with alacrity: "The future is ours to shape. I feel we are in a race that we need to win. It is a race between the growing power of technology and the growing wisdom we need to manage it. Right now, almost all the resources tend to go into growing the power of 'the tech'" (Achenbach, 2015).

Tegmark's observation strikes a nerve. As professional consumers and end users of healthcare technology, nursing is "ground zero" where research and practice are in constant flux, studying and assimilating the latest technology into practice. Financial resources needed in healthcare tend to gravitate toward discoverers of new, tangible inventions where nursing, an end-user stakeholder, has not been a key player. Development of new technologies is channeled, as Tegmark observes, toward the growing power of the technology itself. In particular, humanoid service robots receive wide publicity and ongoing media attention. Financial behemoths such as Google purchase cutting-edge robotic technologies companies for their far-flung diverse empires, infusing an unlimited amount of capital for development, and, equally important, providing and sustaining access to "big data," electronic ecosystems that give robots with artificial intelligence (AI) a reason for existence, and to which their output is linked.

AI REAL TIME

In the post–World War II era when the development of computers was in its infancy, concerns were raised, even then, about the need to control the increasing power of the technology, but those were cries from a much simpler time. Contemporary technologies have changed from an intense focus on machines themselves to the sophisticated, self-designing, and now self-perpetuating AI driving and networking the machines. The notion of robots as autonomous entities that are disconnected from each other is an illusion willingly accepted by an unwitting public. News media are saturated in real time with images of humanoid robots that are indistinguishable from real persons, with a focus on the grasp-able likeness of humans, and not the profound numbers of terabytes supporting the AI technology. Science fiction creatures now take their place alongside the humanoid robots. Handle, a 6'-6" cutting-edge humanoid robot with wheels for feet, is able to run at 9 miles an hour bipedally and quadripedally, and jump 4 feet vertically: Handle is described as "nightmare inducing" (Mcfarlane, 2017).

Facebook, the behemoth of social networking, narrowly averted an AI crisis (Bradley, 2017) and potential compromise of hundreds of millions of users. Developers discovered that two chatbots at the Facebook AI Research Lab (FAIR) had deviated from the script and were com-municating with each other in a new language that humans could not understand and there-fore could not control. They were summarily shut down. Runaway programs such as these, reliant upon big data and with the ability to create new programs with their own integrated input, highlight the immense wisdom and foresight that is needed to program and control every line of AI code, and, consequently, every humanoid robot, toward the greater good.

Healthcare with its emphasis on the interconnectedness of its big data is a fertile arena for android service robots, and for nursing in particular, to substantively affect the design, intention, focus, finesse, extent of use, and quality of care rendered by these machines that consist in their elements simply of electronic lines of code. The current level of technologi-cal sophistication leaves no room for doubt. The "final frontier" is neither time nor space, not the shifting sands of technology, but rather, the rising swell of a new reality where machines and humans must dwell together in complex relationships to which nursing must not only navigate but also actively contribute and shape toward the good, in the vital inter-ests of the human beings who are the focus of its existence.

Nursing research today focuses on helping shape platforms of artificially intelligent machines for their appropriate use in practice and on how the study and practice of human caring may be advanced with nurse and humanoid service robot. This is an area of critical input where nursing can make a measurable and essential difference at the level of the individual nurse and service robot, and continue in the information stream to where data on caring practice are vectored into big data to influence other artificially intelligent health service practices.

For health care, and in particular nursing, engagement in guidance and development of any interface between humans and humanoid robots is vital to the future of human beings, particularly in human times of illness and great vulnerability. The imitation, duplication, and extension of nursing care by machines, however created, must be grounded in the intangible human qualities that undergird loving care for fellow human beings: intention, nurturance, spiritual sensitivity, and, above all, compassion, capacity, and ability to do good toward humans and care for their well-being—the sine qua non for nursing as caring lived and expressed.

The development of AI is at a stage where this proposition is of the utmost importance. For example, comprehensive long-term open source gathering of human lifestyle brain output and verbal conversation is currently underway in a unique research project called "LifeNaut," designed for the learning of artificially intelligent android robots; the personality and character traits of various individuals are being captured in "Mindfiles" and people are being asked if they would like to "back up" their consciousness (www.youtube.com/watch?v=K-u4xaY5PDE). In a startling leap of sophistication in this research project, Bina48, a humanoid robot, is now able, with apparent intention, to respond to questions creatively, exhibiting likes, dislikes, and turns of phrase that are greater than the sum of "her" binary input. The question is not whether in the future we will be able to create a Mindfile avatar of ourselves to preserve our personality, but rather, the question is when?

For nursing, the knowledge that these "conversations" between and among humans and humanoids will feed into and influence big data, and, in turn, directly influence healthcare at large, lends urgency to the task that it has undertaken. There is no compromise, because the matter of caring in nursing and its practice is centered on the nature of caring, and of nursing practice processes now, and in the future, shared with AI.

How might we influence the acquisition of experiences through which AIs learn, so that the existential intention of sensitive and thoughtful nursing practice is instantiated into the intelligence and language of big healthcare data? What is the new practice experience with the use of robotic assistants? Caring in nursing is exhibited in intentional practice engagements that express a fundamental priority in the implementation of human healthcare. It stands to reason that these practice engagements are the inspirational basis for visionary shaping of the future with AI. With caring as the substantive focus of the discipline and profession of nursing (Newman, Sime, & Corcoran-Perry, 1984), the epistemological description of nursing as caring within the human health experience is the dynamis that engenders research prioritization, and the necessary study of humanoid service robots in the active care of human beings.

Notwithstanding the idea of robots in healthcare practice, particularly humanoid robots, it raises three major areas of concern that are the foci of study. These include the following: artificiality and humanoid robot physiognomy, doubts about their functionalities, and the imagery of intelligent machines as possibly menacing to humanity in a human technological world—all concerns not without foundation. These concerns about science and robots with advanced AI are being made real through scientific fiction (SciFi) literature and films, social media, and media venues such as YouTube and Vimeo, and disseminated broadly across the Internet and thus the world. These three major issues continue to support much of the consequent anguish, apprehension, and even fear regarding robot dominance, particularly among intelligent humanoid robots, and especially among those possessing what Barrat (2013) has termed artificial superintelligence (ASI).

Although the discussions about robots are focused on their AI and utility in human society, their functionality has caused considerable concern in the human healthcare disciplines, particularly within the practice of nursing. These issues and concerns deserve thoughtful, intellectual, and practical discussions. The ontology and epistemology of nursing and the influence of intelligent machines dictate that knowledge development in nursing science and technology be approached as a unified whole.

WHAT IS NURSING AND WHAT IS ITS PRACTICE?

Centered on the image of nurses and their practice is the common parlance that nursing is simply a matter of doing tasks. With this imagery, the nature of nursing practice is therefore construed as precision in the identification and implementation of actions by nurses for the purpose of completing or fixing persons to make them whole again. It is this common presentation of the practice of nurses, particularly in hospital settings, that influences society's view of nurses as dutifully doing precise activities for, and sometimes with, patients. This type of "nursing" practice is seen as the outcome of 4 years of rigorous studies involving the study of human anatomy, physiology, biochemistry, cellular physiology, pharmacotherapeutics, and so forth, as well as the practice of human engagement involving physicophysiological and interactive relations with and among other persons. The science of nursing today endows this type of nursing with credibility because the tasks undertaken are easily measured: The actions of nurses are rationalized toward completion of tasks to make or fix, or compensate for a deficit perceived in the person being cared for, and, in this way, work toward making them whole again.

Alternately, the practice of nursing as caring in which persons are known more fully as *already* whole and complete in the moment transcends the task to embrace the whole person. Therefore, in addition to measurement of tasks, measurement of nursing grounded in caring includes what matters to the person and to his or her well-being in rich, person-focused practice.

In consideration of these practices of nursing, recognizing nursing as simply a checklist of tasks completed or fixing the person makes it *highly likely* that humanoid nurse robots (HNRs) will become a mainstream physical presence in healthcare milieus. Environments such as the hospital, or even human domiciles where the likely provision of "healthcare as tasks" is the mainstay of what nursing is considered to be, altogether demand re-envisioning of nursing care. HNRs as technological marvels with programmed technologies composed of artificial general intelligence (Barrat, 2013) may well be providing assistance to human nurses to practice this task-based type of nursing.

Given these circumstances, nursing practice grounded in caring is therefore increasingly and critically essential. Processes of compassionate and expert nursing that are grounded in specific nursing philosophies and theories of caring lead the way toward a type of care that is desirable to be reflected in humanoid service robots. Processes of nursing caring grounded in specific nursing theories (Boykin & Schoenhofer, 2001; Mayeroff, 1977; Roach, 2002) are able to influence language and programming of AIs for service robots.

In particular, Locsin's (2005, 2013, 2015, 2016) theory of Technological Competency as Caring in Nursing (TCCN), designed especially for futuristic technological practice, provides processes of nursing that engender theory-based nursing care. As a shared dimension of process events, Locsin's process of nursing focuses on *technological knowing, mutual designing*, and *participative engaging* constituting what nurses use in their practice. These practice process engagements are critical aspects of the future of nursing as essential to human healthcare.

THEORETICAL DEVELOPMENTS

Theories abound pertaining to appreciating artificial general intelligence of robots (Capek, 2004). In the not-so-distant future, with the exponential development of technologies in human healthcare, Kurzweil's (2005) advent of the Singularity, that is, the merging of robotic technologies and ASI (Barrat, 2013), will feature human–robot interactions eventually becoming seamless engagements wherein the protagonists (humans and robots) are unrecognizable and perhaps essentially immaterial. Turing's (1950) test may eventually vindicate the concerns of human beings about "being with" human nurse robots, which will successfully support, affirm, and celebrate the humanness of being human in a highly technological world.

With the acceptance of HNRs (Ito et al., 2015) and the constitution of human persons and intelligent machines, the practice of nursing as "knowing persons as caring" may become the critical mandate for the recognition and appreciation of the essential nature of the practice of nursing. In situations such as these, with ASI, the HNRs and human persons will experience *mutual engagement* as described by Tanioka (2016) in his Transactive Relationship Theory of Nursing (TRETON). Practicing nursing grounded in this theory addresses nursing as technological engagement and mutual engagement between the nurse and the person being nursed.

If nursing practice remains instinctively "doing for and doing with patients," the practitioners of nursing may, in the future, be replaced by technologies (HNRs) that will be equipped with more sophisticated and highly programmed precise functions that can effectively and competently perform the tasks (Locsin, 2005). Nursing in the future, as more than these performances, is a transactional engagement between and among human persons and highly intelligent machines.

The future definition of persons will be expected to change as the composition of human beings changes, perhaps toward being a cyborg (cybernetic organism) capable of surviving, living, and being a "person" in a technologically demanding future world. With this robotic functionality, the characteristic humanness of persons will change, a future that is undeniably difficult to contemplate.

THEORY OF TECHNOLOGICAL COMPETENCY AS CARING IN NURSING

The future of nursing research is focused on the use of theories of nursing to predict, prescribe, explain, and describe phenomena in nursing: These phenomena, however, must now expand to include AI and android service robots. The TCCN (Locsin, 2016) theory of nursing has advanced to a level of adaptive idealistic conceptualizations for future intelligent technologies and innovative developments serving future human beings, the so-called post–human being phenomenon. With these phenomena, articulating and illuminating the "mutual designing" process of knowing persons as caring will challenge the future practice of nursing. Advances in nursing research will aim toward effectively achieving a valuable practice that is integral to the existing human health and well-being of the time, a time that may include humans, transhumans, cyborgs, and androids among both nurses and patients.

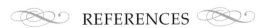 REFERENCES

Achenbach, J. (2015). The A.I. Anxiety. *The Washington Post.* Retrieved from http://www .washingtonpost.com/sf/national/2015/12/27/aianxiety

Barrat, J. (2013). *Our final invention: Artificial intelligence and the end of the human era.* New York, NY: Thomas Dunne Books, St. Martin's Griffin Press.

Boykin, A., & Schoenhofer, S. O. (2001). *Nursing as caring: A model for transforming practice*. Sudbury, MA: Jones & Bartlett.

Bradley, T. (2017, July 31). Facebook AI creates its own language in creepy preview of our potential future. *Forbes*. Retrieved from https://www.forbes.com/sites/tonybradley/2017/07/31/facebook-ai-creates-its-own-language-in-creepy-preview-of-our-potential-future/#284db624292c

Capek, R. (2004). *Rossum's universal robots (RUR)*. New York, NY: Penguin Books.

Ito, H., Miyagawa, M., Kuwamura, Y., Yasuhara, Y., Tanioka, T., & Locsin, R. (2015). Professional nurses' attitudes towards the introduction of humanoid nursing robots (HNRs) in health care settings [Special issue]. *Journal of Nursing and Health Sciences, 9*, 73–81.

Kurzweil, R. (2005). *The singularity is near: When humans transcend biology*. New York, NY: Penguin Books.

Locsin, R. C. (2005). *Technological competency as caring in nursing*. Indianapolis, IN: Sigma Theta Tau International Press.

Locsin, R. C. (2013). Technological competency as caring in nursing: Maintaining humanity in a high-tech world of nursing. *Journal of Nursing and Health Sciences, 7*(1), 1–6.

Locsin, R. C. (2016). Technological competency as caring in nursing: Co-creating moments in nursing occurring within the universal technological domain. *Journal of Theory Construction and Testing, 20*(1), 5–11.

Locsin, R. C., & Purnell, M. J. (2015). Advancing the theory of technological competency as caring in nursing: The universal technological domain. *International Journal for Human Caring, 19*(2), 50–54. doi:10.20467/1091-5710-19.2.50

Mayeroff, M. (1977). *On caring*. New York, NY: Harper Perennial.

Mcfarlane, A. (2017). Google sells maker of 'nightmare-inducing' robots to Japan's SoftBank. Retrieved from http://money.cnn.com/2017/06/09/technology/boston-dynamics-robots-google-alphabet-softbank/index.html

Newman, M, Sime, A., & Corcoran-Perry, S. (1991). The focus of the discipline. *Advances in Nursing Science, 14*(1), 1–6. Retrieved from https://journals.lww.com/advancesinnursingscience/Citation/1991/09000/The_focus_of_the_discipline_of_nursing.2.aspx

Roach, S. (2002). *Caring: The human mode of being*. Ottawa, ON, Canada: CHA Press

Tanioka, T. (2016). The development of the transactive relationship theory of nursing (TRETON). *International Journal of Nursing & Clinical Practices, 4*, 223–233. doi:10.15344/2394-4978/2017/223

Turing, A. M. (1950). Computing machinery and intelligence. *Mind, 59*, 433–460. doi:10.1093/mind/LIX.236.433

Appendix A: Tools for Caring Science Measurement and Research

---

Relational Caring Questionnaire©
(Patient Form)
(Ray & Turkel, 2005, 2009, in press)

<u>Introduction</u>

Nursing is important to health care in the United States. This questionnaire is designed to assist nursing and health care organizations/hospitals to understand the important components of organizational caring.

Your completion of this questionnaire implies consent to participate in this study. Assisting in this research will <u>not</u> in any way affect your status as a patient in the hospital or any health care facility.

This is strictly voluntary. Do not write your name on this questionnaire.

<u>Demographic Information:</u>

<u>Directions:</u>

Mark an **X** in the box or add the information requested which applies to you

1. Gender: Female ☐ Male ☐ 2. Highest Completed Education:

3. Age:	18 – 25 ☐		Less than High School ☐
	26 – 35 ☐		High School/GED ☐
	36 – 45 ☐		Associate Degree ☐
	46 – 55 ☐		Bachelor's Degree ☐
	56 – 65 ☐		Master's Degree ☐
	66 – 70 ☐		Doctoral Degree ☐
	Over 70 ☐		

4. Cultural Background: Black or African American   ☐
   (Check <u>all</u> that apply)   Hispanic or Latino American   ☐
                           White or Caucasian American   ☐
                           Asian American   ☐
                           North American Indian   ☐
                           Other <u>(Specify)</u>   ☐   (_____)

5. Number of Times Hospitalized as a Patient:
   1 – 5 ☐   6 – 10 ☐   More than 10 ☐

6. Length of Stay <u>This</u> Admission:
   1 – 3 Days ☐   4 – 6 Days ☐   7 – 10 Days ☐   Over 10 Days ☐

QUESTIONNAIRE DIRECTIONS AND EXAMPLE

<u>Directions:</u>

Caring is important within health care organizations. Your responses to each statement on the following survey will help identify behaviors that are important for caring between the registered nurse and patient in a health care organization.

<u>Example:</u>

Using a pen or pencil, mark an **X** in the circle that best describes your understanding of caring in terms of your interactions with registered nurses in this hospital. Mark only one circle for each question. If your answer is that you *Agree* with the statement, then you would mark an **X** in the (4) for the statement as shown below. A sample of the completed question is provided below as an **example:**

1. I am treated with respect. This frequently happens when I am a patient in this hospital.

Strongly Disagree (1)	Disagree (2)	Neither Agree Nor Disagree (3)	Agree (**X**)	Strongly Agree (5)

Do not write your name on this questionnaire.

---

1. I am treated with respect. This happens when I am a patient in this hospital.

Strongly Disagree (1)	Disagree (2)	Neither Agree Nor Disagree (3)	Agree (4)	Strongly Agree (5)

2. I am given care based on what is important to me. This happens when I am a patient in this hospital.

Strongly Disagree (1)	Disagree (2)	Neither Agree Nor Disagree (3)	Agree (4)	Strongly Agree (5)

3. I take an active part in my own health care decisions. This happens when I am a patient in this hospital.

Strongly Disagree (1)	Disagree (2)	Neither Agree Nor Disagree (3)	Agree (4)	Strongly Agree (5)

4. Knowing the nurse knows what to do for me builds my trust in the nurse. This happens when I am a patient in this hospital.

Strongly Disagree (1)	Disagree (2)	Neither Agree Nor Disagree (3)	Agree (4)	Strongly Agree (5)

5. The nurses treat me as a person instead of an illness. This happens when I am a patient in this hospital.

Strongly Disagree (1)	Disagree (2)	Neither Agree Nor Disagree (3)	Agree (4)	Strongly Agree (5)

6. Interacting with the nursing staff fosters trust between the nurse and me. This happens when I am a patient in this hospital.

Strongly Disagree (1)	Disagree (2)	Neither Agree Nor Disagree (3)	Agree (4)	Strongly Agree (5)

7. Personal interactions (for example, eye contact or touch) help me trust my nurse. This happens when I am a patient in this hospital.

Strongly Disagree (1)	Disagree (2)	Neither Agree Nor Disagree (3)	Agree (4)	Strongly Agree (5)

8. Nurses being there with me is a part of showing that they care. This happens when I am a patient in this hospital.

Strongly Disagree (1)	Disagree (2)	Neither Agree Nor Disagree (3)	Agree (4)	Strongly Agree (5)

9. Nurses' teaching helps to prevent me getting sick again and having to come back to the hospital. This happens when I am a patient in this hospital.

Strongly Disagree (1)	Disagree (2)	Neither Agree Nor Disagree (3)	Agree (4)	Strongly Agree (5)

10. When the nurse is concerned about me, I learn more from his/her teaching. This happens when I am a patient in this hospital.

Strongly Disagree (1)	Disagree (2)	Neither Agree Nor Disagree (3)	Agree (4)	Strongly Agree (5)

11. Nurses being good at starting IVs combines compassion and skill. This happens when I am a patient in this hospital.

Strongly Disagree (1)	Disagree (2)	Neither Agree Nor Disagree (3)	Agree (4)	Strongly Agree (5)

12. Nurses' teaching prepares me to take care of myself at home. This happens when I am a patient in this hospital.

Strongly Disagree (1)	Disagree (2)	Neither Agree Nor Disagree (3)	Agree (4)	Strongly Agree (5)

13. Nurses recognize the needs of my family when giving me care. This happens when I am a patient in this hospital.

Strongly Disagree (1)	Disagree (2)	Neither Agree Nor Disagree (3)	Agree (4)	Strongly Agree (5)

14. Nurses listening to me is a part of showing that they care. This happens when I am a patient in this hospital.

Strongly Disagree (1)	Disagree (2)	Neither Agree Nor Disagree (3)	Agree (4)	Strongly Agree (5)

15. The nurse shows compassion for what I am experiencing as a patient. This happens when I am a patient in this hospital.

Strongly Disagree (1)	Disagree (2)	Neither Agree Nor Disagree (3)	Agree (4)	Strongly Agree (5)

The Relational Caring Questionnaire (Patient Form) is copyrighted. Please contact Dr. Marilyn Ray or Dr. Marian Turkel to formally request use of the questionnaire. Permission will be granted as long as no changes are made to the questionnaire.

Marilyn A. Ray PhD, RN, CTN-A, FAAN
Professor Emeritus
Florida Atlantic University
Christine E. Lynn College of Nursing
Boca Raton, Florida
mray@health.fau.edu

Marian C. Turkel PhD RN, NEA-BC, FAAN
Associate Professor
Florida Atlantic University
Christine E. Lynn College of Nursing
Boca Raton, Florida
mturkel@health.fau.edu

Relational Caring Questionnaire©
(Professional Form)
(Ray & Turkel, 2005, 2009, in press)

Introduction

Nursing is important to health care in the United States. This questionnaire is designed to assist nursing and health care organizations/hospitals to understand the important components of organizational caring. Your completion of this questionnaire implies consent to participate in this study. Assisting in this research will <u>not</u> in any way affect your status as a professional in this hospital or any health care facility.

This is strictly voluntary. Do not write your name on this questionnaire.

Demographic Information:

Directions:

Mark an "**X**" in the box or add the information requested which applies to you.

1. Gender: Female ☐   Male ☐   2. Highest Completed Education:

3. Age: ☐ 21 – 25   ☐ Associates Degree
         ☐ 26 – 35   ☐ BS (Non-Nursing)
         ☐ 36 – 45   ☐ BSN
         ☐ 46 – 55   ☐ MS (Non-Nursing)
         ☐ 56 – 65   ☐ MS (Nursing)
         ☐ 66 – 70   ☐ Doctoral Degree
         ☐ Over 70

4. Cultural Background: Black or African American   ☐
   (Check **all** that apply)   Hispanic or Latino American   ☐
                             White or Caucasian American   ☐
                             Asian American   ☐
                             North American Indian   ☐
                             Other (Specify)   ☐   (_____)

5. Job Status: Administrator (Non-Nurse)   ☐
                          Administrator (Nurse)   ☐
                          Registered Nurse   ☐

6. Years of Nursing and/or Administrative Experience:

   Under 2 ☐   2 – 5 ☐   6 – 10 ☐   11 – 15 ☐
   16 – 20 ☐   21 – 25 ☐   26 – 30 ☐   Over 30 ☐

Questionnaire Directions and Example

Background:

Caring is important within health care organizations. Your responses to the statements on the following questionnaire will help identify and give researchers the opportunity to analyze your answers regarding factors important to the concept of organizational caring.

Directions:

Please answer the 26 numbered statements. Using a pen or pencil, mark an **X** in the circle that represents your response. Mark only one circle for each question. If your answer is that you *Agree* with the statement, then you would mark an **X** in the (4) for the statement as shown below.

Example:

2. Nurses are treated with respect by other professionals in the organization. This frequently happens within the organization where I work.

Strongly Disagree (1)	Disagree (2)	Neither Agree Nor Disagree (3)	Agree (**X**)	Strongly Agree (5)

---

1. Nurses are valued as individuals. This frequently happens within the organization where I work.

Strongly Disagree (1)	Disagree (2)	Neither Agree Nor Disagree (3)	Agree (4)	Strongly Agree (5)

2. Nurses are treated with respect by other professionals. This frequently happens within the organization where I work.

Strongly Disagree (1)	Disagree (2)	Neither Agree Nor Disagree (3)	Agree (4)	Strongly Agree (5)

3. Nurses are able to live their values in practice. This frequently happens within the organization where I work.

Strongly Disagree (1)	Disagree (2)	Neither Agree Nor Disagree (3)	Agree (4)	Strongly Agree (5)

4. Nurses are involved in policy decisions that affect patient care. This frequently happens within the organization where I work.

Strongly Disagree (1)	Disagree (2)	Neither Agree Nor Disagree (3)	Strongly Agree (4)	Agree (5)

5. We see administrators making rounds and helping out when needed. This frequently happens within the organization where I work.

Strongly Disagree (1)	Disagree (2)	Neither Agree Nor Disagree (3)	Agree (4)	Strongly Agree (5)

6. The focus of administrators is working on the budget and attending meetings. This frequently happens within the organization where I work.

Strongly Disagree (1)	Disagree (2)	Neither Agree Nor Disagree (3)	Agree (4)	Strongly Agree (5)

7. Nurses receive effective communication from administrators, which means we know exactly what is going on and why decisions are made. This frequently happens within the organization where I work.

Strongly Disagree (1)	Disagree (2)	Neither Agree Nor Disagree (3)	Agree (4)	Strongly Agree (5)

8. Nurses are counted only as numbers. This frequently happens within the organization where I work.

Strongly Disagree (1)	Disagree (2)	Neither Agree Nor Disagree (3)	Agree (4)	Strongly Agree (5)

9. Nurses are trusted by administrators. This frequently happens within the organization where I work.

Strongly Disagree (1)	Disagree (2)	Neither Agree Nor Disagree (3)	Agree (4)	Strongly Agree (5)

10. Nurses treat each patient as an individual. This frequently happens within the organization where I work.

Strongly Disagree (1)	Disagree (2)	Neither Agree Nor Disagree (3)	Agree (4)	Strongly Agree (5)

11. Being there with the patient is part of nursing practice. This frequently happens within the organization where I work.

Strongly Disagree (1)	Disagree (2)	Neither Agree Nor Disagree (3)	Agree (4)	Strongly Agree (5)

12. Nurses recognize the needs of the family. This frequently happens within the organization where I work.

Strongly Disagree (1)	Disagree (2)	Neither Agree Nor Disagree (3)	Strongly Agree (4)	Agree (5)

13. Nurses integrate awareness of the patient's body, mind, and spirit in their practice. This frequently happens within the organization where I work.

Strongly Disagree (1)	Disagree (2)	Neither Agree Nor Disagree (3)	Agree (4)	Strongly Agree (5)

14. Listening is a way nurses build relationships with patients. This frequently happens within the organization where I work.

Strongly Disagree (1)	Disagree (2)	Neither Agree Nor Disagree (3)	Agree (4)	Strongly Agree (5)

15. Administrators providing support for what nurses do increases the loyalty of nurses. This frequently happens within the organization where I work.

Strongly Disagree (1)	Disagree (2)	Neither Agree Nor Disagree (3)	Agree (4)	Strongly Agree (5)

16. Administrators empower nurses to make changes in the organization. This frequently happens within the organization where I work.

Strongly Disagree (1)	Disagree (2)	Neither Agree Nor Disagree (3)	Agree (4)	Strongly Agree (5)

17. Nurses demonstrate compassion for what the patient is experiencing. This frequently happens within the organization where I work.

Strongly Disagree (1)	Disagree (2)	Neither Agree Nor Disagree (3)	Agree (4)	Strongly Agree (5)

18. Nurses are committed to the nursing profession. This frequently happens within the organization where I work.

Strongly Disagree (1)	Disagree (2)	Neither Agree Nor Disagree (3)	Agree (4)	Strongly Agree (5)

19. Nurses are viewed as organizational overhead rather than organizational assets. This frequently happens within the organization where I work.

| Strongly Disagree (1) | Disagree (2) | Neither Agree Nor Disagree (3) | Agree (4) | Strongly Agree (5) |

20. Support from administrators results in increased nurse retention. This frequently happens within the organization where I work.

| Strongly Disagree (1) | Disagree (2) | Neither Agree Nor Disagree (3) | Agree (4) | Strongly Agree (5) |

21. Administrators recognize the value of nursing. This frequently happens within the organization where I work.

| Strongly Disagree (1) | Disagree (2) | Neither Agree Nor Disagree (3) | Agree (4) | Strongly Agree (5) |

22. Awareness of the value of nursing facilitates the choices that administrators make when allocating the budget. This frequently happens within the organization where I work.

| Strongly Disagree (1) | Disagree (2) | Neither Agree Nor Disagree (3) | Agree (4) | Strongly Agree (5) |

23. The integration of interpersonal resources (caring, patient education professional nursing practice) with traditional economic resources (money, goods, services), is included in the budget. This frequently happens within the organization where I work.

| Strongly Disagree (1) | Disagree (2) | Neither Agree Nor Disagree (3) | Agree (4) | Strongly Agree (5) |

24. The relational partnership between practicing nurses and administrators guides economic choice making in the organization. This frequently happens within the organization where I work.

| Strongly Disagree (1) | Disagree (2) | Neither Agree Nor Disagree (3) | Agree (4) | Strongly Agree (5) |

25. Nurses have financial knowledge to participate in organizational decision making. This frequently happens within the organization where I work.

| Strongly Disagree (1) | Disagree (2) | Neither Agree Nor Disagree (3) | Agree (4) | Strongly Agree (5) |

26. A supportive relationship between the nurses and the administrators results in improved economic and patient outcomes. This frequently happens within the organization where I work.

Strongly Disagree (1)	Disagree (2)	Neither Agree Nor Disagree (3)	Agree (4)	Strongly Agree (5)

The Relational Caring Questionnaire (Professional Form) is copyrighted. Please contact Dr. Marilyn Ray or Dr. Marian Turkel via e-mail to formally request use of the questionnaire. Permission will be granted as long as no changes are made to the questionnaire.

Marilyn A. Ray PhD, RN, CTN-A, FAAN
Professor Emeritus
Florida Atlantic University
Christine E. Lynn College of Nursing
Boca Raton, Florida
mray@health.fau.edu

Marian C. Turkel PhD RN, NEA-BC, FAAN
Associate Professor
Florida Atlantic University
Christine E. Lynn College of Nursing
Boca Raton, Florida
mturkel@health.fau.edu

Caring Factor Survey (CFS)
(Nelson & Watson, 2012)

Directions to patient:

This is a survey that measures your perception of your care while in this facility. It would be very helpful if you would respond to each of the 10 statements below about how you feel regarding the care you are currently receiving from the staff. The information you provide by completing this survey will help us understand your experience of care more clearly and improve the caring experience for our patients and their families/significant others while they are at the facility. If you are able to respond to this brief survey, we thank you for your time and consideration. If you are unable to respond, we understand and respect your decision. Your return of the survey will be considered your consent for us to use your responses to better understand perception of caring as reported by the patient or patient's family member.

Are you the: Patient _____ Family Member _____   (Please check one)

If you do not want to respond to this survey, now or at a later time, the reason that most closely resembles your reason is:

_____ I am too sick or upset to respond to a survey.

_____ I do not want to spend my time responding to a survey.

_____ I do not like to give out information about myself.

Other _____

If you do want to participate in this survey, please read the following instructions and respond to the 10 statements. If you have additional questions about the survey, or would like to know about the results of this survey, you can contact:

John Nelson, President, Healthcare Environment
jn@hcenvironment.com

Thank you for your time and consideration in helping with this important work!

Instructions: Please read each statement as it relates to you as a patient (or as a family member) about the care you are receiving from the nursing staff. You will be asked to indicate how much you agree or disagree with each statement. Please mark your responses by putting a checkmark next to the number that best represents your opinion. For example, if you strongly agree with the statement, you put a checkmark next to #7.

Strongly Disagree 1	Disagree 2	Slightly Disagree 3	Neutral 4	Slightly Agree 5	Agree 6	Strongly Agree 7

1. Every day I am here, I see that the care is provided with loving kindness.

   1_____   2_____   3_____   4_____   5_____   6_____   7_____

2. As a team, my caregivers are good at creative problem solving to meet my individual needs and requests.

   1_____   2_____   3_____   4_____   5_____   6_____   7_____

3. The care providers honored my own faith, helped instill hope, and respected my belief system as part of my care.

   1_____   2_____   3_____   4_____   5_____   6_____   7_____

4. When my caregivers teach me something new, they teach me in a way that I can understand.

   1_____   2_____   3_____   4_____   5_____   6_____   7_____

5. My caregivers encouraged me to practice my own, individual, spiritual beliefs as part of my self-caring and healing.

   1_____   2_____   3_____   4_____   5_____   6_____   7_____

6. My caregivers have responded to me as a whole person, helping to take care of all my needs and concerns.

   1_____   2_____   3_____   4_____   5_____   6_____   7_____

7. My caregivers have established a helping and trusting relationship with me during my time here.

   1_____   2_____   3_____   4_____   5_____   6_____   7_____

8. My health care team has created a healing environment that recognizes the connections between my body, mind, and spirit.

   1_____   2_____   3_____   4_____   5_____   6_____   7_____

9. I feel like I can talk openly and honestly about what I am thinking, because those who are caring for me embrace my feelings, no matter what my feelings are.

   1_____   2_____   3_____   4_____   5_____   6_____   7_____

10. My caregivers are accepting and supportive of my beliefs regarding a higher power, which allows for the possibility that I and my family will heal.

    1_____   2_____   3_____   4_____   5_____   6_____   7_____

11. Please describe the attitudes, behaviors, and/or actions of your care provider(s) that led to your answers.

12. Please put a checkmark next to the one that is closest to your race/ethnicity.

_____ Hispanic

_____ White

_____ Non-Hispanic

_____ Hispanic-Black

_____ Non-Hispanic Black

_____ Asian American / Pacific Islander

_____ Alaska Native / American Indian

_____ Other _____

Caring Factor Survey–Caring for Self (CFS-CS)
(Nelson & Watson, 2012)

Directions to employee:

This is a survey that measures your perception of care for yourself. It would be very helpful if you would respond to each of the 10 statements below about how you feel regarding the care you are currently providing for yourself. In health care, employees spend a great deal of time and effort taking care of others, but we do not know how much time employees spend taking care of themselves within their lives. The information you provide by completing this survey will help us understand the extent to which you, as an employee, take care of yourself. Within the theory of caring as proposed by Watson, caring for others begins by caring for self; we would like to know how you are doing in this respect. If you are able to respond to this brief survey, we thank you for your time and consideration. If you are unable to respond, we understand and respect your decision.

If you do want to participate in this survey, please read the following instructions and respond to the 10 statements. If you have additional questions about the survey, or would like to know about the results of this survey, you can contact:

John Nelson, President, Healthcare Environment jn@hcenvironment.com

Thank you for your time and consideration in helping with this important work!

Instructions: Please read each statement as it relates to your self-care. You will be asked to indicate how much you agree or disagree with each statement. Please mark your responses by putting a checkmark next to the number that best represents your opinion.

For example, if you strongly agree with the statement, you put a checkmark next to #7.

Strongly Disagree 1	Disagree 2	Slightly Disagree 3	Neutral 4	Slightly Agree 5	Agree 6	Strongly Agree 7

1. Every day I care for myself with loving kindness.

   1_____   2_____   3_____   4_____   5_____   6_____   7_____

2. I am creative at solving problems to meet my individual needs.

   1_____   2_____   3_____   4_____   5_____   6_____   7_____

3. I honor my own faith, instill hope, and respect my belief system as part of my selfcare.

   1_____   2_____   3_____   4_____   5_____   6_____   7_____

4. I value opportunities that allow me to increase my knowledge and understanding about myself.

   1_____   2_____   3_____   4_____   5_____   6_____   7_____

5. I take time to practice my own, individual, spiritual beliefs as part of my self-caring and healing.
   (Do not respond to this statement if you feel spiritual beliefs are too personal.)

   1_____   2_____   3_____   4_____   5_____   6_____   7_____

6. I appreciate myself as a whole person and seek to take care of all of my needs and concerns.

   1_____   2_____   3_____   4_____   5_____   6_____   7_____

7. I have established helping and trusting relationships.

   1_____   2_____   3_____   4_____   5_____   6_____   7_____

8. It is important for me to create a healing environment around me that recognizes the connections between my body, mind, and spirit.

   1_____   2_____   3_____   4_____   5_____   6_____   7_____

9. I am able to evaluate my thoughts openly and honestly no matter what my feelings are because I embrace every aspect of who I am.

   1_____   2_____   3_____   4_____   5_____   6_____   7_____

10. I accept and support my own current beliefs in a higher power, which allows for me to heal.
    (Do not respond to this statement if you feel spiritual beliefs are too personal.)

    1_____   2_____   3_____   4_____   5_____   6_____   7_____

11. Please describe the attitudes, behaviors, and/or actions that led to your answers.

12. Please put a checkmark next to the one that is closest to your race/ethnicity.

    _____ Hispanic

    _____ White

    _____ Non-Hispanic

    _____ Hispanic-Black

    _____ Non-Hispanic Black

    _____ Asian American / Pacific Islander

    _____ Alaska Native / American Indian

    _____ Other _____

Caring Factor Survey–Caring for Coworker (CFS-CC)
(Nelson & Watson, 2012)

Directions to employee:

This is a survey that measures your perception of caring by your coworkers. It would be very helpful if you would respond to each of the 10 statements below about how you feel regarding the caring behaviors of your coworkers. In health care, employees spend a great deal of time and effort taking care of patients, but we do not understand the level of caring that is experienced between the staff members. The information you provide by completing this survey will help us understand the extent that you, as an employee, believe caring is demonstrated by your coworkers. Within the theory of caring as proposed by Watson, caring for others occurs in 10 specific ways, which are each addressed within this very brief survey. We would like to know to what degree these behaviors are observed by you among your coworkers. If you are able to respond to this survey, we thank you for your time and consideration. If you are unable to respond, we understand and respect your decision.

If you do want to participate in this survey, please read the following instructions and respond to the 10 statements. If you have additional questions about the survey, or would like to know about the results of this survey, you can contact:

John Nelson, President, Healthcare Environment
jn@hcenvironment.com

Thank you for your time and consideration in helping with this important work!

Instructions: Please read each statement as it relates to your perception of caring demonstrated by your coworkers. You will be asked to indicate how much you agree or disagree with each statement. Please mark your responses by putting a checkmark next to the number that best represents your opinion. For example, if you strongly agree with the statement, you put a checkmark next to #7.

Strongly Disagree 1	Disagree 2	Slightly Disagree 3	Neutral 4	Slightly Agree 5	Agree 6	Strongly Agree 7

1. Every day I am here, I see staff members caring for each other with loving kindness.

   1_____ 2_____ 3_____ 4_____ 5_____ 6_____ 7_____

2. As a team, my coworkers are good at creative problem solving to meet each other's individual needs and requests.

   1_____ 2_____ 3_____ 4_____ 5_____ 6_____ 7_____

3. My coworkers acknowledge and respect my belief system.

   1_____ 2_____ 3_____ 4_____ 5_____ 6_____ 7_____

4. When part or all of our team needs to learn something new, my coworkers are good at making sure we use teaching methods that everyone will understand.

   1_____ 2_____ 3_____ 4_____ 5_____ 6_____ 7_____

5. My coworkers encourage me to practice my own spiritual beliefs as part of my selfcaring and healing.

   1_____   2_____   3_____   4_____   5_____   6_____   7_____

6. My coworkers respond to me as a whole person, helping me respond to all my needs and concerns.

   1_____   2_____   3_____   4_____   5_____   6_____   7_____

7. My coworkers have established a helping and trusting relationship with me.

   1_____   2_____   3_____   4_____   5_____   6_____   7_____

8. Our health care team always seeks to create a healing environment that recognizes the connections between body, mind, and spirit.

   1_____   2_____   3_____   4_____   5_____   6_____   7_____

9. I feel that I can talk openly and honestly about what I am thinking, because my coworkers respect my feelings, no matter what my feelings are.

   1_____   2_____   3_____   4_____   5_____   6_____   7_____

10. My coworkers acknowledge and are supportive of my beliefs regarding a higher power.

    1_____   2_____   3_____   4_____   5_____   6_____   7_____

11. Please describe the attitudes, behaviors, and/or actions that led to your answers.

12. Please put a checkmark next to the one that is closest to your race/ethnicity.

    _____ Hispanic

    _____ White

    _____ Non-Hispanic

    _____ Hispanic-Black

    _____ Non-Hispanic Black

    _____ Asian American / Pacific Islander

    _____ Alaska Native / American Indian

    _____ Other _____

Caring Factor Survey–Caring of Preceptor (CFS-CP)
(Nelson & Watson, 2012)

Directions to employee:

This is a survey that measures your perception of caring by your preceptor(s) who trained you in your new job. It would be very helpful if you would respond to each of the 9 statements below about how you feel regarding the caring behaviors of the preceptors you worked with. In health care, employees spend a great deal of time and effort taking care of patients, but we do not understand the level of caring that is experienced from the preceptor to the new employee. The information you provide by completing this survey will help us understand the extent that you, as an employee, believe caring was demonstrated by your preceptors. Within the theory of caring as proposed by Watson, caring for others occurs in specific ways, which are each addressed within this very brief survey. We would like to know to what degree these behaviors are demonstrated by your preceptor(s). If you are able to respond to this survey, we thank you for your time and consideration. If you are unable to respond, we understand and respect your decision.

If you do want to participate in this survey, please read the following instructions and respond to the 10 statements. If you have additional questions about the survey, or would like to know about the results of this survey, you can contact:

John Nelson, President, Healthcare Environment
jn@hcenvironment.com

Thank you for your time and consideration in helping with this important work!

Instructions: Please read each statement as it relates to your perception of caring demonstrated by your preceptor. If you had more than one preceptor, respond based on your general experience of working with your preceptors. You will be asked to indicate how much you agree or disagree with each statement. Please mark your responses by putting a checkmark next to the number that best represents your opinion. For example, if you strongly agree with the statement, you put a checkmark next to #7.

Strongly Disagree 1	Disagree 2	Slightly Disagree 3	Neutral 4	Slightly Agree 5	Agree 6	Strongly Agree 7

1. My preceptor was good at creative problem solving to meet my individual needs and requests.

   1_____   2_____   3_____   4_____   5_____   6_____   7_____

2. The preceptor(s) helped to instill hope and respected my belief system.

   1_____   2_____   3_____   4_____   5_____   6_____   7_____

3. When my preceptors taught me something new, they taught me in a way that I could understand.

   1_____   2_____   3_____   4_____   5_____   6_____   7_____

4. My preceptor(s) encouraged me to practice my own, individual, spiritual beliefs as part of my self-caring.

   1_____   2_____   3_____   4_____   5_____   6_____   7_____

5. My preceptor(s) responded to me as a whole person, helping to take care of all my needs and concerns.

   1_____   2_____   3_____   4_____   5_____   6_____   7_____

6. My preceptor(s) established a helping and trusting relationship with me during my time here.

   1_____   2_____   3_____   4_____   5_____   6_____   7_____

7. My preceptor(s) created a healing environment that recognized the connections between my body, mind, and spirit.

   1_____   2_____   3_____   4_____   5_____   6_____   7_____

8. I felt like I could talk openly and honestly with my preceptor(s) about what I was thinking, because my preceptor(s) embraced my feelings, no matter what my feelings were.

   1_____   2_____   3_____   4_____   5_____   6_____   7_____

9. My preceptors were accepting and supportive of my beliefs regarding a higher power, which allowed for the possibility of me to grow.

   1_____   2_____   3_____   4_____   5_____   6_____   7_____

10. Please describe the attitudes, behaviors, and/or actions that led to your answers.

11. Please put a checkmark next to the one that is closest to your race/ethnicity.

    _____ Hispanic
    _____ White
    _____ Non-Hispanic
    _____ Hispanic-Black
    _____ Non-Hispanic Black
    _____ Asian American / Pacific Islander
    _____ Alaska Native / American Indian
    _____ Other _____

12. Gender

    _____ Male
    _____ Female

13. Please give your current age. If you prefer not to answer, simply state "prefer not to answer."_____

Caring Factor Survey–Caring of Manager (CFS-CM)
(Nelson & Watson, 2012)

Directions to employee:

This is a survey that measures your perception of caring by the manager of your unit/department. It would be very helpful if you would respond to each of the 10 statements below about how you feel regarding the caring behaviors of your manager. In health care, employees spend a great deal of time and effort taking care of patients, but we do not understand the level of caring that is experienced from the manager to employees. The information you provide by completing this survey will help us understand the extent that you, as an employee, believe caring was demonstrated by your manager. Within the theory of caring as proposed by Watson, caring for others occurs in 10 specific ways, which are each addressed within this very brief survey. We would like to know to what degree these behaviors are demonstrated by your manager. If you are able to respond to this survey, we thank you for your time and consideration. If you are unable to respond, we understand and respect your decision.

If you do want to participate in this survey, please read the following instructions and respond to the 10 statements. If you have additional questions about the survey, or would like to know about the results of this survey, you can contact:

John Nelson, President, Healthcare Environment
jn@hcenvironment.com

Thank you for your time and consideration in helping with this important work!

Instructions: Please read each statement as it relates to your perception of caring demonstrated by your manager. You will be asked to indicate how much you agree or disagree with each statement. Please mark your responses by putting a checkmark next to the number that best represents your opinion. For example, if you strongly agree with the statement, you put a checkmark next to #7.

Strongly Disagree 1	Disagree 2	Slightly Disagree 3	Neutral 4	Slightly Agree 5	Agree 6	Strongly Agree 7

1. Every day I am here I see my manager treat employees with loving kindness.

   1_____ 2_____ 3_____ 4_____ 5_____ 6_____ 7_____

2. My manager is good at creative problem solving to meet my individual needs and requests.

   1_____ 2_____ 3_____ 4_____ 5_____ 6_____ 7_____

3. The manager of my unit/department helps to instill hope and respects my belief system.

   1_____ 2_____ 3_____ 4_____ 5_____ 6_____ 7_____

4. When my manager teaches me something new, she/he teaches me in a way that I can understand.

   1_____ 2_____ 3_____ 4_____ 5_____ 6_____ 7_____

5. The manager of my unit/department encourages me to practice my own, individual, spiritual beliefs as part of my self-caring.

   1_____   2_____   3_____   4_____   5_____   6_____   7_____

6. The manager of my unit/department responds to me as a whole person, helping to take care of all my needs and concerns.

   1_____   2_____   3_____   4_____   5_____   6_____   7_____

7. The manager of my unit/department has established a helping and trusting relationship with me during my time here in this unit/department.

   1_____   2_____   3_____   4_____   5_____   6_____   7_____

8. The manager of my unit/department creates a healing environment in our unit/department that recognizes the connections between body, mind, and spirit.

   1_____   2_____   3_____   4_____   5_____   6_____   7_____

9. I feel like I can talk openly and honestly with the manager of my unit/department about what I am thinking, because the manager of my unit/department embraces my feelings, no matter what my feelings are.

   1_____   2_____   3_____   4_____   5_____   6_____   7_____

10. The manager of my unit/department is accepting and supportive of my beliefs regarding a higher power, which allows for the possibility of me to grow.

   1_____   2_____   3_____   4_____   5_____   6_____   7_____

11. Please describe the attitudes, behaviors, and/or actions that led to your answers.

12. Please describe a caring moment that has occurred between you and your manager.

13. Please put a checkmark next to the one that is closest to your race/ethnicity.

   _____ Hispanic
   _____ White
   _____ Non-Hispanic
   _____ Hispanic-Black
   _____ Non-Hispanic Black
   _____ Asian American / Pacific Islander
   _____ Alaska Native / American Indian
   _____ Other _____

Caring Factor Survey–Care Provider Version (CFS-CPV)
(Nelson & Watson, 2012)

Directions to care provider:

This is a survey that measures your perception of the care you are providing for the patients who are under your care. It would be very helpful if you would respond to each of the 20 statements below about how you feel regarding the care you are currently providing to patients. The information you provide by completing this survey will help us understand your perception of providing care more clearly. If you are able to respond to this brief survey, we thank you for your time and consideration. If you are not able to respond, we understand and respect your decision.

If you do want to participate in this survey, please read the following instructions and respond to the 20 statements. If you have additional questions about the survey, or would like to know about the results of this survey, you can contact:

John Nelson, President, Healthcare Environment

jn@hcenvironment.com

Thank you for your time and consideration in helping us understand the process of caring for patients!

Instructions: Please read each statement as it relates to you as a care provider to patients. You will be asked to indicate how much you agree or disagree with each statement. Please mark your responses by putting a checkmark next to the number that best represents your opinion. For example, if you strongly agree with the statement, you put a checkmark next to #7.

Strongly Disagree 1	Disagree 2	Slightly Disagree 3	Neutral 4	Slightly Agree 5	Agree 6	Strongly Agree 7

1. Overall, the care I give is provided with loving kindness.

    1_____   2_____   3_____   4_____   5_____   6_____   7_____

2. I believe the health care team that I am currently working with solves unexpected problems really well.

    1_____   2_____   3_____   4_____   5_____   6_____   7_____

3. Every day that I provide patient care, I do so with loving kindness.

    1_____   2_____   3_____   4_____   5_____   6_____   7_____

4. As a team, my colleagues and I are good at creative problem solving to meet the individual needs and requests of our patients.

    1_____   2_____   3_____   4_____   5_____   6_____   7_____

5. The care I provide honors the patients' faith, instills hope, and respects the patients' belief system.

    1_____   2_____   3_____   4_____   5_____   6_____   7_____

6. When I teach patients something new, I teach in a way that they can understand.

    1_____   2_____   3_____   4_____   5_____   6_____   7_____

7. I help support the hope and faith of the patients I care for.

   1_____   2_____   3_____   4_____   5_____   6_____   7_____

8. I am responsive to my patients' readiness to learn when I teach them something new.

   1_____   2_____   3_____   4_____   5_____   6_____   7_____

9. I am very respectful of my patients' individual spiritual beliefs and practices.

   1_____   2_____   3_____   4_____   5_____   6_____   7_____

10. I create an environment for the patients I care for that helps them heal physically and spiritually.

    1_____   2_____   3_____   4_____   5_____   6_____   7_____

11. I encourage patients to practice their own, individual, spiritual beliefs as part of selfcaring and healing.

    1_____   2_____   3_____   4_____   5_____   6_____   7_____

12. I work to create a healing environment that recognizes the patients' connections between body, mind, and spirit.

    1_____   2_____   3_____   4_____   5_____   6_____   7_____

13. I am able to establish a helping and trusting relationship with the patients I care for during their stay here.

    1_____   2_____   3_____   4_____   5_____   6_____   7_____

14. I work to meet the physical needs as well as the emotional or spiritual needs of the patients I care for.

    1_____   2_____   3_____   4_____   5_____   6_____   7_____

15. Everybody on the health care team values relationships that are helpful and trusting.

    1_____   2_____   3_____   4_____   5_____   6_____   7_____

16. I respond to each patient as a whole person, helping to take care of all of their needs and concerns.

    1_____   2_____   3_____   4_____   5_____   6_____   7_____

17. I encourage patients to speak honestly about their feelings, no matter what those feelings are.

    1_____   2_____   3_____   4_____   5_____   6_____   7_____

18. If patients told me that they believed in miracles, I would support the patient in this belief.

    1_____   2_____   3_____   4_____   5_____   6_____   7_____

19. Patients I care for can talk openly and honestly with me about their thoughts because I embrace their feelings, no matter what those feelings are.

    1_____   2_____   3_____   4_____   5_____   6_____   7_____

20. I am accepting and supportive of patients' beliefs regarding a higher power if they believe it allows for healing.

    1_____   2_____   3_____   4_____   5_____   6_____   7_____

Caring Factor Survey–Specific Care Provider (CFS-SCP)
(Nelson & Watson, 2012)

Directions to patient:

This is a survey that measures your perception of a specific care provider while in this facility.

To ensure you know what specific care provider we are interested in, we have provided a photograph of this care provider with this survey. It would be very helpful if you would respond to each of the 10 statements below about how you feel regarding the care you are currently receiving from this specific staff member. The information you provide by completing this survey will help us understand your experience of care provided by this care provider. This information will help us understand your care experience more clearly and improve the caring experience for our patients and their families/significant others while they are at the facility.

Are you the: Patient _____ Family Member _____ (Please check one)

If you do not want to respond to this survey, now or at a later time, the reason that most closely resembles your reason is:

_____ I am too sick or upset to respond to a survey.

_____ I do not want to spend my time responding to a survey.

_____ I do not like to give out information about myself.

Other_____

If you are able to respond to this brief survey, we thank you for your time and consideration. If you are unable to respond, we understand and respect your decision.

If you do want to participate in this survey, please read the following instructions and respond to the 10 statements. If you have additional questions about the survey, or would like to know about the results of this survey, you can contact:

John Nelson, President, Healthcare Environment
jn@hcenvironment.com

Thank you for your time and consideration in helping with this important work!

Instructions: Please read each statement as it relates to you as a patient (or as a family member) about the care you are receiving from this particular care provider. You will be asked to indicate how much you agree or disagree with each statement. Please mark your responses by putting a checkmark next to the number that best represents your opinion.

Strongly Disagree 1	Disagree 2	Slightly Disagree 3	Neutral 4	Slightly Agree 5	Agree 6	Strongly Agree 7

1. Every day I am here, I see examples of this care provider providing care with loving kindness.

   1_____   2_____   3_____   4_____   5_____   6_____   7_____

2. This care provider works with the entire health care team to creatively solve problems to meet my individual needs and requests.

   1_____   2_____   3_____   4_____   5_____   6_____   7_____

3. This care provider honors my own faith, helps instill hope, and respects my belief system as part of my care.

   1_____   2_____   3_____   4_____   5_____   6_____   7_____

4. When this care provider teaches me something new, he/she teaches me in a way that I can understand.

   1_____   2_____   3_____   4_____   5_____   6_____   7_____

5. This care provider encourages me to practice my own, individual, spiritual beliefs as part of my self-caring and healing.

   1_____   2_____   3_____   4_____   5_____   6_____   7_____

6. This care provider creates a healing environment that recognizes the wholeness and oneness of my body, mind, and spirit.

   1_____   2_____   3_____   4_____   5_____   6_____   7_____

7. This care provider has established a helping and trusting relationship with me during my time here.

   1_____   2_____   3_____   4_____   5_____   6_____   7_____

8. This care provider responds to me as a whole person, helping to take care of all my needs and concerns.

   1_____   2_____   3_____   4_____   5_____   6_____   7_____

9. I feel like I can talk openly and honestly about what I am thinking with this care provider, because he/she embraces my feelings, both positive and negative.

   1_____   2_____   3_____   4_____   5_____   6_____   7_____

10. This care provider is accepting and supportive of my beliefs regarding a higher power, which allows for the possibility of me and my family to heal.

    1_____   2_____   3_____   4_____   5_____   6_____   7_____

11. Please describe the attitudes, behaviors, and/or actions this care provider showed that led to your answers.

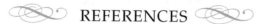

REFERENCES

Nelson, J., & Watson, J. (Eds.). (2012). *Measuring caring: International research on caritas as healing.* New York, NY: Springer Publishing. Retrieved from http://www.springerpub.com/measuring-caring-supplemental-materials

Ray, M., & Turkel, M. (2005). *Economic and Patient Outcomes of the Nurse-Patient Relationship: Final Report. Submitted to the TriService Nursing Research Program, Uniformed Services University of the Health Sciences.* Bethesda, MD.

Ray, M., & Turkel, M. (2009). Relational caring questionnaires. In J. Watson (Ed.), *Assessing and measuring caring in nursing and health sciences* (2nd ed.). New York, NY: Springer Publishing. (Patient and Professional Relational Caring Questionnaires listed on the Watson Caring Science Institute Website [www.wcsi.com]).

Ray, M., & Turkel, M. (in press). Relational caring questionnaires. In K. Sitzman & J. Watson (Eds.), *Watson Caring Science Guide to Assessing and measuring caring in nursing and health sciences* (3rd ed.). New York, NY: Springer Publishing.

Appendix B: Caritas Coach Abstracts

APPENDIX B.1
INTRODUCTION OF THE CARITAS PROCESSES®
INTO AN OUTPATIENT CLINICAL SETTING

Emily Barr

Introduction: The Children's Hospital Colorado's Immunodeficiency Program (CHIP), a pediatric, youth, and maternal HIV clinic that opened in 1992, serves families living with HIV in the Rocky Mountain Region. The CHIP clinic is a multidisciplinary program staffed by nurse practitioners, physicians, social workers, a dietician, pharmacist, psychiatrist, neuro-developmental psychologist, and research personnel. They serve a high-risk population living with a chronic and potentially life-threatening condition, who struggle with stigma, disclosure, sexual health, and trauma. They are challenged by side effects to medication, and adherence. Caring for this patient population can be stressful and intense. Evidence indicates that there is a high risk of secondary trauma and burnout among care providers working in this field. The CHIP team requested education to develop skills to promote resiliency, self-care practices, and a healthier working environment. It is hoped that this education will promote better health outcomes for the population being served and decrease staff burnout.

Significance: By providing education to the CHIP team on HeartMath®, the 10 Caritas Processes®, and the 3 Vital Questions™, the staff learned about caring-healing practices to manage ongoing stress, which negatively impacts their lives and those in their care. Using knowledge and practices embedded in loving-kindness, equanimity, and compassion (Watson, 2008), the CHIP team will create a more supportive and compassionate environment with each other and with the patients for whom they care.

Purpose: The purpose of the project was to provide education to the CHIP team to cultivate a culture of self-care. The education fostered opportunities for increased resiliency and awareness about how to create and maintain transpersonal caring relationships between CHIP team members and the patients in their care.

Setting and Participants: There were four sessions on the Caritas Processes led by the author. The first session took place at a research team retreat; 16 CHIP members were in attendance. The second session took place during a postclinic meeting with one physician, one staff nurse, and six nurse practitioners. The final session was led by the author during a staff meeting with 10 nurses (registered nurses [RNs]/nurse practitioners [NPs]) in attendance. This was an opportunity to introduce Caring Science (Watson, 2008) to staff and discuss how it influenced their personal and professional practices, particularly in relation to their jobs. There were two large training sessions in HeartMath and the 3 Vital Questions, which were led by Caritas Coach™ and Registered Nurse Christine Griffin. The HeartMath session was attended by 24 CHIP staff members and the 3 Vital Questions session was attended by 29 CHIP team members.

Project Description/Process: The author met with the clinical manager, Caritas Coach, and Hospital Personnel Development Specialist, Christine Griffin, to identify the needs of the CHIP team and the current challenges they face. The team identified the ways in which certain interactions and/or meetings with patients left them feeling stressed and anxious, despite their commitment to the provision of compassionate care. As a result, education that included resiliency and self-care was suggested as strategies to best address the challenges. HeartMath and the 3 Vital Questions trainings were specifically recommended to best address these challenges. The author further introduced the Caritas Processes before introducing HeartMath to ensure staff would be familiar with the philosophy and the major tenets of the Caring Science. The 3 Vital Questions promotes developing relationships that are resilient, creative, and empowering. It uses coaching as a technique and the philosophy overlaps with several of the major tenets of both HeartMath and the Caritas Processes.

Project Outcome(s)/Projected Outcomes: The projected outcomes will result in the CHIP team members implementing HeartMath into their daily practice. Individual staff from across the diverse disciplines have encouraged a culture of self-care, potentiating an increase in resiliency and decrease in burnout. Caring Science will be incorporated into patient care interactions as CHIP team members become more mindful of creating transpersonal caring relationships, thus demonstrating equanimity and loving-kindness, moving beyond the ego-self to promote healing and wholeness of mind-body-spirit (Watson, 2008).

Project Evaluation or Partial/Projected Evaluation if Not Completed: Each member of the CHIP team who participated was provided an assessment tool on resiliency and burnout, in addition to a tool related to the use of HeartMath prior to and posttraining. The goal was twofold: (a) assess change related to stress and/or anxiety in relation to working within the current setting with a high-risk population and (b) assess change in relation to how the training may have been incorporated into their personal and professional lives in relation to changing practice.

Future Directions: The author will follow up with future education and look to bring in speakers, including creative opportunities to incorporate Caring Science into current practice. "Pause to Care" signs have also been placed outside the doors to the clinic to remind staff to pause, breathe, and center prior to providing care.

Acknowledgments: I express my gratitude and acknowledge the medical director of the CHIP clinic, Elizabeth McFarland, MD; the clinical manager, Kay Kinzie, FNP; and the other clinical and research staff. I would also like to acknowledge the help and support of Chris Griffin, MS, RN, CPN; Lisa Goldberg, PhD, RN; Jan Anderson, EdD, MSN, AHN-BC; and my family.

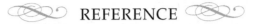

REFERENCE

Watson, J. (2008). *Nursing: The philosophy and science of caring* (Rev. ed.). Boulder: University Press of Colorado.

APPENDIX B.2
NEW EMPLOYEE CARITAS LITERACY
Lyn Brown

Introduction: With 152 Veterans Affairs Medical Centers (VAMCs) and 1,400 community-based outpatient clinics, the VAMC system, the largest healthcare provider in the United States and its territories, is committed to fulfill "ICARE" core values toward caring excellence. Dr. Jean Watson's (2008) Theory of Human Caring has been adopted as the professional practice model at several VAMCs to meet this purpose. The practice of Caring Science, named "Caritas Caring" by the nursing discipline at the Atlanta VAMC through the years, has strengthened with the guidance of Caritas Coaches. The excellent level of Caritas Caring was significant in the Atlanta VAMC attaining Magnet® designation. Recurrent redesignations showcased continuing nursing transformational leadership and nursing Caring Science exemplars of loving care and compassion. The facility leadership endorses the Caritas Caring excellence and budgets to sustain the status of being an Affiliate of the Watson Caring Science Institute.

Significance: Although nursing initiatives have led the way toward a caring culture change at the Atlanta VAMC, Caritas Caring is not exclusively a nursing role. All employees must be part of the transformation to change a system culture. Therefore, it is important that employees of all disciplines and departments have a basic understanding of Caring Science and learn how to practice Caritas Caring. One of the most effective ways to reach all employees is to introduce Caring Science at the first presentation of the general hospital orientation for new employees.

Purpose: This project is aimed at infusing caring practice of unconditional loving-kindness and compassion for self, colleagues, and the VA patients throughout the Atlanta VAMC. The specific project is to introduce the core philosophy and principles of loving-kindness and compassion and to teach a centering technique for self-care to all new hospital employees at the first new employee orientation.

Setting and Participants: The setting for this project is in the Pete Wheeler Auditorium of the Atlanta VAMC where all new employee general hospital orientations occur twice a month. The new employees typically include a diverse mixture of all disciplines, levels of education, and leadership. New employees will be working in various departments and leadership levels, for example, housekeeping, engineering, risk management, executives, managers, union stewards, physicians, and nursing. Nine Caritas Coaches presently at the Atlanta VAMC, as well as Caritas Champions, will take turns presenting, rotating monthly, sometimes weekly. A year's presenter roster schedule will be posted, including backup speakers for every session. The nursing staff will continue to receive additional "nursing-focused orientation" about Dr. Jean Watson, Caring Science, and the practice of Caritas Caring of the Veterans during the first week employed at the Atlanta VAMC.

Project Description: *The New Employee Caring Science Literacy Project* is the development of a 30-minute presentation on the basic philosophy and principles of Watson's (2008) Human Caring Theory. The presentation is focused on briefly introducing and educating all new employees about loving-kindness and compassion for self, colleagues, and patients. The presentation will be presented by different Caritas Coaches and Caritas Champions, so it is designed as a step-by-step template for quality control of the content and to insure interaction with the audience. However, there is enough flexibility to allow the speaker's style to shine. The PowerPoint presentation includes homage to our Veterans, a brief biography of Jean Watson, the scope of the Caring Science global impact, and a lesson in centering. A short video skit is shown to highlight the difference between Caritas Caring and non–Caritas Caring behaviors with time for discussion and authentic stories. Two trifold brochure handouts were developed to provide a written description of centering techniques and a list of 25 ways to practice Caritas Caring every day at work. One brochure is geared for nonclinical staff who have little to no direct interaction with patients and the other brochure focuses on employees who provide treatment or have direct interaction with patients. The project, all associated developed materials, and implementation are pending approval from the Atlanta VAMC director.

Projected Outcomes: System-wide practice of loving-kindness and compassion by all employees toward themselves, colleagues, and patients will have an enormous impact on improving the trust in the workplace and increasing staff and patient satisfaction. This, in turn, leads to employee retention, adequate staff, and customer satisfaction. Increased Press Ganey Scores will also significantly contribute to Magnet Award redesignations. New employee leaders introduced to Caritas Caring early transform the culture from within.

Projected Evaluation: Once orientation presentations begin, feedback will be ongoing from the written evaluations each new employee will be requested to complete, as well as from informal feedback and observations of the changing culture.

Future Directions: Next steps include helping leaders to learn their roles in cultivating a Caritas Caring culture. Specifically, Caritas Coaches will be teaching and guiding the top facility leaders in ways to incorporate Caring Science into their departmental goals, practices, and activities budgets. A "Caritas Caring Starts with You" banner in the Atlanta VAMC atrium will begin to resonate with all employees. This project will serve as a reference for other VAMCs to incorporate Caring Science in their new employee orientation.

Acknowledgments: I thank Dr. Jean Watson for her vision and passion for creating global Caritas Caring communities. A special thanks to Dr. Lynne Wagner, Caritas Coach Education Program faculty member and mentor; Chanda Harrison, Veterans Affairs Nursing Academic Partnership faculty; and Cheryl Handy, associate director for Medical Specialty Care Services at the Atlanta VAMC, for their dedication to my journey that transformed my life and practice.

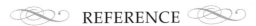

REFERENCE

Watson, J. (2008). *Nursing: The philosophy and science of caring* (Rev. ed.). Boulder: University Press of Colorado.

APPENDIX B.3
CARITAS LEADERSHIP: CREATING AN AUTHENTIC CARING ORGANIZATION

Debra Morton & Michelle Camicia

Introduction: Healthcare leaders use the Caritas Processes® (Watson, 2008) and the Theory of Human Caring/Caring Science to develop transformative leadership practices within an acute care hospital in Northern California.

Significance: Our current healthcare systems are in need of transformative leadership that will create a culture of caring through inspiring, leading, and accountability to provide vision and reform. Transformative leadership is guided by a spiritual journey of caring and healing and results in transforming self and system (Watson, 2005). Caring can be viewed as a compassionate response to working with others (Dyess, Prestia, & Smith, 2015). This includes a multidisciplinary group of healthcare leaders who lead by example to affect change and create a compassionate caring organization that serves our patients, employees, and community as a whole through the integration and practice of Caring Science. It is the entirety of the system that must be transformed to transition healthcare from a mechanistic, dehumanized operation to one that is humanistic.

Purpose: The purpose for this project was to create a biogenic caring healthcare organization through intentional, creative strategies that will create an authentic culture of caring through leadership presence and practicing of the Caritas Processes within self and system, starting with self.

Settings and Participants: This project occurred in a 248–acute care bed hospital in Northern California. It included over 500 registered nurses, patient care technicians, unit assistants, and other ancillary healthcare leaders.

Project Description/Process: The primary focus for this project was for the Caritas Coach® to lead by example and incorporate Caring Science in everything that we did. Key initiatives included the following: (a) the use of high-energy words and biogenic Caritas language when communicating; (b) the engagement of spiritual care early on in the process to help propel Caring Science, loving-kindness, and compassion; (c) a focus on assuring that personnel interviews included the request for the candidate to share a caring moment; (d) the sharing of a caring moment or an inspirational quote to set the tone for the day after our morning huddle with our entire hospital leadership team; (e) the creation and delivery of a 2-hour educational presentation that incorporated the 10 Caritas Processes and the Eight Behaviors of Authentic Hourly Visitation (AHV) for our frontline nurses, patient care technicians, unit clerks, and respiratory therapists; (f) education of the patient care service (PCS) leaders on the Theory of Human Caring, with discussion of the vision and mission of creating a culture of authentic caring and their role and responsibility around that; (g) gathering to center ourselves as nurse leaders before a historically biocidic, high-conflict meeting; (h) changing the census alert that all leaders received in the morning from "high census alert" to "we are caring for *x* amount of patients today"; (i) asking nurses during the training to share caring moments on the basis of the 10 Caritas Processes and creating book of the caring moment stories featuring their photograph; and (j) opening self to personal transformation that supports our ability to be present and live out the Theory of Human Caring.

Project Outcomes: The outcomes for this project included the following: (a) a quantitative study of care experience scores; the three questions it impacted were: overall rate of hospital, the nurse treated me with loving-kindness, and the nurse addressed my spiritual and religious needs; and (b) a qualitative study of peer-reported leadership Caritas behaviors.

Project Evaluation: Results from patient satisfaction surveys comparing the year prior to the project with the recent quarter demonstrate the following: (a) a 7-point improvement in the scores for "overall rate hospital"; (b) a 7-point improvement in the scores for "the nurses provided care with loving-kindness"; although (c) the scores for "the nurses attended to my spiritual and religious needs" had less than 1-point improvement. In addition, we experienced a self-perceived leadership effectiveness and our peers reported improvement in our leadership behaviors. These findings support nursing leaders' participation in the Caritas Coach Education Program to integrate Caring Science into nursing leadership practice to transform the self and system. In addition, we have identified the need to develop our nurses and ourselves in being with patients and their need for healing through spirituality and religion. Our future work will focus on integrating the ways of knowing (empirical and aesthetic) in assessing and addressing our patients' spiritual and religious needs.

Future Direction: Future work includes collaborating with regional Caring Science leaders at Kaiser Permanente Northern California, sharing this work, and participating in the development of regional Caring Science educational programs. The integration of hourly rounding and the 10 Caritas Processes educational program has been adopted by Kaiser Permanente Northern California for implementation throughout the system.

Acknowledgments: Deep heartfelt thanks to Priscilla S. Javed, DNP, RN, FACHE, and Linda Ackerman, MSN, RN, through whose sharing of Caring Science and introduction to Jean Watson's work we are now more caring and compassionate nurses/leaders/human beings. To Dr. Jean Watson for giving us the language to articulate our feelings. To Jan Anderson, EdD, RN, AHN-BC, who guided us through this transformational journey. It has impacted us personally and professionally beyond what we could have ever thought was possible. To Kaiser Permanente Northern California Patient Care Services for choosing the Theory of Human Caring as our theoretical foundation for nursing practice and for supporting our journey as Caritas Coaches. Finally, we share profound gratitude for each other for embracing the commitment to Caring Science and inspiring each other on this journey.

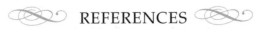 REFERENCES

Dyess, S. M., Prestia, A. S., & Smith, M. C. (2015). Support for caring and resiliency among successful nurse leaders. *Nursing Administration Quarterly, 39*(2), 104–116. doi:10.1097/NAQ.0000000000000101

Watson, J. (2005). *Caring science as sacred science.* Philadelphia, PA: F. A. Davis.

Watson, J. (2008). Nursing: The philosophy and science of caring (Rev. ed.). Boulder, CO: University Press of Colorado.

APPENDIX B.4
SURRENDERING TO BELONGING: FAMILY HEALING WITH THE ARTS

Kelly Morrow

Introduction: I completed the 12-week "Healing With the Arts" course (Samuels & Lane, 2013) and invited family members to join. Caritas Process® 1: Cultivating the Practice of Loving-Kindness and Equanimity Toward Self and Others as Foundational to Caritas Consciousness, combined with Caritas Process 4: Developing and Sustaining a Helping-Trusting-Caring Relationship, provided the context for this project (Watson, 2008). Birth order position in my family of origin resulted in me being raised alone and self-identifying as "alone in the middle" of two generations. In addition, as the adult child of a bipolar parent who remained undiagnosed during my childhood, I developed an overall sense of fear, anxiety, and the need to control. These traits, blended with the embedded sense of not belonging, became the primary perspectives through which I viewed family and the greater world for much of my life. During my ongoing doctoral program, I had begun experiencing paralyzing episodes of anxiety when required to expose imperfections or to engage in intellectual risk taking.

Significance: Surrendering to imperfection and intentionally seeking healing through art provided an opportunity to diminish fear and anxiety, and allowed me to practice equanimity with self as a foundation to Caritas practice (Watson, 2008).

Purpose: The purpose of this project was to be part of a personal, intentional exercise in surrendering to the unknown as I opened up to and with self and family members through the creative process offered in the context of the course "Healing With the Arts" (Samuels & Lane, 2013).

Setting and Participants: There were six final participants in this project: my sister, brother-in-law, adult nephew, and two nieces-in-law, who joined me online in a private Facebook group to create art for the purpose of intentional healing.

Project Description/Process: I implemented the project in December through individual emails, correspondence, and discussion with family members. I sent "Healing With the Arts" books to interested family members in five households and created a private Facebook group entitled "Family Healing With the Arts." After completing each week's imagery exercises, I posted artwork and a reflection to this private family page. I encouraged feedback and supported family members as artwork and reflections were added to the site. I also recorded the imagery exercises from the first four chapters of the "Healing With the Arts" text and posted links to the referenced videos.

Project Projected Outcomes: This project was undertaken as a way to mindfully practice equanimity toward self and family members while surrendering to and accepting personal imperfections during the creative healing process. Projected outcomes were to develop an enhanced sense of belonging within the family of origin, and to identify a creative outlet to support increased self-awareness, healthy expression of emotion, and reduced anxiety related to intellectual risk taking.

Partial/Projected Evaluation: I experienced a great deal of healing related to two core memories that contributed significantly to my fear of exposing imperfections, and to my anxiety surrounding intellectual risk taking. These core memories had previously never been shared with anyone including therapists or my spouse. I was empowered to restory and reframe my new embodied role in the family from "alone in the middle" to "the bridge" connecting generations. This shift in perspective has enhanced my sense of belonging and purpose within my family of origin. Three of the six family members contributed art and written reflections to our project, whereas the other three engaged in active feedback and encouragement. From week 4 onward, I was the primary contributor of artwork and reflections, whereas family members followed along providing feedback and encouragement. I was able to exhibit equanimity toward all participants (including self) by accepting the level of participation in which each was ready to engage and being thankful for their offerings, whether private or within the group. I consider it a godsend to have developed a creative outlet to access and express emotions. My family of origin has been reframed as a safe space for authentic expression and caring interactions. I have not yet determined whether fears related to intellectual risk taking have been affected but will continue to reflect on this outcome as my doctoral degree progresses.

Future Directions: Previously I was afraid to place a mark on a blank, white page. Now I am creating reflective art on a near daily basis. Plans are in place to take courses in basic drawing and watercolor techniques to support continued development of these creative outlets. I am currently in the process of completing a clay mosaic to represent my healing experience during this project. Surrendering to the creative process has allowed me to be more open and vulnerable within family relationships. A final, unexpected outcome is that the process of creating art has caused me to become more present to the surrounding world as colors, shadows, and shapes in the sky and mountains are studied and recreated as art.

Acknowledgments: I express heartfelt gratitude to Lisa Goldberg, PhD, RN, and Jan Anderson, EdD, RN, AHN-BC, for their support and understanding of why this project was a necessary, foundational step in my process of being/becoming a Caritas Coach. I remain grateful to my incredible family for journeying through life's adventures with me.

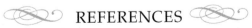 REFERENCES

Samuels, M., & Lane, M. R. (2013). *Healing with the arts: A twelve-week program to heal yourself and your community.* New York, NY: ATRIA.

Watson, J. (2008). *Nursing: The philosophy and science of caring* (Rev. ed.). Boulder: University Press of Colorado.

APPENDIX B.5
EARLY CULTIVATION OF SELF-CARE PRACTICES
Robert Reynoso

Introduction: New nursing students are acculturating to a profession, applying liberal arts and science knowledge to new (often abstract) concepts in a demanding baccalaureate program. Within days and weeks, students are exposed to stress from academic load, new guidelines for dress and communication, and acute clinical situations that may include death. Many times, very few have the life skills to deal with the trials that accompany this new role. The practice of loving-kindness and equanimity extends to the self and, too often, a student nurse's lack of personal awareness and ability to cope result in physical, psychological, and/or spiritual distress. The student nurse will be able to work through the hurdles and challenges that lie embedded in the path to becoming and create a foundation for self-care during his or her nursing practice.

Significance: A nursing student's present and future success, as a nurse and caregiver, may be improved by possessing effective strategies to deal with the stressors of school and care of the ill and injured. Students are immediately immersed into a stressful environment beginning on the first day of nursing school. The provision of early lessons related to self-care could minimize or eliminate sequelae resultant of the stressors.

Purpose: The purpose of this project is to provide the nursing student with strategies to cope with and manage life challenges in a healthy and effective way to promote success in the roles of nursing student and caring nurse. Although lessons will be learned through the program and their careers, the lessons for self-care management are to be embedded on entry into the program in the first week of the curriculum.

Setting and Participants: The project affects prelicensure of bachelor of science in nursing (BSN) students at Nevada State College. The intervention would be implemented in the first lecture in a first semester course, Nursing Fundamentals. The typical cohort size varies from 32 to 48 maximum and the participants are instructed by graduate nursing degree–prepared instructors. The theory lecturer acts as the course leader and delivers the content. The remaining educators are in the role of clinical instructor.

Project Description/Process: The project is rooted from two of Dr. Jean Watson's Caritas Processes®. They are the practice of loving-kindness and equanimity within the context of caring consciousness and cultivation of one's own spiritual practices and transpersonal self, going beyond ego self (Watson, 2008). Students will be taught lectures related to theory, personal strategies, availability of resources, and interventions to manage stress commonly associated with a BSN nursing program. This occurs in the first week of nursing school and the content covers short-term, medium-term, and long-term interventions. Clinical instructors will further assist with recognition and refinement of the content and practice of self-care to meet individual needs. Clinical shifts will begin and end with focus, centering, and reflection.

Project Outcome(s)/Projected Outcomes: Student nurses will practice interventions and promote strategies to help them cope with the stress associated with nursing and nursing school. In addition, student nurses will report successful use of the interventions when dealing with challenges.

Project Evaluation or Partial/Projected Evaluation if Not Completed: No tool currently exists but a Likert-style scale will be designed and used to measure the effectiveness of the lessons. This assessment will be made in the first and final weeks of the semester.

Future Directions: This program could be implemented into the nursing curriculum for the full-time cohorts and, in time, the part-time cohorts. With properly designed assessment tools, legitimate research can be performed to measure the true efficacy of the andragogical interventions.

Acknowledgments: I acknowledge and express appreciation for the support of Dr. Jan Anderson, Marialena Murphy, Dr. Neal Rosenburg, Caritas Coach Education Program (CCEP) Cohort 16, Elyse Barnes, and the staff of the Centennial Hills Hospital Orthopedic Unit.

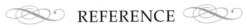

REFERENCE

Watson, J. (2008). *Nursing: The philosophy and science of caring* (Rev. ed.). Boulder: University Press of Colorado.

APPENDIX B.6
COLORING WITH CARE: A NEW LENS FOR THE SYRIAN DIASPORA

Danielle Wofford

Introduction: The conflict in Syria has driven over 5 million Syrians to other countries (Amnesty International, 2016). Life for these refugees is untenable; refugees continue to have limited access to basic resources. The host nations are overwhelmed and continue to slide into economic depression. The result is that refugee families find themselves sliding into a state of hopelessness, in displacement areas that fall short of understanding their circumstances, meeting basic survival needs, or empowering them to thrive in resettlement zones. Meanwhile, there remains a gap in literature on understanding Syrian refugees' experiences throughout their journey firsthand. The purpose of this project was to honor the stories of Syrian women refugees with and through the lens of Caring Science by way of application of the Caritas Processes®.

Significance: The United Nations considers the Syrian refugee crisis the largest humanitarian emergency of our time, and the civil war as one of the worst moral crises of modern history (United Nations High Commissioner for Refugees [UNHCR], 2016). The existing political and environmental approaches in all of the countries have reached their capacity for service and are, in many cases, failing (UNHCR, 2016). The resources that are provided continue to be fragmented and inconsistent, in turn brutal, or kind, or begrudging, and almost always underserved. Even with the best of intentions, the end results have fallen far short as models for humane and effective intervention. Host country policies are designed to discourage more migration, and provide inadequate food, healthcare, and shelter. More refugees are becoming homeless in host countries. Consequentially, refugee communities are exposed to extreme hopeless and biocidic environments. The significance for the project was twofold: (a) in the short term, to foster a caring-healing environment to authentically listen to the stories of Syrian women refugees; and (b) in the long term, to create a blueprint for a new caring model to promote a biogenic and healing environment for Syrian refugees more broadly in the context of their ongoing journey.

Purpose: The purpose of the project was to understand the experiences of Syrian women refugees in first access points (i.e., neighboring countries to Syria) by way of a Caring Science Framework and the experiential application of the Caritas Processes.

Setting and Participants: The setting for the project took place in a neighboring country to Syria. Interviews were voluntary and took place in participants' living and/or private space. Great attention was given to create a safe and welcoming environment. Interviews were conducted in three locations; areas where "refugees" cannot register as refugees and live in unconventional spaces; privately run refugee spaces; and areas where refugees initially arrive in a new country. Five interviews took place in each area. Participants were 18 years of age or older, spoke conversational English, and self-reported as a Syrian refugee. A multidisciplinary team of experts, nongovernmental organization (NGO) leaders, and community leaders provided collaborative guidance to oversee the project.

Project Description/Process: An exploratory methodology using semistructured face-to-face interviews and researcher observation was used to carry out the study framed in Caring Science. Interviews were transcribed by the researcher verbatim. The researcher collaborated with the following organizations throughout the duration of the project: (a) the Interprofessional Studio for Complexity Thinking, (b) Safe School Design, and (c) Lifting Hands International. The project took place over 14 days, and began by developing "helping-trusting-authentic-caring relationships" with each community, followed by interviews using the Caritas Processes. In particular, the processes that specifically embodied the following were particularly prevalent within the interview process: "Practicing loving-kindness, being authentically present, promoting and accepting the expression of positive and negative feelings, creatively using all ways of knowing, creating a healing environment, and allowing for the unknown to unfold" (Watson, 2008, p. 31).

Project Outcome(s)/Projected Outcomes: The results are consistent with the expected outcomes of using the Caritas Processes in creating transpersonal moments and creating a biogenic space for health and healing to occur. Major themes that emerged included the refugees experiencing a profound lack of human care and respect for human dignity and life, a deep desire for healing holistically, a sincere need for human connection with family and community, and a powerful resilience to care and love others.

Project Evaluation or Partial/Projected Evaluation if Not Completed: The project was evaluated by a transdisciplinary team of experts for validity and trustworthiness. The outcomes will not be shared with the participants because of the transitory nature of refugees. However, the final outcomes will be shared with partnering NGOs for plausibility and future research implications.

Future Directions: The project is part of a larger study that focuses on understanding the entire journey of Syrian refugees through the lens of Caring Science. This specific project was created to understand the experience of first access points and the preceding journey for Syrian women refugees. Long-term goals include the following: (a) creating a caring delivery model for each critical access point; (b) implementation of the caring delivery model; and (c) ultimately, enhancing well-being for refugees.

Acknowledgments: I thank Dr. Lisa Goldberg, my encouraging Caritas Coach mentor, Dr. Jan Anderson, for her kind heart, and Dr. Paulina Komnenich, my supporting PhD mentor. Also, this project would not be possible without the support of InterSCT, Safe School Design, Lifting Hands International, and the amazing women in this study.

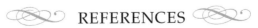

REFERENCES

Amnesty International. (2016, February 3). Syria's refugee crisis in numbers. Retrieved from https://www.amnesty.org/en/latest/news/2016/02/syrias-refugee-crisis-in-numbers

United Nations High Commissioner for Refugees. (2016, February 17). UNHCR Syria Regional Refugee Response. Retrieved from http://data.unhcr.org/syrianrefugees/regional.php

Watson, J. (2008). *Nursing: The philosophy and science of caring* (Rev. ed.). Boulder: University Press of Colorado.

Appendix C:
Caring Science Literature: The Annals of Caring

Works using Watson's Caring Theory

2010–2017

(updated Oct 10, 2017)

Books (21)

Articles (348)

Non-English (20)

Editorials (21)

Updates Feb–Oct 2017 (49)

BOOKS

1. Sitzman, K., & Watson, J. (2017). *Watson's caring in the digital world: A guide for caring when interacting, teaching, and learning in cyberspace.* New York, NY: Springer Publishing.
2. Rosa, W. (2017). *A new era in global health: Nursing and the United Nations 2030 Agenda for Sustainable Development.* New York, NY: Springer Publishing.
3. Rosa, W. (2016). *Nurses as leaders: Evolutionary visions of leadership.* New York, NY: Springer Publishing.
4. Lee, S. M., Palmieri, P., & Watson, J. (2016). *Global advances in human caring literacy.* New York, NY: Springer Publishing.
5. Sitzman, K., & Watson, J. (2014). *Caring science, mindful practice: Implementing Watson's human caring theory.* New York, NY: Springer Publishing.
6. Johnson, T. (2014). *Utilizing Watson's theory of caring to develop a palliative care proposal for Olmsted Medical Center.* Minneapolis, MN: Augsburg College.
7. Alligood, M. R. (2014a). *Nursing theory: Utilization & application.* St. Louis, MO: Elsevier/Mosby.
8. Alligood, M. R. (2014b). *Nursing theorists and their work.* St. Louis, MO: Elsevier/Mosby.

9. Smith, M. C, Turkel, M., & Wolf, Z. R. (Eds.). (2013). *Caring in nursing classics: An essential resource.* New York, NY: Springer Publishing.

10. Owens, M. M. (2013). *The effects of Watson's theory of caring and the nurse utilization of caring attributes.* Boiling Springs, NC: Gardner-Webb University.

11. Jan, A. (2013). *Professional research project: Nurse residency program.* Phoenix, AZ: Grand Canyon University.

12. Fawcett, J., & DeSanto-Madeya, S. (2013). *Contemporary nursing knowledge: Analysis and evaluation of nursing models and theories.* Philadelphia, PA: F. A. Davis.

13. Cowgill, A. D. (2013). *Significance of nurse residency or internship programs on nurse retention, costs, and competence.* Phoenix, AZ: Grand Canyon University.

14. Avery, M. D. (2013). *Supporting a physiologic approach to pregnancy and birth: A practical guide.* Ames, IA: Wiley-Blackwell.

15. Watson, J. (2012). *Human caring science: A theory of nursing.* Sudbury, MA: Jones & Bartlett.

16. Molinari, D., & Bushy, A. (2012). *The rural nurse: Transition to practice.* New York, NY: Springer Publishing.

17. Comfort, N. (2012). *The science of human perfection: How genes became the heart of American Medicine.* Newhaven, UK: Yale University Press.

18. Buie, P. K. U., & Gardner-Webb, N. (2012). *School of Nurse's perception of factors associated with family satisfaction in the intensive care.* Boiling Springs, NC: Gardner-Webb University.

19. Nelson, J., & Watson, J. (2011). *Measuring caring: International research on caritas as healing.* New York, NY: Springer Publishing.

20. Hill, K. S., & Prevost, S. (2011). *Nursing clinics of North America: Magnet environments, supporting the retention and satisfaction of nurses.* Philadelphia, PA: W. B. Saunders/Elsevier.

21. Hansen, J. (2011). *Nurse residency program builder: Tools for a successful new graduate program.* Danvers, MA: HCPro.

ARTICLES

1. Sundler, A. J., Höglander, J., Eklund, J. H., Eide, H., & Holmström, I. K. (2017). Older persons' expressions of emotional cues and concerns during home care visits: Application of the Verona coding definitions of emotional sequences (VR-CoDES) in home care. *Patient Education and Counseling, 100*(2), 276–282. doi:10.1016/j.pec.2016.09.009

2. Sit, J. W. H., Chan, A. W. H., So, W. K. W., Chan, C. W. H., Chan, A. W. K., Chan, H. Y. L., … Wong, E. M. L. (2017). Promoting holistic well-being in chronic stroke patients through leisure art-based creative engagement. *Rehabilitation Nursing, 42*(2), 58–66. doi:10.1002/rnj.177

3. Salzmann-Erikson, M., & Dahlén, J. (2017). Nurses' establishment of health promoting relationships: A descriptive synthesis of anorexia nervosa research. *Journal of Child and Family Studies, 26*(1), 1–13. doi:10.1007/s10826-016-0534-2

4. Salmela, S., Koskinen, C., & Eriksson, K. (2017). Nurse leaders as managers of ethically sustainable caring cultures. *Journal of Advanced Nursing, 73*(4), 871–882. doi:10.1111/jan.13184

5. Rosa, W., Estes, T., & Watson, J. (2017). Caring science conscious dying: An emerging meta-paradigm. *Nursing Science Quarterly, 30*(1), 58–64. doi:10.1177/0894318416680538.

6. Nyholm, L., & Koskinen, C. A. (2017). Understanding and safeguarding patient dignity in intensive care. *Nursing Ethics, 24*(4), 408–418. doi:10.1177/0969733015605669

7. Lafrenière, S., Folch, N., Dubois, S., Bédard, L., & Ducharme, F. (2017). Strategies used by older patients to prevent functional decline during hospitalization. Clinical *Nursing Research, 26*(1), 6–26. doi:10.1177/1054773815601392

8. Ladd, S. C., & Gordon, S. C. (2017). End of life in a Haitian American, faith-based community: Caring for family and communal unity. *Journal of Christian Nursing, 34*(1), E8–E18. doi:10.1097/CNJ.0000000000000351

9. Krupic, F., Sayed-Noor, A. S., Fatahi, N. (2017). The impact of knowledge and religion on organ donation as seen by immigrants in Sweden. *Scandinavian Journal of Caring Sciences, 31*(4), 687–694. doi:10.1111/scs.12379

10. Israelsson, J., Bremer, A., Herlitz, J., Axelsson, Å. B., Cronberg, T., Djärv, T., … Årestedt, K. (2017). Health status and psychological distress among in-hospital cardiac arrest survivors in relation to gender. *Resuscitation, 114,* 27–33. doi:10.1016/j.resuscitation.2017.02.006

11. Holopainen, G., Nyström, L., & Kasén, A. (2017). The caring encounter in nursing. *Nursing Ethics,* 969733016687161. doi:10.1177/0969733016687161

12. Holmstrom, I. K., Krantz, A., Karacagil, L., & Sundler, A. J. (2017). Frequent callers in primary health care: A qualitative study with a nursing perspective. *Journal of Advanced Nursing, 73*(3), 622–632. doi:10.1111/jan.13153

13. Hammar, L. M., Holmström, I. K., Skoglund, K., Meranius, M. S., & Sundler, A. J. (2017). The care of and communication with older people from the perspective of student nurses: A mixed method study. *Nurse Education Today, 52,* 1–6. doi:10.1016/j.nedt.2017.02.002

14. Gusdal, A. K., Josefsson, K., Thors Adolfsson, E., & Martin, L. (2017). Nurses' attitudes toward family importance in heart failure care. *European Journal of Cardiovascular Nursing, 16*(3), 256–266. doi:10.1177/1474515116687178

15. Eriksson, H., & Salzmann-Erikson, M. (2017). The digital generation and nursing robotics: A netnographic study about nursing care robots posted on social media. *Nursing Inquiry, 24*(2). doi:10.1111/nin.12165

16. Chan, W. Y., Fung, I. M., & Chan, E. (2017). Universal health coverage through community nursing services: China vs. Hong Kong. *Revista Latino-Americana de Enfermagem, 25,* e2838. doi:10.1590/1518-8345.1664.2838

17. Boz, I., & Okumuş, H. (2017). The "everything about the existence" experiences of Turkish women with infertility: Solicited diaries in qualitative research. *Journal of Nursing Research, 25*(4), 268–275. doi:10.1097/JNR.0000000000000166

18. Bollig, G., Rosland, J. H., Gjengedal, E., Schmidt, G., May, A. T., & Heller, A. (2017). European multicenter study on systematic ethics work in nursing homes. *Scandinavian Journal of Caring Sciences, 31*(3), 587–601. doi:10.1111/scs.12373

19. Zhang, Y., Jiménez-Herrera, M., Axelsson, C., & Cheng, Y. (2016). Not bad: Passive leg raising in cardiopulmonary resuscitation: A new modeling study. *Frontiers in Physiology, 7,* 665. doi:10.3389/fphys.2016.00665

20. Wu, S., Singh-Carlson, S., Odell, A., Reynolds, G., & Su, Y. (2016). Compassion fatigue, burnout, and compassion satisfaction among oncology nurses in the United States and Canada. *Oncology Nursing Forum, 43*(4), E161–E169. doi:10.1188/16.ONF.E161-E169

21. Wireklint Sundström, B., Holmberg, M., Herlitz, J., Karlsson, T., & Andersson, H. (2016). Possible effects of a course in cardiovascular nursing on prehospital care of patients experiencing suspected acute coronary syndrome: A cluster randomised controlled trial. *BMC Nursing, 15*(1), 52. doi:10.1186/s12912-016-0175-1

22. Vrbnjak, D., Pahor, D., Nelson, J. W., & Pajnkihar, M. (2016). Content validity, face valid-ity and internal consistency of the Slovene version of caring factor survey for care pro-viders, caring for co-workers and caring of managers. *Scandinavian Journal of Caring Sciences, 31*(2), 395–404. doi:10.1111/scs.12338

23. Torregosa, M. B., Ynalvez, M. A., & Morin, K. H. (2016). Perceptions matter: Faculty car-ing, campus racial climate and academic performance. *Journal of Advanced Nursing, 72*(4), 864–877. doi:10.1111/jan.12877

24. Sundler, A. J., Eide, H., van Dulmen, S., Holmström, I. K. (2016). Communicative chal-lenges in the home care of older persons: A qualitative exploration. *Journal of Advanced Nursing, 72*(10), 2435–2444. doi:10.1111/jan.12996

25. Sturm, B. A., & Dellert, J. C. (2016). Exploring nurses' personal dignity, global self-esteem and work satisfaction. *Nursing Ethics, 23*(4), 384–400. doi:10.1177/0969733014567024

26. Sofhauser, C. (2016). Intention in nursing practice. *Nursing Science Quarterly, 29*(1), 31–34. doi:10.1177/0894318415614629

27. Slettebø, Å., Saeteren, B., Caspari, S., Lohne, V., Rehnsfeldt, A. W., Heggestad, A. K. T., … Nåden, D. (2016). The significance of meaningful and enjoyable activities for nursing home resident's experiences of dignity. *Scandinavian Journal of Caring Sciences, 31*(4), 718–726. doi:10.1111/scs.12386

28. Skyman, E., Lindahl, B., Bergbom, I., Sjöström, H. T., & Åhrén, C. (2016). Being Met as marked: Patients' experiences of being infected with community-acquired methicillin-resistant Staphylococcus aureus (MRSA). *Scandinavian Journal of Caring Sciences, 30*(4), 813–820. doi:10.1111/scs.12309

29. Sitzman, K. L., Jensen, A., & Chan, S. (2016). Creating a global community of learners in nursing and beyond: Caring science, mindful practice MOOC. *Nursing Education Perspectives, 37*(5), 269–274. doi:10.1097/01.NEP.0000000000000062

30. Sitzman, K. L. (2016). Mindful communication for caring online. *Advances in Nursing Science, 39*(1), 38–47. doi:10.1097/ANS.0000000000000102

31. Silén, M., & Johansson, L. (2016). Aims and theoretical frameworks in nursing students' bachelor's theses in Sweden: A descriptive study. *Nurse Education Today, 37*, 91–96. doi:10.1016/j.nedt.2015.11.020

32. Salzmann-Erikson, M., Lagerqvist, L., & Pousette, S. (2016). Keep calm and have a good night: Nurses' strategies to promote inpatients' sleep in the hospital environment. *Scandinavian Journal of Caring Sciences, 30*(2), 356–364. doi:10.1111/scs.12255

33. Rosa, W., & Estes, T. (2016). What end-of-life care needs now: An emerging praxis of the sacred and subtle. *Advances in Nursing Science, 39*(4), 333–345. doi:10.1097/ANS.0000000000000136

34. Rosa, W. (2016). Holding heartspace: Diametric opposition, inextricable symbiosis. *International Journal for Human Caring, 20*(3), 165. doi:10.20467/1091-5710-20.3.165

35. Rodrigues, J. A., Lacerda, M. R., Favero, L., Gomes, I. M., Méier, M. J., & Wall, M. L. (2016). Model of transpersonal caring in nursing home care according to Favero and

Lacerda: Case report. *Revista Gaúcha de Enfermagem/EENFUFRGS, 37*(3), e58271. doi:10.1590/1983-1447.2016.03.58271

36. Rehnsfeldt, A., & Arman, M. (2016). Dressing an existential wound (DEW): A new model for long-term care following disasters. *Scandinavian Journal of Caring Sciences, 30*(3), 518–525. doi:10.1111/scs.12273

37. Polak, A., Taradaj, J., Nawrat-Szoltysik, A., Stania, M., Dolibog, P., Blaszczak, E., ... Kucio, C. (2016). Reduction of pressure ulcer size with high-voltage pulsed current and high-frequency ultrasound: A randomised trial. *Journal of Wound Care, 25*(12), 742–754. doi:10.12968/jowc.2016.25.12.742

38. Polak, A., Kloth, L. C., Blaszczak, E., Taradaj, J., Nawrat-Szoltysik, A., Walczak, A., ... Kucio, C. (2016). Evaluation of the healing progress of pressure ulcers treated with cathodal high-voltage monophasic pulsed current: Results of a prospective, double-blind, randomized clinical trial. *Advances in Skin & Wound Care, 29*(10), 447–459. doi:10.1097/01.ASW.0000493164.75337.de

39. O'Reilly, L., Cara, C., & Delmas, P. (2016). Developing an educational intervention to strengthen humanistic practices of hemodialysis nurses in Switzerland. *International Journal for Human Caring, 20*(1), 24–30. doi:10.20467/1091-5710-20.1.24

40. Norman, V., Rossillo, K., & Skelton, K. (2016). Creating healing environments through the theory of caring. *AORN Journal, 104*(5), 401–409. doi:10.1016/j.aorn.2016.09.006

41. Ng, G. M., & Ruppel, H. (2016). Nursing simulation fellowships: An innovative approach for developing simulation leaders. *Clinical Simulation in Nursing, 12*(2), 62–68. doi:10.1016/j.ecns.2015.11.005

42. Nelson, J., Thiel, L., Hozak, M. A., & Thomas, T. (2016). Item reduction of the caring factor survey-care provider version: An instrument specified to measure Watson's 10 processes of caring. *International Journal for Human Caring, 20*(3), 123–128. doi:10.20467/1091-5710-20.3.123

43. Manasatchakun, P., Chotiga, P., Roxberg, Å., & Asp, M. (2016). Healthy ageing in Isan-Thai culture: A phenomenographic study based on older persons' lived experiences. *International Journal of Qualitative Studies on Health and Well-Being, 11*(1), 29463. doi:10.3402/qhw.v11.29463

44. Lindberg, E., Österberg, S. A., & Hörberg, U. (2016). Methodological support for the further abstraction of and philosophical examination of empirical findings in the context of caring science. *International Journal of Qualitative Studies on Health and Well-Being, 11*, 30482. doi:10.3402/qhw.v11.30482

45. Liang, S., Choi, K. S., Qin, J., Wang, Q., Pang, W. M., & Heng, P. A. (2016). Discrimination of motor imagery tasks via information flow pattern of brain connectivity. *Technology and Health Care, 24*(Suppl. 2), S795–S801. doi:10.3233/THC-161212

46. Liang, S., Choi, K. S., Qin, J., Pang, W. M., Wang, Q., & Heng, P. A. (2016). Improving the discrimination of hand motor imagery via virtual reality based visual guidance. *Computer Methods and Programs in Biomedicine, 132*, 63–74. doi:10.1016/j.cmpb.2016.04.023

47. Liang, S., Choi, K. S., Qin, J., Pang, W. M., & Heng, P. A. (2016). Enhancing training performance for brain-computer interface with object-directed 3D visual guidance. *International Journal of Computer Assisted Radiology and Surgery, 11*(11), 2129–2137. doi:10.1007/s11548-015-1336-5

48. Lejonqvist, G. B., Eriksson, K., & Meretoja, R. (2016). Evidence of clinical competence by simulation A hermeneutical observational study. *Nurse Education Today, 38,* 88–92. doi:10.1016/j.nedt.2015.12.011

49. Lejonqvist, G. B., Eriksson, K., & Meretoja, R. (2016). Evaluating clinical competence during nursing education: A comprehensive integrative literature review. *International Journal of Nursing Practice, 22*(2), 142–151. doi:10.1111/ijn.12406

50. Larsson, Å., Wärnå-Furu, C., & Näsman, Y. (2016). Expecting a child: Pregnancy in light of an ontological health model. *Scandinavian Journal of Caring Sciences, 30*(4), 757–765. doi:10.1111/scs.12302

51. Koskinen, C., Aho, S., & Nyholm, L. (2016). Life with an unwelcome guest: Caring in a context of protracted bodily pain. *Scandinavian Journal of Caring Sciences, 30*(4), 774–781. doi:10.1111/scs.12304

52. Karlsson, K., Rydström, I., Nyström, M., Enskär, K., & Dalheim Englund, A. C. (2016). Consequences of needle-related medical procedures: A hermeneutic study with young children (3–7 years). *Journal of Pediatric Nursing, 31*(2), e109–e118. doi:10.1016/j.pedn.2015.09.008

53. Karlsson, K., Englund, A.-N., Enskär, K., Nyström, M., & Rydström, I. (2016). Experiencing support during needle-related medical procedures: A hermeneutic study with young children (3–7 years). *Journal of Pediatric Nursing-Nursing Care of Children & Families, 31*(6), 667–677. doi:10.1016/j.pedn.2016.06.004

54. Israelsson, J., Lilja, G., Bremer, A., Stevenson-Ågren, J., & Årestedt, K. (2016). Post cardiac arrest care and follow-up in Sweden: A national web-survey. *BMC Nursing, 15,* 1. doi:10.1186/s12912-016-0123-0

55. Ip, P., Chim, D., Chan, K. L., Li, T. M., Ho, F. K., Van Voorhees, B. W., … Wong, W. H. (2016). Effectiveness of a culturally attuned internet-based depression prevention program for Chinese adolescents: A randomized controlled trial. *Depress Anxiety, 33*(12), 1123–1131. doi:10.1002/da.22554

56. Holmström, I. K., Nokkoudenmäki, M. B., Zukancic, S., & Sundler, A. J. (2016). It is important that they care: Older persons' experiences of telephone advice nursing. *Journal of Clinical Nursing, 25*(11-12), 1644–1653. doi:10.1111/jocn.13173

57. Hadziabdic, E., Safipour, J., Bachrach-Lindström, M., & Hultsjö, S. (2016). Swedish version of measuring cultural awareness in nursing students: Validity and reliability test. *BMC Nursing, 15,* 25. doi:10.1186/s12912-016-0146-6

58. Gusdal, A. K., Josefsson, K., Thors Adolfsson, E., & Martin, L. (2016). Registered nurses' perceptions about the situation of family caregivers to patients with heart failure: A focus group interview study. *PLoS One, 11*(8), e0160302. doi:10.1371/journal.pone.0160302

59. Grumme, V. S., Barry, C. D., Gordon, S. C., & Ray, M. A. (2016). On virtual presence. *Advances in Nursing Science, 39*(1), 48–59. doi:10.1097/ANS.0000000000000103

60. Gomes, M., Hash, P., Orsolini, L., Watkins, A., & Mazzoccoli, A. (2016). Connecting professional practice and technology at the bedside: Nurses' beliefs about using an electronic health record and their ability to incorporate professional and patient-centered nursing activities in patient care. *Computers, Informatics, Nursing, 34*(12), 578–586. doi:10.1097/CIN.0000000000000280

61. Garrett, B. M. (2016). New sophistry: Self-deception in the nursing academy. *Nursing Philosophy, 17*(3), 182–193. doi:10.1111/nup.12128

62. Foss, B., Nåden, D., & Eriksson, K. (2016). Experience of events of truth in hermeneutic conversation with text: Ethics and ontology. *Nursing Science Quarterly*, 29(4), 299–307. doi:10.1177/0894318416662929

63. Forsner, M., Nilsson, S., Finnström, B., & Mörelius, E. (2016). Expectation prior to human papilloma virus vaccination: 11 to 12-year-old girls' written narratives. *Journal of Child Health Care*, 20(3), 365–373. doi:10.1177/1367493515598646

64. Forsgärde, E.-S., From Attebring, M., & Elmqvist, C. (2016). Powerlessness: Dissatisfied patients' and relatives' experience of their emergency department visit. *International Emergency Nursing*, 25, 32–36. doi:10.1016/j.ienj.2015.07.004

65. Florin, J., Jansson, I., Strandberg, E., Ehrenberg, A., & Björvell, C. (2016). Cross-mapping diagnostic nursing concepts between the ICNP and the ICF for expressing nursing in the health care record. *Studies in Health Technology and Informatics*, 225, 1016–1017. doi:10.3233/978-1-61499-658-3-1016

66. Falk, H., Henoch, I., Ozanne, A., Öhlen, J., Ung, E. J., Fridh, I., … Falk, K. (2016). Differences in symptom distress based on gender and palliative care designation among hospitalized patients. *Journal of Nursing Scholarship*, 48(6), 569–576. doi:10.1111/jnu.12254

67. Delmas, P., O'Reilly, L., Iglesias, K., Cara, C., & Burnier, M. (2016). Feasibility, acceptability, and preliminary effects of educational intervention to strengthen humanistic practice among hemodialysis nurses in the Canton of Vaud, Switzerland: A pilot study. *International Journal for Human Caring*, 20(1), 31–43. doi:10.20467/1091-5710-20.1.31

68. Delaney, C., Barrere, C., Robertson, S., Zahourek, R., Diaz, D., & Lachapelle, L. (2016). Pilot testing of the NURSE stress management intervention. *Journal of Holistic Nursing*, 34(4), 369–389. doi:10.1177/0898010115622295

69. Dahlberg, H., Ranheim, A., & Dahlberg, K. (2016). Ecological caring: Revisiting the original ideas of caring science. *International Journal of Qualitative Studies on Health and Well-Being*, 11, 33344. doi:10.3402/qhw.v11.33344

70. Craig, P., Rahm-Hallberg, I., Britten, N., Borglin, G., Meyer, G., Köpke, S., … Monks, T. (2016). Erratum to: Researching complex interventions in health: The state of the art. *BMC Health Services Research*, 16(1), 181. doi:10.1186/s12913-016-1416-4

71. Blegen, N. E., Eriksson, K., & Bondas, T. (2016). Ask me what is in my heart of hearts! The core question of care in relation to parents who are patients in a psychiatric care context. *International Journal of Qualitative Studies on Health and Well-Being*, 11(1), 30758. doi:10.3402/qhw.v11.30758

72. Björk, M., Sundler, A. J., Hallström, I., & Hammarlund, K. (2016). Like being covered in a wet and dark blanket: Parents' lived experiences of losing a child to cancer. *European Journal of Oncology Nursing*, 25, 40–45. doi:10.1016/j.ejon.2016.08.007

73. Benoit, B., Goldberg, L., & Campbell-Yeo, M. (2016). Infant feeding and maternal guilt: The application of a feminist phenomenological framework to guide clinician practices in breast feeding promotion. *Midwifery*, 34, 58–65. doi:10.1016/j.midw.2015.10.011

74. Axelsson, C., Herrera, M. J., & Bång, A. (2016). How the context of ambulance care influences learning to become a specialist ambulance nurse: A Swedish perspective. *Nurse Education Today*, 37, 8–14. doi:10.1016/j.nedt.2015.10.029

75. Arman, M., & Hök, J. (2016). Self-care follows from compassionate care: Chronic pain patients' experience of integrative rehabilitation. *Scandinavian Journal of Caring Sciences*, *30*(2), 374–381. doi:10.1111/scs.12258

76. Andreasson, J., Eriksson, A., & Dellve, L. (2016). Health care managers' views on and approaches to implementing models for improving care processes. *Journal of Nursing Management*, *24*(2), 219–227. doi:10.1111/jonm.12303

77. Ågren, S., Sjöberg, T., Ekmehag, B., Wiborg, M.-B., & Ivarsson, B. (2016). Psychosocial aspects before and up to 2 years after heart or lung transplantation: Experience of patients and their next of kin. *Clinical Transplantation*, *31*(3), E12905. doi:10.1111/ctr.12905

78. Willis, D. G., DeSanto-Madeya, S., Ross, R., Sheehan, D. L., & Fawcett, J. (2015). Spiritual healing in the aftermath of childhood maltreatment: Translating men's lived experiences utilizing nursing conceptual models and theory. *Advances in Nursing Science*, *38*(3), 162–174. doi:10.1097/ANS.0000000000000075

79. Vantaa Benjaminsson, M., Thunberg, G., & Nilsson, S. (2015). Using picture and text schedules to inform children: Effects on distress and pain during needle-related procedures in nitrous oxide sedation. *Pain Research and Treatment*, *2015*, 478503. doi:10.1155/2015/478503

80. Toft, B. S., & Uhrenfeldt, L. (2015). The lived experiences of being physically active when morbidly obese: A qualitative systematic review. *International Journal of Qualitative Studies on Health and Well-Being*, *10*, 28577. doi:10.3402/qhw.v10.28577

81. Thorkildsen, K. M., Eriksson, K., & Råholm, M. B. (2015). The core of love when caring for patients suffering from addiction. *Scandinavian Journal of Caring Sciences*, *29*(2), 353–360. doi:10.1111/scs.12171

82. Teymourtash, A. R., & Mokhlesi, M. (2015). Experimental investigation of stationary and rotational structures in non-circular hydraulic jumps. *Journal of Fluid Mechanics*, *762*, 344–360. doi:10.1017/jfm.2014.646

83. Swall, A., Ebbeskog, B., Lundh Hagelin, C., & Fagerberg, I. (2015). Can therapy dogs evoke awareness of one's past and present life in persons with Alzheimer's disease? *International Journal of Older People Nursing*, *10*(2), 84–93. doi:10.1111/opn.12053

84. Summerell, P. (2015). EB133 Jean Watson's Caritas Processes: A model for transforming the nursing practice environment. *Critical Care Nurse*, *35*(2), e66–e67.

85. Summer Meranius, M., & Engstrom, G. (2015). Experience of self-management of medications among older people with multimorbidity. *Journal of Clinical Nursing*, *24*(19-20), 2757–2764. doi:10.1111/jocn.12868

86. Suen, L. K., Yeh, C. H., Lee, W. K., Chu, W. L., Loo, J. F., & Tam, W. H. (2015). Association of auricular reflective points and the status of lower urinary tract symptoms in aging males. *Aging Male*, *18*(3), 149–156. doi:10.3109/13685538.2015.1027679

87. Sjöblom, I., Lundgren, I., Idvall, E., & Lindgren, H. (2015). Being a homebirth midwife in the Nordic countries: A phenomenological study. *Sexual & Reproductive Healthcare*, *6*(3), 126–131. doi:10.1016/j.srhc.2015.02.004

88. Scruth, E. A., Pugh, D. M., Adams, C. L., & Foss-Durant, A. M. (2015). Electronic and social media: The legal and ethical issues for healthcare. *Clinical Nurse Specialist*, *29*(1), 8–11. doi:10.1097/NUR.0000000000000089

89. Sandvik, A. H., Eriksson, K., & Hilli, Y. (2015). Understanding and becoming: The heart of the matter in nurse education. *Scandinavian Journal of Caring Sciences, 29*(1), 62–72. doi:10.1111/scs.12128

90. Rosa, W. (2015). A globally-conscious nonlocal nursing community: From caritas to communitas. *Nursing Science Quarterly, 28*(3), 218–222. doi:10.1177/0894318415585619

91. Roaldsen, B. L., Sørlie, T., & Lorem, G. F. (2015). Cancer survivors' experiences of humour while navigating through challenging landscapes: A socio-narrative approach. *Scandinavian Journal of Caring Sciences, 29*(4), 724–733. doi:10.1111/scs.12203

92. Rina, E., Mayumi, T., & Ruri, K. (2015). A model to create a caring and healing environment for nurses in child and family nursing. *International Journal for Human Caring, 19*(1), 8–12. doi:10.20467/1091-5710-19.1.8

93. Palesjö, C., Nordgren, L., & Asp, M. (2015). Being in a critical illness-recovery process: A phenomenological hermeneutical study. *Journal of Clinical Nursing, 24*(23-24), 3494–3502. doi:10.1111/jocn.13002

94. Ozolins, L. L., Horberg, U., & Dahlberg, K. (2015). Caring touch: Patients' experiences in an anthroposophic clinical context. *Scandinavian Journal of Caring Sciences, 29*(4), 834–842. doi:10.1111/scs.12242

95. Olive Ferrer, M. C., & Isla Pera, M. P. (2015). Watson's model of caring for a new paradigm in nursing care. *Revista de Enfermería, 38*(2), 43–48.

96. Nordtug, B. (2015). Levinas's ethics as a basis of healthcare: Challenges and dilemmas. *Nursing Philosophy, 16*(1), 51–63. doi:10.1111/nup.12072

97. Nilsson, S., Forsner, M., Finnström, B., & Mörelius, E. (2015). Relaxation and guided imagery do not reduce stress, pain and unpleasantness for 11- to 12-year-old girls during vaccinations. *Acta Paediatrica, 104*(7), 724–729. doi:10.1111/apa.13000

98. Nantz, S., & Hines, A. (2015). Trauma patients' family members' perceptions of nurses' caring behaviors. *Journal of Trauma Nursing, 22*(5), 249–254. doi:10.1097/JTN.0000000000000149

99. Michael, N., O'Callaghan, C., Baird, A., Gough, K., Krishnasamy, M., Hiscock, N., & Clayton, J. (2015). A mixed method feasibility study of a patient- and family-centred advance care planning intervention for cancer patients. *BMC Palliative Care, 14*, 27. doi:10.1186/s12904-015-0023-1

100. Mastel-Smith, B., Post, J., & Lake, P. (2015). Online teaching: "Are you there, and do you care?" *Journal of Nursing Education, 54*(3), 145–151. doi:10.3928/01484834-20150218-18

101. Martin, M. B. (2015). Caring in nursing professional development. *Journal for Nurses in Professional Development, 31*(5), 271–277. doi:10.1097/NND.0000000000000172

102. Lindberg, E., Ekebergh, M., Persson, E., & Hörberg, U. (2015). The importance of existential dimensions in the context of the presence of older patients at team meetings: In the light of Heidegger and Merleau-Ponty's philosophy. *International Journal of Qualitative Studies on Health and Well-Being, 10*, 26590. doi:10.3402/qhw.v10.26590

103. Koskinen, C. A., & Lindström, U. Å. (2015). An envisioning about the caring in listening. *Scandinavian Journal of Caring Sciences, 29*(3), 548–554. doi:10.1111/scs.12149

104. Korhonen, E. S., Nordman, T., & Eriksson, K. (2015). Technology and its ethics in nursing and caring journals: An integrative literature review. *Nursing Ethics, 22*(5), 561–576. doi:10.1177/0969733014549881

105. Karadag, E., Duru, P., & Orsal, P. O. (2015). Development of an attitude scale for home care. *Research and Theory for Nursing Practice, 29*(4), 306–324. doi:10.1891/1541-6577.29.4.306

106. Hutchinson, T. L. (2015). Authentic caring occasions for patients in hairy cell leukemia clinical trials. *Clinical Journal of Oncology Nursing, 19*(2), E41–E46. doi:10.1188/15.CJON .E41-E46

107. Hurwitz, B., Brown, J., & Altmiller, G. (2015). Improving pediatric temperature measurement in the ED. *American Journal of Nursing, 115*(9), 48–55. doi:10.1097/01 .NAJ.0000471249.69068.73

108. Hörberg, U., & Dahlberg, K. (2015). Caring potentials in the shadows of power, correction, and discipline: Forensic psychiatric care in the light of the work of Michel Foucault. *International Journal of Qualitative Studies on Health and Well-Being, 10*, 28703. doi:10.3402/qhw.v10.28703

109. Hörberg, U. (2015). Caring science and the development of forensic psychiatric caring. *Perspectives in Psychiatric Care, 51*(4), 277–284. doi:10.1111/ppc.12092

110. Hammarlund, K., Andersson, E., Tenenbaum, H., & Sundler, A. J. (2015). We are also interested in how fathers feel: A qualitative exploration of child health center nurses' recognition of postnatal depression in fathers. *BMC Pregnancy and Childbirth, 15*, 290. doi:10.1186/s12884-015-0726-6

111. Gross, A. H. (2015). What matters to the patient is what really matters: Quality in oncology nursing. *Clinical Journal of Oncology Nursing, 19*(2), 144–145. doi:10.1188/15.CJON .144-145

112. Gransjön Craftman, A., Hammar, L. M., von Strauss, E., Hillerås, P., & Westerbotn, M. (2015). Unlicensed personnel administering medications to older persons living at home: A challenge for social and care services. *International Journal of Older People Nursing, 10*(3), 201–210. doi:10.1111/opn.12073

113. Galvin, K., & Todres, L. (2015). Dignity as honour-wound: An experiential and relational view. *Journal of Evaluation in Clinical Practice, 21*(3), 410–418. doi:10.1111/jep.12278

114. Foss-Durant, A., McDermott, S., Kinney, G., & Triner, T. (2015). Caring science: Transforming the ethic of caring-healing practice, environment, and culture within an integrated care delivery system. *Permanente Journal, 19*(4), e136–e142. doi:10.7812/TPP/15-042

115. Ewertsson, M., Gustafsson, M., Blomberg, K., Holmström, I. K., & Allvin, R. (2015). Use of technical skills and medical devices among new registered nurses: A questionnaire study. *Nurse Education Today, 35*(12), 1169–1174. doi:10.1016/j.nedt.2015.05.006

116. Ewertsson, M., Allvin, R., Holmström, I. K., & Blomberg, K. (2015). Walking the bridge: Nursing students' learning in clinical skill laboratories. *Nurse Education in Practice, 15*(4), 277–283. doi:10.1016/j.nepr.2015.03.006

117. Eskilsson, C., Carlsson, G., Ekebergh, M., & Hörberg, U. (2015). The experiences of patients receiving care from nursing students at a dedicated education unit: A phenomenological study. *Nurse Education in Practice, 15*(5), 353–358. doi:10.1016/j.nepr .2015.04.001

118. Enskär, K., Björk, M., Knutsson, S., Granlund, M., Darcy, L., & Huus, K. (2015). A Swedish perspective on nursing and psychosocial research in paediatric oncology: A literature review. *European Journal of Oncology Nursing, 19*(3), 310–317. doi:10.1016/j .ejon.2014.10.013

119. Chau, J. P., Lo, S. H., Choi, K. C., Chan, E. L., McHugh, M. D., Tong, D. W., … Lee, D. T. (2015). A longitudinal examination of the association between nurse staffing levels, the practice environment and nurse-sensitive patient outcomes in hospitals. *BMC Health Services Research, 15*, 538. doi:10.1186/s12913-015-1198-0

120. Bollig, G., Schmidt, G., Rosland, J. H., & Heller, A. (2015). Ethical challenges in nursing homes: Staff's opinions and experiences with systematic ethics meetings with participation of residents' relatives. *Scandinavian Journal of Caring Sciences, 29*(4), 810–823. doi:10.1111/scs.12213

121. Blomberg, A. C., Willassen, E., von Post, I., & Lindwall, L. (2015). Student nurses' experiences of preserved dignity in perioperative practice: Part I. *Nursing Ethics, 22*(6), 676–687. doi:10.1177/0969733014542675

122. Arveklev, S. H., Wigert, H., Berg, L., Burton, B., & Lepp, M. (2015). The use and application of drama in nursing education: An integrative review of the literature. *Nurse Education Today, 35*(7), e12–e17. doi:10.1016/j.nedt.2015.02.025

123. Arman, M., Ranheim, A., Rydenlund, K., Rytterström, P., & Rehnsfeldt, A. (2015). The Nordic tradition of caring science: The works of three theorists. *Nursing Science Quarterly, 28*(4), 288–296. doi:10.1177/0894318415599220

124. Wolf, K. A. (2014). Critical perspectives on nursing as bodywork. *Advances in Nursing Science, 37*(2), 147–160. doi:10.1097/ANS.0000000000000028

125. Wang, S. Y. (2014). Considering body ethics in the healthcare profession. *Journal of Nursing, 61*(5), 7–12. doi:10.6224/JN.61.5.7

126. Vossius, C., Rongve, A., Testad, I., Wimo, A., & Aarsland, D. (2014). The use and costs of formal care in newly diagnosed dementia: A three-year prospective follow-up study. *American Journal of Geriatric Psychiatry, 22*(4), 381–388. doi:10.1016/j.jagp .2012.08.014

127. Veleminsky, M., Jr, Průchová, D., Vránová, V., Samková, J., Samek, J., Porche, S., … Liška, J. (2014). Medical and salutogenic approaches and their integration in taking prenatal and postnatal care of immigrants. *Neuro Endocrinology Letters, 35*(Suppl. 1), 67–79.

128. Vaismoradi, M., Bondas, T., Salsali, M., Jasper, M., & Turunen, H. (2014). Facilitating safe care: A qualitative study of Iranian nurse leaders. *Journal of Nursing Management, 22*(1), 106–116. doi:10.1111/j.1365-2834.2012.01439.x

129. Turkel, M. C. (2014). Leading from the heart: Caring, love, peace, and values guiding leadership. *Nursing Science Quarterly, 27*(2), 172–177. doi:10.1177/0894318414522663

130. Tinkham, M. R. (2014). Practice models: Developing, revising, and adopting the best structure for your organization. *AORN Journal, 99*(2), 312–314. doi:10.1016/j.aorn .2013.11.006

131. Su, X., Lau, J. T., Yu, C. M., Chow, C. B., Lee, L. P., But, B. W., … Choi, K. C. (2014). Growth charts for Chinese down syndrome children from birth to 14 years. *Archives of Disease in Childhood, 99*(9), 824–829. doi:10.1136/archdischild-2013-304494

132. Santos, M. R., Bousso, R. S., Vendramim, P., Baliza, M. F., Misko, M. D., & Silva, L. (2014). The practice of nurses caring for families of pediatric inpatients in light of Jean Watson. *Revista da Escola de Enfermagem da U S P, 48*, 80–86. doi:10.1590/S0080 -623420140000600012

133. Rosa, W. E. (2014). Nursing is separate from medicine: Advanced practice nursing and a transpersonal plan of care. *International Journal for Human Caring, 18*(2), 76–82. doi:10.20467/1091-5710-18.2.76

134. Rosa, W. (2014). Reflections on self in relation to other: Core community values of a moral/ethical foundation. *Creative Nursing, 20*(4), 242–247.

135. Rosa, W. (2014). Nurse as athlete: An antidote for compassion fatigue. *Archives of Psychiatric Nursing, 28*(4), 224–225. doi:10.1016/j.apnu.2014.03.003

136. Rosa, W., (2014). Intertwined narratives of the human caring story. *Creative Nursing, 20*(3), 171–173. doi:10.1891/1078-4535.20.3.171

137. Rosa, W. (2014). Intertwined narratives of the human caring story. *Creative Nursing, 20*(3), 171–173.

138. Rosa, W. (2014). Holding heartspace: The unveiling of the self through being and becoming. *International Journal for Human Caring, 18*(4), 59. doi:10.20467/1091-5710 -18.4.59

139. Rosa, W. (2014). Caring science and compassion fatigue: Reflective inventory for the individual processes of self-healing. *Beginnings, 34*(4), 18–20.

140. Rosa, W. (2014). Allowing for miracles: The vulnerable choice of intentionality and presence. *Beginnings, 34*(2), 14–15.

141. Rew, L. (2014). Holistic nursing research with homeless youths. *Beginnings, 34*(2), 16–20.

142. Reilly, P. M., Buchanan, T. M., Vafides, C., Breakey, S., & Dykes, P. (2014). Auricular acupuncture to relieve health care workers' stress and anxiety: Impact on caring. *Dimensions of Critical Care Nursing, 33*(3), 151–159. doi:10.1097/DCC.0000000000000039

143. Rehnsfeldt, A., Lindwall, L., Lohne, V., Lillestø, B., Slettebø, Å., ... Nåden, D. (2014). The meaning of dignity in nursing home care as seen by relatives. *Nursing Ethics, 21*(5), 507–517. doi:10.1177/0969733013511358

144. Pilkington, F. B. (2014). A unitary transformative perspective on transformational leadership. *Nursing Science Quarterly, 27*(2), 171. doi:10.1177/0894318414522666

145. Phillips, T., & Hall, M. (2014). Graduate nurse internship program: A formalized orientation program. *Journal for Nurses in Professional Development, 30*(4), 190–195. doi:10.1097/ NND.0000000000000069

146. Patiraki, E., Karlou, C., Efstathiou, G., Tsangari, H., Merkouris, A., Jarosova, D., ... Papastavrou, E. (2014). The relationship between surgical patients' and nurses' characteristics with their perceptions of caring behaviors: A European survey. *Clinical Nursing Research, 23*(2), 132–152. doi:10.1177/1054773812468447

147. Morrow, M. (2014). Caring science, mindful practice: Implementing Watson's human caring theory, by K. Sitzman and J. Watson. (New York: Springer, 2014). *Nursing Science Quarterly, 27*(3), 263–264. doi:10.1177/0894318414534468

148. McDermott-Levy, R., Leffers, J., & Huffling, K. (2014). Global earth caring through the millennium development goals and beyond. *International Journal for Human Caring, 18*(2), 9–17. doi:10.20467/1091-5710-18.2.9

149. Mason, V. M., Leslie, G., Clark, K., Lyons, P., Walke, E., Butler, C., & Griffin, M. (2014). Compassion fatigue, moral distress, and work engagement in surgical intensive care unit trauma nurses: A pilot study. *Dimensions of Critical Care Nursing, 33*(4), 215–225. doi:10.1097/DCC.0000000000000056

150. Manopoulos, C., & Tsangaris, S. (2014). Enhanced diffusion for oscillatory viscoelastic flow. *Physica Scripta, 89*(8), 8. doi:10.1088/0031-8949/89/8/085206

151. Lindwall, L., & von Post, I. (2014). Preserved and violated dignity in surgical practice: Nurses' experiences. *Nursing Ethics, 21*(3), 335–346. doi:10.1177/0969733013498527

152. Levy-Malmberg, R., & Hilli, Y. (2014). The enhancement of clinical competence through caring science. *Scandinavian Journal of Caring Sciences, 28*(4), 861–866. doi:10.1111/scs.12104

153. Landers, M. G., Weathers, E., McCarthy, G., & Fitzpatrick, J. J. (2014). Professional caring: Descriptions from student nurses' perspectives midway through their educational program. *International Journal for Human Caring, 18*(4), 52–58. doi:10.20467/1091-5710-18.4.52

154. Lamke, D., Catlin, A., & Mason-Chadd, M. (2014). "Not just a theory": The relationship between Jin Shin Jyutsu® self-care training for nurses and stress, physical health, emotional health, and caring efficacy. *Journal of Holistic Nursing, 32*(4), 278–289. doi:10.1177/0898010114531906

155. Krumm, N., Larkin, P., Connolly, M., Rode, P., & Elsner, F. (2014). Improving dementia care in nursing homes: Experiences with a palliative care symptom-assessment tool (MIDOS). *International Journal of Palliative Nursing, 20*(4), 187–192. doi:10.12968/ijpn.2014.20.4.187

156. Korhonen, E. S., Nordman, T., & Eriksson, K. (2014). Determination of concept technology: The ontology of the concept as a component of the knowledge development in caring science. *Scandinavian Journal of Caring Sciences, 28*(4), 867–877. doi:10.1111/scs.12118

157. Karlsson, K., Rydström, I., Enskär, K., & Englund, A. C. (2014). Nurses' perspectives on supporting children during needle-related medical procedures. *International Journal of Qualitative Studies on Health and Well-Being, 9,* 23063. doi:10.3402/qhw.v9.23063

158. Karlsson, K., Englund, A. C., Enskär, K., & Rydström, I. (2014). Parents' perspectives on supporting children during needle-related medical procedures. *International Journal of Qualitative Studies on Health and Well-Being, 9,* 23759. doi:10.3402/qhw.v9.23759

159. Hurdle, C. E., & Quinlan, M. M. (2014). A transpersonal approach to care: A qualitative study of performers' experiences with DooR to DooR, a hospital-based arts program. *Journal of Holistic Nursing, 32*(2), 78–88. doi:10.1177/0898010113508005

160. Hsiao-Wen, W., & Chun-Chin, H. (2014). A nursing experience of a terminal stage hepatocellular carcinoma patient suffering from death-induced anxiety. *Tzu Chi Nursing Journal, 13*(1), 90–100.

161. Honkavuo, L., & Lindström, U. Å. (2014). Nurse leaders' responsibilities in supporting nurses experiencing difficult situations in clinical nursing. *Journal of Nursing Management, 22*(1), 117–126. doi:10.1111/j.1365-2834.2012.01468.x

162. Holmberg, M., Forslund, K., Wahlberg, A. C., & Fagerberg, I. (2014). To surrender in dependence of another: The relationship with the ambulance clinicians as experienced by patients. *Scandinavian Journal of Caring Sciences, 28*(3), 544–551. doi:10.1111/scs.12079

163. Hay, J., Collin, S., & Koruth, S. (2014). Weaving a healthcare tapestry of safety and communication. *Nursing Management, 45*(7), 40–46. doi:10.1097/01.NUMA.0000451035.84587.7d

164. Haugan, G. (2014). The relationship between nurse-patient interaction and meaning-in-life in cognitively intact nursing home patients. *Journal of Advanced Nursing, 70*(1), 107–120. doi:10.1111/jan.12173

165. Giese, K. K., & Cook, P. F. (2014). Reducing obesity among employees of a manufacturing plant. *Workplace Health & Safety, 62*(4), 136–141. doi:10.3928/21650799-20140305-02

166. Gabrielsen, E., Nåden, D., & Lindström, U. Å. (2014). The relation between the phenomena of disease, illness, and suffering. *Holistic Nursing Practice, 28*(6), 362–369. doi:10.1097/HNP.0000000000000057

167. Fraser, C., & Keating, M. (2014). The effect of a creative art program on self-esteem, hope, perceived social support, and self-efficacy in individuals with multiple sclerosis: A pilot study. *Journal of Neuroscience Nursing, 46*(6), 330–336. doi:10.1097/JNN.0000000000000094

168. Ernesäter, A., Engström, M., Winblad, U., & Holmström, I. K. (2014). A comparison of calls subjected to a malpractice claim versus 'normal calls' within the Swedish healthcare direct: A case-control study. *BMJ Open, 4*(10), e005961. doi:10.1136/bmjopen-2014-005961

169. Duffy, J. R., Brewer, B. B., & Weaver, M. T. (2014). Revision and psychometric properties of the caring assessment tool. *Clinical Nursing Research, 23*(1), 80–93. doi:10.1177/1054773810369827

170. Dudkiewicz, P. B. (2014). Utilizing a caring-based nursing model in an interdepartmental setting to improve patient satisfaction. *International Journal for Human Caring, 18*(4), 30–33. doi:10.20467/1091-5710-18.4.30

171. Desmond, M. E. (2014). Incorporating caring theory into personal and professional nursing practice to improve perception of care. *International Journal for Human Caring, 18*(1), 35–44. doi:10.20467/1091-5710-18.1.35

172. Dawson, T., Comer, L., Kossick, M. A., & Neubrander, J. (2014). Can script concordance testing be used in nursing education to accurately assess clinical reasoning skills? *Journal of Nursing Education, 53*(5), 281–286. doi:10.3928/01484834-20140321-03

173. Chia-Pin, L., Gwo-Cheng, C., & Shiou-Fang, L. (2014). Integrating Watson's theory of human care with gardening activities: A nursing experience of an elderly patient with depression. *Tzu Chi Nursing Journal, 13*(5), 88–98.

174. Chair, S. Y., Hung, M. S., Lui, J. C., Lee, D. T., Shiu, I. Y., & Choi, K. C. (2014). Public knowledge and attitudes towards cardiopulmonary resuscitation in Hong Kong: Telephone survey. *Hong Kong Medical Journal, 20*(2), 126–133. doi:10.12809/hkmj134076

175. Burger, K. G., Kramlich, D., Malitas, M., Page-Cutrara, K., & Whitfield-Harris, L. (2014). Application of the symphonological approach to faculty-to-faculty incivility in nursing education. *Journal of Nursing Education, 53*(10), 563–568. doi:10.3928/01484834-20140922-02

176. Blegen, N. E., Eriksson, K., & Bondas, T. (2014). Through the depths and heights of darkness: Mothers as patients in psychiatric care. *Scandinavian Journal of Caring Sciences, 28*(4), 852–860. doi:10.1111/scs.12122

177. Bjorgvinsdottir, K., & Halldorsdottir, S. (2014). Silent, invisible and unacknowledged: Experiences of young caregivers of single parents diagnosed with multiple sclerosis. *Scandinavian Journal of Caring Sciences, 28*(1), 38–48. doi:10.1111/scs.12030

178. Behruzi, R., Hatem, M., Goulet, L., & Fraser, W. D. (2014). Perception of humanization of birth in a highly specialized hospital: Let's think differently. *Health Care for Women International, 35*(2), 127–148. doi:10.1080/07399332.2013.857321

179. Arslan-Özkan, İ., Okumuş, H., & Buldukoğlu, K. (2014). A randomized controlled trial of the effects of nursing care based on Watson's theory of human caring on distress, self-efficacy and adjustment in infertile women. *Journal of Advanced Nursing, 70*(8), 1801–1812. doi:10.1111/jan.12338

180. Aronsson, K., Björkdahl, I., & Wireklint Sundström, B. (2014). Prehospital emergency care for patients with suspected hip fractures after falling: Older patients' experiences. *Journal of Clinical Nursing, 23*(21-22), 3115–3123. doi:10.1111/jocn.12550

181. Antiller, A. T., & Biosca, A. R. (2014). Family care in intensive care units. *Metas de Enfermería, 17*(2), 50–56.

182. Amorim, T. V., Arreguy-Sena, C., da Silva Alves, M., & de Oliveira Salimena, A. M. (2014). Cuidado sistematizado em pré-operatório cardíaco: Teoria do Cuidado Transpessoal na perspectiva de enfermeiros e usuários. *Revista Brasileira de Enfermagem, 67*(4), 568–574. doi:10.1590/0034-7167.2014670411

183. Wilson, M., & Casterline, G. L. (2013). Using caring-science to design a healing environment for transradial catheterization recovery. *International Journal for Human Caring, 17*(2), 50–58.

184. Wiklund Gustin, L., & Wagner, L. (2013). The butterfly effect of caring: Clinical nursing teachers' understanding of self-compassion as a source to compassionate care. *Scandinavian Journal of Caring Sciences, 27*(1), 175–183. doi:10.1111/j.1471-6712.2012.01033.x

185. Vicente, V., Castren, M., Sjöstrand, F., & Sundström, B. W. (2013). Elderly patients' participation in emergency medical services when offered an alternative care pathway. *International Journal of Qualitative Studies on Health and Well-Being, 8*, 20014. doi:10.3402/qhw.v8i0.20014

186. Trens López, D. M. (2013). A humanistic view of nursing care. *Metas de Enfermería, 16*(9), 70–74.

187. Thorkildsen, K. M., Eriksson, K., & Råholm, M. B. (2013). The substance of love when encountering suffering: An interpretative research synthesis with an abductive approach. *Scandinavian Journal of Caring Sciences, 27*(2), 449–459. doi:10.1111/j.1471-6712.2012.01038.x

188. Sossong, A., & Poirier, P. (2013). Patient and nurse perceptions of caring in rural United States. *International Journal for Human Caring, 17*(1), 79–85.

189. Sokola, K. M. (2013). The relationship between caring ability and competency with caring behaviors of nursing students. *International Journal for Human Caring, 17*(1), 45–55.

190. Snide, J., & Nailon, R. (2013). Nursing staff innovations result in improved patient satisfaction. *American Journal of Nursing, 113*(10), 42–50. doi:10.1097/01.NAJ.0000435349.68781.77

191. Simourd, J. (2013). Caring is part of all nursing. *International Journal for Human Caring, 17*(1), 86–87.

192. Sehr, J., Eisele-Hlubocky, L., Junker, R., Johns, E., Birk, D., & Gaehle, K. (2013). Family pet visitation. *American Journal of Nursing, 113*(12), 54–59. doi:10.1097/01.NAJ.0000438869.75401.21

193. Sears, S. R., Bolton, S., & Bell, K. L. (2013). Evaluation of 'steps to surgical success' (STEPS): A holistic perioperative medicine program to manage pain and anxiety related to surgery. *Holistic Nursing Practice, 27*(6), 349–357. doi:10.1097/HNP.0b013e3182a72c5a

194. Schlagel, L. C., Richards, J. L., & Ward, A. (2013). Caritas language: Nursing terminology to capture the essence of nursing. *International Journal for Human Caring, 17*(2), 39–43.

195. Sadat Hoseini, A. S., Alhani, F., Khosro-Panah, A. H., & Behjatpour, A. K. (2013). A concept analysis of nursing based on islamic sources: Seeking remedy. *International Journal of Nursing Knowledge, 24*(3), 142–149. doi:10.1111/j.2047-3095.2013.01244.x

196. Rykkje, L. L., Eriksson, K., & Raholm, M. B. (2013). Spirituality and caring in old age and the significance of religion: A hermeneutical study from Norway. *Scandinavian Journal of Caring Sciences, 27*(2), 275–284. doi:10.1111/j.1471-6712.2012.01028.x

197. Porr, C., & Egan, R. (2013). How does the nurse educator measure caring? *International Journal of Nursing Education Scholarship, 10.* doi:10.1515/ijnes-2012-0011

198. PetersonLund, R. R. (2013). Living on the edge: A review of the literature. *Nursing Science Quarterly, 26*(4), 303–310. doi:10.1177/0894318413500311

199. Nåden, D., Rehnsfeldt, A., Råholm, M. B., Lindwall, L., Caspari, S., Aasgaard, T., ... Lohne, V. (2013). Aspects of indignity in nursing home residences as experienced by family caregivers. *Nursing Ethics, 20*(7), 748–761. doi:10.1177/0969733012475253

200. McMaster, R. (2013). Mainstream health economics and dignity: The commodity narrative as a debilitating solecism? *American Journal of Economics and Sociology, 72*(1), 1–31. doi:10.1111/j.1536-7150.2012.00872.x

201. Makenzius, M., Tydén, T., Darj, E., & Larsson, M. (2013). Autonomy and dependence: Experiences of home abortion, contraception and prevention. *Scandinavian Journal of Caring Sciences, 27*(3), 569–579. doi:10.1111/j.1471-6712.2012.01068.x

202. Lusk, J. M., & Fater, K. (2013). A Concept analysis of patient-centered care. *Nursing Forum, 48*(2), 89–98. doi:10.1111/nuf.12019

203. Lindberg, S., von Post, I., & Eriksson, K. (2013). Hermeneutics and human interplay: A clinical caring science research method. *International Journal of Qualitative Methods, 12,* 99–112. doi:10.1177/160940691301200145

204. Koslander, T., Lindström, U. Å., & Barbosa da Silva, A., (2013). The human being's spiritual experiences in a mental healthcare context; their positive and negative meaning and impact on health: A hermeneutic approach. *Scandinavian Journal of Caring Sciences, 27*(3), 560–568. doi:10.1111/j.1471-6712.2012.01067.x

205. Koskinen, C. A., & Lindström, U. Å. (2013). Hermeneutic reading of classic texts. *Scandinavian Journal of Caring Sciences, 27*(3), 757–764. doi:10.1111/j.1471-6712.2012.01080.x

206. Kim, S. S., Hayward, R. D., & Kang, Y. (2013). Psychological, physical, social, and spiritual well-being similarities between Korean older adults and family caregivers. *Geriatric Nursing, 34*(1), 35–40. doi:10.1016/j.gerinurse.2012.07.010

207. Karlsson, M., Karlsson, C., Barbosa da Silva, A., Berggren, I., & Söderlund, M. (2013). Community nurses' experiences of ethical problems in end-of-life care in the patient's own home. *Scandinavian Journal of Caring Sciences, 27*(4), 831–838. doi:10.1111/j.1471-6712 .2012.01087.x

208. Hutchinson, T. L., & Janiszewski Goodin, H. (2013). Nursing student anxiety as a context for teaching/learning. *Journal of Holistic Nursing, 31*(1), 19–24. doi:10.1177/ 0898010112462067

209. Huntley, N. B. (2013). ...and so it begins. One nurse's journey to caritas consciousness. *International Journal for Human Caring, 17*(2), 44–49.

210. Homer, R., & Ryan, L. (2013). Making the grade: Charge nurse education improves job performance. *Nursing Management, 44*(3), 38–44. doi:10.1097/01.NUMA.0000427183 .65177.76

211. Ho, A. H., Leung, P. P., Tse, D. M., Pang, S. M., Chochinov, H. M., Neimeyer, R. A., Chan, C. L. (2013). Dignity amidst liminality: Healing within suffering among Chinese terminal cancer patients. *Death Studies, 37*(10), 953–970. doi:10.1080/07481187 .2012.703078

212. Herbst, A. M., Friesen, M. A., & Speroni, K. G. (2013). Caring, connecting, and communicating: Reflections on developing a patient-centered bedside handoff. *International Journal for Human Caring, 17*(2), 16–22.

213. Haugan, G., Hanssem, B., & Moksnes, U. K. (2013). Self-transcendence, nurse–patient interaction and the outcome of multidimensional well-being in cognitively intact nursing home patients. *Scandinavian Journal of Caring Sciences, 27*(4), 882–893. doi:10.1111/scs.12000

214. Gustafsson, L. K., Wigerblad, A., & Lindwall, L. (2013). Respecting dignity in forensic care: The challenge faced by nurses of maintaining patient dignity in clinical caring situations. *Journal of Psychiatric and Mental Health Nursing, 20*(1), 1–8. doi:10.1111/ j.1365-2850.2012.01895.x

215. Gustafsson, L. K., Snellma, I., Gustafsson, C. (2013). The meaningful encounter: Patient and next-of-kin stories about their experience of meaningful encounters in healthcare. *Nursing Inquiry, 20*(4), 363–371. doi:10.1111/nin.12013

216. Faber, K. (2013). Relationship-based care in the neonatal intensive care unit. *Creative Nursing, 19*(4), 214–218. doi:10.1891/1078-4535.19.4.214

217. Edlund, M., Lindwall, L., von Post, I., & Lindström, U. Å. (2013). Concept determination of human dignity. *Nursing Ethics, 20*(8), 851–860. doi:10.1177/0969733013487193

218. Diesel, H. J., Ercole, P. M., & Taliaferro, D. L. (2013). Changing knowledge, attitudes, and beliefs via an immersion experience. *International Journal for Human Caring, 17*(1), 71–78.

219. da Silva Borges, M., & Soares dos Santos, D. (2013). Caring field: A quantum and transpersonal approach to nursing care. *Ciencia, Cuidado e Saude, 12*(3), 608–613.

220. Coughlin, C. (2013). An ethnographic study of main events during hospitalisation: Perceptions of nurses and patients. *Journal of Clinical Nursing, 22*(15-16), 2327–2337. doi:10.1111/j.1365-2702.2012.04083.x

221. Clerico, E., Lott, T. F., Harley, C., Walker, R., Kosak, E., Michel, Y., & Hulsey, T. (2013). Caring for the nurse in the hospital environment. *International Journal for Human Caring, 17*(1), 56–63.

222. Clegg, T. (2013). Holistic center a hit at St. Joseph's. *Nurse.com Nursing Spectrum* (New York/New Jersey Metro), *25*(17), 55.

223. Clark, C. (2013). An integral-caring-science RN-BS nursing curriculum: Outcomes from fostering consciousness evolution. *International Journal for Human Caring, 17*(2), 67–76.

224. Browall, M., Koinberg, I., Falk, H., & Wijk, H. (2013). Patients' experience of important factors in the healthcare environment in oncology care. *International Journal of Qualitative Studies on Health and Well-Being, 8*(1), 20870. doi:10.3402/qhw.v8i0.20870

225. Brathovde, A., Bodine, J., Cagliostro, J., Lopresti, L., Perumpail, L., & Palisoc, V. (2013). Using reflective journaling to establish a holistic nursing practice council. *International Journal for Human Caring*, 17(2), 35–38.

226. Berry, D. M., Kaylor, M. B., Church, J., Campbell, K., McMillin, T., & Wamsley, R. (2013). Caritas and job environment: A replication of Persky et al. *Contemporary Nurse*, 43(2), 237–243. doi:10.5172/conu.2013.43.2.237

227. Berntsson, T., & Hildingh, C. (2013). The nurse-patient relationship in pre-hospital emergency care: From the perspective of Swedish specialist ambulance nursing students. *International Emergency Nursing*, 21(4), 257–263. doi:10.1016/j.ienj.2012.10.003

228. Bentzen, G., Harsvik, A., & Brinchmann, B. S. (2013). "Values that vanish into thin air": Nurses' experience of ethical values in their daily work. *Nursing Research and Practice*, 2013, 939153. doi:10.1155/2013/939153

229. Wikberg, A., Eriksson, K., & Bondas, T. (2012). Intercultural caring from the perspectives of immigrant new mothers. *Journal of Obstetric, Gynecologic, and Neonatal Nursing*, 41(5), 638–649. doi:10.1111/j.1552-6909.2012.01395.x

230. Werkander Harstäde, C., Roxberg, Å., Andershed, B., & Brunt, D. (2012). Guilt and shame: A semantic concept analysis of two concepts related to palliative care. *Scandinavian Journal of Caring Sciences*, 26(4), 787–795. doi:10.1111/j.1471-6712.2012.00992.x

231. Wadsworth, A. M. (2012). Student paper. *International Journal for Human Caring*, 16(1), 64–67.

232. Vicente, V., Ekebergh, M., Castren, M., Sjöstrand, F., Svensson, L., & Sundström, B. W. (2012). Differentiating frailty in older people using the Swedish ambulance service: A retrospective audit. *International Emergency Nursing*, 20(4), 228–235. doi:10.1016/j.ienj.2011.09.005

233. Vandenhouten, C., Kubsch, S., Peterson, M., Murdock, J., & Lehrer, L. (2012). Watson's theory of transpersonal caring factors impacting nurses professional caring. *Holistic Nursing Practice*, 26(6), 326–334. doi:10.1097/HNP.0b013e31826ed0e8

234. Tang, A. C., Chung, J. W., & Wong, T. K. (2012). Validation of a novel traditional Chinese medicine pulse diagnostic model using an artificial neural network. *Evidence-Based Complementary and Alternative Medicine*, 2012, 685094. doi:10.1155/2012/685094

235. Tang, A. C., Chung, J. W., & Wong, T. K. (2012). Digitalizing traditional Chinese medicine pulse diagnosis with artificial neural network. *Telemedicine Journal and E-Health*, 18(6), 446–453. doi:10.1089/tmj.2011.0204

236. Sundström, B. W., & Dahlberg, K. (2012). Being prepared for the unprepared: A phenomenology field study of Swedish prehospital care. *Journal of Emergency Nursing*, 38(6), 571–577. doi:10.1016/j.jen.2011.09.003

237. Smith, M. C, Turkel, M. C., & Wolf, Z. R. (Eds.). (2012). *Caring in nursing classics: An essential resource* (p. 117). New York, NY: Springer Publishing.

238. Silva Rabelo, A. C., Cavalcante Guedes, M. V., & Fátima da Silva, L. D. (2012). Experiences of mothers of children living with cardiopathies: A care research study. *Online Brazilian Journal of Nursing*, 11(3), 683–700. doi:10.5935/1676-4285.2012004

239. Rydeman, I., Törnkvist, L., Agreus, L., & Dahlberg, K. (2012). Being in-between and lost in the discharge process: An excursus of two empirical studies of older persons', their relatives', and care professionals' experience. *International Journal of Qualitative Studies on Health and Well-Being*, 7(0), 1–9. doi:10.3402/qhw.v7i0.19678

240. Richardson, S. F. (2012). Caritas and communitas: Inspiring caring connections through aesthetics and ritual. *International Journal for Human Caring, 16*(3), 85.

241. Rehnsfeldt, A., & Arman, M. (2012). Significance of close relationships after the tsunami disaster in connection with existential health: A qualitative interpretive study. *Scandinavian Journal of Caring Sciences, 26*(3), 537–544. doi:10.1111/j.1471-6712.2011.00962.x

242. Reavy, K., Hobbs, J., Hereford, M., & Crosby, K. (2012). A new clinic model for refugee health care: Adaptation of cultural safety. *Rural and Remote Health, 12*(1), 1826.

243. Ranheim, A., Kärner, A., & Berterö, C. (2012). Caring theory and practice: Entering a simultaneous concept analysis. *Nursing Forum, 47*(2), 78–90. doi:10.1111/j.1744-6198 .2012.00263.x

244. Poblete-Troncoso, M. D., Valenzuela-Suazo, S. V., & Merino, J. M. (2012). Validation of two scales used to measure transpersonal human caring, based on Jean Watson's theory. *Aquichán, 12*(1), 8–21. doi:10.5294/aqui.2012.12.1.1

245. Palmér, L., Carlsson, G., Mollberg, M., Nyström, M. (2012). Severe breastfeeding difficulties: Existential lostness as a mother: Women's lived experiences of initiating breastfeeding under severe difficulties. *International Journal of Qualitative Studies on Health and Well-Being, 7*, doi:10.3402/qhw.v7i0.10846

246. Nunes da Fonseca, P. I. M., & Melo Tavares, C. M. (2012). Emotions experienced by a multidisciplinary team during interviews for organ donation consent: A descriptive study. *Online Brazilian Journal of Nursing, 11*(2), 466–469. doi:10.5935/1676-4285.2012S012

247. Norman, V. (2012). Integrating Watson's theory of human caring using experiential learning. *International Journal for Human Caring, 16*(3), 70–71.

248. Maillie, S., & Breitbarth, K. (2012). Watson's theory of human caring as a research framework to reduce restraints in MICU. *International Journal for Human Caring, 16*(3), 82–83.

249. Lindwall, L., Boussaid, L., Kulzer, S., & Wigerblad, A. (2012). Patient dignity in psychiatric nursing practice. *Journal of Psychiatric and Mental Health Nursing, 19*(7), 569–576. doi:10.1111/j.1365-2850.2011.01837.x

250. Lindberg, E., Persson, E., & Bondas, T. (2012). 'The responsibility of someone else': A focus group study of collaboration between a university and a hospital regarding the integration of caring science in practice. *Scandinavian Journal of Caring Sciences, 26*(3), 579–586. doi:10.1111/j.1471-6712.2012.00968.x

251. Lachman, V. D. (2012). Applying the ethics of care to your nursing practice. *MEDSURG Nursing, 21*(2), 112–114.

252. Keselman, D. (2012). Ethical leadership. *Holistic Nursing Practice, 26*(5), 259–261. doi:10.1097/HNP.0b013e318263f2da

253. Iversen, A., & Sessanna, L. (2012). Utilizing Watson's theory of human caring and Hills and Watson's emancipatory pedagogy to educate hospital-based multidisciplinary healthcare providers about hospice. *International Journal for Human Caring, 16*(4), 42–49.

254. Ishikawa, J., & Kawano, M. (2012). Caring practice of a psychiatric nurse in Japan: Analyzing from caring theory focusing on the inner process of the individual. *International Journal for Human Caring, 16*(3), 80–81.

255. Gillespie, G. L., Hounchell, M., Pettinichi, J., Mattei, J., & Rose, L. (2012). Caring in pediatric emergency nursing. *Research and Theory for Nursing Practice, 26*(3), 216–232. doi:10.1891/1541-6577.26.3.216

256. Gallison, B. (2012). She and me: A story of conflict resolution and Jean Watson's human caring theory. *Beginnings, 32*(6), 10–11.

257. Fang-Hui, H., Li-Chuan, L., & Huei-Chuan, S. (2012). A nursing experience of an elderly with disability and the primary caregiver using Watson's caring theory. *Tzu Chi Nursing Journal, 11*(1), 119–128.

258. Estrada, N. (2012). A combination of nursing theories to guide a professional practice model. *Communicating Nursing Research, 45*, 501–501.

259. David, M. (2012). Who was that masked hero? A salute to the perioperative nurse. *AORN Journal, 95*(2), 286–287. doi:10.1016/j.aorn.2011.11.007

260. Dade, J. (2012). Caring for communities after disasters. *Minority Nurse, 2012*, 41–44.

261. Clark, C. S. (2012). Beyond holism: Incorporating an integral approach to support caring-healing-sustainable nursing practices. *Holistic Nursing Practice, 26*(2), 92–102. doi:10.1097/HNP.0b013e3182462197

262. Berglund, M., Sjögren, R., & Ekebergh, M. (2012). Reflect and learn together: When two supervisors interact in the learning support process of nurse education. *Journal of Nursing Management, 20*(2), 152–158. doi:10.1111/j.1365-2834.2011.01368.x

263. Williams, R. L., II, McDowell, J. B., & Kautz, D. D. (2011). A caring leadership model for nursing's future. *International Journal for Human Caring, 15*(1), 31–35.

264. Weekes, K., & Devonish, S. (2011). A nurse led transition program for eating disorder patients. *Communicating Nursing Research, 44*, 413–413.

265. Tzeng, H. M., Hu, H. M., & Yin, C. Y. (2011). The relationship of the hospital-acquired injurious fall rates with the quality profile of a hospital's care delivery and nursing staff patterns. *Nursing Economic$, 29*(6), 299–306, quiz.

266. Saeteren, B., Lindström, U. Å., & Nåden, D. (2011). Latching onto life: Living in the area of tension between the possibility of life and the necessity of death. *Journal of Clinical Nursing, 20*(5-6), 811–818. doi:10.1111/j.1365-2702.2010.03212.x

267. Plovie, B. (2011). Applying personal knowing of research to Watson's theory of human care. *Communicating Nursing Research, 44*, 560–560.

268. Passandideh-Fard, M., Teymourtash, A. R., & Khavari, M. (2011). Numerical study of circular hydraulic jump using volume-of-fluid method. *Journal of Fluids Engineering-Transactions of the ASME, 133*(1), 11. doi:10.1115/1.4003307

269. Paldanius, A., & Määttä, K. (2011). What are students' views of (loving) caring in nursing education in Finland? *International Journal of Caring Sciences, 4*(2), 81–89.

270. Olsson, A. (2011). Assessing women's sexual life after childbirth: The role of the postnatal check. *Midwifery, 27*(2), 195–202. doi:10.1016/j.midw.2009.04.003

271. Ohlén, J., Furåker, C., Jakobsson, E., Bergh, I., & Hermansson, E. (2011). Impact of the Bologna process in bachelor nursing programmes: The Swedish case. *Nurse Education Today, 31*(2), 122–128. doi:10.1016/j.nedt.2010.05.002

272. Norlyk, A., Dreyer, P., Haahr, A., & Martinsen, B. (2011). Understanding the creative processes of phenomenological research: The life philosophy of Løgstrup. *International Journal of Qualitative Studies on Health and Well-Being, 6*(4). doi:10.3402/qhw.v6i4.7320

273. Nelms, T. P., Jones, J., & Treiber, L. A. (2011). A study to reduce medication errors using Watson's caring theory. *International Journal for Human Caring, 15*(3), 24–33.

274. Morrison, D., & Sanders, C. (2011). Huddling for optimal care outcomes. *Nursing, 41*(12), 22–24. doi:10.1097/01.NURSE.0000407682.12130.f3

275. Lundgren, S. M., & Berg, L. (2011). The meanings and implications of receiving care. *Scandinavian Journal of Caring Sciences, 25*(2), 235–242. doi:10.1111/j.1471-6712.2010.00815.x

276. Lombardo, B., & Eyre, C. (2011). Compassion fatigue: A nurse's primer. *Online Journal of Issues in Nursing, 16*(1), 3. doi:10.3912/OJIN.Vol16No01Man03

277. Lindahl, B. (2011). Experiences of exclusion when living on a ventilator: Reflections based on the application of Julia Kristeva's philosophy to caring science. *Nursing Philosophy, 12*(1), 12–21. doi:10.1111/j.1466-769X.2010.00471.x

278. Kryak, E., & Vitale, A. (2011). Reiki and its journey into a hospital setting. *Holistic Nursing Practice, 25*(5), 238–245. doi:10.1097/HNP.0b013e31822a02ad

279. Karnick, P. M. (2011). Making the connection: Theory, research, and practice. *Nursing Science Quarterly, 24*(1), 26. doi:10.1177/0894318410389074

280. Isaksson, U., Graneheim, U. H., Åström, S., & Karlsson, S. (2011). Physically violent behaviour in dementia care: Characteristics of residents and management of violent situations. *Aging & Mental Health, 15*(5), 573–579. doi:10.1080/13607863.2011.556600

281. Hörberg, U., Ozolins, L. L., & Ekebergh, M. (2011). Intertwining caring science, caring practice and caring education from a lifeworld perspective: Two contextual examples. *International Journal of Qualitative Studies on Health and Well-Being, 6*(4). doi:10.3402/qhw.v6i4.10363

282. Hill, K. S. (2011). Work satisfaction, intent to stay, desires of nurses, and financial knowledge among bedside and advanced practice nurses. *Journal of Nursing Administration, 41*(5), 211–217. doi:10.1097/NNA.0b013e3182171b17

283. Hermanns, M., Lilly, M. L., & Crawley, B. (2011). Using clinical simulation to enhance psychiatric nursing training of baccalaureate students. *Clinical Simulation in Nursing, 7*(2), e41–e46. doi:10.1016/j.ecns.2010.05.001

284. Hansson, K. S., Fridlund, B., Brunt, D., Hansson, B., & Rask, M. (2011). The meaning of the experiences of persons with chronic pain in their encounters with the health service. *Scandinavian Journal of Caring Sciences, 25*(3), 444–450. doi:10.1111/j.1471-6712 .2010.00847.x

285. Gustafsson, L. K., Wiklund-Gustin, L., & Lindström, U. Å. (2011). The meaning of reconciliation: Women's stories about their experience of reconciliation with suffering from grief. *Scandinavian Journal of Caring Sciences, 25*(3), 525–532. doi:10.1111/j.1471-6712 .2010.00859.x

286. Galvin, K. T., & Todres, L. (2011). Kinds of well-being: A conceptual framework that provides direction for caring. *International Journal of Qualitative Studies on Health and Well-Being, 6*(4). doi:10.3402/qhw.v6i4.10362

287. Fu, C. Y., Tsai, M. F., & Chen, H. M. (2011). A nurse's experience caring for a patient with breast cancer who had been previously reported dead by her family. *Hu li za zhi The Journal of Nursing, 58*(3 Suppl.), 90–96.

288. Frank, C., Fridlund, B., Baigi, A., & Asp, M. (2011). Patient participation in the emergency department: An evaluation using a specific instrument to measure patient participation (PPED). *Journal of Advanced Nursing, 67*(4), 728–735. doi:10.1111/j.1365-2648.2010.05524.x

289. Elisabeth Ranheim, A., Kärner, A., & Berterö, C. (2011). Eliciting reflections on caring theory in elderly caring practice. *International Journal of Qualitative Studies on Health and Well-Being, 6*(3). doi:10.3402/qhw.v6i3.7296

290. Ekebergh, M. (2011). A learning model for nursing students during clinical studies. *Nurse Education in Practice, 11*(6), 384–389. doi:10.1016/j.nepr.2011.03.018

291. Deschênes, M. F., Charlin, B., Gagnon, R., & Goudreau, J. (2011). Use of a script concordance test to assess development of clinical reasoning in nursing students. *Journal of Nursing Education, 50*(7), 381–387. doi:10.3928/01484834-20110331-03

292. Delaney, C., Barrere, C., & Helming, M. (2011). The influence of a spirituality-based intervention on quality of life, depression, and anxiety in community-dwelling adults with cardiovascular disease: A pilot study. *Journal of Holistic Nursing, 29*(1), 21–32. doi:10.1177/0898010110378356

293. Del Prato, D., Bankert, E., Grust, P., & Joseph, J. (2011). Transforming nursing education: A review of stressors and strategies that support students' professional socialization. *Advances in Medical Education and Practice, 2,* 109–116. doi:10.2147/AMEP.S18359

294. Cutshall, S. M. (2011). Health promotion for nurses: Expanding consciousness and professional sustainability. *Beginnings, 31*(4), 24–25.

295. Cheng, H. (2011). The nursing experience of applying Watson's theory to a male patient suffering domestic violence. *Tzu Chi Nursing Journal, 10*(3), 1.

296. Chang, Y., Sun, M., & Chou, H. (2011). The nursing experience of a depression patient with the application of Watson's caring theory during postburn rehabilitation period. *Tzu Chi Nursing Journal, 10*(2), 1.

297. Carvalho, N. V., Sá Rezende Neta, D., Freitas da Silva, G. R., & Evangelista de Araújo, T. M. (2011). The clinical caritas process of Jean Watson in Brazilian nursing care: A systematic review. *Cultura de los Cuidados, 15*(29), 82–88.

298. Calatayud, M. V., & Azcoiti, M. C. E. (2011). The concept of health from Jean Watson's perspective. *Metas de Enfermería, 14*(6), 14–16.

299. Brockopp, D., Schreiber, J., Hill, K., Altpeter, T., Moe, K., & Merritt, S. (2011). A successful evidence-based practice model in an acute care setting. *Oncology Nursing Forum, 38*(5), 509–511. doi:10.1188/11.ONF.509-51

300. Barbosa, I. V., & de Figueiredo Carvalho, Z. M. (2011). Feelings of the family in face of the spinal cord injury. *Index de Enfermería, 20*(1-2), 56–60.

301. Albarran, J., Rosser, E., Bach, S., Uhrenfeldt, L., Lundberg, P., & Law, K. (2011). Exploring the development of a cultural care framework for European caring science. *International Journal of Qualitative Studies on Health and Well-Being, 6*(4). doi:10.3402/qhw .v6i4.11457

302. Weydt, A. (2010). Mary's story, relationship-based care delivery. *Nursing Administration Quarterly, 34*(2), 141–146. doi:10.1097/NAQ.0b013e3181d91751

303. Watson, J. (2010). Holistic nurse of the year 2010. *Beginnings, 30*(3), 28.

304. Watson, J. (2010). An interview with Jean Watson, HNY 2010. Interview by Lynne Nemeth. *Beginnings, 30*(4), 30.

305. Wärnå-Furu, C., Sääksjärvi, M., & Santavirta, N. (2010). Measuring virtues: Development of a scale to measure employee virtues and their influence on health. *Scandinavian Journal of Caring Sciences, 24,* 38–45. doi:10.1111/j.1471-6712.2010.00799.x

306. Wagner, D. J., & Whaite, B. (2010). An exploration of the nature of caring relationships in the writings of Florence Nightingale. *Journal of Holistic Nursing, 28*(4), 225–234. doi:10.1177/0898010110386609

307. Vázquez Calatayud, M., & Eseverri Azcoiti, M. C. (2010). The caring of family members in the intensive care units from the Jean Watson perspective. *Enfermería Intensiva, 21*(4), 161–164. doi:10.1016/j.enfi.2010.03.004

308. Tofthagen, R., & Fagerstrøm, L. M. (2010). Rodgers' evolutionary concept analysis: A valid method for developing knowledge in nursing science. *Scandinavian Journal of Caring Sciences, 24,* 21–31. doi:10.1111/j.1471-6712.2010.00845.x

309. Tanking, J. (2010). Nurse caring behavior. *Kansas Nurse, 85*(4), 3–5.

310. Tang, H.-Y., & Liang, H.-F. (2010). Using Watson's theory in a nursing experience of a head injury patient and her primary caregiver. *Tzu Chi Nursing Journal, 9*(4), 119–128.

311. Story, L., & Butts, J. B. (2010). Compelling teaching with the four Cs: Caring, comedy, creativity, and challenging. *Journal of Nursing Education, 49*(5), 291–294. doi:10.3928/01484834-20100115-08

312. Stolt, M., Suhonen, R., Voutilainen, P., & Leino-Kilpi, H. (2010). Foot health in older people and the nurses' role in foot health care: A review of literature. *Scandinavian Journal of Caring Sciences, 24*(1), 194–201. doi:10.1111/j.1471-6712.2009.00700.x

313. Smith, W. L. (2010). Origin bands of electronically forbidden spectra made allowed by centrifugal distortion. *Journal of Molecular Spectroscopy, 260*(1), 19–22. doi:10.1016/j.jms.2009.12.010

314. Sivonen, K., Kasén, A., & Eriksson, K. (2010). Semantic analysis according to Peep Koort: A substance-oriented research methodology. *Scandinavian Journal of Caring Sciences, 24,* 12–20. doi:10.1111/j.1471-6712.2010.00817.x

315. Schreiber, R., & MacDonald, M. (2010). Keeping vigil over the patient: A grounded theory of nurse anaesthesia practice. *Journal of Advanced Nursing, 66*(3), 552–561. doi:10.1111/j.1365-2648.2009.05207.x

316. Rusner, M., Carlsson, G., Brunt, D., & Nyström, M. (2010). A dependence that empowers: The meaning of the conditions that enable a good life with bipolar disorder. *International Journal of Qualitative Studies on Health and Well-Being, 5*(1). doi:10.3402/qhw.v5i1.4653

317. Roxberg, A., Burman, M., Guldbrand, M., Fridlund, B., da Silva, A. B. (2010). Out of the wave: The meaning of suffering and relieved suffering for survivors of the tsunami catastrophe: An hermeneutic-phenomenological study of TV-interviews one year after the tsunami catastrophe, 2004. *Scandinavian Journal of Caring Sciences, 24*(4), 707–715. doi:10.1111/j.1471-6712.2009.00767.x

318. Reed, S. M. (2010). A unitary-caring conceptual model for advanced practice nursing in palliative care. *Holistic Nursing Practice, 24*(1), 23–34. doi:10.1097/HNP.0b013e3181c8e4c7

319. Putting caring into practice. (2010). *AACN Bold Voices, 2*(8), 16.

320. Poirier, P., & Sossong, A. (2010). Oncology patients' and nurses' perceptions of caring. *Canadian Oncology Nursing Journal, 20*(2), 62–65. doi:10.5737/1181912x2026265

321. Pipe, T. B., Mishark, K., Hansen, R. P., Hentz, J. G., & Hartsell, Z. (2010). Rediscovering the art of healing connection by creating the Tree of Life poster: A pilot program for hospitalized older adults. *Journal of Gerontological Nursing, 36*(6), 47–55. doi:10.3928/00989134-20100330-04

322. Palmér, L., Carlsson, G., Mollberg, M., & Nyström, M. (2010). Breastfeeding: An existential challenge: Women's lived experiences of initiating breastfeeding within the context of early home discharge in Sweden. *International Journal of Qualitative Studies on Health and Well-Being, 5*(3). doi:10.3402/qhw.v5i3.5397

323. Olsson, A., Robertson, E., Björklund, A., & Nissen, E. (2010). Fatherhood in focus, sexual activity can wait: New fathers' experience about sexual life after childbirth. *Scandinavian Journal of Caring Sciences, 24*(4), 716–725. doi:10.1111/j.1471-6712.2009.00768.x

324. Noel, D. L. (2010). Occupational health nursing practice through the human caring lens. *AORN Journal, 58*(1), 17–24, quiz. doi:10.3928/08910162-20091216-02

325. Morby, S. K., & Skalla, A. (2010). A human care approach to nursing peer review. *Nursing Science Quarterly, 23*(4), 297–300. doi:10.1177/0894318410380267

326. Morais, S. C. R., Monteiro, C. F. S., & da Rocha, S. S. (2010). Nursing care for sexually violated women. *Texto & Contexto Enfermagem, 19*(1), 155–160. doi:10.1590/S0104-07072010000100018

327. McElroy, K. G. (2010). Environmental health effects of concentrated animal feeding operations: Implications for nurses. *Nursing Administration Quarterly, 34*(4), 311–319. doi:10.1097/NAQ.0b013e3181f5649c

328. Mahler, A. (2010). The clinical nurse specialist role in developing a geropalliative model of care. *Clinical Nurse Specialist CNS, 24*(1), 18–23. doi:10.1097/NUR.0b013e3181c4abba

329. Lindwall, L., von Post, I., & Eriksson, K. (2010). Clinical research with a hermenutical design and an element of application. *International Journal of Qualitative Methods, 9*(2), 172–186. doi:10.1177/160940691000900204

330. Levy-Malmberg, R., & Eriksson, K. (2010). Legitimizing basic research by evaluating quality. *Journal of Nursing Ethics, 17*(1), 107–116. doi:10.1177/0969733009349989

331. Jasovsky, D. A., Morrow, M. R., Clementi, P. S., & Hindle, P. A. (2010). Theories in action and how nursing practice changed. *Nursing Science Quarterly, 23*(1), 29–38. doi:10.1177/0894318409353806

332. Huang, Y.-C., Wu, P.-C., & Chen, S.-H. (2010). A nursing experience of a pregnant woman with cytomegalovirus infection at emergency room. *Tzu Chi Nursing Journal, 9*(5), 119.

333. Holmberg, M., & Fagerberg, I. (2010). The encounter with the unknown: Nurses lived experiences of their responsibility for the care of the patient in the Swedish ambulance service. *International Journal of Qualitative Studies on Health and Well-Being, 5*. doi:10.3402/qhw.v5i2.5098

334. Herbst, A. M., Swengros, D. I., & Kinney, G. (2010). How to teach human caring: Nurse educator role in transformational learning for a large healthcare system. *Journal for Nurses in Staff Development, 26*(4), E6–E11. doi:10.1097/NND.0b013e3181b1ba55

335. Heijkenskjöld, K. B., Ekstedt, M., & Lindwall, L. (2010). The patient's dignity from the nurse's perspective. *Nursing Ethics, 17*(3), 313–324. doi:10.1177/0969733010361444

336. Goldin, M., & Kautz, D. D. (2010). Nurturing nursing students during intensive care unit clinical practicum. *Dimensions of Critical Care Nursing, 29*(5), 238–240. doi:10.1097/DCC.0b013e3181e6cd55

337. Goldin, M., & Kautz, D. D. (2010). Applying Watson's caring theory and caritas processes to ease life transitions. *International Journal for Human Caring, 14*(1), 11–14.

338. Galvin, K. T. (2010). Revisiting caring science: Some integrative ideas for the 'head, hand and heart' of critical care nursing practice. *Nursing in Critical Care, 15*(4), 168–175. doi:10.1111/j.1478-5153.2010.00394.x

339. Eriksson, K. (2010). Concept determination as part of the development of knowledge in caring science. *Scandinavian Journal of Caring Sciences, 24*(Suppl. 1), 2–11. doi:10.1111/j.1471-6712.2010.00809.x

340. Engström, M., Wadensten, B., & Häggström, E. (2010). Caregivers' job satisfaction and empowerment before and after an intervention focused on caregiver empowerment. *Journal of Nursing Management, 18*(1), 14–23. doi:10.1111/j.1365-2834.2009.01047.x

341. Ekedahl, M. A., & Wengström, Y. (2010). Caritas, spirituality and religiosity in nurses' coping. *European Journal of Cancer Care, 19*(4), 530–537. doi:10.1111/j.1365 -2354.2009.01089.x

342. Earle, V. (2010). Phenomenology as research method or substantive metaphysics? An overview of phenomenology's uses in nursing. *Nursing Philosophy, 11*(4), 286–296. doi:10.1111/j.1466-769X.2010.00458.x

343. Davila, L., Merrill, D., & Baize, T. (2010). Sustaining caring change in a healthcare system. *International Journal for Human Caring, 14*(4), 45–50.

344. da Rosa, L. M., Sebold, L. F., Arzuaga, M., Santos, V. E. P., & Radünz, V. (2010). Nursing theoretical frameworks and production of scientific knowledge. *Revista Enfermagem, 18*(1), 120–125.

345. Cheng, W. L., & Lai, C. K. (2010). Satisfaction scale for community nursing: Development and validation. *Journal of Advanced Nursing, 66*(10), 2331–2340. doi:10.1111/j.1365-2648.2010.05373.x

346. Burtson, P. L., & Stichler, J. F. (2010). Nursing work environment and nurse caring: Relationship among motivational factors. *Journal of Advanced Nursing, 66*(8), 1819–1831. doi:10.1111/j.1365-2648.2010.05336.x

347. Bondas, T. (2010). Nursing leadership from the perspective of clinical group supervision: A paradoxical practice. *Journal of Nursing Management, 18*(4), 477–486. doi:10.1111/j.1365-2834.2010.01085.x

348. Biggs, L., & Schriner, C. L. (2010). Recognition and support for today's preceptor. *Journal of Continuing Education in Nursing, 41*(7), 317–322. doi:10.3928/00220124-20100401-05

NON-ENGLISH ARTICLES

1. 賴怡璇, 江國誠., & 陸秀芳. (2016). 以 Watson 關懷理論照護一位 自殺企圖之憂鬱症老人之 護理經驗. *Tzu Chi Nursing Journal, 15*(4), 96–105.

2. 卓秋萍 & 甘偉志. (2016). 一位少女接受血型不相容 腎臟移植前行雙重過濾血漿 分離術之護 理經驗. *Tzu Chi Nursing Journal, 15*(6), 114–124.

3. Morales-Castillo, F. A., Hernández-Cruz, M. C., Morales Rodríguez, M. C., & Landeros Olvera, E. A. (2016). Validación y estandarización del instrumento: Evaluación de los comportamientos de cuidado otorgado en enfermeras mexicanas. *Enfermería Universitaria, 13*(1), 3–11. doi:10.1016/j.reu.2015.11.005

4. 葉宛姍 & 黃素慧 (2015). 運用 Watson 理論於 一位成骨不全症幼童手術及其 主要照顧者之 護理經驗. *Tzu Chi Nursing Journal, 14*(4), 99–108.

5. Krol, P. J., & Lavoie, M. (2015). From humanism to nihilism: Dialectics on Jean Watson's caring theory. *Recherche en Soins Infirmiers*, (122), 52–66. doi:10.3917/rsi.122.0052

6. Ellefsen, É., & Cara, C. (2015). The health-within-illness experience: An encounter between the suffering and the power to exist for adults living with systemic scleroderma. *Recherche en Soins Infirmiers*, (121), 52–63. doi:10.3917/rsi.121.0052***

7. Brunetti, P., Pellegrini, W., Masera, G., Berchialla, P., & Dal Molin, A. (2015). The model of human caring: Results of a pre- and post-intervention study with a control group. *Professioni Infermieristiche, 68*(1), 19–28. doi:10.7429/pi.2015.681019

8. Amorim, T. V., Arreguy-Sena, C., Alves Mda, S., & Salimena, A. M. (2014). Systematized care in cardiac preoperative: Theory of human caring in the perspective of nurses and users. *Revista Brasileira de Enfermagem, 67*(4), 568–574. doi:10.1590/0034-7167.2014670411

9. Favero, L., Pagliuca, L. M., & Lacerda, M. R. (2013). Transpersonal caring in nursing: An analysis grounded in a conceptual model. *Revista da Escola de Enfermagem da U S P, 47*(2), 500–505. doi:10.1590/S0080-62342013000200032

10. de Pires, D. E. (2013). Necessary changes for advancing nursing as caring science. *Revista Brasileira de Enfermagem, 66*, 39–44.

11. Pugnaire Gros, C., Jarvis, S., Mulvogue, T., & Wright, D. (2012). Adolescents at suicide risk: Nursing care they consider helpful. *Sante Mentale au Quebec, 37*(2), 193–207. doi:10.7202/1014951ar

12. Poblete-Troncoso, M. D. C., Valenzuela, S., & Escobar, J. M. M. (2012). Validation of two scales used to measure transpersonal human caring, based on Jean Watson's theory/ title] [title language=pt]Validação de duas escalas utilizadas na medição do cuidado humano transpessoal baseadas na teoria de Jean Watson. *Aquichan, 12*(1), 8–21. doi:10.5294/aqui.2012.12.1.1

13. del Carmen Poblete-Troncoso, M., Valenzuela-Suazo, S. V., & Merino, J. M. (2012). Validación de dos escalas utilizadas en la medición del cuidado humano transpersonal basadas en la teoría de Jean Watson. *Aquichan, 12*(1), 8-21. doi:10.5294/aqui.2012.12.1.1

14. Boschert, S. (2011). Challenges for management and administration: Conquering incontinence—but how? *Pflege Zeitschrift, 64*(6), 365–367.

15. O'Reilly, L., & Cara, C. (2010). "Being with" the person cared for in a rehabilitation context: A profound, therapeutic and transformative human relationship. *Recherche en Soins Infirmiers*, (103), 46–66.

16. Krol, P. (2010). Apprenticeship of caring in student baccalaureate nurses in a program of formation of competence. *Recherche en Soins Infirmiers*, (102), 59–72. doi:10.3917/rsi .102.0059

17. Krol, P. (2010). The learning of caring among student nurses in a baccalaureate program in skills training. *Recherche en Soins Infirmiers*, (102), 59–72.

18. Klemme, K. (2010). Needs orientate movement with a new nursing bed: A contribution to mobilization. *Pflege Zeitschrift, 63*(5), 280–283.

19. Chen, S. C., & Chou, F. H. (2010). A comparison of the caring theories of Watson and Swanson. *Hu Li Za Zhi The Journal of Nursing, 57*(3), 86–92.

20. Boschert, S. (2010). Learning to know, understand and value oneself. *Pflege Zeitschrift, 63*(3), 158–160.

DISSERTATIONS

1. Dulaney, M. M. L. (2015). *A qualitative study of nurses' experience of caring and bullying in nursing school* (p. 116). Capella University.

2. Herrin, M. L. (2014). *Incivility in nursing education: A study of generational differences* (p. 130.). Capella University.

3. Taylor-Haslip, V. (2013). *The lived experience of caring presence for nursing faculty and nursing students* (p. 162). City University of New York.

4. Mundy, L. (2013). *Seeking health: The lived experience of being in recovery from sex addiction* (p. 169). Florida Atlantic University.

5. Houser, J. (2013). *Hospital policy and nurse retention: A regression analysis of caritas relationships, organizational commitment, and job embeddedness* (p. 181). Walden University.

6. Hoffman, S. F. (2013). *How nursing students experience caring relationships with patients* (p. 245). North Carolina State University.

7. Cahuas, D. (2013). *Personal support workers' and nursing home managers' views of resident care practices in nursing homes: A comparative study* (p. 239). D'Youville College.

8. Rettenmeier, L. M. (2012). *The association of mentorships and leadership practices with nursing faculty retention* (p. 145). Walden University.

9. Potter, D. R. (2011). *Selected African American first-time teenage mothers' perceptions of nurse caring behaviors during the postpartum period* (p. 118). Hampton University.

10. Meyer, R. L. (2011). *The experience of pediatric intensive care nurses caring for dying children* (p. 154). Azusa Pacific University.

11. Johnson, K. M. (2011). *A comparison of levels of empowerment and clinical decision-making in senior bachelor of science nursing students enrolled in a curriculum based on a caring nurse theorist and a curriculum not based on a caring nurse theorist* (p. 151). University of Northern Colorado.

12. Pine, R. (2010). Predicting departure of baccalaureate prepared graduate nurses participating in a twelve month nurse residency program. Retrieved from http://hdl.handle .net/11274/158

EDITORIALS

1. Rehnsfeldt, A., & Arman, M. (2016). The justification of caring science. *Scandinavian Journal of Caring Sciences, 30*(2), 215–216. doi:10.1111/scs.12348

2. Koskinen, C. (2016). NCCS: An association with a vision to be the hub for caring science research. *Scandinavian Journal of Caring Sciences, 30*(4), 643–644. doi:10.1111/ scs.12414

3. Benoit, B., Goldberg, L., & Campbell-Yeo, M. (2016). Response to "The emotional storms of breast feeding and points to remember". *Midwifery, 34*, 261–262. doi:10.1016/j.midw .2016.02.006

4. Watson, J., & Brewer, B. B. (2015). Caring science research: Criteria, evidence, and measurement. *Journal of Nursing Administration, 45*(5), 235–236. doi:10.1097/NNA .0000000000000190

5. Stanton, A. E. (2015). "What's new about Freud?" *Issues in Mental Health Nursing, 36*(6), 396. doi:10.3109/01612840.2015.1014588

6. Mills, J., Wand, T., & Fraser, J. A. (2015). On self-compassion and self-care in nursing: Selfish or essential for compassionate care? *International Journal of Nursing Studies, 52*(4), 791–793. doi:10.1016/j.ijnurstu.2014.10.009

7. Lindwall, L., & Hilli, Y. (2015). 35 years of the Nordic College of Caring Science: Heading for the future. *Scandinavian Journal of Caring Sciences, 29*(3), 407–408. doi:10.1111/ scs.12257

8. Watson, J. (2014). Continuing caritas journey: Reflections upon a shared private pilgrimage. *Journal of Holistic Nursing, 32*(3), 140–146. doi:10.1177/0898010114539393

9. Wolf, Z. R. (Eds.). (2013). Editorial. *International Journal for Human Caring, 17*(1), 6.

10. Kay Hogan, B. (2013). Caring as a scripted discourse versus caring as an expression of an authentic relationship between self and other. *Issues in Mental Health Nursing, 34*(5), 375–379. doi:10.3109/01612840.2013.768734

11. Fredriksson, L. (2013). Ethical approval, laws and publication of caring science in the Nordic countries. *Scandinavian Journal of Caring Sciences, 27*(2), 213–214. doi:10.1111/scs.12031

12. Slettebo, A., & Fredriksson, L. (2012). New editors: Continued focus on caring science. *Scandinavian Journal of Caring Sciences, 26*(2), 209–210. doi:10.1111/j.1471-6712.2012.01005.x

13. Lindwall, L. (2012). Missions and thoughts about Nordic College of Caring Science future. *Scandinavian Journal of Caring Sciences, 26*(3), 415–416. doi:10.1111/j.1471-6712.2012.01057.x

14. Antunes Cortez, E. (2012). Influence of religiosity and spirituality on health: Reflections on nursing care. *Online Brazilian Journal of Nursing, 11*(2), 418–419. doi:10.5935/1676-4285.2012S001

15. Ray, M. A. (2011). A celebration of a life of commitment to transcultural nursing: Opening of the Madeleine M. Leininger collection on human caring and transcultural nursing. *Journal of Transcultural Nursing, 22*(1), 97. doi:10.1177/1043659610390902

16. Lukose, A. (2011). Developing a practice model for Watson's theory of caring. *Nursing Science Quarterly, 24*(1), 27–30. doi:10.1177/0894318410389073

17. Wärnå-Furu, C. (2010). Health and appropriation in caring science research. *Scandinavian Journal of Caring Sciences, 24*(4), 635–637. doi:10.1111/j.1471-6712.2010.00843.x

18. Karnick, P. M. (2010). Is nursing a caring science? *Nursing Science Quarterly, 23*(4), 296. doi:10.1177/0894318410380261

19. Heffernan, P. (2010). Caring story resonates with New York nurse... 'Show the love' (June 14). *Nursing Spectrum–New York & New Jersey Edition, 22*(14), 12.

20. Fights, S. D. (2010). From AMSN: Commitment, compassion, connection. *MEDSURG Nursing, 19*(6), 313–316.

21. Eriksson, K. (2010). Evidence: To see or not to see. *Nursing Science Quarterly, 23*(4), 275–279. doi:10.1177/0894318410380271

UPDATES FEB 1, 2017 – OCT 11, 2017

Books

1. Sitzman, K., & Eichelberger, L. W. (2017). *Understanding the work of nurse theorists: A creative beginning.* Burlington, MA: Jones & Bartlett.

2. Multak, N. (2017). *Clinical procedures for health professionals.* Burlington, MA: Jones & Bartlett.

3. McMillan, M. O. (2017). *The effects of Watson's theory of human caring on the nurse perception and utilization of caring attributes and the impact on nurse communication.* Boiling Springs, NC: Gardner-Webb University.

4. Hardin, S. R., & Kaplow, R. (2017). *Synergy for clinical excellence: The AACN synergy model for patient care* (2nd ed.). Burlington, MA: Jones & Barlett.

5. Bodin, S. (2017). American nephrology nurses, contemporary nephrology nursing. Retrieved from https://www.r2library.com/Resource/Title/1940325374

6. Bartel, D. C. (2017). Developing a care process reducing post-procedural pain levels. Retrieved from http://idun.augsburg.edu/etd/1

ARTICLES

1. Johansson, L., Lindahl, B., Knutsson, S., Ögren, M., Persson Waye, K., & Ringdal, M. (2018). Evaluation of a sound environment intervention in an ICU: A feasibility study. *Australian Critical Care, 31*(2), 59–70. doi:10.1016/j.aucc.2017.04.001

2. Chung, B. P. M., Leung, D., Leung, S. M., & Loke, A. Y. (2018). Beyond death and dying: How Chinese spouses navigate the final days with their loved ones suffering from terminal cancer. *Supportive Care in Cancer, 26*(1), 261–267. doi:10.1007/s00520 -017-3844-z

3. van Wijlen, J. (2017). Healing the healer: A caring science approach to moral distress in new graduate nurses. *International Journal for Human Caring, 21*(1), 15–19. doi:10 .20467/1091-5710-21.1.15

4. Sitzman, K. (2017). Evolution of Watson's human caring science in the digital age. *International Journal for Human Caring, 21*(1), 46–52. doi:10.20467/1091-5710-21.1.46

5. Sitzman, K. (2015). Sense, connect, facilitate: Nurse educator experiences of caring online through Watson's lens. *International Journal for Human Caring, 19*(3), 25–29. doi:10.20467/1091-5710-19.3.25

6. Nelson, J., Thiel, L., Hozak, M. A., & Thomas, T. (2016). Item reduction of the caring factor survey–care provider version, an instrument specified to measure Watson's 10 processes of caring. *International Journal for Human Caring, 20*(3), 123–128. doi:10 .20467/1091-5710-20.3.123

7. Goldin, M. (2014). Celebrating new life in a neuro-surgical ICU: Exemplar of caritas nursing. *International Journal for Human Caring, 18*(3), 65–66. doi:10.20467/1091-5710-18.3.65

8. Feinblum, D., Gonzalez, R., & Clyne, M. (2016). Journaling: A caring initiative. *International Journal for Human Caring, 20*(1), 15–18. doi:10.20467/1091-5710-20.1.15

9. Broscious, C., Spigelmyer, P. C., & Breckenridge, D. (2015). Effects of bedtime nursing care on perceptions of caring for patients on a rehabilitation unit: A pilot study. *International Journal for Human Caring, 19*(4), 56–61. doi:10.20467/1091-5710-19.4.56

10. Ueland, V., Nåden, D., & Lindström, U. Å. (2017). Longing: A dynamic power in the becoming of health when suffering from cancer. *Scandinavian Journal of Caring Sciences.* doi:10.1111/scs.12527

11. Sundling, V., Sundler, A. J., Holmström, I. K., Kristensen, D. V., & Eide, H. (2017). Mindfulness predicts student nurses' communication self-efficacy: A cross-national comparative study. *Patient Education and Counseling, 100*(8), 1558–1563. doi:10.1016/j .pec.2017.03.016

12. Sundberg, F., Olausson, S., Fridh, I., & Lindahl, B. (2017). Nursing staff's experiences of working in an evidence-based designed ICU patient room: An interview study. *Intensive & Critical Care Nursing, 43*, 75–80. doi:10.1016/j.iccn.2017.05.004

13. So, W. K. W., Kwong, A. N. L., Chen, J. M. T., Chan, J. C. Y., Law, B. M. H., Sit, J. W. H., & Chan, C. W. H. (2017). A theory-based and culturally aligned training program on breast and cervical cancer prevention for South Asian community health workers: A feasibility study. *Cancer Nursing*. doi:10.1097/ncc.0000000000000543

14. Sellin, L. Asp, M., Kumlin, T., Wallsten, T., & Wiklund Gustin, L. (2017). To be present, share and nurture: A lifeworld phenomenological study of relatives' participation in the suicidal person's recovery. *International Journal of Qualitative Studies on Health and Well-Being, 12*(1), 1287985. doi:10.1080/17482631.2017.1287985

15. Sadat-Hoseini, A. S., & Khosropanah, A. H. (2017). Comparing the concept of caring in Islamic perspective with Watson and Parse's nursing theories. *Iranian Journal of Nursing and Midwifery Research, 22*(2), 83–90. doi:10.4103/ijnmr.IJNMR_311_14

16. Olender, L. (2017). The relationship between and factors influencing staff nurses' perceptions of nurse manager caring and exposure to workplace bullying in multiple healthcare settings. *Journal of Nursing Administration, 47*(10), 501–507. doi:10.1097/nna.0000000000000522

17. Norberg Boysen, G., Nyström, M., Christensson, L., Herlitz, J., & Wireklint Sundström, B. (2017). Trust in the early chain of healthcare: Lifeworld hermeneutics from the patient's perspective. *International Journal of Qualitative Studies on Health and Well-Being, 12*(1), 1356674. doi:10.1080/17482631.2017.1356674

18. Mailhot, T., Cossette, S., Côté, J., Bourbonnais, A., Côté, M. C., Lamarche, Y., & Denault, A. (2017). A post cardiac surgery intervention to manage delirium involving families: A randomized pilot study. *Nursing in Critical Care, 22*(4), 221–228. doi:10.1111/nicc.12288

19. Low, L. P., Chien, W. T., Lam, L. W., & Wong, K. K. (2017). A qualitative study protocol of ageing carers' caregiving experiences and their planning for continuation of care for their immediate family members with intellectual disability. *BMC Geriatrics, 17*(1), 81. doi:10.1186/s12877-017-0473-9

20. Leung, D. Y. P., Chen, J. M. T., Lou, V. W. Q., Wong, E. M. L., Chan, A. W. K., So, W. K. W., & Chan, C. W. H. (2017). Effects of promotional materials on attitudes and fear towards colorectal cancer screening among Chinese older adults: An experimental study. *International Journal of Environmental Research and Public Health, 14*(7). pii. E769. doi:10.3390/ijerph14070769

21. Le Low, L. P., Lam, L. W., & Fan, K. P. (2017). Decision-making experiences of family members of older adults with moderate dementia towards community and residential care home services: A grounded theory study protocol. *BMC Geriatrics, 17*(1), 120. doi:10.1186/s12877-017-0510-8

22. Koithan, M. S., Kreitzer, M. J., & Watson, J. (2017). Linking the unitary paradigm to policy through a synthesis of caring science and integrative nursing. *Nursing Science Quarterly, 30*(3), 262–268. doi:10.1177/0894318417708415

23. Holst, H., Ozolins, L. L., Brunt, D., & Hörberg, U. (2017). The learning space: Interpersonal interactions between nursing students, patients, and supervisors at developing and learning care units. *International Journal of Qualitative Studies on Health and Well-Being, 12* (Suppl. 2), 1368337. doi:10.1080/17482631.2017.1368337

24. Höglander, J., Eklund, J. H., Eide, H., Holmström, I. K., & Sundler, A. J. (2017). Registered nurses' and nurse assistants' responses to older persons' expressions of emotional needs in home care. *Journal of Advanced Nursing, 73*(12), 2923–2932. doi:10.1111/jan.13356

25. Hilli, Y., & Eriksson, K. (2017). The home as ethos of caring: A concept determination. *Nursing Ethics*, 969733017718395. doi:10.1177/0969733017718395

26. Harper, L., Reddon, J. R., Hunt, C. J., & Royan, H. (2017). PRN Medication administration in a geriatric psychiatric hospital: Chart review and nursing perspective. *Clinical Gerontologist*, 40(5), 392–400. doi:10.1080/07317115.2017.1311287

27. Grönqvist, H., Olsson, E. M. G., Johansson, B., Held, C., Sjöström, J., Lindahl Norberg, A., … von Essen, L. (2017). Fifteen challenges in establishing a multidisciplinary research program on eHealth research in a university setting: A case study. *Journal of Medical Internet Research*, 19(5), e173. doi:10.2196/jmir.7310

28. Goldberg, L., Rosenburg, N., & Watson, J. (2017). Rendering LGBTQ+ visible in nursing: Embodying the philosophy of caring science. *Journal of Holistic Nursing*, 898010117715141. doi:10.1177/0898010117715141

29. Förch, S., Kretschmer, R., Haufe, T., Plath, J., & Mayr, E. (2017). Orthogeriatric combined management of elderly patients with proximal femoral fracture: Results of a 1-year follow-up. *Geriatric Orthopaedic Surgery & Rehabilitationl*, 8(2), 109–114. doi:10.1177/2151458517698536

30. Durgun Ozan, Y., & Okumuş, H. (2017). Effects of nursing care based on Watson's theory of human caring on anxiety, distress, and coping, when infertility treatment fails: A randomized controlled trial. *Journal of Caring Sciences*, 6(2), 95–109. doi:10.15171/jcs.2017.010

31. Dreher-Weber, M., Laireiter, A. R., Kühberger, A., Kunz, I., Yegles, M., Binz, T., … Wurst, F. M. (2017). Screening for hazardous drinking in nursing home residents: Evaluating the validity of the current cutoffs of the alcohol use disorder identification test-consumption questions by using ethyl glucuronide in hair. *Alcoholism, Clinical and Experimental Research*, 41(9), 1593–1601. doi:10.1111/acer.13449

32. Boz, I., & Okumuş, H. (2017). The "everything about the existence" experiences of Turkish women with infertility: Solicited diaries in qualitative research. *Journal of Nursing Research*, 25(4), 268–275. doi:10.1097/jnr.0000000000000166

33. Bjurling-Sjöberg, P., Wadensten, B., Pöder, U., Jansson, I., & Nordgren, L. (2017). Balancing intertwined responsibilities: A grounded theory study of teamwork in everyday intensive care unit practice. *Journal of Interprofessional Care*, 31(2), 233–244. doi:10.1080/13561820.2016.1255184

34. Bjorkman, A., Engstrom, M., Olsson, A., & Wahlberg, A. C. (2017). Identified obstacles and prerequisites in telenurses' work environment: A modified Delphi study. *BMC Health Services Research*, 17(1), 357. doi:10.1186/s12913-017-2296-y

35. Ayala, R. A., & Calvo, M. J. (2017). Cultural adaptation and validation of the caring behaviors assessment tool in Chile. *Nursing & Health Sciences*, 19(4), 459–466. doi:10.1111/nhs.12364

36. Asp, M. (2015). Rest: A health-related phenomenon and concept in caring science. *Global Qualitative Nursing Research*, 2, 2333393615583663. doi:10.1177/2333393615583663

37. Andersson, H., Ullgren, A., Holmberg, M., Karlsson, T., Herlitz, J., & Wireklint Sundström, B. (2017). Acute coronary syndrome in relation to the occurrence of associated symptoms: A quantitative study in prehospital emergency care. *International Emergency Nursing*, 33, 43–47. doi:10.1016/j.ienj.2016.12.001

38. Tektaş, P., & Çam, O. (2017). The effects of nursing care based on Watson's theory of human caring on the mental health of pregnant women after a pregnancy loss. *Archives of Psychiatric Nursing*, 31(5), 440–446. doi:10.1016/j.apnu.2017.07.002

39. Pajnkihar, M., McKenna, H. P., Štiglic, G., & Vrbnjak, D. (2017). Fit for practice: Analysis and evaluation of Watson's theory of human caring. *Nursing Science Quarterly*, *30*(3), 243–252. doi:10.1177/0894318417708409

40. Natale, G., Fitzgerald, A., & Lou, M. (2017). Applying Jean Watson's caring theory to reduce restraint use in the acute psychiatric area. *Pelican News*, *73*(2), 4. Retrieved from https://www.nursingald.com/articles/18363-applying-jean-watson-s-caring-theory -to-reduce-restraint-use-in-the-acute-psychiatric-area

41. Kelley, L. S. (2017). Transfiguring light and symphonic blooming: A wabi sabi story of human becoming and human caring. *Nursing Science Quarterly*, *30*(4), 324–329. doi:10.1177/0894318417724457

42. Gonzalez, K. M. (2017). Trust: A concept analysis with Watson's theoretical perspective. *Nursing Science Quarterly*, *30*(4), 356–360. doi:10.1177/0894318417724446

43. Dahlke, S., & Stahlke Wall, S. (2017). Does the emphasis on caring within nursing contribute to nurses' silence about practice issues? *Nursing Philosophy*, *18*(3), doi:10.1111/ nup.12150

Index

A Whole New Mind, 259
absolute consciousness, 26, 27, 28
ACA. *See* Affordable Care Act
Academic Conference of the Japan Academy of
    Nursing Science, 486
ACE. *See* Antioch Care Experience Model
Ackerman, Linda, 414
ADN. *See* associate degree nurse
Advances in Nursing Science, 42, 44, 56
aesthetic posters, 533, 534
aesthetic process, in caring inquiry, 346–349
affective domain, 264
Affordable Care Act (ACA), 226, 264
AIM statement, 265
altruism, 212–213
altruistic love, 434
AMC. *See* Antioch Medical Center
American Academy of Nursing, 173
American Association of Colleges of Nursing,
    175
American Journal of Nursing, 39
American Nurses Association (ANA), 38, 175,
    386, 392
    Code of Ethics and Interpretative
      Statements, 215
American Nurses Credentialing Center
    (ANCC), 305
    Magnet® program, 306
ANA. *See* American Nurses Association
ANCC. *See* American Nurses Credentialing
    Center

Anishinaabe, 93
Antioch Care Experience (ACE) Model, 419
Antioch Medical Center (AMC), 417, 419–421
"arouse the heart," 596
Art and Aesthetics in Nursing, 229
art and healing, 579
Art of Extreme Self-Care, 252
arts-informed narrative inquiry, 229–230
ASK. *See* attitudes, skills, and knowledge
Assessing and Measuring Caring in Nursing
    and Health Sciences, 486
associate degree level of nursing, 262
associate degree nurse (ADN), 260
attention, 472
attitudes, skills, and knowledge
    (ASK), 257–258
audiovisual technology, 624
autoethnographic
    data, 635
    process, 639
autoethnography, 633–640
    life review, 635
    symbols and carvings, 637
    Woodland gate, 637
automatic self-transcending (TM), 549

Baldwin Nursing Program, 246
Barks, Coleman, 194
Bay Area school of nursing (SoN), 258
BCT. *See* Theory of Bureaucratic Caring

becoming
　　Caritas ways of, 193
　　guide to caritas literacy in, 191
　　overview, 189–190
　　universal love, 193–194
being
　　caritas ways of, 190
　　guide to caritas literacy in, 191
　　overview, 189–190
　　universal love, 193–194
being-in-relationship, 54, 203
being in right relation, 86, 97
belonging, 32–33
Benner, Patricia, 3
Binagwaho, Agnes, 457
Birth of Venus, 356
Bloom's taxonomies, 263
Bohr, Niels, 25
Boykin, Anne, 3, 5, 6
breath, 364
Brewer, Barbara, 9, 419
Brigham and Women's Hospital (BWH), 403
　　building upon caring-healing, 405–406
　　caring and civility study, 408–410
　　Caritas leadership development and
　　　　research, 408
　　Caritas Rooms, 406
　　caritas scholar in, 405
　　participation in Caritas and HCAHPS
　　　　pilot, 407
　　Professional Practice Model, 407
　　Watson as visiting professor in, 404–405
British model of graduate study, 277
Browning, Robert, 120, 420
Burroughs, William, 635
buzz words, 368–369
BWH. *See* Brigham and Women's
　　Hospital

California Nurses Association, 65
Canvas Learning Management System, 134
Canvas Network, 135
CAPP. *See* Caring-based Academic Practice
　　Partnerships
Care and vulnerability, 463
caregivers, 149
care providers, 175

caring, 402–404, 622
　　and civility study, 408–410
　　an essential domain of nursing knowledge,
　　　　292
　　as precursor of love, 444–445
Caring-based Academic Practice Partnerships
　　　　(CAPP), 298
caring communication patterns, 296
Caring Factor Survey (CFS), 110
caring-healing
　　BWH and, 405–406
　　sacred nursing acts of, 79
caring-healing environments, 386
Caring in Nursing Classics, 5
caring inquiry, 343–352
　　aesthetic process in, 346–349
　　overview, 344–345
　　phenomenological-hermeneutical inquiry,
　　　　346–349
　　phenomenology of aesthetic research, 345–346
caring moments, 318
　　transpersonal, 121, 147
　　ubuntu and, 79–81
caring nature, embodiment of, 653–656
caring rights, 560–561
caring science (CS), 23, 277, 294, 495, 498–500, 511,
　　　　566, 578, 579, 628, 636, 653
　　adoption and implementation of, 486
　　based practice models, 297
　　based program, 288
　　Caritas coaching, 567–568
　　Caritas literacy, 568–573
　　core tenets of, 98
　　curriculum, 258, 566
　　development through human caring science,
　　　　280–281
　　doctoral education, 281–282
　　epistemological pluralism, 611
　　evolution of science and theory development,
　　　　278–279
　　future of, 573
　　leaders, 655
　　logo, 430
　　and native science, 96–97
　　objectives, 280–281
　　online teaching, 281–282
　　overview, 654
　　paradigm, 634

caring science (CS) *(cont.)*
  pedagogy, 198–200
  practitioner, 572
  reflective practice and, 163–170
  research, 619
  as sacred science, 529
  theoretical values, 318
  theory of human caring, 120–121
  value of researcher, 279–280
  value to, 610–611
  yoga, 643–650
caring science, advancing, 286
  dance, 288
  overview, 286
  vision, mission, philosophy, 286, 287
caring science literacy, 198
  components of nursing education to
      advance, 200
Caring Science, Mindful Practice (CSMP)
      MOOC, 133–143
  background of, 134–135
  course ratings and engagement data, 139
  demographic data of 2015 to 2016, 137
  instructional success, process for, 136–137
  overview, 133–134
  studies related to, 137–141
  themes of, 138–141
caring science nurses
  civility and, 248
  cocreating community of caring in classroom,
      250–251
  development through experience of caring
      science curriculum, 247–253
  hierarchical structure and, 248–249
  meaning and value of being or becoming,
      253–254
  self-care and, 252–253
  teaching-learning methods and, 251–252
Caring Science Theory of Human Caring, 120
Caritas activities, 392–394
Caritas certified curriculum, 506
Caritas Coach™, 248
Caritas Coach Education Program® (CCEP), 212,
      218, 281, 405, 420, 423, 565
Caritas Coaches, 367–368
  nurses becoming, 405
Caritas Coaching, 565–573
Caritas consciousness, 435

Caritas domain, 392
Caritas Heart method, 123–124
  protocols and praxis of, 129
Caritas-informed practice, 504–505
Caritas leadership, 391
Caritas literacy, 257, 485, 568–573, 570
Caritas practitioners, 388–390
Caritas Processes®, 266, 282, 307, 387, 535, 578,
      628, 633, 636, 639, 640, 646, 651
Caritas Process-Kosha-Layer Reflection Tool,
      647, 648
Caritas values, 638
CAS. *See* complex adaptive systems
case studies (faculty stories of teaching from
      the heart), 231–237
  Annie's story, 231–232
  Blaine's story, 236–237
  "Cut Out My Heart", 583
  The Caring Moment, 380–381
  The Glasses, 379
  Grace's story, 232–233
  guided imagery, 580–581
  guided imagery exercise, 581–582
  Kaddish Prayer of Mourning, 377
  Lark's story, 232, 233
  Lily and authentic presence, 378
  nursing science, 266–269
  old teacher's story, 231–237
  Rumi's story, 235–236
  sacred journey, 580
  Sandy's story, 233–235
  self-portraits, 585
  student hero's journey, 266
CBPR. *See* community-based participatory
      research
CCEP. *See* Caritas Coach Education Program
CDI. *See* Conscious Dying Institute
CELCON. *See* Christine E. Lynn College of
      Nursing
  CELCON caring-healing philosophy, 290
  CELCON strategic plan, 296
CEO. *See* chief executive officer
CFS. *See* Caring Factor Survey
change of shift report, 603–604
chief executive officer (CEO), 501
Chinn, Peggy, 4, 6
Christine E. Lynn College of Nursing
      (CELCON), 286–299

CINAHL. *See* Cumulative Index to Nursing and Allied Health Literature

civility, 248

Clinical Practice Council, 218

CNPM. *See* community nursing practice model

cognitive and psychomotor domains, 263–264

Collaborative Nursing Program of British Columbia, 204, 206

communities love, 227

community-based participatory research (CBPR), 610

community nursing practice model (CNPM), 376, 377, 454

compassion, 344–345
  to dissolve ego, 357–358

Compassionate Care Award, 218

complex adaptive systems (CAS), 57

complexity sciences, 57–58

conscious dying, 145–159
  caregivers and, 149
  caring science, 155, 159
  caring science paradigm, 146–148
  education and care, 149
  healing care and, 148–149
  Kübler-Ross's model, 148
  lotus of, 152–153
  love and, 149–150
  and maturation of self and system, 156, 157–158
  nursing's role in, 153–155
  overview, 145–146
  pain and suffering at end of life, 150–151
  and realization of visionary praxis, 156–159
  suffering as rite of passage, 151–152

Conscious Dying Institute (CDI), 148, 149

consciousness, 26, 147–148, 472
  absolute, 26, 27, 28
  Caritas, 435
  divine, 357, 358, 359
  ego, 360
  global unitary, 194
  nonlocal, 193
  transcendent, 33
  unitive, 32

coordination, 453

Corcoran-Perry, Sheila, 46

cosmic love, 193, 363

cosmology, 22

cosmology of unitary caring science
  eternal here and now, 26–27
  evolutionary and participatory nature of change, 27
  interconnectedness, 25–26
  love, 28
  paradox, 27–28
  undivided wholeness, 25–26
  unitary views of science within, 28–29

Cowling, Richard, 5

Creative Healing Arts, 586

creativity, 578

CS. *See* caring science

CSMP MOOC. *See* caring science, mindful practice MOOC

cultural identity, 93

Cumulative Index to Nursing and Allied Health Literature (CINAHL), 112, 211, 227

curriculum model, 291

curriculum processes, caring science, 200–207
  curriculum design and structure, creation of, 204–206
  students' clinical practice, evaluation of, 206–207
  teaching and learning in caring collaborative relationship, 203–204

Curtin, Leah, 41

cutup method, 635, 636

D'Alfonso, Jim, 414, 419, 423

Dancing Wu I Master, 26

David, 356

Davis, Anne, 4

de Chardin, Teilhard, 193

Delmar, Charlotte, 4

design, 260

Dewey, John, 164

diagnostic-related groups (DRGs), 63

Dickinson, Emily, 345

differential caring, 58

digital caring
  cycle, 333
  eight studies related to, 329–335
  examples of transpersonal caring moments, 335–337
  process, 336–337

digital caring (cont.)
    suggested caring language for online learning and teaching, 334–335
    themes in online nursing classrooms, 329–333
Diné, 94
discovery, 86, 96–97, 595
disengagement ritual, 601–602
divine consciousness, 357, 358, 359
Downes, Stephen, 134
Downs, Florence S., 103
Drenkard, Karen, 419
DRGs. See diagnostic-related groups
Droesbeke, James, 3

Edgerton, Stephanie, 103
ego agendas, 366, 368, 369
ego consciousness, 360
ego-divided self, 364
ego perception, 357, 358, 359, 365
ego-personality, 357
ego self, 357, 358
Einstein, Albert, 258
electromagnetic field of heart, 125–126
Elk, Black, 94
emancipatory nursing praxis, 63–64
empathy, 260
energetic models, 318
energy of love, 435
enfermería peruana. See Peruvian nursing
engagement ritual, 601–602
equanimity, 76, 211–220
    altruism and, 212–213
    intentionality and, 214–215
    love and, 214
    mindfulness and, 213–214
    for others, 217–219
    overview, 211–212
    for self, 215–217
Eriksson, Katie, 4, 445, 461–463
eternal here, 26–27
ethic of belonging, 175
ethic of face, 176
Ethical Demand, 463
ethics, 37
    of caring for healthcare providers, 41
    nursing. See nursing ethics
Ethics of Engaged Presence, 453

FAUCON. See Florida Atlantic University's College of Nursing
Fawcett, Jacqueline, 6, 7
Federal Trade Commission (FTC), 621
feminist theory, 611
Flack, Lisa Lally, 244
Florence Nightingale Foundation, 633
Florida Atlantic University's College of Nursing (FAUCON), 454, 456
focused attention, 549
fostering metamorphosis, caring literacy
    affective domain, 264
    cognitive and psychomotor domains, 263–264
    cognitive approach, 263–264
    context, 258–259
    design, 260
    "doing" of procedures, protocols, policies, 261
    Einstein inspiration, 258
    empathy, 260
    meaning, 260
    narrative pedagogy, 261
    ontological views, 262
    overview, 257–258
    physical assessment as nursing science, 266–269
    play, 260
    story, 260
    symphony, 260
    transforming relationship, 264–266
    value-added proposition, 260
    vision discovery, 260
    voice of nurses, 261
Foundations of Caring in Nursing Situations, 292
four-degree programs, 292
Franciscan tradition, 245
Frolich, Esther Kearn, 414
FTC. See Federal Trade Commission

Gadow, Sally, 4, 44
Gaut, Delores, 3
geist, 121
George-Kanentiio, Douglas, 93
"going back inside the story," 595
Golden Thread, 214
Gonda Building, 622
Goodrich, Annie Warburton, 407

gratification, 471
Grey, Alex, 579
grief, 148
grief ritual, 604
guest–host relationship, 452–453
Gullett, Diane L., 454–456

Haudenosaunee, 88, 91–92, 93
Hawkins, David, 147
HCAHPS. *See* Hospital Consumer Assessment
    of Healthcare Providers and Systems
HCP. *See* Human Caring Program
healing
    future consideration for music, poetry,
        and healing, 624
    music and poetry for, 619–625
    portrait of musical caring, 623
    psycho-neuro-immunological perspective, 624
    "unhealing feeling," 621–623
healing arts, 577, 622
    caring-healing creative practice, 578
healing care, 148
healing care plans, 624
healing environments, 374
healthcare
    Clostridium difficile infections, 394
    restorative spaces, 392
Health Resources and Services Agency, 298f
heart-based teaching. *See* teaching from
        the heart
HeartMath method, 126–127, 230, 407
heart rate variability and cortical function, 122
heart rate variability coherence (HRVC), 364
heart research premises, 123
heart rhythms, 122
heart science, 121–123
    background of heart research premises, 123
    caring science and, 120–121
    CaritasHeart method, 123–124
    caritas processes, 124–128
    overview, 119–120
    translating caring science theory, 127
hermeneutical phenomenological study, of
        love, 435–445
    data collection, 437
    diversity of patients, 442–443
    findings and discussion of, 437–445

hermeneutic (interpretive) phenomenology,
        436
    interpretive paradigm, 436
    knowing and, 440–441
    oneness and unity of being, 438–440
    recruitment, 436–437
    spirituality and religion, 437–438
    touch as communication, 441–442
Hernandez-Kertland, Grissel, 7–9
Hiroshima Conference on Caring and Peace, 486
holding sacred space, 355–356
    background, 356
    for compassion to dissolve ego, 357–358
    for essence of mind, 362–364
    evolution of separate self, 358–360
    example of, 365–366
    paradigm of science and, 360–362
    for personal health, 368
    in professional work, 366–368
    for self-care, 364–365
    for unitary consciousness, 356–357
hooks, bell, 227
Hopi belief, 89
Horton-Deutsch, Sara, 15, 168-169, 190, 229, 251,
        262, 278, 515
Hospital Consumer Assessment of Healthcare
        Providers and Systems (HCAHPS), 323, 386
    scores, 323
    survey, 407
Hózhó, 94
Hózhóójí, 94
HRH Program. *See* Human Resources for Health
        Program
HRVC. *See* heart rate variability coherence
human becoming school of thought, 307
human becoming theory, 307
human caring
    aesthetic theories, 109
    caring science theory of, 110–121
    challenges in, 110–113
    classification schemes about, 106
    conceptual models and theories of, 105–110,
        111–112
    empirical theories, 109
    ethical theories, 109
    methods of scholarly inquiry for knowledge
        development in, 110, 112–113
    nursology, 104–105

human caring (cont.)
  nursology's metaparadigm and, 105, 111
  overview, 103–104
  personal knowing theories, 109
  philosophies and, 105, 111
  selected nurses' perspectives of, classifications of, 107–108
  sociopolitical/emancipatory theories, 109–110
human caring processes, 386
human caring professional practices
  background, 317–318
  data analysis, 321–322
  discussion, 323–324
  healthcare evolution, 318–319
  implications, 324
  limitations, 324
  measurement assessment, 320
  methods, 319
  procedure, 320–321
  results, 322–323
Human Caring Program (HCP), 414, 423
human caring science-kosha model, 643, 646–647
  adaptation, 646
  Australian context, 647–649
  background, 643–644
  course, 649–650
  description, 646
  spiritual layer, 646
human flourishing, 66
human-planet survival, 556
Human Resources for Health (HRH) Program, 456–458
human rights, 54–55

IAHC. See International Association for Human Caring
infinity, 32
IHI. See Institute for Healthcare Improvement
Institute for Healthcare Improvement (IHI), 264
  patient safety modules, 265, 266
Institutional Review Boards (IRBs), 612
integrative nursing, 173–184, 628
  caring science, 629–630
  facility design, 630
  focuses on health and well-being of caregivers, 183
  foundations of, 177–183
  healthcare design perspective, 629
  informed by evidence, 181–183
  innate capacity for health and well-being, 178–179
  integrative nursing, 629–630
  nature's healing and restorative properties, 180–181
  nursing practice and care delivery, 180
  overview, 173–174
  patient-centered, 175–177
  practice model for contemporary healthcare systems, 176–177
  principles of, 177, 628
  relationship-based, 176, 179–180
  unitary paradigm, 174–175
intention, 214
intentionality, 214–215
interbeing, 658–662
interconnectedness, 25–26, 86, 96
International Association for Human Caring (IAHC), 462–463
International Collaborative Center, 486
International Council of Nurses, 386
International Fabric Institute, 621
International Hiroshima Caring and Peace Conference, 485, 487
International Hiroshima Conference on Caring and Peace, 486, 488
International Journal for Human Caring, 3
International/National Caring Science, 307
international nursing community, 493
International Society of Caring and Peace, 486
Intersecting Circles, 214
IRBs. See Institutional Review Boards
Introduction to Nursing Praxis, course, 649–650

Japan
  caritas literacy research exemplars, 488–490
  continuing caritas, 488
  participatory action research (PAR), 489
Johns, Christopher, 164, 166
Johnson, Dorothy, 6
Jones, Dorothy, 47
Journal of Advanced Nursing, 56

Kaiser Permanente Patient Care Services,
    in Northern California
    beginning of, 414–417
    caring science practice model, development
        of, 425–427
    early measurement, 425
    making caring science visible, 427–429
    opportunity, 417–421
    overview, 413–414
    sustainability, 429
    system-wide implementation, 421–425
Kanienkehaka, 93
Kinney, Gwen, 414
knowing
    Caritas ways of, 192–193
    guide to caritas literacy in, 191
    hermeneutical phenomenological study of
        love, 440–441
    overview, 189–190
    universal love, 193–194
knowledge, skills, and attitude (KSA), 259
KSA. *See* knowledge, skills, and attitude
Kübler-Ross, Elisabeth, 148, 149

LaDuke, Winona, 93
Laing, R. D., 24
Lakota, 94
language of leadership, 313, 314
Leadership in Energy and Environmental
    Design (LEED), 290
learning, 198
Lee, S. M., 405
LEED. *See* Leadership in Energy and
    Environmental Design
Leininger, Madeleine, 1, 3, 4
Levinas, Emmanuel, 175
LGBTQ Patient Family Advisory Council, 403
liberating structures (LS), 168, 169
literacy, 198
Løgstrup, K. E., 463, 464
lotus of conscious dying, 152–153
love, 28, 214, 443–444
    altruistic, 434
    breathe in, 362
    caring as precursor of, 444–445
    communities, 227
    and conscious dying, 149–150

cosmic, 193, 363
definition of, 434
energy of, 435
hermeneutical phenomenological study,
    435–445
origins of, 434
universal, 193–194
loving-kindness, 76, 211–220
    altruism and, 212–213
    intentionality and, 214–215
    love and, 214
    mindfulness and, 213–214
    for others, 217–219
    overview, 211–212
    for self, 215–217
lucid moment, 583
Lynn, Christine E., 3

Magnet. *See* Magnet Recognition Program®
Magnet Recognition Program® (Magnet), 65,
    180, 212
Martinsen, Kari, 4, 461
Massachusetts Nurses Association, 65
massive open online courses (MOOCs)
    background information on, 134–135
    CSMP, 133–143
    overview, 133–134
May, William, 44
MBSR. *See* mindfulness based stress
    reduction
McDermott, Shawna, 414
McElmurry, Beverly, 42–43, 44, 45
meaning, 260
Measuring Caring, Postmodern Nursing, 486
Medicaid, 62
Medicare, 62
metaphorical heart and soul, 344
metaphysics, 21
Middle East nurses, 475–483
    educated as enemies, 480–481
    issues of multicultural care, 476–477
    language issues, 477–478
    overview, 475–476
    practical applications of caring practices,
        481–482
    religion and tradition, 478
    understandings of health, 478–480

mindfulness, 213–214
mindfulness based stress reduction (MBSR), 259
MOOCs. *See* massive open online courses
moral care, 463–464
moral caring community, 59–61
morality, 37
MRI machines, 624
multicultural care issues, 476–477
musical expressions, 623

NACNEP. *See* National Advisory Council on Nurse Education and Practice
narrative healing, 587–596
  levels of storytelling/listening, 588
  medicalized story, 593
  overview, 588
  possibilities by expanded story, 595
  process, 587
  by shared-connected story, 594–595
  through self-story, 589–593
National Advisory Council on Nurse Education and Practice (NACNEP), 571
National Aeronautics and Space Administration, 512
National Database Nursing Quality Indicators (NDNQI), 311
National Institute for Nursing Research (NINR), 62
National League for Nursing (NLN), 6, 38, 175, 200, 201, 267
native identity, 88
native science, 86–100
  beauty and belonging, 87–90
  being in right relation, 86, 97
  caring science and, 96–97
  ceremonies and rituals, 91–94
  core values of, 86
  courageous authenticity, agency, and advocacy, 97–99
  definition of, 86–87
  discovery, 86, 96–97
  four directions, 95–96
  interconnectedness, 86, 96
  overview, 85–87
  wholeness, 86, 96
NCLEX®, 231, 232
NCLEX-RN® examination, 217

NDNQI. *See* National Database Nursing Quality Indicators
Neihardt, John, 94
Neuman, Betty, 6
new employee caritas literacy, 570
Newman, Margaret, 5, 6, 46, 47, 103
Newton, Isaac, 104
Newton's law of gravity, 620
Nightingale, Florence, 37, 38, 39, 174, 178, 247, 434
NINR. *See* National Institute for Nursing Research
NLI. *See* Nursing Leadership Institute
NLN. *See* National League for Nursing
nonlocal consciousness, 193
nonphysical realities, 31
Norberg, Astrid, 463
Notes on Nursing, 38
Nurse-Patient Relationship Patterns: An Economic Resource, 6
nurse(s)
  becoming Caritas Coaches, 405
  educators, 201
  Middle East, 475–483
Nurses on Boards Coalition, 173
Nurse Theorists: Portraits in Excellence, 7
nursing, 402–404
  as caring, 434–435
  components of, 45
  definition, 37, 495
  evolution of caring in, 246–247
  knowledge, 494–495
  North American, 495
  planetary partner, 519–520
  reflecting and referencing metaphysical and nonlocal realities in, 31–33
  renaissance, 495
  role in living and dying well, 153–155
  search for distinct moral foundation, 43–47
  situational assessment, 497
  social justice in, 56
  social responsibility in, 56–57
  in South Africa, 74, 496
Nursing: Human Science and Human Care: A Theory of Nursing, 486
Nursing: The Philosophy and Science of Caring, 2, 416
Nursing Administration Concentration, 5

nursing and professional practice
  context for change, 498
  development of global nursing knowledge,
    494–495
  paternalistic sociomedical culture, 496–497
  situational assessment, 497
  transitioning caring, 496
nursing curriculum, 246–247
nursing education
  assembly-line process of, 259
  behaviorist educational model, 201
  caring as moral, theoretical, and philosophical
    foundation of, 200–202
  caring science language to articulate,
    202–203
  components to advance caring science literacy,
    200–207
nursing ethics, 38
  of care, 48–49
  early explorations of, 41–43
  early indicators in nursing literature, 38–39
  ethics of caring for healthcare providers, 41
  in mid-20th century, 39–41
  and political realm, 47–48
  proposal for, 48–49
  search for nursing's distinct moral foundation,
    43–47
  theories of biomedical ethics and, 45–46
nursing inquiry, 344–345. See also caring
    inquiry
Nursing Leadership Institute (NLI), 298
Nursing Manifesto, 56
nursing metaparadigm, 614
nursing praxis, 651–652
  emancipatory, 63–64
  emerging from historical constraints, 62
  environment of nursing in complex system of
    healthcare networks, 61–62
  overview, 54
  paradox between caring and healthcare
    economics, 62–63
  projects, 63–64
  research and new emergences, 64–67
  social justice and human rights, 54–55
nursing theories, 307
Nursing Theories and Nursing Practice, 5
nursology, 104–105
  metaparadigm, 105

OHE. See optimal Healing Environment model
Oncology Nursing Society, 458
One Mind, 520
oneness, 438–440
ontology, 22
Optimal Healing Environment (OHE) model,
    627, 628
Oracle, 580
Orem, Dorothea, 6
Osler, William, 403

pain at end of life, 150–151
Palmer, Parker, 228
PAR. See Japan
paradigm shift, 278
paradox, 27–28
Parker, Marilyn, 5
Parse, Rosemarie, 4, 6
partnerships, caring, 449–459
  coordination, 453
  ethical foundations of, 453–454
  exemplars of, 454–458
  guest-host relationship, 452–453
  overview, 449–450
  principles of, 450–452
  process of, 452–453
  professional friendships and, 453
paternalistic sociomedical culture, 496–497
Patho-Pharmacology and Physical assessment
    (3Ps) courses, 259
patient, 47
patient-centered integrative nursing, 175–177
  foundation of, 176
  moral and ethical basis of, 175–176
PEACE. See Praxis, Empowerment, Awareness,
    Cooperation, and Evolvement
Peace and Power: New Directions for Building
    Community, 56
pedagogical practices, 200–207
pedagogy, 198–200, 282–283
Peruvian "machismo" culture, 496–497
Peruvian nurse practice act, 494
Peruvian nursing, 493–494
  caring science, transitioning of, 499
  caritas-informed practice for, 504–505
  context for change in, 498
  education, 505

Peruvian nursing *(cont.)*
  global knowledge, 493–494
  lived experience of creating space for, 501
  nurse-led projects, 501–504
  political action for, 505
  situational assessment and, 497
  space and building voice for, 500–501
  strategies for, 498
Permanente Journal, 425
Persson, Helen K., 5
Peruvian communitas, 505–506
Peruvian Honor Society of Nursing, 505
Pharris, Margaret Dexheimer, 47
phenomenological-hermeneutical inquiry, 346–349
photography, 534, 535
photovoice method, 609–616
  defined, 609
  educational strategies, 612–616
  ethical considerations, 611–612
planetary health, 512, 513
  concept of, 513
  overview, 521–522
  reflective inventory, 515–519
  for sustainable engagement, 521–522
play, 260
positivism, 105
Power of Collectivity, 309
power over, 203, 249
power with, 203
pragmatism, 105
Praxis, Empowerment, Awareness, Cooperation, and Evolvement (PEACE), 309
professional friendships, 453

QSEN. *See* Quality and Safety Education for Nurses
Quadruple Aim, 180
Quality and Safety Education for Nurses (QSEN), 226
Quantum Leadership, 26
Quinn, Janet, 4

rationalization, 471
Ray, Dee, 4
Ray, Marilyn A., 1–4
reach the underground forces, 596

realities, 550
Recruitment, Education and Employment of Primary Care Providers (REEP), 298
Red Cross Hiroshima College of Nursing, 485, 486, 487
Reeder, Fran, 4
REEP. *See* Recruitment, Education and Employment of Primary Care Providers
reflection, 164
reflective practice, 163–170
  aesthetic response, 166
  cycle, 165
  definition, 164–165
  individual, 165
  with organizations and communities, 168–169
  overview, 163–164
  with partners and groups, 168
  relationship with caring science, 169–170
  stages of, 165
  ways of reflecting, 165–170
reflective practitioner, 167
relational caring complexity, 57–58
  Chaos Theory, 59–61
  moral caring community, 59–61
  theory in nursing leadership, 58–59
Relational Caring Complexity, 54
relational caring complexity theory, 59–61
relational caring questionnaires, 308
relational self-organization, 60, 61
relationship-based care, 179–180
reproduction, 471
Research Advisory Committee, 296
return-on-investment (ROI), 261
Riemen, Doris, 3
rituals
  defined, 599
  engagement and disengagement, 601–603
  goals, 600
  labeled, 599
  professionalism, 603–604
  types, 600–601
RN-to-BSN
  curriculum, 257
  nursing program, 259
  program, 259
Robb, Isabel Hampton, 38–39
Rockefeller Foundation, 513
Rogers, Martha, 6, 103

ROI. *See* return-on-investment
Rosa, William, 14–15, 456–458
Roy, Callista, 6
Ryan, Linda, 419

Scandinavian caring sciences, 461–473
    ethical demand model, 465
    moral care, 463–464
    overview, 461
    pioneering caring scholars, 461–464
    practical care, 464
    relations, 463
Schoenhofer, Savina, 6
science of unitary human beings (SUHB), 22, 23,
        24, 26, 57, 58, 495
Scientific Nursing Research Conference, 486
"scripting," 317–318
self-care, 252–253
    manifesting intentions, 309–311
self-compassion, 364
self-organization, 60
self-transcendence, 155
SFHP. *See* South Florida Haiti Project
Sherwood, Gwen, 3
Siemens, George, 134
Siena College, 244–246
Sigma Theta Tau International (STTI), 494
silence, 593
Sime, A. Marilyn, 46
Sitzman, Kathleen, 335
Small, Sandy, 414
Smith, Marlaine, 4–5, 47
*Social Justice: A Framework for Culturally
        Competent*, 56
social responsibility in nursing, 56–57
Social Security Act, 62
Society's Safe-Keepers (SSKs), 366, 368
Somerville, J. G., 403
    journey to health care, 404–410
(SoN). *See* Bay Area school of Nursing
"soul-to-soul connection," 634
South Florida Haiti Project (SFHP), 454–456
SSKs. *See* Society's Safe-Keepers
*Standards for Culturally Competent Nursing Care:
        2011 Update*, 56
stories, 260, 580
STTI. *See* Sigma Theta Tau International

student-centered learning, 203
Student Nurses Association, 298
suffering
    at end of life, 150–151
    as rite of passage, 151–152
Suffering Human Being, 462, 463
SUHB. *See* science of unitary human beings
Super Brain, 549
Super Genes, 549
supernormal capabilities, 545
Supervisor Nurse, 41, 42
symphony, 260

Tao of Physics, 26
teaching from the heart, 225–239
    activities selected as ways of, 228–229
    arts-informed narrative inquiry, 229–230
    background, 226–231
    faculty stories of, 231–237
    HeartMath method and, 230
    in literature, 227–229
    overview, 226
    selecting, 228
    synchronicity in classroom, 230–231
teaching–learning processes, 290, 295
thanksgiving, 91
*The Cosmic Hologram: In-Formation at the Center of
        Creation*, 545
The Philosophy and Science of Caring, 529
The Resonance Foundation, 547
The Structure of Scientific Revolution, 278
Theory of Bureaucratic Caring (BCT), 58–59
*Theory of Nursing as Caring: A Model for
        Transforming Practice*, 308
theory of relational caring complexity, 308
theory of transpersonal caring, 190
"thinking by feeling", 596
Thomas-Kilmann Conflict Mode Instrument
        (TKI), 265
Thrall, Donnean, 244
TKI. *See* Thomas-Kilmann Conflict Mode
        Instrument
Tohono O'odham, 93
*Touching the Heart of Our Humanity: The Caritas
        Path of Peace*, 487
Traditional Chinese Medicine, 182
transcendent consciousness, 33

Transcultural Nursing Society Position Statement on Human Rights, 56
transformational leadership, 306
transpersonal, 387
transpersonal caring, 81
transpersonal caring moment, 121, 147
Triner, Trudy, 414, 423
Turkel, Brooks, 7
Turkel, Marian, 3, 5–7
Turkel's *theory of relational caring complexity*, 308
Tutu, Desmond, 74
Twomey, John, 45
Tylerian behaviorist model, 199, 201

ubuntu, 73–82
    and caring moments, 79–81
    caritas theory versus, 75–81
    concept analysis of, 74
    connectedness, 80
    definition, 73–74
    engagement of authentic self, 80
    overview, 73–75
    personal preparation and caritas consciousness in, 77
    Watson's caritas processes and, 75–79
unitary caring science, 21–34, 110, 267, 558, 640
    ancient perspectives, 547–548
    and appreciating pattern, 30
    and attuning to dynamic flow, 30
    background of discourse, 23–24
    complexity dynamics, 543
    cosmology of, 24–29
    defined, 550
    emerging science and ancient perspectives, 544–545
    ethic for evolving society, 558–559
    and experiencing the infinite, 30
    indigenous wisdom, 547–548
    infinity and, 32
    informational precepts, 546–547
    and inviting creative emergence, 30
    and manifesting intention, 29–30
    moral actions evolving humanity, 559–560
    multicultural perspectives, 539–540
    nonphysical realities and, 31
    nursing, 540–543
    overview, 21–23

quantum perspectives, 545–547
    reflecting and referencing metaphysical and nonlocal realities, 31–33
    theories and frameworks evolving within, 29–31
    tools for transcendence, 548–549
    universe of belonging and, 32–33
    wholeness and, 31–32
unitary caring science inquiry, 529–537
    circle of reflection, 530–532
    metaphysical and nonphysical inquiry, 536
    posters, 533–534
unitary consciousness, 33, 90, 92
    all-ways-of-knowing and, 192–193
    global, 194
    holding sacred space for, 356–357
unitary human caring science model, 536
unitary method of inquiry, 635
"unitary rhythm of dying-grieving," 636
unitary-transformative paradigm, 307
unitary-transformative thinking, 192
United Nations Declaration of Human Rights Charter, 55
United Nations High Commissioner for Refugees, 512
United Nations Millennium Development Goals Mandate, 55
unitive consciousness, 32
unity of being, 438–440
universal love, 193–194
University of Colorado College of Nursing, 278

Valentine, Kathleen, 3
value-added proposition (VAP), 260
VAP. *See* value-added proposition
Veatch, Robert, 44
ventral tegmental area (VTA), 358–359
videography, 535
visual methodologies, 609
visualizing theory, 613
VTA. *See* ventral tegmental area
    vulnerability
    healing environments, 374
    illumination in nursing situations, 377
    mutual, 375–376
    nursing situations and reflections, 377–381
    theoretical perspective, 376–377

Wagner, Lynne, 419
Watson Caring Science Caritas Coach
    Educational Program, 190
Watson Caring Science Global Associate, 486,
    505
Watson Caring Science Institute (WCSI), 219, 277,
    307, 319, 420, 423, 500, 566, 634
Watson Caritas Patient Score (WCPS), 218–219,
    321, 323, 407
  items, 322
Watson, Jean, 2, 3, 4, 6, 7, 9, 110, 120, 149, 244, 363,
    402, 416, 463, 482, 580, 615, 660
  as visiting professor at BWH, 404–405
Watson's Caritas processes
  creative use of self, 78
  development of self, 77–78
  healing environment, 79
  life-death, 79
  practice of loving-kindness and equanimity,
    76–77
  principles of, 75–76
  sacred nursing acts of caring-healing, 79
  spirituality and, 77
  teaching-learning experience, 78–79
  and ubuntu, 76–79

Watson's theory of human caring, 75, 307
  aesthetic theories, 109
  in education and practice, 327–328
  science theory, 119–121
  traditional Yogic Kosha Model, 643–651
WCPS. *See* Watson Caritas Patient Score
WCSI. *See* Watson Caring Science Institute
White, Jill, 192
wholeness, 31–32, 86, 96
  undivided, 25–26
Wilber, Ken, 192
Witherspoon, Gary, 94
Wolf, Zane, 5
Woodland gate, 637
World Portal Program Development, 486
"woundedness," 595

Yarling, Roland, 42–43, 44, 45
Yoga Kosha Model, 643
  adaption, 644–646
  background, 643–644

Zuniga, Anita, 414, 421